The Neuropsychology of Anxiety

OXFORD PSYCHOLOGY SERIES

1. *The Neuropsychology of Anxiety* J. A. Gray
2. *Elements of Episodic Memory* E. Tulving
3. *Conditioning and Associative Learning* N. J. Mackintosh
4. *Visual Masking* B. G. Breitmeyer
5. *The Musical Mind* J. A. Sloboda
6. *Elements of Psychophysical Theory* J.- C. Falmagne
7. *Animal Intelligence* L. Weiskrantz
8. *Response Times* R. D. Luce
9. *Mental Representations* A. Paivio
10. *Memory, Imprinting, and the Brain* G. Horn
11. *Working Memory* A. Baddeley
12. *Blindsight* L. Weiskrantz
13. *Profile Analysis* D. M. Green
14. *Spatial Vision* R. L. DeValois and K. K. DeValois
15. *The Neural and Behavioural Organization of Goal-Directed Movements* M. Jeannerod
16. *Visual Pattern Analyzers* N. V. S. Graham
17. *Cognitive Foundations of Musical Pitch* C. L. Krumhansl
18. *Perceptual and Associative Learning* G. Hall
19. *Implicit Learning and Tacit Knowledge* A. S. Reber
20. *Neuromotor Mechanisms in Human Communication* D. Kimura
21. *The Frontal Lobes and Voluntary Action* R. Passingham
22. *Classification and Cognition* W. K. Estes
23. *Vowel Perception and Production* B. S. Rosner and J. B. Pickering
24. *Visual Stress* A. Wilkins
25. *Electrophysiology of Mind* Edited by M. D. Rugg and M. G. H. Coles
26. *Attention and Memory* N. Cowan
27. *The Visual Brain in Action* A. D. Milner and M. A. Goodale
28. *Perceptual Consequences of Cochlear Damage* B. C. J. Moore
29. *Binocular Vision and Stereopsis* I. P. Howard and B. J. Rogers
30. *The Measurement of Sensation* D. Laming
31. *Conditioned Taste Aversion* J. Bures, F. Bermúdez—Rattoni, and T. Yamamoto
32. *The Developing Visual Brain* J. Atkinson
33. *The Neuropsychology of Anxiety, 2e* J. A. Gray and N. McNaughton
34. *Looking Down on Human Intelligence* I. J. Deary
35. *From Conditioning to Conscious Recollection* H. Eichenbaum and N. J. Cohen
36. *Understanding Figurative Language* S. Glucksberg
37. *Active Vision* J. M. Findlay and I. D. Gilchrist
38. *The Science of False Memory* C. J. Brainerd and V. F. Reyna
39. *The Case for Mental Imagery* S. M. Kosslyn, W. L. Thompson, and G. Ganis
40. *Seeing Black and White* A. Gilchrist
41. *Visual Masking, 2e* B. Breitmeyer and H. Oğmen
42. *Motor Cognition* M. Jeannerod
43. *The Visual Brain in Action* A. D. Milner and M. A. Goodale
44. *The Continuity of Mind* M. Spivey
45. *Working Memory, Thought, and Action* A. Baddeley
46. *What Is Special about the Human Brain?* R. Passingham
47. *Visual Reflections* M. McCloskey
48. *Principles of Visual Attention* C. Bundesen and T. Habekost
49. *Major Issues in Cognitive Aging* T. A. Salthouse
50. *Perceiving in Depth* Ian P. Howard
51. *The Neurobiology of the Prefrontal Cortex: Anatomy, Evolution, and the Origin of Insight* Richard E. Passingham and Steven P. Wise
52. *The Evolution of Memory Systems: Ancestors, Anatomy, and Adaptations* Elisabeth A. Murray, Steven P. Wise, and Kim S. Graham
53. *Understanding the Prefrontal Cortex: Selective advantage, connectivity, and neural operations* Richard E. Passingham
54. *Remembering: An Activity of Mind and Brain* Fergus I. M. Craik

UN COUP DE DÉS

JAMAIS

N'ABOLIRA LAE HASARD

Toute Pensée émet un Coup de Dés

Stéphane Mallarmé

The Neuropsychology of Anxiety

An Enquiry into the Functions of the Septo-Hippocampal System

Third Edition

Neil McNaughton
Department of Psychology, Brain Health Research Centre, University of Otago, Dunedin, New Zealand

and

Jeffrey A. Gray
Deceased

OXFORD
UNIVERSITY PRESS

OXFORD
UNIVERSITY PRESS

Great Clarendon Street, Oxford, OX2 6DP,
United Kingdom

Oxford University Press is a department of the University of Oxford.
It furthers the University's objective of excellence in research, scholarship,
and education by publishing worldwide. Oxford is a registered trade mark of
Oxford University Press in the UK and in certain other countries

Published in the United States of America by Oxford University Press
198 Madison Avenue, New York, NY 10016, United States of America

British Library Cataloguing in Publication Data

Data available

Library of Congress Control Number: 2023947343

ISBN 978–0–19–884331–3

DOI: 10.1093/oso/9780198843313.001.0001

Printed in the UK by
Bell & Bain Ltd., Glasgow

For Venus, without whom this book could not have been written; for Julie, without whom it could not have been rewritten; for Catriona who waited patiently for decades for her turn; and in memory of Jeffrey, without whom this edition had to be written, but whose influence pervades it.

Preface

This third edition of 'The Neuropsychology of Anxiety' provides a further updated theory of septo-hippocampal function combined with an updated theory of anxiety. We believe these components are each superior to their domain-specific competitors; and their combination is a unique single wholistic account for normal anxiety and generalized anxiety disorder and normal memory and clinical amnesia.

Correct use of the theory has proved to depend on highly specific factual details and specific precise definitions of its terms. Our view of the data often differs from conventional views. (For example, we argue at length that the firing of a hippocampal cell never represents a 'place field' in any normal sense; and our use of 'anxiety' is much more specific and restricted than in current psychiatric classifications.) So, for the whole theory, one must read the whole main text (and the supporting material for completeness). Critically, applying Occam's Razor, competing theories must be judged for their capacity to account for *all* of the data that we include. We see our theory as unique in the extent (albeit still incomplete) to which it integrates *all* of these data.

The book is also nearly unique in its attempt to integrate data across so many different domains of the literature. This led to a logistical problem with the second edition: it became very large. So, the main text laid out the basic argument with minimal supporting detail. We provided 10 electronic appendices that are 'reprinted' in the current edition as PDF files at http://dx.doi.org/10.17605/OSF.IO/YW32K. For the current edition, we also provide a list of detailed supporting published reviews, with URLs. Lists of both the appendices and the reviews are provided on pages xxix–xxxi.

To keep our detailed argument under control the book has three layers. The first layer is Chapter 1, which contains an overview of the entire argument. The second layer is Chapters 2–14, which expand on the arguments of Chapter 1 in what we hope is sufficient depth for the majority of readers. The third layer is Appendices 1–10 and the detailed published reviews, which provide additional detail of a type that we expect will only be required piecemeal by those wanting the full detail of some specific argument—and so we would not expect these to be read in full by most readers. These horizontal layers also allow some vertical division.

For those reading this book from a purely hippocampal or memorial perspective it may be advantageous to start with Chapters 6–10 and read the hippocampally-oriented appendices (4–10) as necessary. Chapter 8 deals with the nature of temporal lobe amnesia and attempts to resolve the conflict between the different current views of 'types of memory' that are sensitive or insensitive to hippocampal formation damage. Hopefully our hippocampal analysis will then persuade them to read the rest of the book.

For those interested in anxiety, we recommend that they start at the beginning and we hope that they will then find themselves sufficiently impressed by our arguments for the importance of the septo-hippocampal system to read Chapters 6–10. The key arguments with respect to the clinical aspects of anxiety are presented in Chapter 9. However, for a less neural perspective, skipping from Chapter 5 to Chapters 12–14 will retain the main high-level ideas.

For those, like Joe LeDoux, who feel that in the past we ignored important contributions to anxiety from the frontal cortex, we now provide Chapter 11. This also extends our neurology of the Goal Inhibition System to the insula.

Despite the advances of the last 20 years, our theory still does not claim to be a complete one. So, within certain artificially limited data domains (e.g. the effects of hippocampal lesions on tests that are supposedly specific to certain types of memory function) aficionados may feel that certain other theories are superior or at least more parsimonious. As will be seen in the various sections of this book, we believe our theory to be at least the equal of the opposition even within each of these specialized domains. However, we feel that comparative judgements between the theories should be made over the *whole* range of the available data and here we believe our theory is clearly superior. No other theory of hippocampal function explains (or even tries to explain) the highly specific effects of all known classes of anti-anxiety drugs on the hippocampal formation; and no other theory of anxiety explains why anxiolytic drugs have effects on supposed tests of reference memory function. We would ask our readers, therefore, not to judge our theory solely on its capacity to beat their favoured hypothesis with respect to some small subset of the data covered in this book, but rather to look at the success (or even applicability) of their alternative hypothesis over the whole range of data integrated here.

The core of the theory (presented in a brief article, Gray, 1970a) has stood for half a century. This is probably the best reason for taking both the psychological and neural aspects of it seriously. The core of the theory presented in this edition is the same as in the first and second. Nonetheless, as was the case with the second edition, much of what is said in detail in this edition is new. We have needed to bring more than two decades of new data into register with the theory; contrasting it with recent new theories; and, in particular, in rephrasing many of the arguments and redefining terms in an attempt to eliminate the misunderstandings of the past. For example, we try to make clearer that the Goal Inhibition System (renamed from 'Behavioural Inhibition System' to deal with some recent definitional problems with personality scales) is neither involved in all inhibition of behaviour (particularly action stopping) nor involved solely in behavioural *inhibition*—indeed a theoretically fundamental property is its engagement in *active* risk analysis behaviour. This was stated in the first edition, emphasized more in the second edition, and remains core in the current edition.

Thus, the uniqueness of our view of anxiety derives from analysis of the neuropsychology and neurophysiology of the septo-hippocampal system. Likewise, the uniqueness of our view of the septo-hippocampal system derives from our analysis of the neural, psychological, and ethological effects of anxiolytic drugs. Despite these linkages, *neither in the first edition nor here do we equate anxiety with hippocampal function nor, especially, anxiety disorder with hippocampal dysfunction.* Rather, we view the hippocampus as including in its information processing capacities certain operations that are crucial for the maintenance and elaboration of anxiety. In particular, in the present edition, we see anxiety as resulting, in its most fundamental form, from interaction between the septo-hippocampal system and the amygdala in the control of decisions and between the amygdala and insula for the control of arousal and attention.

Emotion and temporal lobe function are still arguably the most important areas currently requiring clarification for psychology and neurology, respectively. We believe the theory presented in this book successfully reconciles the older 'emotion' view of the temporal lobe with the more recent 'memory' view, presenting a new view of parallel Papez circuits

(McNaughton and Vann, 2022). Its arguments, therefore, are relevant to both emotion and memory in general as well as to anxiety in particular and are relevant to temporal lobe function in general as well as the hippocampal formation in particular.

As with our reason for giving the theory credence, the main reason for producing this third edition is that the original theory has withstood the test of time. This was based on similarities between the effects of anxiolytic drugs and hippocampal lesions. These similarities are more remarkable now. The original theory was also based on the fact that anxiolytic drugs change hippocampal electrical activity. Recent drugs (e.g. pregabalin and ketamine) have shown that this is both more general and more firmly established. Likewise, the early theory emphasized the role of monoamine systems in hippocampal function, anxiety, and the relation between them. We show that this role continues to become clearer, more pervasive, and perhaps coherent.

While the core of the theory remains unchanged, it would be strange if more than two decades of experimental and theoretical advances did not require some modification of the details and arguments presented in the second edition.

First, recent data have greatly strengthened the crucial original hypothesis that anxiolytic drugs achieve important clinical effects through the septo-hippocampal system. They have also given us a much clearer idea of the neurophysiological basis for these effects. But, even more than the second edition, while confirming our original emphasis on hippocampal function as being a crucial mediator of action of anxiolytic drug action, the new data further expand the list of other key structures of the Goal Inhibition System (entorhinal cortex, posterior cingulate cortex, and amygdala) to include the periaqueductal grey in the subcortical direction and the insula and orbital frontal cortex in the cortical direction.

Second, many details of the theory were expanded and adjusted in the second edition to bring it into line with the analysis of clinical anxiety, the neurology of obsessive-compulsive disorder, and the role of the hippocampus and prefrontal cortex in memory—this expansion has continued in the current edition. Conversely, the role of the temporal end of the hippocampus in anxiety has become generally accepted. Despite this alignment with some accepted data on hippocampal function, our theory of memory is in one sense the antithesis of theories that see the hippocampal system as supporting the formation of memories or which see it as some type of intermediate store (see Eichenbaum et al., 1994; Koster et al., 2018). We offer, as before, a view of the hippocampus (including its septal end) as a primarily inhibitory organ suppressing noise more than enhancing signal. In the present edition the precise role of this inhibition in the control of inappropriate memories is more extensively explicated as a special case of the more general functions of the hippocampal formation. We also emphasize the role of the hippocampus in the generation of active behaviour designed to gain the information with which to resolve a conflict.

We have, between us, studied anxiety, septo-hippocampal function, and the relation between them, for a total of more than 70 person-years. As before, this edition must include many ideas that we jointly or separately expressed previously. It has also borrowed extensively and sometimes wholesale from many others. Despite this, and despite the fact that the core of the theory remains essentially unchanged, we believe that this edition presents a new, more detailed, synthesis of work on anxiety and hippocampal function. It shows, more clearly than ever before, that the two must be treated as related, but not identical, topics; and that cortical rhythmicity homologous with rat hippocampal rhythmicity may now provide us with a biomarker that can unlock anxiety and anxiety disorder, as we have defined them.

Acknowledgements

Third Edition

It is not usual to acknowledge one of the authors, but I feel that this is an appropriate place to record my personal intellectual debt to the late Jeffrey Gray. His undergraduate lectures on learning theory sparked my continuing interest in psychology and gave me the strong belief that we must always use behaviour as the fundamental evidence; but that appropriate experiments can and should deduce internal processes within the Conceptual Nervous System. He was the supervisor of my third year undergraduate research project on the effects of an anxiolytic on behavioural inhibition; the primary question of which still remains unanswered. He kindly agreed to act as an unofficial mentor of my PhD work in Southampton; and was my post-doctoral employer for more than a decade. He was the editor of my first book, *Biology and Emotion*; and did me the honour of asking me to rewrite *Neuropsychology of Anxiety*, when the publisher requested a second edition. It is inevitable that his abiding influence has shaped the thoughts and writing of this third edition even when the words are not his verbatim original. I am also grateful to his estate for agreement to a third edition.

I have received much advice and help on specific issues that I hope is suitably acknowledged in the text; where I have failed to do so, I apologize. A large number of people made a more substantial intellectual contribution, in some cases over many years. In particular, the new material on personality in Chapter 12 owes much to my training in personality theory by Philip Corr, Colin DeYoung, and Luke Smillie. In addition, I thank the following (in alphabetical order). Caroline Blanchard for many years of useful comment and, in particular, detailed feedback on the content of Chapter 2. Philip Corr raised questions, immediately after the appearance of the second edition, that he and I have attempted to answer in what became a series of papers over the intervening years. He read and provided detailed comment on multiple chapters (1–5, 12) and I apologize for having neither the time nor the skill to produce the kind of text he suggested. Colin DeYoung has also provided much comment over the years and provided detailed feedback on Chapters 11 and 12. He also introduced me to the word cryptomnesia when I proposed to him a 'new' aspect of the theory that he pointed out he had originally suggested to me and published some years earlier. Paul Glue has collaborated with me on our biomarker development and has led the work on ketamine and anxiety that I cite (and which led to our 'double hit' hypothesis). He also checked Chapter 14 for psychiatric errors, suggesting a number of missing citations. Olivia Harrison checked content in Chapter 6. Frederico Graeff continued to supply advice and comment and also hospitality when I visited Ribeirão Preto en route to presenting a keynote address in his honour at the first annual reunion of the Instituto Brasilero de Neuropsicologia e Compartamento (Brasilian Institute of Neuropsychology and Behaviour) in Rio de Janeiro (see McNaughton, 2011, for the requested 'bit of history'). Gavan McNally checked the amine-related content in Chapter 6. Lynne Nadel provided useful comment on recent theories of amnesia (Chapter 8). Luděk Nerad commented on §11.7. Daniela Espinoza Oyarce and Nicolas Cherbuin provided joint comments on Chapters 11 and 12. Richie Poulton checked the content of Chapter 13. Luke Smillie provided detailed comment on and discussion of Chapter 1. Peter Somogyi has provided extensive email interactions over the years on theta, the septum, and hippocampal inhibition—introducing me to Teevra neurons among much else. I also appreciated the face-to-face discussions with him when he visited Dunedin; not to mention the recipe for *Paprikás Csirke* provided by Karla. This also seems an appropriate place to thank Johnathan Williams for many decades of general issue raising, discussion and critique and, in particular, for his reminders about the importance of septal elicitation of theta. Gordon Winocur provided a succinct tutorial bringing me up to speed on recent theories of amnesia (Chapter 8). Calvin Young has provided many years of extensive critical discussion of, and collaboration on, rhythmicity and, in particular, provided a critique of §9.2. Hélio Zangrossi has provided over the years extensive insight into animal models of anxiety (McNaughton and Zangrossi, 2008) and has been my go-to source for information on serotonergic drugs. He kindly hosted a visit to Ribeirão Preto that allowed me to learn about the periaqueductal grey from the experts there. Finally, I would like to thank the PhD students who did the heavy lifting for several detailed reviews: Wei-Xing Pan, Damon Mitchell, Matt Stevenson, Ralph Frost (Man Chung Fung), Carlos Silva.

Neil McNaughton

Second Edition

I am grateful to all my students who, over the years I have been preparing this second edition, have not only put up with its distraction of me from their work but have helped me with comments, ideas, and friendship. I must also thank the University of Otago and my head of Department Professor Geoffrey White for their permitting me 6 months of prolonged research time without which this edition would have appeared many years later than it has. Len Jarrard is owed special thanks for providing Jeffrey and myself with a haven at Washington and Lee University where, for several days halfway round the world from each of our places of work, we could meet and thrash out the final details of the present edition.

In producing this second edition, I owe a particular intellectual debt to Robert and Caroline Blanchard, Fred Graeff, Ray Kesner, Ian Kirk, and Olga Vinogradova. Many of the modifications to the original theory arose out of discussions with them, making it difficult to acknowledge their precise contribution in the text. Others who have discussed their ideas with me, and who I hope will forgive me for what I have done with them, are Carol Barnes, Rob Berman, Brian Bland, Michael Davis, Joe Le Doux, Joaquin Fuster, Charlie Gross, Len Jarrard, Bruce McNaughton, Sheri Mizumori, Tony Phillips, Bob Sainsbury, Bob Vertes, and Tony Wright. I have tried to acknowledge their contributions in the text but in case I have failed to fully acknowledge my borrowings, I thank them here.

I am also most grateful for those who provided detailed comment on draft chapters: Cliff Abraham, Carol Barnes, Rob Berman, Stuart Checkley, Fred Graeff, Ray Kesner, Ian Kirk, Brian Young, and Sidney Wiener. Here, particular thanks must go to Carol Barnes and Sidney Wiener for their extensive criticism of my analysis of single cell recordings which has resulted in major changes—and, I hope they will think, improvements.

Moana Theodore and Marlane Bronstring gave me extensive help with the references. Very many others, far too numerous to mention, have kindly sent us reprints and preprints of their work over the last few years, we thank them for their help here and have acknowledged their work by citation in the text. Joe Ledoux's courier delivery of his book *The Emotional Brain* to us was particularly appreciated, as was Bob Vertes's hand delivery of a draft of his major review with Bernat Kocsis of 'brainstem-diencephalo-septohippocampal systems controlling the theta rhythm of the hippocampus'. We are also very grateful to those who responded heroically to a last minute request for preprints and papers which I wished to cite directly but lacked a copy: Robert Adamec, John Aggleton, Efrain Azmitia, David Barlow, Bob and Caroline Blanchard, Brian Bland, Randy Commissaris, John Dalrymple-Alford, Phillip Best, Elena Brazhnik, Sam Deadwyler, William Deakin, Howard Eichenbaum, Don Fowles, Steven Fox, Tamas Freund, Sandra File, Mike Gabriel, Patricia Goldman-Rakic, Donald Klein, George Koob, Serge Laroche, Joe Ledoux, Isaac Marks, Paul Monmaur, Richard Morris, Elizabeth Murray, Lynn Nadel, Tim Otto, Michael Petrides, Tony Phillips, Trevor Robbins, Edmund Rolls, Bob Sainsbury, Larry Squire, Dallas Treit, Case Vanderwolf.

The updating of this second edition over the last few years has been greatly aided by the immensely supportive environment of the Department of Psychology at the University of Otago and by the sheer number of laboratories in the Department working directly on the hippocampus, memory, and plasticity, each from their own perspective. Thanks for many unacknowledged inputs go to Cliff Abraham (LTP/LTD), David Bilkey (theta/memory), Mike Colombo (single cells/memory), Cynthia Darlington and Paul Smith (pituitary adrenal hormones and plasticity), Bob Knight (amnesic syndromes), Brian Young (single cells) and Geoff White (signal detection models of memory).

Neil McNaughton

First Edition

I am deeply grateful to Professor Jean Scherrer for the kindness and hospitality he extended to me during my stay in his laboratory in the Faculté de Médicine, Université de Paris VI, in 1979–1980, when the first edition of this book was written. My thanks are also due to the Nuffield Foundation for the award of a Social Science Research Fellowship which, in 1975–1976, allowed me to start working on the book, and for help in the preparation of the manuscript. I am indebted to all of my colleagues and students at Oxford for innumerable ideas and points of information which have influenced my thinking over the years. Particular thanks are due to Marianne Fillenz, for educating me in the mysteries of the noradrenergic neuron; to Dr Nicholas Rawlins, for clarifying many points in hippocampal physiology; to Mrs S. Digby-Firth and Mrs M. Penning-Rowsell for their care in preparing the manuscript; and to my sons, Ramin and Babak, for editorial assistance.

Jeffrey A. Gray

Contents

Abbreviations

AIC	Anterior insular cortex
BAS	Behavioural Approach System
BIS	Behavioural Inhibition System
C&W	Carver & White BIS?BAS scales
CBT	Cognitive Behavioural Therapy
CNS	Central Nervous System
CR	Cognitive restructuring
CR	Conditioned response
CRF	Corticotropin-releasing factor
CS	Conditioned aversive stimuli
CS	Conditioned stimulus
CT	Cognitive Therapy
DR	Dorsal raphe
DRL	Differential Reinforcement of Low Rates
ERK	Extracellular signal-related kinase
FFFS	Fight-Flight-Freeze System
FN	Feedback negativity
GADS	Goldberg Anxiety and Depression Scales
GAS	Goal Attraction System
GCSR	Goal-conflict-specific EEG rhythmicity
GIS	Goal Inhibition System
GRS	Goal Repulsion System
HCN	Hyperpolarization-activated, cation nonselective
HiTOP	Hierarchical Taxonomy of Psychopathology
ILC	Insular limbic cortex
ISAC	Insular somatic association cortex
LTM	Long-term memories
LTP	Long-term potentiation
MDD	Major depressive disorder
MFG	Medial frontal gyrus
MPFC	Medial prefrontal cortex
MS	Medial septum
MTT	Multiple Trace Theory
NMDA	N-methyl-D-aspartate
OCD	Obsessive-Compulsive Disorder
PD	Panic Disorder
PTSD	Post-Traumatic Stress Disorder
RDoC	Research domain criteria
RewP	Reward positivity
ROI	Regions of interest
RPE	Reward prediction error
RSA	Rhythmic slow activity
RST	Reinforcement sensitivity theory

SDAT	Senile dementia of the Alzheimer type
SHS	Septo-hippocampal system
SSRI	Specific serotonin reuptake inhibitors
SST	Stop signal task
STAI	State-Trait Anxiety Inventory
TMAS	Taylor's Manifest Anxiety Scale
TR	Treatment resistance
TTT	Trace Transformation Theory
US	Unconditioned stimulus
VBS	Visible Burrow System
VR	Virtual reality

List of online appendices and reviews

LIST OF APPENDICES

Folder available at http://dx.doi.org/10.17605/OSF.IO/YW32K

Appendix 1: The behavioural profile of anxiolytic drugs
Appendix 2: The periaqueductal grey, medial hypothalamus, and amygdala
Appendix 3: The prefrontal cortex and cingulate cortex
Appendix 4: Anatomy of the septo-hippocampal system
Appendix 5: Electrophysiology and pharmacology of the septo-hippocampal system
Appendix 6: Electrical activity of the septo-hippocampal system and behaviour
Appendix 7: Electrical stimulation of the septo-hippocampal system, behaviour, and sleep
Appendix 8: Behavioural effects of large septo-hippocampal lesions
Appendix 9: Dissecting the septo-hippocampal syndrome
Appendix 10: Ascending modulatory systems

LIST OF SUPPORTING REVIEWS

Corr, P. J., DeYoung, C. G. & McNaughton, N. 2013. Motivation and Personality: A Neuropsychological Perspective. *Social and Personality Psychology Compass,* 7, 158-175 https://doi.org/10.1111/spc3.12016

Corr, P. J. & McNaughton, N. 2012. Neuroscience and approach/avoidance personality traits: A two stage (valuation-motivation) approach. *Neuroscience & Biobehavioral Reviews,* 36, 2339-2354. https://doi.org/10.1016/j.neubiorev.2012.09.013

Corr, P. J. & McNaughton, N. 2016. Neural Mechanisms of low trait anxiety and risk for externalizing behaviour. *In:* Beauchaine, T. P. & Hinshaw, S. P. (eds.) *The Oxford Handbook of Externalizing Spectrum Disorders.* Oxford Handbooks Online: Oxford University Press. https://doi.org/10.1093/oxfordhb/9780199324675.013.1.

Frost, R. & McNaughton, N. 2017. The neural basis of delay discounting: A review and preliminary model. *Neuroscience & Biobehavioral Reviews,* 79, 48-65. https://doi.org/10.1016/j.neubiorev.2017.04.022

Gray, J. A. 1971. *The psychology of fear and stress,* London, Weidenfeld and Nicolson.

Gray, J. A. 1975. Elements of a two-process theory of learning, London, Academic Press.

Gray, J. A. 1977. Drug effects on fear and frustration: Possible limbic site of action of minor tranquilizers. *In:* Iversen, L. L., Iversen, S. D. & Snyder, S. H. (eds.) *Handbook of psychopharmacology. Vol 8: Drugs, neurotransmitters and behaviour.* New York: Plenum Press.

Gray, J. A. 1987. *The psychology of fear and stress,* London, Cambridge University Press.

Gray, J. A. & McNaughton, N. 1983. Comparison between the behavioural effect of septal and hippocampal lesions: a review. *Neuroscience & Biobehavioral Reviews,* 7, 119-188. https://doi.org/10.1016/0149-7634(83)90014-3

McNaughton, N. 1989. Biology and Emotion, Cambridge, Cambridge University Press.

McNaughton, N. 1993. Stress and behavioural inhibition. *In:* Stanford, S. C. & Salmon, P. (eds.) *Stress: an integrated approach.* Academic Press.

McNaughton, N. 2011. Fear, anxiety and their disorders: past, present and future neural theories. *Psychology & Neuroscience,* 4, 173-181. https://doi.org/10.3922/j.psns.2011.2.002

McNaughton, N. & Bannerman, D. 2024. The homogenous hippocampus: How hippocampal cells process goals. OSF, preprint. https://doi.org/10.31219/osf.io/a458n

McNaughton, N. & Corr, P. J. 2004. A two-dimensional neuropsychology of defense: Fear/anxiety and defensive distance. *Neuroscience & Biobehavioral Reviews,* 28, 285-305. https://doi.org/10.1016/j.neubiorev.2004.03.005

McNaughton, N. & Corr, P. J. 2008a. Animal cognition and human personality. *In:* Corr, P. J. (ed.) *The Reinforcement Theory of Personality.* Cambridge: Cambridge University Press. http://www.philipcorr.net/uploads/downloads/41.pdf.

McNaughton, N. & Corr, P. J. 2008b. The neuropsychology of fear and anxiety: A foundation for Reinforcement Sensitivity Theory. *In:* Corr, P. J. (ed.) *The Reinforcement Theory of Personality.* Cambridge: Cambridge University Press. http://doi.org/10.1017/CBO978051 1819384.003.

McNaughton, N. & Corr, P. J. 2009. Central theories of motivation and emotion. *In:* Berntson, G. G. & Cacioppo, J. T. (eds.) *Handbook of Neuroscience for the Behavioural Sciences.* Hoboken, New Jersey: John Wiley & Sons Inc. https://doi.org/10.1002/9780470478509.neubb00203.

McNaughton, N. & Corr, P. J. 2014. Approach, avoidance, and their conflict: the problem of anchoring. *Frontiers in Systems Neuroscience,* 8, A0124. https://doi.org/10.3389/fnsys.2014.00124

McNaughton, N. & Corr, P. J. 2016. Mechanisms of comorbidity, continuity, and discontinuity in anxiety-related disorders. *Development and Psychopathology,* 28, 1053-1069. https://doi.org/10.1017/S0954579416000699

McNaughton, N. & Corr, P. J. 2018. Survival circuits and risk assessment. *Current Opinion in Behavioral Sciences,* 24, 14-20. https://doi.org/10.1016/j.cobeha.2018.01.018

McNaughton, N. & Corr, P. J. 2022. The non-human perspective on the neurobiology of temperament, personality, and psychopathology: What's next? *Current Opinion in Behavioral Sciences,* 43, 255-262. https://doi.org/10.1016/j.cobeha.2021.11.005

McNaughton, N., DeYoung, C. G. & Corr, P. J. 2016. Approach/avoidance. *In:* Absher, J. R. & Cloutier, J. (eds.) *Neuroimaging personality, social cognition and character.* San Diego: Elsevier. https://doi.org/10.1016/B978-0-12-800935-2.00002-6

McNaughton, N. & Glue, P. 2020. Ketamine and neuroticism: a double-hit hypothesis of internalizing disorders. *Personality Neuroscience,* 3, e2. https://doi.org/10.1017/pen.2020.2

McNaughton, N., Kocsis, B. & Hajós, M. 2007. Elicited hippocampal theta rhythm: a screen for anxiolytic and procognitive drugs through changes in hippocampal function? *Behavioural Pharmacology,* 18, 329-346. https://doi.org/10.1097/FBP.0b013e3282ee82e3

McNaughton, N. & Mason, S. T. 1980. The neuropsychology and neuropharmacology of the dorsal ascending noradrenergic bundle - a review. *Progress in Neurobiology,* 14, 157-219. https://doi.org/10.1016/0301-0082(80)90021-0

McNaughton, N. & Smillie, L. D. 2018. Some metatheoretical principles for personality neuroscience. *Personality Neuroscience,* 1, e11. https://doi.org/10.1017/pen.2018.9

McNaughton, N. & Vann, S. D. 2022. Construction of complex memories via parallel distributed cortical-subcortical iterative integration *Trends in Neurosciences,* 45, 550-562. https://doi.org/10.1016/j.tins.2022.04.006

McNaughton, N. & Wickens, J. 2003. Hebb, pandemonium and catastrophic hypermnesia: The hippocampus as a suppressor of inappropriate associations. *Cortex,* 39, 1139-1163. https://doi.org/10.1016/S0010-9452(08)70882-7

McNaughton, N. & Zangrossi, H. 2008. Theoretical approaches to the modeling of anxiety in animals. *In:* Blanchard, R. J., Blanchard, D. C., Griebel, G. & Nutt, D. J. (eds.) *Handbook of Anxiety and Fear,* Oxford, UK: Elsevier B.V. https://ddoi.org/10.1016/S1569-7339(07)00002-1.

Mitchell, D. J., McNaughton, N., Flanagan, D. & Kirk, I. J. 2008. Frontal-midline theta from the perspective of hippocampal "theta". *Progress in Neurobiology,* 86, 156-185. https://doi.org/10.1016/j.pneurobio.2008.09.005

Pan, W.-X. & McNaughton, N. 2004. The supramammillary area: its organization, functions and relationship to the hippocampus. *Progress in Neurobiology,* 74, 127-166. https://doi.org/10.1016/j.pneurobio.2004.09.003

Silva, C. & McNaughton, N. 2019. Are periaqueductal gray and dorsal raphe the foundation of appetitive and aversive control? A comprehensive review. *Progress in Neurobiology,* 177, 33-72. https://doi.org/https://doi.org/10.1016/j.pneurobio.2019.02.001

Stevenson, M. & McNaughton, N. 2013. A comparison of phenylketonuria with attention deficit hyperactivity disorder: Do markedly different aetiologies deliver common phenotypes? *Brain Research Bulletin,* 99, 63-83. https://doi.org/10.1016/j.brainresbull.2013.10.003

1
Overview

The hippocampus—an organ of hesitation and doubt

P.V. Simonov (1974)

1.1 Content and structure

1.1.1 A convergent integration

This book argues that 'anxiety' should be defined via the action of selective anxiolytic drugs (making it distinct from fear). Such anxiety has evolved to allow cautious approach to danger (and so involves conflict between attractive and repulsive goals); while fear evolved to allow simple removal from danger. Anxiety acts to inhibit incorrect goals ('hesitation') and to allow risk assessment to select correct goals ('doubt').

Conceptually, anxiety is controlled by a Goal Inhibition System (GIS[1]) that has the septo-hippocampal system (SHS; see §1.10) at the core of its central nervous system components. The hippocampus is involved in the motivated suppression of unwanted engrams (i.e. interference) not the formation of wanted engrams; with damage to it producing not amnesia but catastrophic hypermnesia (excessive engram activation that, tip-of-the-tongue fashion, blocks correct recall). The GIS is activated when activation of a Goal Attraction System (GAS[1]) and a Goal Repulsion System (GRS[1]) conflict with each other. The neuropsychology of these three systems provides a map for motivation-related personality traits, for defensive disorders (extremes of traits) in psychiatry, for comorbidity, and for the different actions of drugs and cognitive therapies used to treat these disorders. The book as a whole is supported by supplementary appendices and reviews (DOIs listed on pages xxix–xxxi) and provides a detailed, integrated, perspective on all these topics.

We[2] provide, here, a unique account both of the neuropsychology of anxiety (including other defensive emotions) and of SHS function. We *integrate* these two domains (as well as adaptive function, disorder, and personality) by a fundamental and consistent appeal to the actions of *selective* anxiolytic drugs: those that affect clinical anxiety *but do not affect panic.* Our neurology extends from the periaqueductal grey to prefrontal cortex and insula; and our psychology accounts not only for healthy defensive reactions but for the family of neurotic disorders and for variations among them. We believe that the depth of detail and extent of coverage of the theory are important for its scientific validity. We know

[1] Renamed from the Behavioural Inhibition System (BIS), ditto for GAS, GRS; see §1.7 and Table 1.1.

[2] 'We' is often retained from the text of the previous edition. With many new elements of the current text, as in this case, I intend 'we' to include Jeffrey in spirit. NMcN.

The Neuropsychology of Anxiety, Third Edition. Neil McNaughton and Jeffrey A. Gray, Oxford University Press.
 DOI: 10.1093/oso/9780198843313.003.0001

of no other theory that integrates the same volume of data—and we would argue that, in each individual area that we review, our theory is at least as successful as the simpler theories often preferred within those areas. Critically, we believe it is much simpler than any competitor when applied to the data as a whole and so best satisfies Occam's rule[3] for deciding between theories.

Our theory also has longevity and predictive validity. The core elements (Gray, 1969; Gray, 1970b) and their elaboration (Gray, 1982) were retained when the theory was updated with two decades of new data and ideas (Gray and McNaughton, 2000). In the subsequent two decades, the world has continued to change. We now have sLORETA and fMRI to identify the source of anxiety biomarkers; and know the identity of H.M. (Chapter 8). Machine learning and convolutional neural nets entangle all areas (even us, Wang et al., 2019). COVID-19 has arrived with increased rates of neurotic disorder (Tucker and Czapla, 2020; Taquet et al., 2021; Ferber et al., 2021; see Harper et al., 2021, on fear and positive behaviour change). As a result, the theory presented here has, again, grown but its bedrock has not changed and in several areas the growth has allowed higher order simplification. Importantly, we can now integrate disparate views of anxiety and its neural basis; and disparate views of hippocampal function (Chapter 8). We weave together a plethora of prior separate views into a convergent integration.

1.1.2 Structure

This book is intended to be read straight through from start to finish. But given the range of topics covered, we suspect many readers would prefer to skip to the chapter of most relevance to them (e.g. Chapter 7 for those interested in hippocampal function and Chapter 12 for those interested in reinforcement sensitivity theory) and then expand their view to other chapters for the full picture or the appendices and supplementary reviews as necessary for further detail.

This first chapter provides an overview of our entire argument. Subsequent chapters provide detailed discussion and justification. More extensive evidence for more contentious points is provided in separate appendices and published reviews (listed on pages xxix–xxxi).

The main chapters start with the evolutionary functions of fear and anxiety (Chapter 2), their differences in terms of learning theory (Chapter 3), and most importantly their distinct pharmacology (Chapter 4)—leading to an initial picture (Chapter 5) of an anxiolytic-sensitive portion of the 'Conceptual Nervous System' (Hebb, 1955) that is specific to conflict resolution and distinct from systems that are specific to positive and negative (see §1.12.4) goals, respectively.

We then present a hierarchical, two-dimensional, neurology of the underlying defence control systems (Chapter 6) that includes the hippocampus as a key node in the control of anxiety. This leads us to deeper consideration of the nature of the information 'coded' by hippocampal cells (Chapter 7) and the nature of hippocampal-sensitive 'types' of memory (Chapter 8). Chapter 9 then presents and justifies key fundamental principles derived from Chapters 1–8; with Chapter 10 presenting the basic, subcortical, core of the

[3] 'Pluralitas non est ponenda sine necessitate' Gulielmus de Occam: Quodlibeta, V, Q.i (in Boehner, 1957).

septo-hippocampal theory. This core, and the material in Chapter 6, is then extended to include prefrontal cortex (Chapter 11).

Finally, we extend the state neuropsychology of the theory to personality traits (Chapter 12), anxiety disorder syndromes (Chapter 13), and implications for treatment (Chapter 14). Our theory of anxious personality (Chapter 12) sees dysfunction (Chapters 13, 14) as driven by extremes of otherwise adaptive traits (and so integrates healthy personality and psychopathology). We offer a 'double hit' hypothesis of neurotic disorders (McNaughton and Glue, 2020) that sees these as resulting from the interactions of the extremes of two or more traits (with neuroticism as a general factor coupled with one or more disorder-specific traits). The picture of personality presented also allows a convergence of a more recent detailed neurological picture of different defensive traits with an older simple view of 'reward' and 'punishment' sensitivity, respectively.

Our key difference from many psychologists and psychiatrists is that we have always anchored our theory objectively (rather than 'rationally' or 'lexically') by defining 'anxiety' via the action of those anxiolytic drugs that are *not* also panicolytic and antidepressant (Chapter 4). We, therefore, distinguish anxiety from fear/phobia, panic, obsession, and depression. We also now make a key distinction (Chapter 3) between reinforce**ment** (particularly in the guise of reward prediction error and future behaviour change) and reinfor**cers** (attractors and repulsors that elicit upcoming current behaviour).

We see anxiety as the result of goal conflict detected by a GIS that has the SHS at its centre. So, we emphasize both motivational (goal-related) aspects of memory processing and, conversely, memorial aspects of anxiety disorders. We differ from at least older neuropsychological theories in seeing the whole SHS as a key system that detects goal conflict and generates outputs that lead to conflict resolution (Chapters 9, 10). During consolidation and retrieval of goal-related information, this conflict resolution is crucial for memory if interference is present—with SHS inhibition suppressing incorrect (noise) goal engrams not enhancing correct (signal) goal engrams. We argue that interference is the key property distinguishing the many supposed 'types' of hippocampal-sensitive memory (Chapter 8). Negative affective engram tagging is, then, the basis for the chronic condition of anxiety disorder and the slow rate of its correction by anxiolytic drugs.

1.2 Why anxiety? Why neuropsychology? Why the hippocampus?

Why is a 'neuropsychology of anxiety' needed? We believe it provides solutions to an important set of modern problems.

'Anxiety' (in its colloquial meaning) is common in modern societies. It is a frequent unwanted experience in our day-to-day life when we are faced with conflicting work or social choices. It is more serious when it becomes chronic and dysfunctional. 'Anxiety disorders' (as labelled by psychiatrists) are the most prevalent in psychiatry (Kessler et al., 2005; Kessler et al., 2012) and the sixth worst in terms of generating disability (Baxter et al., 2014). They account for about 1 in 10 suicides (Baxter et al., 2014); and are a serious and ever-increasing burden on healthcare resources (Cryan and Sweeney, 2011; Maron and Nutt, 2017; Kessler, 2007). Most strikingly, 'anxiety disorders' tend to start early in life (Cryan and Sweeney, 2011; Maron and Nutt, 2017) and often result in chronic impairment (Meyer, 2017).

Despite its importance, 'anxiety' is poorly understood. Definitions of 'anxiety' are various and contradictory, which has forced us to provide our own definition (see §1.4 based on McNaughton, 2018). With no clear biological definition, psychiatric diagnosis is weak. Diagnostic systems are forced to use lists of signs and symptoms (American Psychiatric Association, 2013; World Health Organization, 2021). Thus, psychiatry's labels are equivalent to 'high temperature coughing disease' and not linked to a fundamental underlying mechanism of dysfunction (Insel et al., 2010). Psychiatry lacks names like COVID-19, which has the SARS-CoV-2 virus as its known cause. So, anxiety treatment is poorly targeted, creating high costs and extensive societal impact (Maron and Nutt, 2017)—conventional treatments take a long time to act, and fail completely in about one-third of patients (Roy-Byrne, 2015).

Doctors cannot be blamed when basic science is lacking. We believe that our job is to replace the current symptom-list systems with diagnoses based on neuropsychology (i.e. a detailed integration of neuroscience and psychology). We agree with the Director of the National Institute of Health, Thomas Insel that 'mental disorders are biological disorders involving brain circuits that implicate specific domains of cognition, emotion, or behaviour' (Insel, 2013). Clinicians need a single system based on the aetiology and pathophysiology of disorders (Insel et al., 2010) if they are to diagnose and treat them effectively (Cryan and Sweeney, 2011; Markou and Cryan, 2012). But we also agree that

> personality neuroscience is at the forefront of developments when it manages to integrate personality and neural approaches and not implicitly (or explicitly) privilege one over the other. This relies on deep theoretical integration – a challenge in itself. This need is seen, for example, with the NIMH approach going awry by privileging the neural over the psychological, at least according to its former director, Thomas Insel (2022[4]). We see this critique in other representative reviews of standard practices in psychiatry.
>
> (Corr and Mobbs, 2023, p. 3)

This book updates our broad-ranging neuropsychology of anxiety, which provides a detailed theoretical basis for: 1) understanding defensive reactions; 2) the development of diagnoses of their distinct disorders; and, 3) seeing the disorders as extremes of biologically-based motivation-related personality traits. It includes a preliminary example of the development of a theoretically-based biomarker for such a personality trait that also acts (at extreme values) as a biomarker for an 'anxiety' disorder.

Why is this book also 'an enquiry into the functions of the septo-hippocampal system'? Using anxiolytic drugs to define anxiety (§1.6) means that our neuropsychology is necessarily, and uniquely, entwined with a theory of the functions of the SHS. Thus, we provide a theory of SHS function that we believe is more comprehensive than the available alternatives. The current edition involves updates of both the data and theory of our previous editions that further strengthen the idea that the SHS is the core of a system that controls goal conflict processing, with goal inhibition contributing as much to anxiety (as opposed to fear) as it does to memory processing (Chapters 7–10) but not completely reflecting either.

This edition provides more detailed neural maps than before of not only anxiety systems (in the sense of systems that process goal conflicts) but also goal repulsion (see §1.12.4) systems (that control panic, phobia, and some aspects of obsession) and, for the first time,

[4] Cited as Insel, T. (2022). *Healing: Our path from mental illness to mental health.* New York: Penguin Press.

provides a matching map of goal attraction systems (that control approach, including impulsiveness). In addition, the anxiety and memory strands of the theory are now interwoven with a theory of the functions of prefrontal cortex (including the insula) and its interactions with the SHS. Despite this expansion, and the many modifications of specific details, the updated theory rests on the same foundations as the original theory, while having a conceptually simpler, more systematic, superstructure.

1.3 Some departures from conventional views

Our theory has always been unconventional. But over the years there has been some convergence: with the temporal end of the hippocampus now generally seen by others as involved in anxiety; and our view of anxiety *disorder*[5] now emphasizing memory consolidation. In this section we will highlight some remaining departures from conventional views for those who care about this past history.

1.3.1 The homogenous hippocampus

To be clear, we hold and always have, that ***all*** aspects of the hippocampus contribute to the resolution of 'hesitation and doubt' (Simonov, 1974; Simonov, 1997). We still hold that the SHS detects conflict between concurrently active goals; that it resolves this conflict by increasing the weight given to affectively negative information by goal processing areas; and that this bias towards negative affect increases anxiety in some tasks while reducing the effects of interference on memory in others. 'Space' or 'memory' in rodent research are among a number of ways of generating the goal conflict that gives rise to hesitation and doubt. Fear without such conflict does not require the SHS but does require areas like the amygdala. Space or memory without such conflict (i.e. without interference, see Chapter 8) does not require the SHS but does require neocortex.

Critically, which may seem cantankerous, we still insist, that the hippocampus is homogenous, with *a single, fundamental, computational function* reflected in its consistent lamellar structure. A slice taken across the hippocampus is anatomically similar along its entire length and across mammalian species, including humans; and the electrophysiology of an isolated slice in an organ bath is essentially identical across all these cases. It is true that the mainstream has come to accept anxiety-related aspects of hippocampal function; but only for its large temporal end[6]; with space/memory-related aspects of hippocampal function 'that operate in parallel' at the small septal end (Wells et al., 2013, p. 8650). We still hold that even the septal end of the hippocampus has a fundamental role in goal conflict, and so anxiety; and that it has only a tangential (although symptomatically consequential) role in space or memory. We see the SHS as processing inputs from goals (compounds of situation and motivation, §1.12.4), with these being coded concurrently by the dorsal ('where') and ventral ('what')

[5] The use of 'anxiety' to *mean* disorder is one of many sources of confusion. Clearly, a thing cannot be its own disorder!

[6] Hence, 'hippocampus' = seahorse (visualized upside down). Note that this end has *most* expanded phylogenetically in humans. Human dorsal hippocampus is probably no bigger functionally than that of a rat. Rat hippocampus is shaped like a banana so it should really be the 'musa' if you are not anthropocentric.

processing streams, which connect with dorsal (septal) and ventral (temporal) hippocampus, respectively (but with some mixing in the entorhinal cortex; Nilssen et al., 2019). As a result, the hippocampus carries out the same computations (see McNaughton & Bannerman, 2024) but on different 'where' and 'what' aspects of the goal at its two ends (with more complex where + what processing in the midsection, §10.5).

1.3.2 The prospective prefrontal cortex

The earliest statement of the core elements of the theory held that 'there is reason to suppose that the frontal orbital cortex acts as the cortical representation of the septo-hippocampal system' (Gray, 1970b, p. 479). Nonetheless, our previous account was both limited and *ad hoc* in dealing with anxiolytic-resistant anxiety (see §13.2.2) and its sensitivity to prefrontal and cingulate lesions (see §11.1). Joe LeDoux (2002 p. 288) explicitly disagreed with our emphasis on the hippocampus and said 'in my opinion, [the second edition] still gives the septum and hippocampus too prominent a role, at the expense of the amygdala and prefrontal cortex'. There are now both new data and theoretical developments on the role of prefrontal cortex (including the insula) in anxiety. Here, therefore, we have embedded prefrontal cortex fully within our theory (§1.12.10; Chapter 11; Fig. 11.15) but without giving it primacy.

We now include rostromedial orbital frontal cortex and parts of the insula in the system that controls anxiety (with lateral orbital frontal cortex included in the fear system). The insula, importantly, *now accounts* (with the basolateral amygdala and perhaps orbital cortex) for the *arousal and attention outputs* of the GIS. Critically (see Fig. 1.8), we see the bulk of the dorsal and ventral trends of prefrontal cortex as controlling the forward planning of goals and resolving conflicts in their *serial sequencing* using 'horizontal' recycling in loops with posterior cortex; whereas anxiety systems resolve conflicts in *concurrent choice* between them using 'vertical' iterative calculation in the Papez circuits that loop from hippocampus via mamillary bodies and anterior thalamus and back to hippocampus via frontal and temporal cortex (for details see Fig. 9.9).

1.3.3 Theoretical change and lack of it

The current edition shows some movement from our earlier departures from convention but not major reversal. Are we just stubborn? Or, worse, are we constitutionally perverse?

If we are stubborn, it is justified by half a century of new data consistent with the basics of the original theory (Gray, 1969; Gray, 1970b). More importantly, the cornerstone data that continue to support our theory are still *unaccounted for and, until recently, unmentioned by other theories of the SHS*. For over five decades, our competitors have largely ignored that:

1) What are now called the 'classical' anxiolytic drugs (e.g. barbiturates, benzodiazepines) have effects on behaviour like those of SHS lesions (Gray, 1977). By the time of the 2nd edition (Gray and McNaughton, 2000), this parallel had proved to be *predictive* for the 'novel' anxiolytics (e.g. buspirone and serotonergic antidepressants). Unlike the classical drugs, novel anxiolytics do not act via $GABA_A$ receptors but through $5HT_{1A}$; and they do not share any of the side effects (anticonvulsant, sedative, hypnotic, and

addictive) of the classical anxiolytics. Despite these mechanistic differences, the parallel with SHS lesion effects extends, for both classical and novel anxiolytics, to distinctively 'hippocampal' tests (McNaughton and Morris, 1992; McNaughton and Morris, 1987). Anxiety and spatial processing are superficially different aspects of SHS function that appear to reflect a single class of neural process (i.e. goal conflict).

2) The classical anti-anxiety drugs produce specific impairments (Gray, 1982) in the control of Rhythmical Slow Activity (RSA/'theta' also called 'theta'[7] or 'hippocampal theta'). This is a characteristic phasic pattern of firing of cells in the hippocampus and related structures. It is controlled by pacemaker cells in the medial septal area and, because many cells fire synchronously, can give rise to an easily recorded gross extracellular rhythm. Importantly: (a) similar impairments in the control of RSA/'theta' are produced by all clinically effective anti-anxiety drugs (§9.1), including the novel anxiolytics (including pregabalin, Baldwin et al., 2013; Siok et al., 2009; Field et al., 2001), anxiolytic antidepressants such as imipramine, and anxiolytic psychedelics such as ketamine (Engin et al., 2009); (b) this is so far true *only* for drugs known to be clinically effective in treating generalized anxiety disorder as compared to, say, schizophrenia; and (c) these impairments in hippocampal electrophysiology—when produced by manipulations confined to the specific brain nuclei controlling them—produce behavioural effects equivalent in many respects to those of systemic administration of anxiolytics. The effects of these compounds on hippocampal electrophysiology can therefore account, in principle, for the bulk of the critical anxiolytic-induced changes in behaviour shared by SHS lesions. We now know that the rhythmicity of RSA/'theta', in and of itself, is important for hippocampal function (McNaughton et al., 2006b) and intracranial injections of an anxiolytic can produce similar changes in RSA/'theta' and behaviour to systemic injections (Woodnorth and McNaughton, 2002b). Gray's 1969, and particularly 1977, versions of the theory remain predictive (McNaughton et al., 2007).

What of our perversity? Since 1982, there has been evolution of our theory, other theories of the SHS, other theories of the neural basis of anxiety, and theories of the psychological nature of generalized anxiety. Our second edition (Gray and McNaughton, 2000) saw these evolutions as convergent, reducing (though not eliminating) our unconventionality. This trend has continued.

Our theory differs from the others—most notably in attempting to combine them. But, in several cases, it differs only semantically, particularly as a result of a specific analysis that we offer of the distinction between 'fear' and 'anxiety'. Critically, we define 'anxiety' via anxiolytic action. This requires adjustment of the various (§1.4) psychologically oriented/everyday uses of the word. So, we will try to persuade you that many still-current orthodoxies are, in critical respects incomplete, when they are not totally wrong; and that here we have moved towards and so captured the common centre towards which all of the theories continue to converge. Crucially, our theory's competitors are usually applied only to limited parts of the data set that we incorporate. Our theory may appear somewhat more complex in its explanation in a

[7] RSA/'theta' was discovered in species where it is in the 4–7 Hz (human EEG theta) band. However, in rats RSA/'theta' spans the human theta and alpha (8–12 Hz) bands. Importantly, we have found (see McNaughton, 2018) an anxiolytic-sensitive rhythm in the human EEG that also spans theta + alpha and so, following Vanderwolf (1969); Vanderwolf (2003, Note 8 p. 22), we will use RSA/'theta' for both human and rat 2–12 Hz and restrict theta to 4–7 Hz.

limited domain such as hippocampal 'place fields' (Chapter 7), but even there we believe we capture those specific data better (McNaughton & Bannerman, 2024).

In summary, we argue that the role of the SHS in the control of memory is indirect, it resolves conflicts between similarly, and highly, activated concurrent goals (and, so, their engrams). In memory paradigms (and consolidation), this reduces interference. Critically for the relationship of memory to the control of anxiety, we postulate that the SHS resolves goal conflict, and so memory interference, by *amplifying negative affective goal associations*. So, in our view, 'amnesia' resulting from hippocampal damage could more properly be described as 'catastrophic hypermnesia' (McNaughton and Wickens, 2003). This double-negative view is consistent with reports of apparent failure to retrieve correct items because of intrusion errors (i.e. retrieval of items that were previously correct but are now incorrect). As we will detail in Chapter 8, it is the variety of ways in which the specific methodological features of a memory test can generate conflict between correct and incorrect items that has given rise to the profusion of dichotomies of 'types of memory' supposedly supported (but occasionally not), by the hippocampal formation.

Our perspective also accounts for the fact that the hippocampus is clearly not a long-term memory store, and for the problems with seeing a structure that has become relatively over 30 times smaller than neocortex with encephalization (Stephan and Andy, 1969) as a temporary store for memories that are then somehow copied to other areas—or even as a store for higher order forms of memory (see §8.2.10). Likewise, while recent 'memory index' ideas (Goode et al., 2020) may account for relatively small size, they do not account for hippocampal lesion effects on unlearned responses, nor the *lack* of hippocampal effects on learning from which interference has been eliminated (Chapter 8).

We see the same basic SHS mechanisms, when hyperactive or hypersensitive, as giving rise to something akin to generalized anxiety disorder. Increases in the valence of affectively negative associations cause not only current goals to be judged as more threatening than normal, but also a consequential bias towards the storage of more threatening associations of those goals (Eysenck et al., 2007; Eysenck and Derakshan, 2011). Thus, anxiety has not only an emotional component, but also a unique cognitive component. We shall argue that, while the amygdala is indeed necessary for the expression of many emotional aspects of anxiety, it is so because of its interactions with the SHS; the latter remains the central subcortical structure for the specific cognitive components of anxiety and also the *principal* mediator of the behavioural effects of the anti-anxiety drugs. That said, we will also include aspects of prefrontal cortex, particularly the insula, in the systems that resolve goal conflicts—particularly in the control of arousal and attention.

1.4 What is 'anxiety'?

Our departures from convention are in part simply semantic. We differ, not on the experimental facts (most of which are not in dispute), but on decisions as to which facts are to be included as explicanda, what inferences are to be drawn from them, and which words should be used to summarize them. Word choice is particularly important since we use theory to restrict our meanings of several words. It becomes particularly acute when dealing with the lexical jungle of personality (Chapter 12).

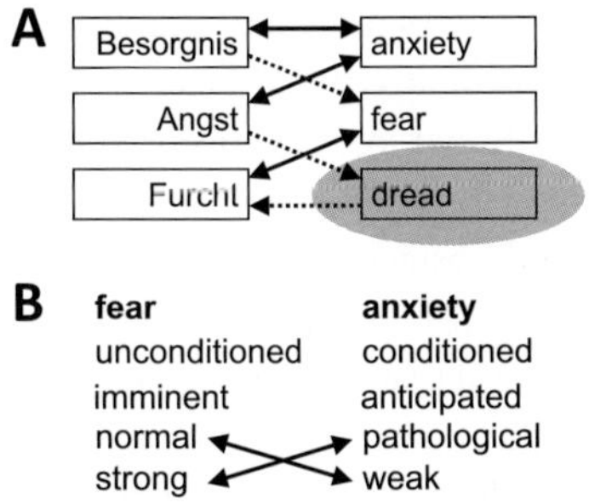

Fig. 1.1 What are the meanings of "fear" and "anxiety"? A. Translation paths between anxiety-related words in German and English using Collins German Dictionary (from McNaughton, 2018, with permission). B. Common bases for distinguishing between fear and anxiety in scientific or common English. Grey arrows are cases of significant meaning discrepancies—see text.

There are two problems with the word 'anxiety'. The first is one with everyday usage: it is not clear what 'anxiety' means and, in particular, in how it differs from 'fear'. There is also no clear scientific consensus (for a 'roundtable' discussion, see Grogans et al., 2023). The second problem is scientific: both 'anxiety' and 'fear' (whatever we take them to mean) normally refer to internal experiences that are not easily accessible to objective measurement. Our strategy will be to bootstrap from a range of objective measurements to scientific (functional, evolutionary) definitions and then show that these new definitions map quite well to some of the current other usages.

The usage problem is exemplified in Fig. 1.1[8]. One way to investigate meaning is to check translations in a dictionary (we used an older Collins German Dictionary for Fig. 1.1A, other dictionaries would give somewhat different results). Students of Freud will be unsurprised that 'anxiety' translates as 'Angst' and vice versa. There is, in principle, no problem with the fact that 'anxiety' also translates as 'Besorgnis' (so Angst and Besorgnis would be types of anxiety) but then we find that 'Besorgnis' translates as 'fear' (but not vice versa) and 'Angst' translates as 'dread' (but not vice versa). Besorgnis/dread translate to fear/Furcht but not vice versa and, more surprisingly, Besorgnis and dread do not translate to each other.

A second way to investigate meaning is to look at the key factors people use to distinguish the words (Fig. 1.1B). Psychologists, including our first edition (Gray, 1971; Gray, 1982), have distinguished fear and anxiety as being unconditioned and conditioned, respectively. The most recent major edition of the 'Diagnostic and Statistical Manual of mental disorders' of the American Psychiatric Association sees fear as a response to imminent threat and anxiety as a response to anticipated future threat (American Psychiatric Association, 2013, p 826; text revision in American Psychiatric Association, 2022)[9]. Many would see fear as normal but anxiety as pathological. Conversely, others would see fear as strong and anxiety as weak. These distinctions do not map to each other and the last two, effectively, contradict each other as pathological (= anxiety) would be expected to be strong (= fear). As a result there is a plenitude of partially overlapping definitions of 'anxiety' and 'fear' with a large number of meanings spread among different people (Davitz, 1969). Definitional uncertainty

[8] Part A of this figure and the bulk of the argument that follows are taken from McNaughton (2018).
[9] Imminent/anticipated is much the same distinction as certain/potential, see Chapter 2.

remains even within a discipline such as psychiatry. '*Some* definitions of anxiety distinguish it from fear . . . The manifestations of anxiety and fear are the same' (American Psychiatric Association, 1987, p392, our emphasis). 'Anxiety disorders include disorders . . . of excessive fear' (American Psychiatric Association, 2013, p 826).

There is a second fundamental obstacle for construction of any neuropsychological account of 'anxiety': the most immediate referent for the state of anxiety is our own personal experience. Not only can we not know if that experience maps directly to someone else's, but the bulk of available neuropsychological data are from non-human animal experiments where we expect the experience not to be identical with our own.

But there is, nonetheless, a way to proceed that we have previously suggested as a general approach to all emotions.

> We allow any and every meaning of the word . . . to outline an approximate area of observations and experiment. We then attempt to account for as much of the data as possible with some small number of assumptions. Some part of the resultant theory may then be found to map back to our original conception of [the] emotion, providing a scientific definition of the term. On the other hand, it may not, in which case . . . scientifically speaking there is no such thing. (McNaughton, 1989b, p. 4)

1.5 Fear versus anxiety—ethoexperimental analysis

One scientific way to account for fear/anxiety-related behaviours is to ask about their adaptive functions. This can be done particularly conveniently with ethoexperimental and ethopharmacological analysis; where experiments are conducted in a laboratory but ethology rather than behaviour analysis takes centre stage (Blanchard and Blanchard, 1990a; Blanchard et al., 1993). Importantly the emphasis on adaptive function focuses on rich behaviour sets provided by the animal (rather than limiting responses to a single arbitrary manipulandum chosen by the experimenter). This will help us define expected inputs to the key goal control systems of our theory.

The crucial point (see Chapter 2 for a full discussion) is that what a rat must do to leave an area where there *is* a cat is quite different from when it must do (to gain food or water) to safely enter an area where a cat has been or might be. Cats and cat odour, respectively, have the advantage of being stimuli that can release these two different classes of behaviour without the need for prior training; but it is the form of behaviour that is important in this context, not the type of stimulus that elicits it. Also important is the concept of defensive distance. Different forms of behaviour are appropriate at different distances from the cat (e.g. fight is only appropriate or, indeed, possible when the cat is close), but this 'intensity' variable is independent of the cat/cat odour distinction. (Defensive distance also determines whether a human will receive help from others; Vieira et al., 2020). The Blanchards included the cat-related behaviours in a 'fear defence battery' and the cat-odour-related behaviours in an 'anxiety defence battery'. Having already distinguished 'fear' and 'anxiety' on purely ethological grounds, they then showed that the 'anxiety' *but not* the 'fear' behaviours are affected by drugs defined as 'anxiolytic' on purely clinical grounds. They thus linked one functional set of rat behaviour to human clinical dysfunction. (Note that simple phobia in people is also insensitive to anxiolytics; Sartory et al., 1990.)

The Blanchards themselves suggested that the categorical distinction between fear and anxiety depended on whether the predator is *actually* or only *potentially* present (echoing the DSM-5 imminent/anticipated distinction mentioned earlier). However, behaviour analysis (Chapter 3) shows that the key adaptation is to remove the animal *from,* or to facilitate entry *into,* a dangerous situation. Whether the danger is clear and present or only presumed, the question is: Is active or passive avoidance involved? If active, fear is involved; if passive, anxiety. This categorical dimension, of 'defensive direction', is quite distinct from the smoothly graded dimension of 'defensive distance' considered earlier (McNaughton and Corr, 2004). Crucially (Chapter 3), it will allow us to include in our analysis of fear versus anxiety the events of both loss and omission of gain, as well as stimuli related to these events.

The two distinctions, of defensive direction and defensive distance, are theoretically independent of one another: an animal may be engaged in approach to, or escape from, danger for any intensity of danger. The greater the danger, the more intense will be the degree of activation of the active or passive avoidance system and the stronger the corresponding emotional state (anxiety during the need to approach to danger, fear during escape from it).

The two dimensions are not, however, independent in experimental practice. Given a fixed appetitive motivation conflicting with the danger, the closer the animal is to the point of danger, the more likely it is that escape will take precedence over anxious approach. In the straight alley, as exemplified in Neal Miller's classic studies of approach-avoidance conflict (e.g. Miller, 1944; see Gray, 1987b; McNaughton et al., 2016), the animal approaches the goal and then oscillates back and forth at a point where the decrease in defensive distance is such that the approach and avoidance tendencies are just in balance (Fig. 1.2). 'So, if the rat shown in [Fig. 1.2] is treated with an anxiolytic drug, it will no longer dither and will approach closer to, and sometimes reach, the goal box (Bailey and Miller, 1952; Barry and Miller, 1965)—since the drug affects the passive avoidance generated by goal conflict but not basic approach or basic active avoidance tendencies (Gray, 1977)' (McNaughton et al., 2016, p. 30).

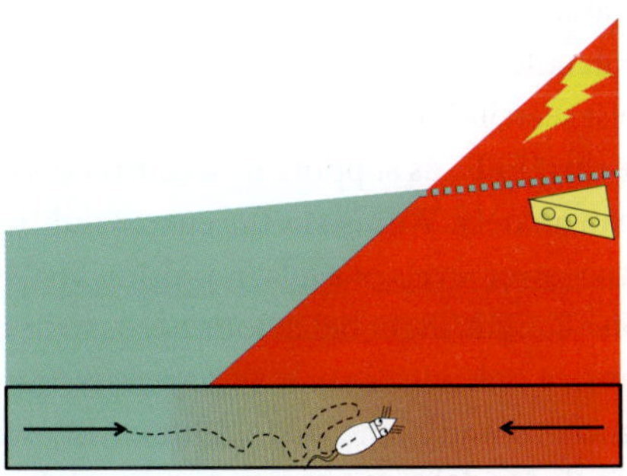

Fig. 1.2 Interaction of approach and avoidance gradients and the generation of conflict. Positive goals (e.g., cheese for a hungry rat) have an effect on behaviour that decreases slowly with distance (green). Negative ones (e.g., shock) have a steeper gradient (red). Their interaction (graded color in bottom panel) means a rat will initially run toward food but then will stop part way and dither if there is a shock. Figure and legend from McNaughton et al. (2016) with permission.

It should be noted, also, that defensive distance, as defined by the Blanchards, is a *cognitive* construct. For any particular individual in a specific situation, defensive distance does depend on physical (or temporal) distance from the danger; but it also depends on the perceived amount of threat: the greater the perceived threat, the greater is the physical distance from it that combines with perceived threat to produce a particular value of defensive distance. The strength of this perception will vary both with the external physical intensity of the threat and with the personality of the individual (Chapter 12). A particularly tough rat will attempt to, and often succeed, in seeing off a cat that a meek rat will not.

These data suggest that there are at least two functional neural systems—one controlling 'fear' and one 'anxiety', with each being hierarchically organized (§1.14) to control behaviours appropriate to different defensive distances. But where are these systems in the brain?

1.6 Starting points for a neuropsychology of anxiety

At least four different starting points have been used by scientists attempting to bridge the gap between the human experience of anxiety and animal (including human) brain systems. Not surprisingly, these different starting points gave rise to different initial conclusions. The available state analyses also do not map neatly to the various biologically-inspired attempts to produce trait scales. The trait scales, and problems with their rational rather than neural derivation, are reviewed in McNaughton (2020) and also Chapter 12.

The first, and most direct, starting point is electrical stimulation of the brain that elicits various forms of defensive behaviour—and so may be eliciting a matching central state. Both escape behaviour ('flight') and defensive aggression ('fight') can be elicited from the medial hypothalamus and from the periaqueductal grey (Flynn, 1967; Flynn, 1969; Panksepp, 1982; Graeff, 1991; Davis and Panksepp, 2018). Human patients, stimulated in the periaqueductal grey, 'expressed strong emotions referring to feelings of death, fear, terror and impending doom. … these feelings were real and terrifying to the patients' (Iacono and Nashold, 1982, p 276). The stimulation is clearly generating a central state in rats (not just eliciting a behaviour): the same stimulation will produce fight or flight depending on environmental conditions. Roughly speaking, if escape is possible, that is the dominant response; if it is not, but something that can be attacked is present in the test chamber, then defensive aggression is seen. In both cases the detailed behaviour is directed appropriately to the current situation. The stimulation is best seen, then, as activating a unified emergency 'fight/flight/freeze system' (!FFFS); but we see this !FFFS as supporting a central state linked to human fear, particularly panic, not to human anxiety. We also in the current edition (Table 1.1) see the !FFFS proper as occupying only the lower levels of a fear/repulsion system[10].

As emphasized in Chapter 2, fight/flight behaviour needs to be categorically distinguished from other classes of defensive behaviour such as risk assessment even in rats (Blanchard and Blanchard, 1990b; Blanchard and Blanchard, 1990c). Also, while fight/flight is sensitive to anti-panic ('panicolytic') drugs, it is not sensitive to anxiolytic drugs (Blanchard et al., 1997b). Conversely, 'the hypothalamic-pituitary-adrenal axis is activated by anticipatory anxiety but not by panic attack nor by electrical stimulation of the rat periaqueductal grey' (Graeff and Del-Ben, 2008, p. 1326).

[10] This change of use being flagged by the '!'.

A second possible starting point is the effects of brain lesions in man. In the past, with what appeared to be extreme cases of anxiety, resistant to both psychological treatment and classic anxiolytics, lesions of the cingulate or prefrontal cortex could appear helpful. So cingulate and prefrontal cortex might mediate extreme (Marks et al., 1966) or complex anxiety. Against this, we will argue (Chapter 13) that cases of obsessive-compulsive disorder reflect fear rather than anxiety (Rapoport, 1989). However, a major addition to our new theoretical superstructure (Chapter 11) expands our theory to include orbital frontal cortex and the insula. In particular, we suggest that anxiety, can involve both cortical and subcortical structures together or separately under different circumstances.

A third, particularly productive, starting point has been detailed neuroscientific analysis of fear conditioning. This has given rise to a continuing orthodoxy that locates anxiety in the amygdala. As is well known, if an initially neutral stimulus (e.g. a light flash or a brief tone) is paired, in a standard Pavlovian conditioning paradigm, as a conditioned stimulus (CS) with a painful unconditioned stimulus (UCS) such as electric foot-shock, the CS comes to elicit a variety of conditioned responses (CRs) interpreted as signs of fear (e.g. freezing/immobility, increased heart rate, defecation, increased readiness to startle, etc.). Extensive experimental work, especially in the laboratories of Joe LeDoux (1992; 1994; Schafe et al., 2005; Lamprecht et al., 2009; Doyère et al., 2007) and Michael Davis (1992a; 1992b; 1992c; Davis, 2002) located formation of such CRs to plasticity in the amygdala. We do not dispute the observations but suggest that simple conditioned fear of this kind is more closely (but not entirely) related to human clinical phobia than anxiety. However, we will argue that other aspects of the amygdala are also, separately, involved in anxiety (as with contextual 'fear' conditioning) and, likewise, in positive affect. We also see this tri-partite functional division as starting at lower levels particularly in the periaqueductal grey (Silva and McNaughton, 2019; Chapter 6).

The fourth starting point, which we particularly favour, is the effects of anti-anxiety drugs. 'Anxiolytics' in the sense that we will use the word are classes of drug that reduce self-reported or physician-assessed anxiety in the clinic (particularly generalized anxiety) and which ***as a class do not affect panic, phobia, or obsession*** (nor, *as a class*, have side effects like addiction or anticonvulsant action).There is no getting round this selectivity; and our labelling takes account of it.

No drug is a 'magic bullet' with only the one desired action. But, as indicated earlier, the anxiolytic approach is now extremely powerful with the availability of two distinct classes ($5HT_{1A}$, calcium channel) of novel anxiolytics to triangulate on the previously known effects of the classical anxiolytics ($GABA_A$). These different chemical classes share clinical anxiolytic action but have radically different mechanisms of direct pharmacological action and non-overlapping side effects. Neural or behavioural effects shared by all three classes of anxiolytic drug have, therefore, a high probability of delineating processes involved in clinical anxiety or in its amelioration. Our approach is to use the *common* ultimate actions of *all* clinically well-established *specific* anxiolytic drugs to *define* anxiety itself. Remarkably, this emphasis on common ultimate action has led to no major changes in our original presumed behavioural profile for anxiolytics in general (Gray, 1977) despite this profile having been based originally only on data from the classical anxiolytic drugs, usually sodium amytal[11]. It has also not led us to abandon the core neural elements of the original theory—although each

[11] A barbiturate also known as sodium amylobarbitone or sodium amobarbital.

edition (including this one) has made significant additions to that original core in both the cortical and subcortical directions.

1.7 Anxiolytics, goal conflict, and the goal inhibition system

Early study of the effects of classical anxiolytics on the behaviour of experimental animals, especially in paradigms derived from animal learning theory, gave rise to the concept of a 'Behavioural Inhibition System'/BIS (Gray, 1976). This system was held to account for the detailed behavioural profile of anxiolytic drug action (Gray, 1977). The theory of the anxiolytic BIS was expounded in detail in our first edition (Gray, 1982) and our second edition (Gray and McNaughton, 2000) provided a functional account of its effective inputs via integration of ethoexperimental analysis (§ 1.2, Chapter 2) with learning-theory (Chapter 3). Importantly, ethopharmacology validated the ethological approach in the context of our original anxiolytic-based theory. So, while the drugs still had primacy, their effects could be rephrased in simple functional terms. This functional perspective has, so far, stood the test of time; but the drugs remain primary and provide the only validity test of biomarkers (e.g. McNaughton et al., 2013; Shadli et al., 2015; Shadli et al., 2016; Shadli et al., 2020a).

The BIS was named, within a learning theory context, for its most obvious distinguishing characteristic (suppression of ongoing goal-directed responding). But this name can lead to a number of misunderstandings. The BIS is neither the sole source of inhibition of goal-directed behaviour nor is it directly related to action stopping, which is insensitive to anxiolytic drugs (McNaughton et al., 2013; Shadli et al., 2015). Within the reinforcement sensitivity theory (RST) of personality (see, Corr, 2008b) there has been misunderstanding both of the role of the BIS and of its relationship to the !FFFS. The name also does not hint at its primary function: to *resolve conflict* between goals. In relation to conflict resolution, inhibition of pre-potent behaviour is just a first enabling step and changes in arousal, attention, negative bias, risk assessment, and information gathering (which have always been included in the BIS theory) are at least as important.

Here, we adopt a renaming of this anxiolytic-defined system to the 'Goal Inhibition System'/GIS (introduced and justified in more detail in McNaughton, 2020). Provided you are clear as to our original concept of the BIS, this is a superficial change. However, with respect to RST, this is a substantive change since the existing widely used BIS/BAS scales (Carver and White, 1994) cannot be taken to measure the sensitivity of the GIS and, in any case, the BIS scale appears to measure worry not 'behavioural inhibition' (§12.8.4). In Chapter 12 we discuss means of developing a true GIS scale using biomarkers not 'rational' or 'lexical' assumptions. The key is to emphasize the goal-related (as opposed to action-related) nature of the system. Similar issues for RST arise with our renaming of the other systems in terms of attraction and repulsion (see Corr and McNaughton, 2012).

Similarly, we propose a renaming of our original fear-related system from the FFFS to the 'Goal Repulsion System'/GRS. We retain !FFFS as a label for the original set of proximal survival circuits (LeDoux, 2012) within the lower levels of the GRS that control *undirected* fight, flight, and freezing. But we provide the higher levels that control all non-specific behaviours directed away from any repulsive goal (§1.12.4) with a new, more appropriate designation.

In particular we discuss the issue that 'fight' as included or rejected by a range of current 'rational' questionnaires is not !FIGHT (§12.13).

Likewise, we propose a renaming of the original Behavioural Approach System (BAS) to 'Goal Attraction System'/GAS. Again, in many cases this will appear a simple superficial change but, in relation to RST, it should be clear that a *single* GAS sensitivity measure cannot be identified directly with any one of the *three* existing BAS scales (Carver and White, 1994)—although these may in fact be mono-factorial (Maack and Ebesutani, 2018). We also argue (Chapter 12), using neural measures, that the BAS scales are more related to dopaminergic systems and 'reward prediction error' (§12.7.2; Schultz, 2016; Schultz et al., 2017). Here, the good news is that this dopaminergic perspective re-generates the original 'reward'/ 'punishment' perspective but with new nuances and in parallel with the GAS, GRS[!FFFS], and GIS systems.

The key features of the GAS, GIS, and GRS, taken as the three major goal control systems of the brain, are shown in Table 1.1. What is meant by goal, attractor, repulsor, negative bias and conflict resolution is summarized in §1.12.4 and will be dealt with in detail in later chapters. An important point, driven by the neurology of the next section, is that the lowest level of all three systems can be seen as involving sets of survival circuits (LeDoux, 2012) that control proximal stimulus-specific behaviours. So, the lowest levels of the repulsion system contain the structures that were first identified with the !FFFS as well as structures controlling disgust, for example; and equivalent components of the attraction system control eating, lordosis, etc. Importantly all three systems include stationary 'behaviour' that nonetheless fulfils the required adaptive function: lordosis, defensive quiescence (often labelled freezing or conditioned freezing), and freezing (proper). These can all be distinguished by specific body postures in the rat that match the adaptive function.

The basic concepts of the GIS are shown in Fig. 1.3 with progressively more complex versions in Figs. 3.2 and Fig. 5.1. The GIS is activated by goal conflict. In the simplest cases, this occurs when an action directed towards a prepotent positive goal encounters a negative consequence. When activated, the GIS is held to stop or enhance existing stopping of ongoing behaviour, increase vigilance, increase arousal, and increase negative valence (so increasing the inhibition of approach relative to avoidance behaviour). Lesion data (Gray, 1970b; Gray, 1977; Gray and McNaughton, 1983; Gray and McNaughton, 2000) have established that the SHS is a key element in the GIS. All anxiolytics, most discovered since construction of the original theory, impair the control of hippocampal RSA/'theta' (McNaughton et al., 2007) as well as hippocampal-sensitive behaviour.[12] We also now know that RSA/'theta' frequency rhythmicity in and of itself is important for hippocampal function (McNaughton et al., 2006b) and that anxiolytics injected into a nucleus that controls RSA/'theta' frequency alter both frequency and behaviour to the same extent as systemic administration (Woodnorth and McNaughton, 2002).

[12] The effects of the novel anxiolytics on both animal behaviour and in the clinic appear to show U shaped dose response curves; to require long-term administration for clear effects; and to show some other minor differences from classical anxiolytics. We will resolve this apparent difficulty by appeal to evidence that this is due to their opposite effects on the pituitary adrenal axis to those of classical anxiolytics. But note that, in any case, the similarity of the animal behaviour and human clinical response in this regard supports rather than weakens the theory.

Table 1.1 A new nomenclature for the primary goal control systems (from McNaughton, 2020). Note that GRS replaces the previous FFFS, while !FFFS is retained as a subsystem of GRS. The ! flags the behaviours as specific elicited response not general goal-oriented tendencies

	The three major goal (situation + motivation) control systems		
New name	Goal **Attraction** System	Goal **Inhibition** System	Goal **Repulsion** System
Abbreviation	GAS	GIS	GRS
Originally	BAS	BIS	FFFS
Goal type	Attractor	Multiple conflicting	repulsor
Reinforcer type	Positive	Increased negative bias or decreased positive bias	negative
Distal behaviour	Attraction	Inhibition	repulsion*
Motivation type	Appetitive	Informative	aversive
Survival function	Consumption	Conflict resolution	Defence
Proximal stimulus-specific behaviours**	Social aggression*** Eat (inc. Predation***) Drink Affiliate (e.g. groom) Mate (e.g. lordosis), etc.	Defensive quiescence**** Rear risk assess, etc.	*!Fight****** *!Freeze******* *Flight* [!FFFS] *Disgust,* *etc.*

Notes:

1 Systems are fronto-limbic-hypothalamic and distinct from motor (action) control.

2 GIS defined by anxiolytic drugs.

3 Proximal GRS includes basic FFS as defined by Gray 1971/1987.

4 GIS activated by upcoming goal conflict; GRS by negative outcome conflict.

5 Survival circuits as in Ledoux (2012); see also *Current Opinion in Behavioral Sciences* 2018, 24, pp. 1–180.

* 'avoidance' (active = GRS/passive = GIS) and 'withdrawal' are ambiguous.

** trait control generally includes proximal-specific as well as distal-general behaviours.

***! Added to distinguish from 'Fight' - previously including social aggression and predation.

****! Added to distinguish from 'Freeze' previously including defensive quiescence.

Thanks to Johnathan Williams, Colin Deyoung, and Philip Gable for discussion.

1.8 Fear versus anxiety—neurology

Our four basic starting points give us multiple candidates for the 'seat of anxiety' and/or 'the seat of fear': the PAG; hypothalamus; amygdala; SHS; and cingulate and frontal cortices. Can all these inferences be correct? Clearly, each of these regions plays some kind of a role in defensive behaviour and the associated emotional states. And, since the brain is a single coordinated (albeit highly differentiated) system, these multifarious regions must interact to coordinate the control of defence. It is also clear that, underlying the whole gamut of neurotic disorders, we need to postulate at least two separate neuropsychological systems (see Chapter 13). The critical evidence is a pharmacological dissociation: there are drugs which alleviate self-reported anticipatory anxiety but not panic attacks, and others that can

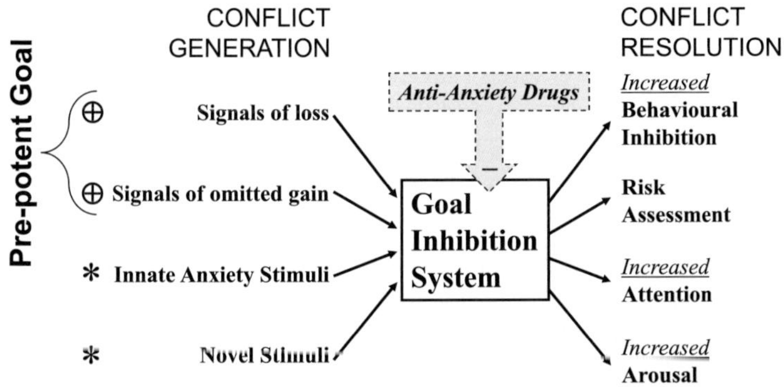

Fig. 1.3 The Goal Inhibition System (GIS). This responds to any of its adequate inputs (CONFLICT GENERATION) with all of its outputs (CONFLICT RESOLUTION). It is defined as the substrate on which all anxiolytics act (Chapters 2-4). The key feature of the input stimuli is that they generate goal conflict. A pre-potent goal must be in conflict with similarly activated incompatible goals (Chapter 3). Novel stimuli and innate anxiety stimuli are held to automatically elicit incompatible goals (*). Thus, where a to-be-punished response is weak or where a novel stimulus elicits only approach tendencies uncontaminated with avoidance, the GIS will *not* be engaged. Output includes increased behavioural inhibition (see chapter 3), arousal, and attention (including risk assessment behaviour, which is now shown separately). Renamed and adapted from the Behavioural Inhibition System of Gray (1982).

alleviate panic as well as, independently, anxiety (Table 4.1; see also Blanchard et al., 1997b). Importantly, anxiolytics not only do not have effects comparable to those of panicolytic drugs, but actually increase the degree of fight/flight behaviour elicited by stimulation of the central grey (Graeff, 1994).

Ethoexperimental analysis (§1.5; Chapter 2) suggests that defensive distance and defensive direction combine to determine the appropriate behaviour. Both behaviour and stimulus analysis can range from 'slow and sophisticated', where there is room and time to manoeuvre, to 'quick and dirty' (LeDoux, 1994), when danger is immediate. Variation in defensive distance, then, creates variation in functional requirements, which more detailed neural analysis (Chapter 6) suggests map to a hierarchy (§1.14) of defence system structures (e.g. Graeff, 1994) in which the lowest level, the periaqueductal grey, coordinates undirected escape (Graeff and Del-Ben, 2008); the medial hypothalamus coordinates directed escape (Canteras and Graeff, 2014); the amygdala coordinates simple active avoidance (Calder et al., 1996; Morris et al., 1996a; Phillips et al., 1997; Phillips et al., 1998); the anterior cingulate cortex coordinates more complex active avoidance (Rapoport, 1989); and the orbital frontal cortex coordinate more long-term planned avoidance (Chapter 11).

What of defensive direction? The same detailed neural analysis (Chapter 6, Chapter 11) shows that in parallel with the structures that control defensive avoidance, there are structures within the same general neural complexes that control defensive (careful, risky) approach. Critically, each of these parts of the defensive approach system responds to injections of anxiolytic drugs and shows local RSA/'theta'. We have, then, a symmetrical, hierarchical, two-dimensional subcortical defence system (McNaughton and Corr, 2004). Since the GIS requires approach-avoidance (or other equivalent) goal conflict, our current subcortical and cortical goal control (and arousal and attention control) models include matching details of the approach system. Note that the prefrontal cortex ('planning circuits') may sometimes operate independently of lower levels ('survival circuits'). Both the key structures involved and their functions are complex new additions to the theory and will be discussed in detail later and are shown in Fig. 6.5 (lower-level goal control survival circuits only) and Fig. 11.15 (lower- and higher-level goal and arousal/attention circuits).

Although identified as just one of a range of structures included in the GIS (see also Calhoon and Tye, 2015), the hippocampus is for both historical and neural reasons the one that we see as central to our neuropsychology of anxiety. It is also the one where our current view is at greatest divergence from the conventional space/memory view, particularly of the septal part of the hippocampus. A further important feature is that our theory is not just of the hippocampus but, because of the central role of RSA/'theta' in anxiolytic action, our theory is of an extended SHS. It is to this we now turn in somewhat more detail.

1.9 Anxiolytics, the septo-hippocampal system, and RSA/'theta'

In sections 1.10–1.12, we will make clear what structures are included in the SHS, summarize what the SHS does, and present a new computationally-oriented model of how the SHS functions. But first we will emphasize four reasons for linking anxiolytic action to the SHS.

1.9.1 Why link anxiolytic action to the SHS? #1 drugs and lesions

First, the parallel between the behavioural effects of the anxiolytic drugs and those of experimental lesions to the SHS is strikingly strong (see Chapter 4 and particularly Table 4.2). We speak here of lesions to the 'septo-hippocampal system' because the parallel in fact has three limbs. We first pick out those effects of lesions to the hippocampal formation that are matched by similar effects of lesions to the parts of the septal area that are most closely connected to the hippocampus: the medial septal area, which projects to the hippocampus; and the lateral septal area, which receives return projections from the hippocampus. These *joint* effects of hippocampal and septal lesions are found to resemble closely the effects of anxiolytic drugs.

This parallel was first pointed out by Gray (1970b) on the basis of very limited data—mainly the effects of sodium amytal and a small number of lesion experiments. This then (Gray, 1982) proved predictive for all (Gray, 1977) the classical ($GABA_A$) anxiolytic drugs (barbiturates, benzodiazepines and ethanol) as well as several hundred lesion studies (Gray and McNaughton, 1983). Later (Gray and McNaughton, 2000), the prediction was found to extend to novel anxiolytics, especially agonists at the serotonin/5-hydroxtryptamine 1A receptor ($5HT_{1A}$) such as buspirone. So, this cornerstone of our theory not only has an immense volume of data supporting it but has now shown predictive validity for half a century, and across drug types with no known common direct actions on the nervous system and no common clinical effects other than the relief of anxiety in at least some patients.

1.9.2 Why link anxiolytic action to the SHS? #2 drugs and RSA/'theta'

Second, early experiments from our laboratories using the classical $GABA_A$ anxiolytics demonstrated (Gray, 1982) that these all have in common two electrophysiological 'signatures' that involve hippocampal RSA/'theta' – signatures that, taken together, are not shared with any drugs shown not to be anxiolytic in the clinic. This pattern has also proved predictive.

As noted briefly already, RSA/'theta' is a rhythmic burst firing pattern of neurones in the hippocampus and related structures which, because it is synchronous across very large numbers of cells, often gives rise to a high-voltage quasi-sinusoidal electrographic slow rhythm (approximately 5–10 Hz in the unanaesthetized rat) that can be recorded from the hippocampal formation under a variety of behavioural conditions. RSA/'theta' is controlled by pacemaker cells located in the medial septal area, which themselves receive a frequency-setting input from structures in the midbrain, including importantly the medial supramammillary nucleus (Kirk and McNaughton, 1991; Kirk and McNaughton, 1993). It is possible to drive RSA/'theta' by low-frequency electrical stimulation of the medial septal area (one RSA/'theta' wave being elicited by each pulse) or to elicit it by high-frequency (e.g. 100 Hz) stimulation of the reticular formation (which provides input to the medial supramammillary nucleus, where frequency is encoded and relayed to the medial septum).

The common electrophysiological signatures of the classical anxiolytics are: (1) an elevation of the threshold for septal driving of hippocampal RSA/'theta' that is relatively specific to an intermediate RSA/'theta' frequency of 7.7 Hz (at which, in the undrugged male rat, there is a minimum threshold for RSA/'theta' driving; Fig. 9.1); and (2) a reduction in the frequency of RSA/'theta' elicited by reticular stimulation of given intensity (in both drugged and undrugged animals there is a linear relation between stimulus intensity and elicited RSA/'theta' frequency with no non-linearity in the region of 7.7 Hz; Fig. 9.2). We have been unable to demonstrate both of these signatures together in any other class of drugs (Chapter 9).

The novel anxiolytics offered a stringent test of the predictive generality of these electrophysiological signatures, which (Gray and McNaughton, 2000) they duly passed (see also Chapter 9; Appendix 5). This predictive validity from the clinic to the test has been extended further recently (McNaughton et al., 2007). Predictive validity from the test to acute action on animal behaviour has been reported (Yeung et al., 2012); but this needs to be treated with considerable caution and it should be emphasized that human clinical anxiolytic action requires long-term administration of the drugs (Wheatley, 1990) as does comparability between classical and novel anxiolytics with animal behaviour models (Zhu and McNaughton, 1995b).

1.9.3 Why link anxiolytic action to the SHS? #3 neural control

Third, selectively reproducing parts of the SHS electrographic signatures of the anxiolytic drugs reproduces parts of the behavioural profile that they share with septal and hippocampal lesions. This is an important result: it demonstrates that the electrographic signatures are not just accidental correlates of clinical action, but represent functional effects of the drugs on the SHS that can, in combination, reproduce large parts of the behavioural profile of systemic administration of anxiolytics. Importantly, since both signatures are obtained in response to electrical stimulation, we have shown that it is rhythmicity of an appropriate frequency that is important for hippocampal function, whether this is induced with a natural or artificial pattern of stimulation (McNaughton et al., 2006b).

In early experiments, we were able to show (see Gray, 1982) that the first, septally-elicited, electrophysiological signature of anxiolytic drug action noted earlier could be reproduced by selective lesion of the dorsal ascending noradrenergic bundle (Gray et al., 1975). This pathway arises from the locus coeruleus in the brain stem to innervate most of the forebrain, including the SHS (§6.11). On the basis of these observations we proposed that the action of the anxiolytics on SHS function is in part mediated by the drug-induced reduction of activity in the dorsal bundle shown by Fuxe et al. (1975). For somewhat similar reasons we additionally suggested that anxiolytic drug action is mediated in part also by reduction in activity in the ascending serotonergic pathway that arises in the median raphe nucleus and innervates the SHS. For both of these monoamine pathways, Fuxe et al. (1975) had demonstrated that stress increases release of the relevant transmitter (noradrenaline[13] or serotonin) in the terminal areas, and that anxiolytic drug action, while not affecting basal release, antagonizes this stress-induced increment in release. Furthermore, other experiments, especially from Segal's (Segal and Bloom, 1974; Segal and Bloom, 1976) laboratory, had shown that such increases in monoamine release facilitate the passage of neural information around hippocampal circuits. Thus, by counteracting these monoaminergic effects, the anxiolytics would be expected to impede hippocampal information processing.

The behavioural effects of lesions of the dorsal ascending noradrenergic bundle were interesting (McNaughton and Mason, 1980). For many tasks they did in fact reproduce the effects of anxiolytic drugs, essentially in full. But, for a substantial number of tasks sensitive to anxiolytics and septal and hippocampal lesions, they were totally without effect. Disruption to the ascending serotonergic pathway was effective in some of the noradrenergic-insensitive tasks particular those using painful stimuli (whereas lesions of the dorsal noradrenergic bundle have greater effects in tasks using frustrative non-reward).

In later experiments (see Gray and McNaughton, 2000), we found that our second, reticular-elicited signature of anxiolytic drug action could be reproduced by injections of a benzodiazepine into the medial supramammillary nucleus (mSuM; McNaughton et al., 1995a). mSuM (for review, see Pan and McNaughton, 2004) relays information arising in areas such as the nucleus reticularis pontis oralis, sending it via the medial forebrain bundle to the medial septum. We have shown that it is one site at which RSA/'theta' frequency is actually computed (Kirk and McNaughton, 1991; Kirk and McNaughton, 1993) and that, in a fixed interval task (which is *insensitive* to dorsal noradrenergic bundle lesions) mSuM injections of a classical anxiolytic both reduced RSA/'theta' frequency and affected behaviour to the same extent and in the same way as did systemic injections (Woodnorth and McNaughton, 2002b). Cell-specific lesions of mSuM show that it is involved in other tasks including, importantly for goal inhibition, differential reinforcement of low rates of response and, like hippocampal lesions, affects contextual but not simple fear conditioning but unlike both hippocampal lesions and anxiolytic drugs is not involved in spatial learning (Pan and McNaughton, 2002).

[13] Recent evidence suggests that co-release of dopamine may be important for modulation of hippocampal function by the dorsal bundle (Takeuchi et al., 2016).

1.9.4 Why link anxiolytic action to the SHS? #4 direct action

Fourth, it has now become clear that anxiolytic drugs act directly on the septum and hippocampus, with different anatomical targets producing different parts of the systemic effect. Both benzodiazepine and 5HT1A agonists, injected into the dorsal hippocampus, decrease anxiety-like behaviour in the elevated plus-maze but not defensive burying test (Menard and Treit, 2001; Menard and Treit, 1998). In contrast, a 5HT1A agonist, injected into the septum, decreases anxiety-like behaviour in the defensive burying test but not the elevated plus-maze (Menard and Treit, 1998). There are also difference between GABAA and 5HT1A agonists.

> Inhibition of dorsal hippocampal neuronal function—whether by electrolytic lesions, direct or indirect GABAA receptor agonists, GABA reuptake inhibitors, or TTX blockade of Na+ channels—decreased fear reactions in the elevated plus-maze and social interaction tests ... The effects of 5-HT1A receptor agonists microinfused into the dorsal hippocampus are mixed ..., only the ultrasonic vocalization test reliably detected the anxiolytic effects of 5-HT1A agonists infused into the dorsal hippocampus. In the elevated plus-maze, two studies found anxiolytic effects after dorsal hippocampal infusion of 5-HT1A agonists, while four found no effect. In the social interaction test, 5-HT1A agonists in the dorsal hippocampus had no effect in one study, and anxiogenic effects in another.
>
> Engin and Treit (2008, p. 13)

1.9.5 Why link anxiolytic action to the SHS? Conclusion

Putting together these new observations with the earlier ones, our theory now holds that anxiolytic drugs directly reduce the release of noradrenaline and serotonin into, or reuptake from, the SHS (combining septum and hippocampal actions) *and* directly alter the encoding of RSA/'theta' frequency via areas such as the supramammillary nucleus. These direct effects on modulatory systems then degrade (but do not totally eliminate) information processing in the SHS. In turn, these indirect changes in SHS function (and some direct changes) then account for the bulk of the behavioural effects of all clinically effective, centrally acting, anxiolytic drugs. However, further effects of many of these drugs (especially, as we shall see, on the fear-potentiated startle response) are achieved by additional direct actions on the other GIS structures.

1.10 What is the septo-hippocampal system?

What we have so far rather loosely presented is a hypothesis of anxiolytic drug action that focuses on the SHS but attributes many SHS changes to actions of these drugs on ascending noradrenergic, serotonergic, and GABAergic pathways. These actions block increases that would otherwise have occurred in the signal-to-noise ratio[14] of hippocampal processing.

[14] The amines affect the signal-to-noise ratio of spatial summation in neurones, while the RSA/'theta'-frequency-controlling GABAergic pathway affects the signal to noise ratio of temporal summation; see Appendix 5.

These various subtle changes in the control of hippocampal RSA/'theta' (and hence often in the gross RSA/'theta') result in a reduced acuity of the SHS in its processing of threat signals (and of negative affective valence in memory paradigms). But what is the SHS that is affected by these changes in RSA/'theta'?

The septum and the hippocampus are strongly interlinked and are separated from much of the rest of the brain by the ventricles. As a result, they can fairly easily be removed from the brain by blunt dissection (Fig. 1.4A). This feature of the gross anatomy gives us the first of many reasons for speaking of a unified 'septo-hippocampal system'.

But the primary cell layer of this easily dissected archicortical tissue is continuous with neocortex—so where do we draw the line between SHS and neocortex generally? The central role of RSA/'theta' in our theory of anxiolytic drug action is the basis for our definition of the SHS itself. This explains why our SHS does not completely overlap with what is anatomically the hippocampus proper. For we treat as SHS all those structures that receive direct, RSA/'theta'-activity-controlling, inhibitory-GABAergic input from the medial septal area. The SHS, on current knowledge, therefore includes the entorhinal cortex, the dentate gyrus, the hippocampus proper, the subicular area, and the posterior cingulate cortex. These can be viewed as iteratively connected to frontal cortex by a topographically organized set of parallel 'Papez' circuits (§9.9.2; based on McNaughton and Vann, 2022).

The roles in behaviour of *all* these regions, as well as the ascending systems that control RSA/'theta', are therefore relevant and will accordingly be reviewed in the chapters that follow. In these reviews we shall attempt to strengthen and refine the central parallel, already noted, between, on the one hand, the behavioural effects of lesions to the septal area and hippocampus and, on the other, those of the anxiolytic drugs.

While the SHS, so defined, is anatomically much more extensive than the hippocampus proper, there are two important ways in which the effects of anxiolytic drugs are likely to be more limited than the list of structures comprising the SHS might imply. First, the anxiolytic drugs do not impair all aspects of the control of RSA/'theta'.[15] They are likely therefore to produce only a subset of the behavioural effects that can be produced by total elimination of RSA/'theta'. For example, as noted previously, the effects of destruction of the dorsal ascending noradrenergic bundle appear to cover only a subset of the effects of lesions to the SHS. Second, the anxiolytic drugs, even if they eliminated RSA/'theta', would not produce a complete dysfunction of the SHS. Because, according to our model, they only affect RSA/'theta' (and not other aspects of SHS processing), they only degrade rather than eliminate processing in the SHS. Hence, when they have effects like those of septal or hippocampal lesions, we would expect these effects to be weaker. So, taking these two points together, we would not expect the central parallel between lesions to the septum and hippocampus proper, on the one hand, and anxiolytic drug treatment on the other to be qualitatively or quantitatively exact. What is surprising, under these circumstances, is how very good the parallel in fact is.

Nonetheless, although we suppose the action of anxiolytics on the SHS to be indirect and incomplete, it still follows from the centrality of this action that an account of the neuropsychology of anxiety must be derived from an account of the cognitive functions of the SHS, and particularly the hippocampal formation. We turn now therefore to consider this, our

[15] For example, they do not produce the state-dependent total blockade of RSA/'theta' that is characteristic of reduction in the cholinergic input; see Appendix 5.

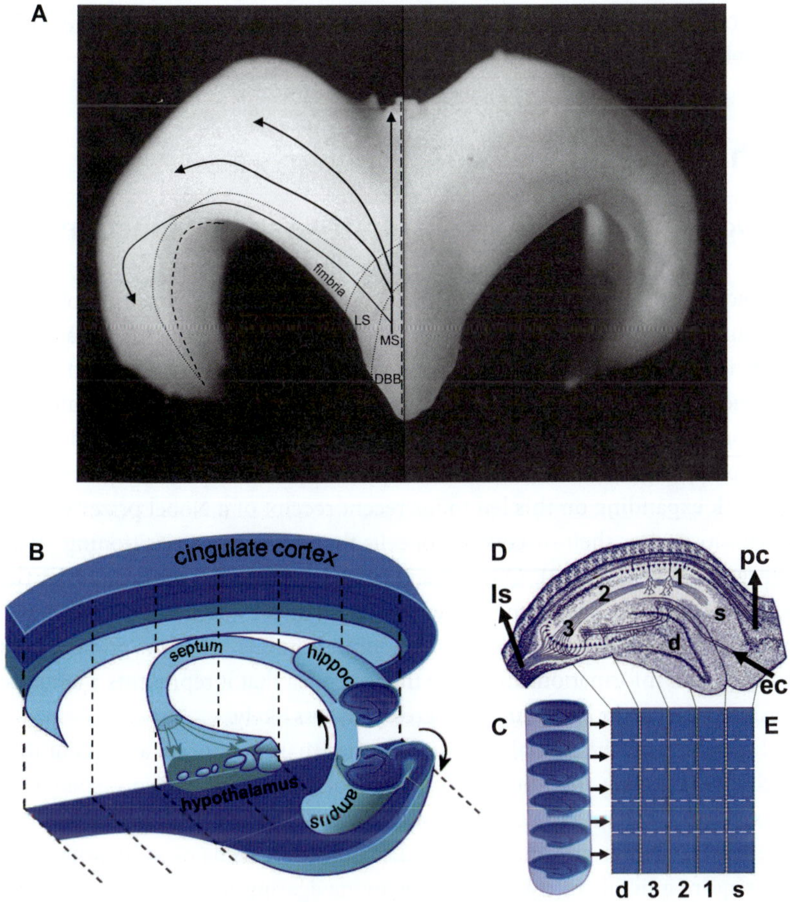

Fig. 1.4 The hippocampal formation and its relation to the septal area. (A) The hippocampal formation and septal area are largely surrounded by ventricle and can be dissected from the brain of a rat. Photograph by J.P. Broad, from Rawlins (1977) with permission. We have roughly indicated the location of the medial septum (MS), diagonal band of Broca (DBB), the lateral septum (LS) and the fimbria. (B) The hippocampal formation, septal area, fornix-fimbria, and connections to the hypothalamus drawn as if partially dissected out of the brain (derived from Gastaut and Lammers, 1961). A segment has been cut out of the middle of the hippocampus showing cell fields of Ammon's Horn (Cornu Ammonis: CA1, CA2, CA3), the subiculum, and the dentate gyrus. Arrows indicate the major sources of outflow, to the subcortex (particularly hypothalamus), and to the cortex. (C) The dissected hippocampus can be viewed as a stack of essentially identical slices, each with the same basic circuitry. (D) Primary circuitry of the mammalian hippocampus. This is essentially repeated in each slice (lamella). Input from the medial and lateral entorhinal cortex (**ec**) enters in the medial and lateral perforant paths, which synapse in middle and outer portions, respectively, of the dendrites of the dentate gyrus (d) granule cells. These send mossy fibres, which synapse on CA3 pyramidal cells (**3**) which, in turn, send output to the lateral septum (ls) and, via the Schaffer collaterals (Sch) to the CA2 (**2**) and CA1 (**1**) pyramids. Area CA1 send a weak projection, via the alveus and fimbria and a stronger projection to the subiculum (**s**) which, in turn, sends projections to areas such as posterior cingulate cortex (**pc**) and, via the alveus and fimbria, to the mammillary bodies. (Modified from an original drawing by D.S. Kerr, with permission.)

other departure from convention: the notion that the functions of the entire hippocampal formation relates to anxiety (as distinct from spatial cognition or memory).

1.11 What does the SHS do?

1.11.1 Does hippocampus contribute to spatial function?

Since the pioneering insight of O'Keefe and Dostrovsky (1971), based on observations of just seven single neurones in the hippocampus of the freely moving rat, it has been repeatedly confirmed that, when the rat is allowed to traverse a spatially extended environment, such neurones display 'place fields', that is, they tend each to fire systematically in one part of the environment but not others. These observations led O'Keefe and Nadel (1978) to propose that the key cognitive function of the hippocampus is to process spatial information. O'Keefe's work expanding on this led to his recent receipt of a Nobel prize (with May-Britt and Edvard Moser) 'for their discoveries of cells that constitute a positioning system in the brain' (Burgess, 2014, p. 1120). O'Keefe and Nadel (1978) also proposed that the hippocampus forms and stores spatial memories, as re-affirmed by Nadel (1991). But, we later argued (Gray and McNaughton, 2000) that the hippocampus does not provide a long-term store of any type of information; and since then the idea that it represents a temporary store with transfer to the cortex has seemed progressively less likely.

So we focus here on the spatial cognition, rather than memorial, aspects of the O'Keefe and Nadel (1978) model: that the hippocampus forms, in non-humans, spatial maps and, in humans, cognitive maps, applicable to sensory and conceptual domains of all kinds. We focus here on the simpler non-human case. Lesion experiments overwhelmingly show that tasks that require animals to solve problems by navigating in spatially extended environments, for example mazes or Morris's (1981; Morris, 1984) widely used swimming pool, are especially sensitive to the deleterious effects of lesions to the hippocampal formation, or to only the hippocampus proper, and usually more so than apparently equivalent non-spatial tasks (Morris et al., 1982; Jarrard, 1983; Morris et al., 1990). Importantly, both novel and classical anxiolytics have qualitatively similar effects to hippocampal lesions in this regard (McNaughton and Morris, 1987; McNaughton and Morris, 1992).

1.11.2 Is hippocampal function exclusively spatial?

What is not so clear is whether, as postulated by O'Keefe and Nadel, the functions of the hippocampus are exclusively (or even directly) to do with spatial cognition. The earliest literature contains numerous instances of clearly non-spatial cognitive deficits in animals after hippocampal damage. But it was usually possible to discount these reports on the grounds that the damage extended well beyond the hippocampus proper into other components of the hippocampal formation, or even regions outside that. (Note, however, that the SHS as defined by our theory encompasses most of the structures which would have been incidentally damaged by old style 'hippocampal' lesions.) This discounting is no longer possible: there are clear instances of damage limited to the hippocampus proper which has led to deficits in non-spatial performance.

For example, Davidson and Jarrard (1993) studied rats with excitotoxic lesions which removed virtually all the hippocampus proper (including the CA1-CA3, dentate granule and hilar regions) but nothing else. These animals failed instrumental conditioning of a clearly non-spatial contextual cue (the state of hunger). Similarly, Ridley et al. (1995) studied marmosets with excitotoxic lesions confined to the CA1 pyramidal cell field of the hippocampus proper. These animals were impaired in conditional but not simple discriminations to an equal extent, whether the dimension along which the discrimination was required was spatial (position) or not (object irrespective of position).

Consistent with these lesion experiments, virtually all of several hundred cells recorded from the hippocampus proper and entorhinal cortex had task-related correlates in a non-spatial timing task (Young and McNaughton, 1997). Most of these 'timing fields' were unique and virtually none were consistent with the coding of a 'place field' by the cell in question. There are also eyeblink fields that seem to support trace but not delay conditioning (see McNaughton & Bannerman, 2024). Likewise, with rats using 'a joystick to manipulate sound along a continuous frequency axis, [cells represent] entire behavioural task, including activity that formed discrete firing fields at particular sound frequencies ... suggesting that common circuit mechanisms in the hippocampal–entorhinal system are used to represent diverse behavioural tasks' (Aronov et al., 2017, p. 719).

1.11.3 Is hippocampal 'spatial' function truly spatial

A related issue is whether the 'spatial' aspects of hippocampal functions are truly spatial. Rats with hippocampal system damage can learn and remember spatial positions perfectly well provided training or testing is conducted suitably (Whishaw et al., 1995; Eichenbaum et al., 1990; Hannesson and Skelton, 1998; Whishaw and Tomie, 1997). This suggests that the problems in spatial tasks could have a non-spatial origin. Similarly, in Appendix 6 (and see Chapter 7), we review extensive data which suggest that 'place fields' do not code unambiguously for places, change with non-spatial changes in the environment, and are not topographically mapped into the hippocampus. Importantly, firing before a choice point (which usually occurs in a place before it) appears to code more the upcoming choice than the current position (§7.4.1). All of these data suggest that the 'placeness' of fields is not the result of uniquely spatial encoding. They also demonstrate that no structure receiving output from the hippocampus could, from that output alone, determine unambiguously and at all times where the animal is within all the spaces it has experienced.

The various non-spatial *memory* hypotheses of hippocampal function grew out of a quite different literature: in the clinic, humans with temporal-lobe damage. Show profound amnesia, Starting with the famous patient, H.M. (Milner et al., 1968)[16], the hippocampus was seen as the prime source of the profound amnesia shown, although the damage almost invariably included many other structures. Memory hypotheses of hippocampal function continue to evolve (see Chapter 8), which is a warning that memory in any simple sense is not the issue. A major role in consolidation or actual storage of long-term memories has morphed to the idea of a temporary store but even that has problems as does the linkage of memory to one

[16] Henry Gustav Mollaison died on 2 December 2008. An extract of his *New York Times* obituary and a photograph are provided at the beginning of Chapter 8. See also Annese et al. (2014).

end of the hippocampus and anxiety to the other: and, clearly, not all memory functions are compromised even with the extensive temporal-lobe damage of H.M. But to say the hippocampus does not provide functions specific to memory is not to say that it is not important for some memory *tasks* (Chapter 8).

To this day, impairments in some memory tests alongside preservation of memory in others or in minor variants of the same paradigm, have spawned a bewildering variety of theoretical dichotomies between hippocampal-dependent and hippocampal-independent forms of memory (Eichenbaum et al., 1994). Some members of this list of dichotomies appear to be largely the same as others, apart from the names used, but in other cases real theoretical divergences are involved (Chapter 8; Table 8.1 lists over 20 different proposed types). Even in the latter cases most are still current. The hippocampus, then, appears superficially to do something related to some specific type of memory.

But, as we did with the spatial hypothesis, we can ask of the memory hypothesis: is this all that the hippocampus does? And, is its involvement in memory tasks due to a specifically memorial function? The evidence from lesion studies is clear: deficits are seen after damage to the SHS in a great variety of tasks that lack any significant memorial component (Gray and McNaughton, 1983). As with other aspects of the various controversies concerning hippocampal function, it can be objected to the great majority of these studies that the damage included much besides the hippocampus proper. However, there are again reports in which lesions confined to the hippocampus proper have given rise to non-memorial changes in behaviour. In one such experiment (Jarrard et al., 1986) rats with excitotoxic lesions of the hippocampus showed increased resistance to extinction of a running response rewarded with food in the straight alley. Since the same animals had shown no difficulty in acquiring the running response, this increased resistance to extinction could not be attributed to a memorial (or, indeed, spatial) deficit.

Conversely, careful analysis of memory-oriented experiments (Chapter 8) suggests that those aspects of a memory task that are regarded by the theoretically minded experimenter as defining its critical class membership (e.g. working vs. reference or procedural vs. episodic memory) are not what give rise to hippocampal sensitivity. Rather, in many cases, sensitivity to hippocampal damage is conferred by the combination of a source of interference in the task *and* a capacity in the control animals to overcome that source of interference (essentially the position taken by Weiskrantz and Warrington, 1975). Taking this together with the fact that amnesics' errors are often intrusions of items which would have been correct in previous trials brings us to the view that hippocampal damage does not prevent subjects from storing correct information. Rather, it prevents them from inhibiting storage or retrieval of incorrect information, which then replaces what would have been a correct response on testing. It is for this reason that we have suggested earlier that 'amnesia' could be more correctly termed 'catastrophic hypermnesia' (McNaughton and Wickens, 2003).

In addition, as already indicated, the lesion literature demonstrates striking parallels to the behavioural effects of the anxiolytic drugs. This drug parallel, too, on at least some fronts extends to experiments in which the lesion is confined to the hippocampus proper, as in the Jarrard et al. (1986) report of increased resistance to extinction (though the literature on selective hippocampal lesions is too sparse to come to any general conclusion on this score). If we ask of this 'anxiolytic-like syndrome', what SHS function does it point to, the answer is necessarily (given the chain of argument we are following) the mediation of some process that is fundamental to anxiety. More specifically, given Fig. 1.3 (deduced from the behavioural effects of the anxiolytics), the SHS is seen as responding to stimuli associated with punishment and non-reward (i.e. to threat) by interrupting ongoing behaviour so as to allow information gathering (the 'attention' output of the GIS). The lesion literature gives ample justification for this view of SHS function (Gray and McNaughton, 1983). In particular, there are many reports after either septal or hippocampal damage of behavioural changes that are best described as reduced behavioural inhibition (the Jarrard et al., 1986, study of extinction of rewarded running is again a good example) rather than impairments in either spatial cognition or memory. Thus, whatever the hippocampus does, its disruption affects spatial cognition, memory, *and* behavioural inhibition, the precise outcome apparently depending largely upon the task the animal is set.

We see as a major virtue of our theory that it attempts to encompass all of these data within a single explanatory framework. We argue that the GIS in general and SHS in particular detect and respond to goal conflict.

1.12 How does the SHS do it? A common computational core

The anatomy of the hippocampus proper is relatively simple (Fig. 1.4c, d). The same basic circuit is repeated over the entire septo-temporal length of this structure in a series of circuit-board-like slices (lamellae, Appendix 4). It cannot have, buried within it, multiple different subsystems, one subserving spatial cognition, one some specific class of memory, one behavioural inhibition, etc. A single core computational function could be discharged by the hippocampus on different types of input-output transaction (involving *inter alia* space, memory, behavioural inhibition, etc.) depending upon the task the animal is required to solve (e.g. Eichenbaum et al., 1994). Most other theorists see the hippocampus as carrying out some desirable computation within its own structure with different classes of input (e.g. to septal and temporal hippocampus) resulting in different classes of output (space and anxiety, respectively). We see it as primarily *suppressing* undesirable computations *in other structures*—and operating on fundamentally the same class of input (a goal, §1.12.4) with apparent variations in functional output depending on the results of its execution of a comparator function.

Conceptually we must think it terms of high-level descriptors, and these are useful as heuristics (but provide only approximate appreciation of the scope of our theory). They can be viewed as emergent properties of more general and fundamental computational processes. Importantly, the nature of the complex heuristics arises not from the SHS itself but from its target structures.

1.12.1 The comparator: a goal conflict detector not engram creator

The key idea is that the SHS acts as a goal comparator[17]. Activations of goal representations in other areas send efference copies to the SHS. Comparison delivers one of two results: match,

[17] Strictly, a hierarchical set of parallel comparators comprising the hippocampal formation, the subicular area, retrosplenial cortex, and the Papez loops that circulate information from via the mammillary bodies, the anteroventral thalamus, the cingulate gyrus, prefrontal cortex, and back to the subiculum, §9.9.2.

i.e. the goals are compatible; or mismatch, i.e. they are incompatible. The comparator system then operates in one of two modes. 'Match' results in 'just checking' mode. There is no goal conflict and control of behaviour is left with motor programming circuits; while the comparator system carries on monitoring efference copies of current goals. 'Mismatch' results in 'control' mode. There is goal conflict (most commonly with ongoing appetitive behaviour facing sudden threat, i.e. a predicted input of pain, or loss); under these conditions, the comparator takes control of behaviour and operates the outputs of the GIS as illustrated in Fig. 1.3. Thus, the comparator is the cognitive or computational heart of the GIS.

In control mode, the output of the comparator circuits must try to solve the problem posed by the goal conflict. The first step is goal inhibition. The previous ongoing motor program is stopped; and the normal output controlled by its goal and the conflicting goal are blocked (while the goals remain active). The blocked goals generate summated arousal and attention, that is further enhanced by the GIS via increased negative cognitive bias and, so, risk aversion. The second step is conflict resolution. GIS output causes the gathering of further information, both from the environment and from scanning of memory stores, in search of alternative descriptions of the perceptual world and/or alternative motor programs that can eliminate the mismatch/circumvent the threat.

During this second step, a period of intensive cognitive processing, the animal may be seen to engage in 'risk assessment' behaviour (the 'increased attention' output of the GIS), e.g. in the rat, adoption of a 'stretched attend' or 'rearing' posture (Blanchard and Blanchard, 1990a). Risk assessment behaviours (and internal memory scanning) are precisely the forms of behaviour that are most sensitive to the action of the anxiolytic drugs.

With increased detection of threat by risk assessment, repulsion from the negative goal (e.g. predator, social embarrassment) will take precedence over attraction from the positive goal (e.g. food, social approval) and will lead to escape or avoidance. With decreased detection of threat or detection of an alternative positive goal attraction to the positive goal will take precedence and will lead to approach and gratification.

1.12.2 Mismatch and contextual tagging

The result of the cognitive processing initiated in this way by mismatch/threat consists in a form of contextual tagging that increases or decreases motivation value goals. Then, on the next choice between goal A (situation A + motivation A) versus goal B (situation B + motivation B) preferences will be changed. Note that 'contextual tagging' would result from the simple operation of association- and reinforcement-based neural plasticity linked to iterative processing in the Papez circuits (Fig. 9.9).

Application of the notion of contextual tagging to the spatial and memorial aspects of hippocampal function is then relatively straightforward. Contextual tagging is not, however, motivationally unbiased—for adaptive reasons it favours more risk aversive tags. So, one of the most common results of activity in the comparator circuits is that a specific positive goal acquires a negative tag, that can be read as 'faulty needs checking'. In consequence the goal produces slower responding and with greater risk assessment on subsequent occasions.

The spatial environment and spatial location constitute the most important forms of context that mammals encounter. Any contextual tagging system, including our originally postulated comparator, must therefore depend critically upon just the kind of spatial mapping function that O'Keefe and Nadel (1978) have attributed to the hippocampus. The converse is also true. The three-dimensional complexity of a spatially extended environment requires for its analysis a system that is capable of determining a detailed contextual specification of the conditions under which different action patterns are correct: if one starts at position P aiming for a goal in location L action pattern A is correct, but if one starts at position Q, action pattern B is correct, etc., for many different possible starting positions (not to mention many different possible goals in the same general environment). Given our general model, therefore, it is unsurprising that hippocampal function is critical for spatial cognition. We differed, and continue to differ, from O'Keefe and Nadel's position, however, in not restricting context to its spatial variety and seeing context as a source of interference.

With regard to memory, here too the role of contextual tagging in the hippocampal contribution is at once apparent. The kind of memory that is 'lost' after damage to the hippocampal formation is precisely that form which, when intact, is tagged for context, not only spatially, but also temporally and in other ways (e.g. gustatory or olfactory), and so made safe from the effects of interference. Destruction of the hippocampus impairs this tagging capacity, so preventing the further memory formation from proceeding correctly but not eliminating memories already stored.

Thus, we found that marmosets with excitotoxic damage to the CA1 cell field could no longer perform a conditional discrimination learned before the lesion or learn new conditional discriminations. After transplantation of a neuroepithelial stem cell line reconstituting the damaged hippocampus (Sinden et al., 1997), however, the marmosets were not only able to solve new conditional discriminations but also successfully retrieved the original discrimination learned prior to the lesion (Virley et al., 1999). This result clearly demonstrates that the lesion-induced impairment affected the handling of stored information, but left that stored information itself intact.

1.12.3 Multiple outputs from goal conflict

So far, the hippocampus appears to carry out a wide range of computations—checking, detecting mismatch, inhibiting, tagging, and so on—and with results that encompass everything from preventing amnesia to generating anxiety. Described in this way these processes are unduly complex for such simple circuitry. Here we resolve these problems through a linked set of ideas: that all inputs to the hippocampus represent perceived or recalled goals (so conflating stimuli, memories, responses, motor programs, and plans); that the hippocampus detects when there is conflict between concurrently active goals (so conflating just checking, comparator, prediction, and mismatch functions); and that, when conflict is detected, the hippocampus produces output that increases the valence of affectively negative stimuli and associations (so conflating the goal inhibition, tagging, risk aversion, and memorial functions).

The hippocampal processes, such as neuroplasticity, are inherently simple, implying a fairly basic transformations of its inputs. The observed differences in its various apparent functions are determined by the structures receiving its output rather than by its performing a range of truly different functions. Importantly, the critical SHS circuitry includes the entorhinal cortex and the posterior cingulate cortex, and we postulate additional logical gates within the SHS that determine its precise outputs under different conditions (Chapter 10).

We thus have a large amount of parallel processing circuitry (Fig. 9.9) all doing what is computationally, if not at the psychological level, a simple job on information packets that are hierarchically ordered in their complexity.

1.12.4 On the nature of a goal

We have been making the concept of a goal do a lot of work. It is now time to look at it in more depth. 'Goal' as an explanatory concept in psychology has always been contentious (George and Johnson, 1985). In particular, the resultant behaviour must be distinguished from that controlled by simple gradients (as with bacteria approaching food). We use it simply in the sense described by Hinde (1998, p. 307; see also Towe and Luschei, 1981):

> Some authors have labeled behaviours as 'directive' or 'goal directed' on the sole criterion that variable means are used to achieve a consummatory situation ... [but if] each type of behaviour is stereotyped, its cessation could be due merely to inhibitory effects consequent upon performances, rather than to error signals ... [In contrast] if rats are subjected to spinal or cerebellar operations so as to interfere with their motor coordination, they may nevertheless use quite novel movements to make errorless runs through a maze. The essential point here is that the new movements are not stereotyped, but selected from variable patterns in such a manner as to bring the animal nearer the goal. Furthermore, the new patterns are 'directly and efficiently substituted without any random activity'.
>
> This leads to a question (McNaughton et al., 2016, pp. 26–27, which see for further elaboration on goals and taxes)
>
> So, what is a goal for an organism? What kind of internal representation is a goal? Imagine you are a hungry rat and you have just been placed in a T maze by an experimenter. If you are hungry and you know from previous experience that there is food and it is at the end of one arm, then that particular food-bearing arm will be a goal for you. The other arm does not have food and so is not a goal for you at the moment. Likewise, if the food is moved to the other arm (and you know that it has been moved), that arm will now become your goal. However, if you are not hungry, even the arm with food will not be a goal, and you will probably decide to curl up in the end of the start arm and have a snooze (experimenters often test rats in the day time, which is the time they normally sleep). A goal, therefore, has both cognitive/identifying and motivational/consummatory properties. Its cognitive properties distinguish it from other places, times, or combinations of stimuli that may have the same motivational properties (we will refer to each specific set of such cognitive properties as a 'situation'). Its motivational properties derive from the organism's current need to acquire some specific stimulus—food, drink, etc.—and the presence of the relevant motivational stimulus in the situation. Importantly, neither the 'situation' nor the 'motivation' by themselves will generate goal-directed behavior. It is their compound 'goal representation' that does so. In contrast, while we can discern 'goals' for behavior in an evolutionary sense (e.g., the goal of random exploration could be said to be the discovery of food), this behavior is not goal-directed in the sense that behavior is controlled by an internal representation of the end point of the behavioral sequence.
>
> To say that an animal has a goal needs some justification. How do we know that a rat's behaviour is not simply the result of taxes or, in the case of complex learned running in a maze,

> simply a long sequence of stimulus-response reactions that act like a string of taxes? In an experiment where a tone predicted a shock it was found that a sheep lifted its leg off the pad that delivered the shock. Had the sheep learned a simple stimulus-response relationship? If the sheep was turned over so its head was on the pad it lifted its head rather than its leg in response to the tone. Even in this very simple case, the sheep has clearly learned the relationship between the two stimuli and has not learned a fixed 'conditioned response' (Cahill et al., 2001).

For our current purposes, the most important feature of the term 'goal' is that it can be distinguished from both 'stimulus' and 'response' in their pure sense—and represents a necessary conflation of higher order variants of the two. The goal of the rat running down the runway has both a situation (in this case, place) component and a motivation (the animal's tendency to run towards it) or response-generating component. Remove either situation or motivation and it would cease to be a goal. As discussed in detail in Chapter 7, we see the firing of hippocampal cells as reflecting information about goals. Goals often have fixed locations in space, hence the place fields often found with hippocampal cells. But they may not, hence the non-spatial fields seen in the majority of cells in non-spatial tasks. Further, they depend on the animal's (as opposed to the experimenter's) intent, hence the changes in the location of place fields when reinforcement contingencies change, their capacity to predict upcoming choices, and the fact that hippocampal cell firing does not always reflect the contingencies that experimenters think that they have embodied in the paradigm.

1.12.5 Positive and negative goals

This section is quoted directly from McNaughton et al. (2016, pp. 27–28)

In all these cases the animals are demonstrating control of behaviour by an internal representation that is a compound of identifying situation and motivating consummatory stimulus, which calls forth whatever behaviours are available to the animal, given the situation, to achieve consummation.

We also need to be clear that, in this sense of situation-motivation compound, there can be two very different types of goals, relating to approach or avoidance, which can conflict with, or reinforce, each other in the control of behaviour. The word 'goal' is typically used in English to signify something we want to achieve in the positive sense. As we have already seen, there can be positive and negative taxes (with the organism moving to increase or decrease the relevant signal, moving up or down its gradient, respectively). Likewise, there can be positive and negative goals; with the goal creating what might be called a 'cognitive gradient' that then determines the animal's specific behaviour. A positive goal is an attractor, something to be included in the desired future state; and a negative goal is a repulsor, something to be excluded or avoided in the desired future state.

In the top left-hand panel of [Fig. 1.5], a shock or some other unpleasant event or object is represented in the bottom left-hand corner. If a rat is aware of this danger it will run directly away—shown by the arrows in the figure—and the tendency to run will decrease as the rat moves away from the object.(Miller, 1944) The object is a repulsor. The red zone represents all the paths that will be taken by any rat, and its grading represents the change in running

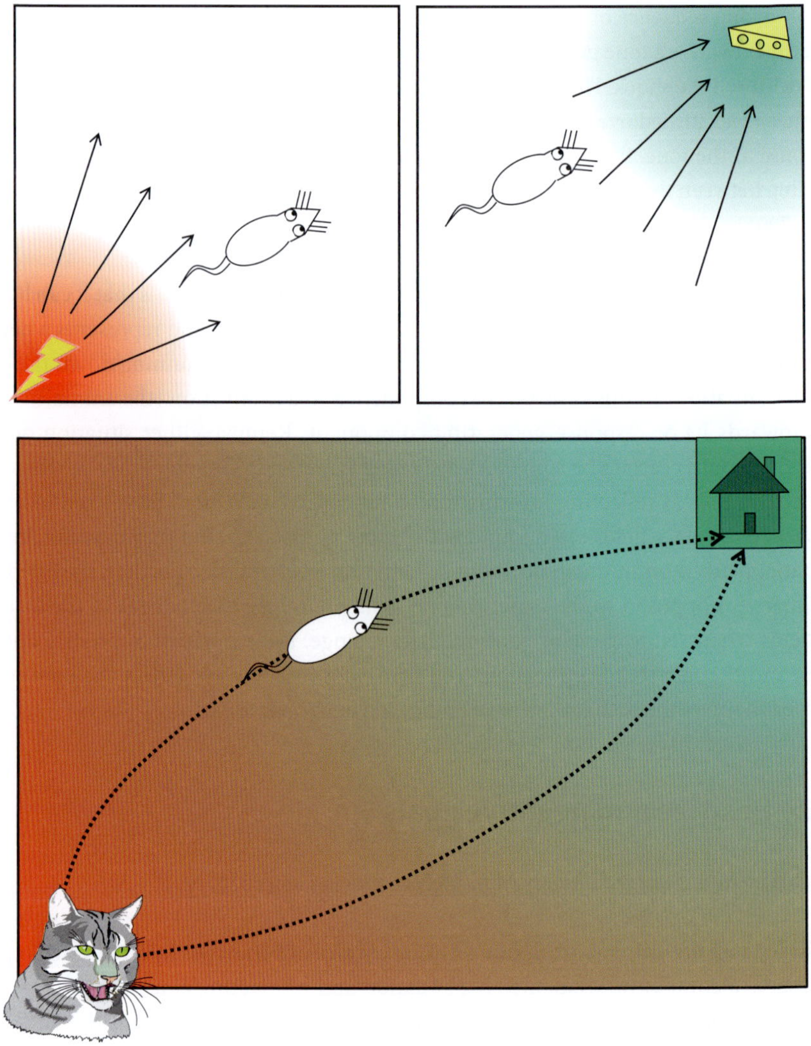

Fig. 1.5 Diagrammatic representation of cognitive gradients created by shock (top left), food (top right) and by the combination of danger and safety (bottom). The solid arrows represent the direction of movement of a rat located at the base of the arrow. The dashed curves represent the path taken by a rat from danger to safety (see text). [From McNaughton et al. (2016) with permission]

strength resulting from the cognitive gradient created by the rat's internal representation of the danger. Conversely, in the top right-hand panel is the equivalent representation of the paths taken by a rat running to food, or some other attractor, that is in the top right-hand corner of the rectangular box. The only substantive difference between the shock and the food is that the direction of movement, relative to the gradient, is opposite—as with positive and negative taxes.

Whether behaviour is controlled by a positive or negative goal can be difficult to determine without careful analysis. It might seem obvious that danger is negative. However, when faced with danger (such as a cat) a rat may be motivated to seek safety (its home burrow), which constitutes a positive goal. In many threatening situations, then, both avoidance of danger and approach to safety can occur. Typically, when close to danger the rat will avoid (moving directly away from the danger because any other path will take it closer to the cat and increase the chance of being caught), and when close to its burrow it will head straight for that. The result ([Fig. 1.5], bottom panel) will be a curvilinear path in the simplest cases with the initial running being avoidance of the negative goal of danger and the later running being approach to the positive goal of safety. With several examples of the same situation and with an animal starting in different positions, we can determine the nature of the controlling goal from the set of trajectories. If they diverge from a point (as in [Fig. 1.5], top left) then they are controlled by a negative goal and if they converge (top right) then they are controlled by a positive goal.

1.12.6 The SHS does not code goals/engrams

It is important to be clear that the SHS does not *code* goals as such. It receives efference copies from brain areas that do code goals and so mirrors the specificity of encoding of those areas (e.g. eye blinks coded in cerebellar circuits, §7.1). However, it receives this efference copy of the true encoding of the goal information only so that it can detect when more than one goal is concurrently highly activated, i.e. when there is goal conflict. For this purpose, the hippocampus itself need only know that there are a number of goals, not precisely what they are. Indeed, the same hippocampal cell could, in principle, respond to a number of different goals (with more goals producing more activity in the cell in question). However, the area from which it receives the information will, at any one time, tend to code for only one goal, giving the hippocampal cell an apparent selectivity of information coding. (This selectivity derives, in our view, from the fact that motor programming areas are topographically mapped into the SHS, producing a mapping of what is essentially 'goal space'; see Appendix 4.)

Goal information comes from all areas that can be concerned with specifically goal-directed behaviour (including areas as diverse as the prefrontal cortex, amygdala, and cerebellum). Note, however, we hold that the serial sequencing of goals that is the true 'planning' function takes place in the prefrontal cortex, perhaps the most prominent area among those that send to the hippocampus information about goals.

Importantly, it is now clear (Chapter 11) that the SHS processes goals (attractors and repulsors), not the potentially conflicting actions linked to them. Thus, in the learning of mirror drawing there is considerable conflict between old and new muscular patterns required to achieve the goal; but there is only one goal and so no goal conflict, and there is motor system rather than hippocampal involvement. That is why someone like H. M., who lacked a hippocampus, could learn mirror drawing as well as anyone else. Similarly, anxiolytic drugs that reduce goal-conflict-specific rhythmicity do not affect action stopping (McNaughton et al., 2013; Shadli et al., 2015; Shadli et al., 2020a).

1.12.7 Control mode iteration

When it receives information about only one prepotent goal, the hippocampal formation is, effectively, in 'just checking mode' (§1.12.1). When, in addition, it receives information about a second conflicting goal, it detects the multiplicity and effectively enters 'control mode' (§1.12.1). Note that no real change in the nature of goal processing occurs between these two modes. At all times information enters the comparator and is integrated but, when the summation of inputs passes some threshold, it also produces output.

The output from the hippocampal formation involves the return of information to those areas whose activity has given rise to conflict—providing a simple, quite general, affectively negative biasing function. The effect is to increase the valence of affectively negative stimuli and associations of stimuli (memories) and, particularly with chronic conflict, reduce the valence of affectively positive stimuli. This output, therefore, shifts approach-avoidance conflict in the avoidance direction on both the current and future occasions (see tagging in §1.12.2). The net result of this process is determined, however, not by the hippocampal formation but by its target structures. The details of how this is achieved determine our interpretation of the functional role of RSA/'theta'.

The mechanism we postulate relies upon the concept of iterative networks. To introduce this concept, we first describe Marr and Poggio's (1976) solution to the global stereopsis problem (summarized and illustrated by Frisby (1979, pp. 150–151). We use their model solely as an analogy but it should, nonetheless, give an idea of the power and apparent sophistication that iteration can produce in the processing of information by even simple parallel networks of the type we postulate as linking the hippocampal formation with goal processing structures.

'Global stereopsis' is the capacity to see depth, and as a result the form of an object, in random dot stereograms presented to the two eyes. The stereograms themselves (Fig. 1.6A) start with black or white squares in a totally random pattern to be presented to one eye. You copy the first and then moving portions to simulate the disparity on the retina of an object above the background.

Alone, each half of the pair is totally random. Viewed as a pair through a stereoscope, the depth, and hence form, of the object coded in the stereogram becomes visible (Fig. 1.6D). At this point, every dot in one stereogram has been matched by some mechanism in the brain to a dot in the other, the specific disparity calculated, and depth deduced. Since the dots themselves are indistinguishable one from the other, this is a daunting computational task when there are many such dots (often taking humans between 30 seconds to 2 minutes to see anything).

Fig. 1.6C shows a diagrammatic representation of a small part of a simple network devised by Marr and Poggio (see Frisby, 1979, p. 150) that solves this computational problem. The key features of this network are: (a) the input patterns from the two eyes are 'clamped' onto the input lines of adjacent sides of the square lattice; (b) lateral facilitation and lateral inhibition within the network then change the activity at each of the nodes where the two types of input line intersect; and, most importantly, (c) the result of this change is, in turn, fed back to the network and the process is *iterated* until the network settles into a stable state. This last step may require a very large number of iterations. If we assume that the human visual system solves the problem in the same way as the network model, and that a single iteration takes, say, 50 ms, then the typical undergraduate in a psychology practical class has a nervous system that requires of the order of 1,000 successive iterations to solve the problem for any new image. However, because these calculations are done iteratively, feeding the output from one calculation back as input for the next, only a few (2 or 3) layers of neurones are required

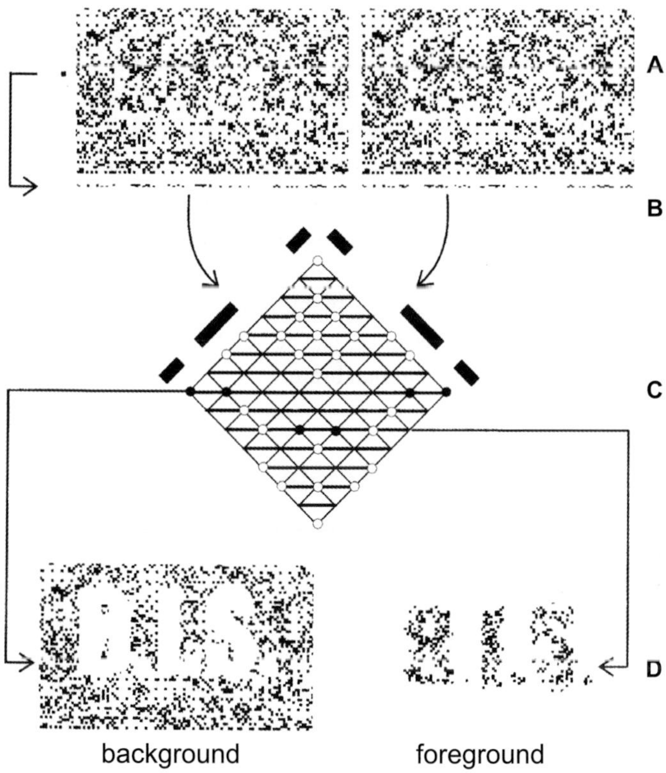

Fig. 1.6 Marr and Poggio's computational solution to the global stereopsis problem (for more detailed description, including simulation outputs, see Frisby, 1979, p. 150-151).
A. Random dot stereograms are constructed by first creating a purely random image (left hand side) and then taking part of it, here an area defined by superimposing the letters B.I.S., and shifting the dots a small amount to one side. Dots in the area shifted to are erased and the blank space created by the shift is filled with more random dots. This creates a second image that, by itself, constitutes random dots (right hand side) but which, taken together with the other half of the stereo pair, defines two areas (B.I.S. and its background) which differ in retinal disparity and hence implied depth when viewed binocularly.
B. A slice taken horizontally at the point marked by the filled square at the left of the left-hand image in A.
C. Small portions of B taken from the equivalent areas for the left and right eye and superimposed as input onto a computational lattice. Each intersection in the lattice represents a cell (or node). Thick lines represent reciprocal excitatory connections between cells, thin lines reciprocal inhibitory connections. The imposed input from the left and right eye will initially cause a large number of nodes to be activated by coincident input from the two eyes. This will include not only cases where a dot in one image is correctly matched to a dot in the other (filled circles) but also cases where an incorrect match, or 'false fusion', occurs (open circles). In terms of analogy with our view of the BIS, it is the presence of these incorrect matches that is the equivalent of conflict. The excitatory and inhibitory connections within the lattice then, over a large number of cycles, eliminate activity in the nodes representing incorrect matches, leaving the activity representing correct matches. Note that it is not the initial level of activity in any node that determines whether it will remain—rather it is the relation between it and the recursive changes in activity within the network.

(Contd.)

for all of these calculations for any particular point in space. We would see the hippocampus as being enmeshed in several parallel loops each with multiple layers (Fig. 9.9).

Lest this detailed treatment of global stereopsis should tempt you to think that the hippocampus, if it works in the same general way, must perform some kind of visual figure-ground calculation, it should be noted that similar iterative circuitry is used by Hinton et al. (1993) for 'clean up' units that adjust discrepancies between words and semantic units in a neural network simulating reading. This matches the global stereopsis model in terms of the fact that iteration is used to resolve differences between conflicting sources of input, but cannot be viewed as a figure-ground computation in any conventional sense. A particularly interesting property of the Hinton et al. model is that it has been constructed in such a way that changes in its behaviour when it is 'lesioned' can account for many of the changes resulting from damage to language areas in the human brain.

1.12.8 Cortical and subcortical loops

The SHS is richly supplied with the means to interact iteratively with both cortical (e.g. Fig. 9.9) and subcortical areas, so as to extract higher order information. It has been something of a puzzle that the cortical and subcortical inputs to the hippocampus appear to carry very similar information (Appendix 3). If, however, the SHS carries out calculations akin to those required for global stereopsis, these various sources of information might well be expected to differ only subtly, as do the images from the left and right eye, or word and semantic code. The SHS might, then, be concerned to extract the higher order basis of the differences (the equivalent of depth for stereograms, or of meaning for the case of reading words). Given the complexity of the circuits in which, as we shall see later in the book, the hippocampus is embedded, we should be prepared for the SHS to be capable of dealing with many different higher order properties of the same input information.

Given the power of iterative networks, what use might the hippocampal system make of them? Our general answer to this question is that the hippocampal system acts so as to increase the valence of adverse outcomes associated with items (locations in space, associative bonds in memory, or motor programs). This 'association' can be innate or acquired. In relation to memory, this general approach makes our position the antithesis of most others (including that of Eichenbaum et al., 1994), with whose views we otherwise have much in common) by supposing that the hippocampal formation acts, not to strengthen associations that are retained, but to weaken those that are discarded—causing the system to avoid their

---

Fig. 1.6 *(continued)*

D. Each horizontal line of nodes in C represents a particular retinal disparity and hence depth. Once activity in the network has stabilized, only the correct matches (filled circles) remain active. Their output is then sent to different arrays, each topographically mapped with respect to the visual world, representing particular depths (see arrows connecting C to D). These have the 'ground' (left) and 'figure' (right) separated one from the other. In terms of the analogy with our view of the GIS, it is the reduction of a very large number of conflicting possibilities (represented by all the matches, correct and incorrect, in C) to the single possibility represented by the right-hand image in D that is the same general class of operation as that carried out by the GIS.

retrieval. Consistent with this position, there is evidence that the errors made in memory tests by patients with hippocampal damage over-represent items that would have been correct under slightly different circumstances (§8.4.1). Such a pattern of errors cannot come from enhanced forgetting, as would be predicted if the role of the hippocampus were simply to facilitate the formation of (correct) memories. It *is* predicted, however, if this role is to eliminate competing (incorrect) memories. Similarly, our theory predicts that hippocampal deficits will be seen only in those tasks in which interference is actually overcome by control subjects, not in those in which interference is present but not overcome by controls.

In summary, then, the common computational core postulated in our model as lying at the heart of hippocampal function, whether this is manifest in spatial cognition, memory, or anxiety, comprises a comparator, to detect conflict between concurrent activation of incompatible goal-seeking mechanisms, coupled to iterative networks that link the SHS to memory stores (in the temporal lobes), complex motor programming circuits (in the basal ganglia and frontal cortex), 'fixed action pattern' circuits (in, e.g. the amygdala and hypothalamus) and thalamocortical perceptual systems, with all of which the SHS interacts so as to increase the weighting of items with greater potentially adverse significance (Fig. 10.4).

The SHS produces such an increase in negative weighting at every cycle of a series of computations that progressively increase bias (and hence suppress goals) until one or other goal is sufficiently predominant to take control of the motor mechanisms. This increase in negative bias has two consequences. It affects current motor output directly, and it affects future motor output indirectly through its biasing of associations (including those that are just being formed). Additionally, while its iterative operations continue to fail to resolve the conflict, the SHS produces additional output that engages exploratory mechanisms designed to resolve the conflict through the obtaining of new information about the environment (thus preventing the animal from getting locked into an impasse). We also presume that during consolidation, and particularly during sleep (Appendix 7), the hippocampus can direct a similar 'internal exploration' (§10.6.3), which in human beings may best be thought of as rumination.

1.12.9 The need for phasic control

In Marr and Poggio's model, since it is carried out on a digital computer, each cycle of computation is quite discrete. However, the effects of opening ion channels on hippocampal neurones can change neuronal excitability for periods of time that equal or exceed the time it takes information to circulate from the hippocampus to its targets and back (Miller, 1991; Miller, 1989). The effect of RSA/'theta' (and particularly the imposition of a regular period of inhibition on hippocampal cells by the septal input) will be to quantize hippocampal processing and thus reduce the chances that the effects of information received on a previous cycle interfere with the comparator's assessment of inputs on the current cycle. From this follows the conclusion that RSA/'theta' will be important, particularly for complex or evenly balanced conflicts; but, since it only increases the acuity of processing in the temporal domain, RSA/'theta' will not be essential for the hippocampus to perform at least some functions where a mere degradation in performance is not crucial.

Here we should note also that the extensive circuitry controlling the frequency of RSA/'theta' (Fig. 9.3–9.7) and gating its occurrence (Fig. 10.3) implies that particular levels of that activity will not be universally beneficial (or RSA/'theta' would occur all the time at a fixed level). Nor, therefore, should we assume that the interaction of the hippocampus with other brain structures will always be beneficial. Certainly, there are some behavioural tasks (e.g. two-way active avoidance in a shuttlebox) where lesions of the SHS produce an improvement in performance in percent correct (if not adaptive) terms.

A final point to note is that goal conflict may result from the activation of quite different response systems (e.g. approach, avoidance) or from the activation of an essentially single response system (e.g. lever pressing) equally by two different stimulus sources (left lever, right lever). While Fig. 1.7 shows a single circuit plan, which can resolve both types of conflict, the full version of our theory (Chapter 10, Fig. 10.4) ascribes the resolution of what can be thought of as response-response (motivation-motivation), stimulus-stimulus (situation-situation) and response-stimulus (orienting) versions of goal conflict to different parts of the overall SHS.

1.12.10 Prefrontal cortex

We have so far dealt with the prefrontal cortex and cingulate cortex (the sites, it will be recalled, at which psychosurgery is practised for the treatment of certain drug-resistant forms of anxiety) quite casually. Encompassing, as they do, a huge portion of the cortical mantle, our exposition[18] of their precise function and organization (and hence their interaction with the SHS) will require all of Chapter 11 (see also Appendix 3).

Briefly, we view them (Fig. 11.2, following, e.g. Barbas and Pandya, 1991) as being hierarchically organized areas that deal (in their successively 'higher' layers) with progressively higher levels of anticipation of action. Thus, the frontal eye fields can be viewed as pre-pre-motor cortex and area 46 (with its role in working memory), as pre-pre-pre-motor cortex (Fig. 11.7).

In the same way, then, that we distinguished the role of the SHS (in resolving concurrent goal–goal conflict) from the role of the defence system and other motor systems in resolving motor program conflicts without goal conflict, so we must distinguish the role of the SHS from that of prefrontal and cingulate cortex. In our view these cortical areas are involved, quite independently of the hippocampus, in the resolution (i.e. ordering) of conflicts between successive subgoals in a task. In the case of prefrontal cortex this amounts to saying that it is concerned with plans more than goals as such. However, where (as is common in certain types of working memory task) there is concurrent goal conflict within such a task, both the SHS and the prefrontal cortex are likely to be involved.

We already noted (§1.3.2) that our theory has responded, albeit incompletely, to theoretical developments in the role of the prefrontal cortex in anxiety. These are largely those of Joe LeDoux (LeDoux, 2014; LeDoux, 2012; LeDoux, 2002; LeDoux, 2000; LeDoux, 2015; see also Stevenson and McNaughton, 2013; Corr and McNaughton, 2016; Paulus and Stein, 2006). We have incorporated much of what LeDoux has to say about frontal cortex and mental disorder. However, we depart from what he has to say in a way that is largely semantic but also

[18] We present a wholistic species-general account of neural organization. Particularly with PFC this may seem to ignore differences between the species. But we see these differences as quantitative and relating to the depth of cortical filtering of information; while fundamental functional organization remains largely conserved (e.g. Rocchi et al., 2021).

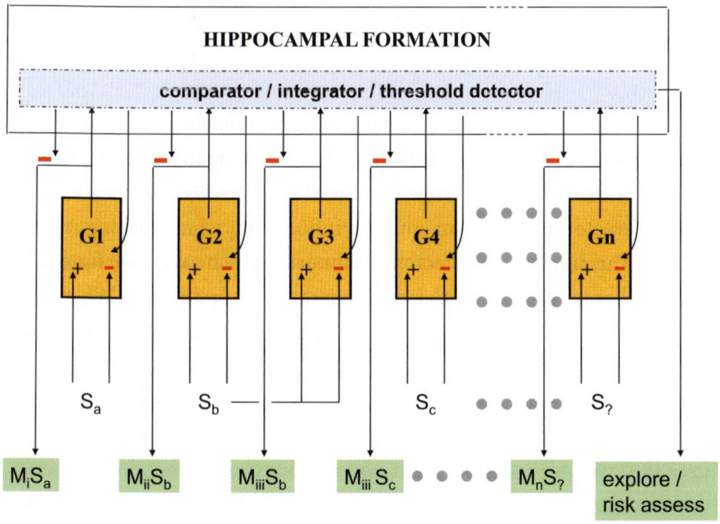

Fig. 1.7 The hippocampal formation as a general device for the resolution of goal conflict. A goal is defined as a particular combination of situation (S) and motivation (M). Often, two goals will differ in both of these attributes (M_iS_a versus $M_{ii}S_b$). However, some situations may activate more than one motivation ($M_{ii}S_b$ versus $M_{iii}S_b$), e.g., a goal box which elicits both approach (because of a prior association with food) and avoidance (because of a prior association with shock). Likewise, some motivations can be activated by more than one situation ($M_{iii}S_b$ versus $M_{iii}S_c$) as in a lever press response for food that may be elicited by either a left or a right lever (or both) depending on the prior history of reinforcement. Any situation (e.g., S_a) is held to activate a particular goal (G1) defined by the conjunction of that stimulus and a particular response (M_iS_a). The strength of activation is determined by integration of the prior affectively positive (+) and affectively negative (-) associations of that goal. In many cases the goal (say G1) will be the only one with sufficient net activation to produce a response or, if another goal is activated, G1 will nonetheless be the clear winner. In this case the motivation (M_i) directs appropriate responses to the relevant situation (S_a). The hippocampal formation will receive an efference copy of the output from G1, but in this case will not react. Conflict is defined as the case when two or more goals (e.g., G1 and G2) are nearly equally and highly activated. The hippocampus as a comparator determines the degree of conflict and the greater this is and (as an integrator) the greater the total motivation of the goals, the greater will be its output. The output has two effects. First, it blocks the output from the areas defining the goals (e.g., G1) to the areas responsible for achieving them (e.g., M_iS_a, $M_{ii}S_a$). Second, it increases the value of any affectively negative associations (including, in humans, inferences) specific to that goal. In many cases this will allow resolution of the conflict in favor of that goal which has the lesser negative associations. Output from the hippocampus is increased, recursively, (as in the global stereopsis model of Fig. 1.6) until conflict is resolved while, at the same time, commanding exploratory/risk assessment activity (including memory scanning) that can provide additional information (either devaluing existing negative or positive information or providing new negative or positive information) that changes the balance between the goals and allows the conflict to be resolved in favor of one of them.

reflects some disagreement at the neural level. The semantic separation starts with his view that anxiety:

> . . . is a cognitive state in which *working memory is monopolized by fretful, worrying thoughts.* The difference between an ordinary state of mind (of working memory) and an anxious one is that, in the latter case, systems involved in emotional processing, such as the amygdala, have detected a threatening situation, and are influencing what working memory attends to and processes. This in turn will affect the manner in which executive functions select information from other cortical networks and from memory systems. . . . When the organism, through working memory, conceives that it is facing a threatening situation and is *uncertain about what is going to happen* or about the best course of action to take, anxiety occurs. (LeDoux, 2002, p. 288, added emphasis)

We would agree that worry (and obsession and rumination) depend on prefrontal mechanisms including working memory (Chapter 11; §11.5.2). However, we will link worry more to neuroticism (a risk factor) than either anxiety or fear *per se* (Chapter 12). We also do not believe that worry is directly linked to clinical anxiety (Meyer et al., 1990) but, instead, is a state that can cause negative thoughts to be retrieved (Borkovec et al., 1983) and so impact not just on state anxiety but on fear. We see it as linked to rumination (iteration of the past)

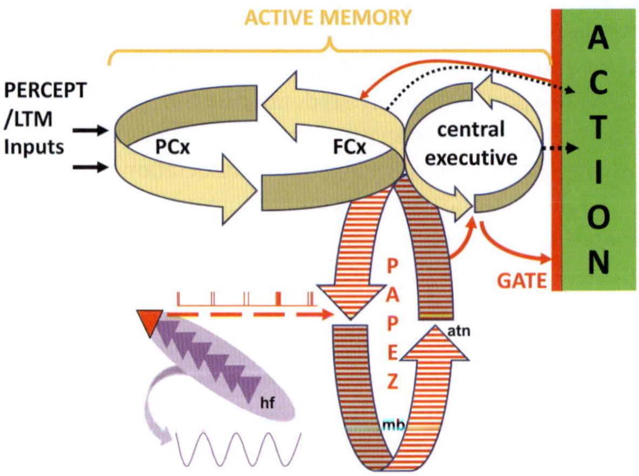

Fig. 1.8 Overall interaction of the 'horizontal' active memory loops (see Fig. 11.5, Fig. 11.6 for more detail) with the multiple 'vertical' parallel Papez circuits (see Fig. 9.9 for more detail). Goal (situation + motivation) in formation is held in active memory by circulation through loops from posterior (PCx) to frontal (FCx) cortex and back again. In frontal cortex this information is processed by the central executive that, in particular, controls sequencing of goals and subgoals to generate action. Efference copies of currently activated goals are sent to the hippocampal formation (hf), which has rhythmic bursts of cell firing with the whole structure showing a local field potential RSA/'theta' rhythm. When goal conflict is detected output from the hf is passed through the mamillary bodies (mb) and anterior thalamic nuclei (atn) and produces *iterative* processing in the Papez circuits connected to anterior limbic and thence more posterior prefrontal cortex before completing the return circuit in the hf. The hippocampus can block action by input to the same prefrontal circuits that control simple stopping via a gate that blocks output from GO circuits that are activated in parallel with STOP circuits (§11.5.4, Fig. 11.8).

and its effects on depression (Nolen-Hoeksema, 2001) and to obsession (iteration of the present)—with worry iterating predictions of the future. Critically, while we think uncertainty can activate worry, we also (Chapters 2 and 3) see uncertainty as just one means of generating goal conflict, with goal conflict being the most important thing for anxiety (both normal and pathological *as we define it, §1.4)*. We believe LeDoux's view applies more to a common factor in the aetiology of what we term the neurotic disorders as a whole than to disorders of anxiety (as opposed to panic, phobia, obsession, etc.) as a trait; and even less to brief periods of adaptive anxiety as a state.

Importantly, orbital frontal, infralimbic, and prelimbic cortex are distinctive in receiving direct inputs from the hippocampus (CA1 and subiculum; Fig. 11.2A) and are ideally placed for iterative interaction via the return side of the Papez circuit (while also receiving indirect input from the hippocampus via the mamillary bodies and anterior thalamus; Fig. 9.9). As noted in §1.3.2, we see these hippocampal, comparator/integrator, loops as operating essentially 'vertically' with prefrontal cortex; while posterior cortex, active memory, loops operate horizontally (Fig. 1.8).

1.13 The amygdala, insula, arousal, and attention

In the past, it has been common to see the amygdala as the seat of 'anxiety' (with this usually conflated with fear). However, the amygdala does both too much and too little to be characterized as a structure that specifically processes anxiety/fear.

First, amygdala action that is too broad. The amygdala forms cue-reinforcer associations not only when the reinforcer is aversive, but also when it is appetitive (Chapter 6). Thus, lesions to the amygdala impair not only conditioned fear (as measured, e.g., by cardio-acceleration) but also active avoidance and rewarded approach behaviour. *Unconditioned* responses such as aggressive and sexual behaviour also depend to a major extent on the amygdala. Given these data, we accept that the amygdala plays a major role in controlling the output (particularly autonomic/arousal) of many, perhaps all, emotion systems. Indeed, as we shall see, we view the amygdala as being one of the structures that is crucial in generating the arousal and autonomic components of anxiety. But there is little reason to attribute to the amygdala a role *specifically* in anxiety. The fact that it is involved in controlling autonomic output and behaviour for so many different classes of emotional stimuli argues that it is, rather, a general controller of emotional output of all types.

Second, a key feature of human anxiety lies in apprehension of the possibility of, not pain or loss, but omission of anticipated gain. There are a number of well-controlled experimental paradigms in which such 'anticipatory frustration' (Amsel, 1962; Amsel, 1992) can be measured in animals; and there is much experimental evidence that anxiolytics weaken this state (Gray, 1977). Studies of behaviour in these paradigms after lesions to the amygdala, however, have usually failed to show the effects that would be expected if such lesions reduce anxiety (Appendix 1).

Lastly, if one does accept the anxiolytic drug starting point for the analysis of the neuropsychology of anxiety, there is a critical lack of concordance between the behavioural effects of these drugs and lesions to the amygdala, respectively (Table 4.2). Amygdala lesions have failed to reproduce the effects of anxiolytic drugs on behaviour in a number of schedules involving reward omission, on two-way active avoidance, in the water maze, in the elevated

+ maze, and on rearing (this last being one of the key components of the Blanchards' anxiety defence test battery). If the amygdala is the 'seat of anxiety', some explanation for this lack of concordance is required.

Conversely, amygdala (but not SHS) lesions reproduce the effects of anxiolytics on single alternation, conditioned suppression, social interaction, and fear-potentiated startle. So, we accept that a full account of the neuropsychology of anxiety requires adequate consideration of the roles played by the amygdala and especially of the interactions between this structure and the SHS.

We also, here, add the insula (§11.7) as a structure generally involved in 'internal monitoring' and so, like the amygdala, in the control of attention and arousal. Also like the amygdala, different parts of the insula appear to deal with different motivational systems; and some parts are not only involved in anxiety as a state but in the control of trait anxiety (Paulus and Stein, 2006).

To the decision-related circuits of the SHS that produce the goal inhibition and risk assessment output of the GIS (Fig. 1.3), therefore, we add arousal/attention-related circuits including the amygdala and insula. A key point to note here is that, in relation to goal conflict, attraction and repulsion compete via subtraction to control decision making; while they summate to elicit arousal. These opposed calculations require separate machinery (Fig. 11.14), the outputs of which are combined in an 'arousal-decision' integration to determine the direction and intensity of behavioural commands (Gray and Smith, 1969).

1.14 Hierarchical organization and parallel processing

We noted in §1.8 that visual inputs to the amygdala are from multiple levels of a hierarchically organized (quick and dirty through slow and sophisticated) sensory system. As discussed in Chapter 6, multiple equivalent levels of other sensory systems are also directly connected to the amygdala. (The main cortical area which does not project to the amygdala is the parietal cortex.) This leads to a very neat account (LeDoux, 1994; §6.1.3) of the functioning of the avoidance system.

Activity at each level of each sensory system is passed to the amygdala directly and in parallel. Note that this is not redundant as, for example, the geniculate codes for a simple CS, while the auditory cortex codes for the discrimination between a CS+ (associated with punishment) and a CS– (associated with the absence of punishment), and so on. In each case, then, a particular type of avoidance response can be produced simply by strengthening (via long-term potentiation; see Appendix 2) the appropriate connection in the amygdala. This can directly link, for example, neurones that code for a simple auditory stimulus in the geniculate to neurones that control avoidance motor programs.

An important corollary of LeDoux's formulation is that each of the nuclei in the hierarchical active defensive system (from the periaqueductal grey to the anterior cingulate; §1.8, Chapter 6) must be presumed to be receiving sensory information at all times. Hence, given adequate stimuli, all of them will be *concurrently* pre-programming a range of quite independent potential responses. This multiplicity of potential responses may seem complicated; but it can easily be controlled by a system that employs release (inhibition of inhibition), rather than activation, to control responses (see, e.g. Chapter 2 of McNaughton, 1989b; Grillner, 2018; Grillner and Robertson, 2016; Grillner and Thompson, 2021). The concurrent high-intensity activation of multiple networks, coupled with control by release from inhibition, allows the sudden dramatic shifts that can be seen in experimental animals between, say, freezing and defensive attack. This can be attributed to a shift of disinhibitory influences from, e.g. a (continuously updated) freezing motor program to a (continuously updated) defensive attack motor program.

As with modern network models of many processes, all of these structures are reciprocally connected. Despite our description of, for example, the dorsal periaqueductal grey as controlling undirected escape behaviour, it is probably much better to view this structure as part of a distributed system, including the hypothalamus, amygdala, anterior cingulate, posterior cingulate and hippocampus, in which certain patterns of activity engage the various fight/flight/freeze nuclei and include them within the effective distributed network. The periaqueductal grey may then be the most important node through which information passes during fight, flight, and freezing, but it would be an error to think of it as the only structure in the defensive system active at that time, or even as the only structure contributing to escape.

Our analysis of the defensive system has, so far, closely followed those of LeDoux and Graeff (see Chapter 6 and Appendix 2). However, we differ from them in thinking that the hippocampus should not be viewed as, say, a source of contextual stimuli which can come to control the amygdala (in which case there should be strong hippocampal-amygdala connections rather than, as is predominantly the case, the other way round). Rather, we think of the hippocampus as a device that can resolve goal conflicts (as outlined previously), not only between separate programs concurrently activated within the amygdala, but also between programs in the amygdala and those outside the defence system. It is important in this context, as with the case of mirror drawing, to emphasize that the SHS is involved in the resolution of goal rather than motor conflict. In LeDoux's and Graeff's formulations the lower levels of the defence system (both for stimulus processing and response production) can be over-ridden by the higher levels. Thus, if a sophisticated avoidance response is being programmed, this prevents the occurrence of counterproductive undirected escape. Resolution of this type of conflict between levels is solely the business of the active defence system (via, e.g. inhibition of the periaqueductal grey by the amygdala). However, where there are two equally attractive (or equally unattractive) alternatives to which to direct incompatible avoidance responses, then interaction between the hippocampus and the amygdala (or other related areas) will be required to resolve the conflict between the different goals.

1.15 The Reinforcement Sensitivity Theory (RST) and anxious personality

Chapter 12, 'Anxiety and personality' links the anxiolytic-derived state neuropsychology of the previous chapters to personality traits. Given our characterization of the state control of anxious behaviour it is a small step to see traits as sensitivities of the structures, goal control systems, and more global modulators of the systems. This provides a foundation for seeing psychiatric disorders as resulting from one or more extremes of trait sensitivities.

While our main focus is anxiety, we also discuss the implications of our hierarchically organized neuropsychology for RST (originally proposed by Gray, 1970a; see McNaughton and Corr, 2019b, for critique; named by Pickering, 1997; see also Corr, 2008b) with additional comment on the, also hierarchically organized, Big 5 (e.g. measured via the NEO-PI,

Costa and McCrae, 1985; or NEO-PI-R, Costa and McCrae, 1995; for a recent overview see DeYoung, 2015). For this, we cover attraction and repulsion as well as conflict resulting from reaction to reinfor**cers** (with comment on the application of our neuropsychology to the 'revised' RST that emerged from our second edition).

Key details of the mapping of our neuropsychology to RST and, in particular, of our renaming of the systems to avoid confusion with prior RST scale labels, were summarized in §1.7. The key features of the systems are detailed in Table 1.1.

We emphasize that attraction and repulsion can each be produced by manipulating gain and loss, depending on the contingency involved. Thus, in addition to sensitivity to attraction, repulsion, and conflict we need to account for trait sensitivities of gain and loss (where the difference between the two is reflected in 'loss aversion'). In addition, we provide a new dopaminergic neurology for reinforce**ment** sensitivity that strongly distinguishes reinforce**ment** from reinfor**cers** and so includes only two traits (positive and negative). We argue that conflation of these different, often orthogonal, traits has created the current difficulties experienced by RST. Importantly for the main subject of this book, we distinguished trait anxiety (as defined by us) both from neuroticism (operating at a higher level in the hierarchy) and from various forms of trait fear (operating at the same level).

In arriving at our picture of motivation-related traits, we had to review issues arising from word meanings, evolution, the need for biomarkers, hierarchical organization, disorders as extremes of traits, and continuity versus discontinuity of disorders. We identify problems with the naming of existing RST scales, and discusses future neural solutions. We also found it necessary to provide recommendation for the application of neuropsychology to personality work, emphasizing the need for biomarkers (with our recently discovered anxiety disorder biomarker as an example) and for extreme care with linguistically derived scales (whether lexical or rational).

1.16 The clinical neuropsychology of anxiety and its treatment

1.16.1 Clinical neuropsychology and diagnosis

Our clinical neuropsychology of what we will term 'neurotic' disorders, is described in detail in Chapter 13. It follows very closely from the hierarchical view of the defence system obtained from animal experiments and distinguishes between anxiety and fear disorders in a way that maps only partially to existing labels at the symptom level and departs further at the syndrome level.

A particular symptom (e.g. panic or obsession) is deemed to result from a high level of activity in the relevant brain site (periaqueductal grey and anterior cingulate, respectively). However, this 'symptom' may be adaptive in response to appropriate (usually extreme) environmental stimuli; or pathological, due to biochemical or neural dysfunction in the site concerned; or (which gives rise to most of the problems of differential diagnosis in the clinic) may in fact be the result of a normal local reaction to input from pathology elsewhere in the system (which has multiple reciprocal connections). Worse still, our theory holds that a high *prevalence* of, say, panic symptoms does not necessarily indicate a disorder of the structures that (proximately) mediate these symptoms. They may be secondary consequences of disorder (or comorbid disorders) in some other part of the defence system.

Our concentration in this part of the argument on identifying specific brain regions involved in the specific symptoms and syndromes of anxiety leads us to emphasize, in Chapter 13, the differences in function between each such region. We argue that what is needed is diagnostic tests of the underlying neural dysfunction giving rise to what may be quite variable symptoms across cases. This emphasis contrasts with the surrounding two chapters, dealing respectively with the personality traits that predispose to and underpin the anxiety disorders, and with the general effectiveness of some recent pharmacological treatments of these disorders.

Data from both these areas of research provide striking evidence that, despite the complexity of the brain systems that underlie the phenomena of anxiety, fear, and the neurotic disorders, there is an underlying unity that binds them together. Our picture of this unity is reflected in a 'double hit' hypothesis of the neurotic disorders (McNaughton and Glue, 2020). As detailed in §13.2.3, we believe it is not high neuroticism or high trait anxiety, *per se*, that generates what we would term anxiety disorder but the combination of the two. As a result, in many cases, either a drug such as ketamine (which ameliorates all the neurotic disorders) or a selective anxiolytic drug (which by definition ameliorates only anxiety) will be effective. The same general/specific distinction can be made for traits underlying panic, phobia, obsession, etc. Importantly, different balances between these factors (potentially including, e.g. comorbidity of anxiety and depression) can lead to sensitivity or resistance to conventional treatments (and likely some cases of resistance to ketamine and other psychedelics as well). We believe that theory-based trait sensitivity biomarkers will allow prediction of appropriate treatment.

1.16.2 Treatment of the neurotic disorders

Chapter 14 discusses the treatment of anxiety and fear disorders via behavioural and cognitive methods in detail (CBT), and consider their impact on the brain, and their integration with drug therapies (pharmacotherapy) to achieve augmentation. It briefly summarizes pharmacotherapy, including drug–drug augmentation, based on the detailed reviews of this in earlier chapters (particularly Chapter 4). Critically, we see all therapies, whatever their modality, as altering reported disorders at the level of the Conceptual Nervous System via changes wrought at the level of the Central Nervous System with hormones, synapses, and circuit dynamics all playing their part. Both levels are important. We are used to chemical changes (as with alcohol) producing mental changes; but in disorders such as post-traumatic stress disorder cognitive changes can result in brain changes. Both in terms of understanding, and treatment, an integrated neuropsychological approach is important.

We conclude with a brief overview of novel psychedelic therapies and their apparent targeting of neuroticism to ameliorate neurotic disorders in general; and use our double hit (neuroticism + disorder-specific trait) model to account for disorders, for treatment resistance, disorder sequencing, and comorbidities—and for the relative therapeutic specificity and slow action of conventional drugs. We expect a bright future with exciting further developments in the separate and combined targeting of neuroticism by psychedelics, novel CBT methods, and novel combinations of older drugs.

1.17 Conclusion

The purpose of this introductory chapter has been to lay out in broad terms the main themes of the book and the main lines of the theory it contains. We have not dismissed alternative theories either of anxiety or the functions of the SHS without careful consideration of their merits and of the evidence in their support. At many points, indeed, rather than dismissing them, we subsume modified versions of these theories into our own model; and in all cases we attempt to incorporate within its explanatory scope the evidence upon which they rest. These efforts to grapple with a wide range of data from many sources and bearing on many specific issues have necessarily made the main text large.

The text includes further areas of research that we have barely mentioned; but is only sufficient expansion to allow the reader to get a full picture of the issues. However, in many cases our interpretations of the data run counter to orthodoxy. We provide further detailed support as appendices and supplementary reviews (with DOIs listed on pages xxix–xxxi). Even in the appendices, we have not tried to be fully comprehensive and have cited reviews rather than primary sources wherever possible.

Despite this, the reader may well feel from time to time, as the authors certainly did, that the wood can get lost for the trees. It may be useful at such moments to return to this chapter to check our final destination: a theory that simultaneously provides an account of the neuropsychology of anxiety and of the cognitive functions of the various brain systems (most centrally the SHS) that jointly contribute to that neuropsychology. In a slogan that the rest of the book seeks to justify: we see the septo-hippocampal system, at the neural level, as being central to an anxiolytic-defined GIS at the psychological level; and we see these systems as giving rise to pathological anxiety when hyperactive, and to amnesia (catastrophic hypermnesia) when hypoactive.

2
Ethology and anxiety

2.1 Why ethology?

We initially (Gray, 1982), derived the adequate stimuli for anxiety (i.e. inputs to the Goal Inhibition System/GIS) largely empirically, with no unifying principle other than drug action. The second edition (Gray and McNaughton, 2000) introduced ethological and ethopharmacological analysis (covered in this chapter) that provided, integrated with operant data (Chapters 3 and 4), just such a principle.

Ethological analysis is a natural starting point for anyone interested in defining anxiety or any other emotion (see, e.g. Ursin, 1985; McNaughton, 1989b). Importantly for our primary approach to anxiety, ethopharmacology provides a cross-check for both rodents (Blanchard and Blanchard, 1990a; Rodgers et al., 1995; Blanchard et al., 1997a; Setem et al., 1999) and humans (Perkins et al., 2009; Lippold et al., 2020); and anchors translation between the species.

In particular, Bob[1] and Caroline Blanchard have argued that the functional significance of behaviour attributed to any emotion must be taken into account; and 'reflects the dynamics of that behaviour in interaction with the ecological systems in which the species has evolved, implying that these dynamics... can be determined far more efficiently when the behaviour is studied under conditions typical of life for the particular species' (Blanchard and Blanchard, 1990c, p. 125). Such functional analysis can transcend species boundaries, since species-specific behaviours can be characterized by their species-general functions (McNaughton, 1989b; Blanchard, 2017; Mobbs and Kim, 2015). The latter shape 'circuits that instantiate functions that allow organisms to survive and thrive by detecting and responding to challenges and opportunities. Included, at a minimum, are circuits involved in defense, maintenance of energy and nutritional supplies, fluid balance, thermoregulation, and reproduction. These survival circuits and their adaptive functions are conserved to a significant degree across mammalian species, including humans' (LeDoux, 2012, p. 654) and support goal-directed behaviour (Sternson, 2013).

The main problem for ethological analysis is to retain enough of the natural environment to elicit the full gamut of a species' defence reactions, but with sufficient control to allow parametric manipulation of stimuli and precise measurement of responses. So, the Blanchards spent many years using 'ethoexperimental' methods (Blanchard and Blanchard, 1988) to analyse the reactions of prey to natural predators: of rats to cats; of wild rats to human beings; and of mice to rats. Critically, what separated their approach from the operant approach described in the next chapter was their concentration on innate responses. They used stimuli that the rat had not previously encountered but to which rats as a species were adapted.

[1] His death in 2013 was a major loss to science. A special issue of *Neuroscience and Biobehavioral Reviews* (Volume 76, Part A, pp. 1–184, May 2017) reporting an international workshop on translational neuroscience and mental disorder celebrates his memory and includes an overview of his neurobiological legacy (Brain, 2017).

The Neuropsychology of Anxiety, Third Edition. Neil McNaughton and Jeffrey A. Gray, Oxford University Press.
 DOI: 10.1093/oso/9780198843313.003.0002

Importantly, unlike pure field ethology, they used experimental methods so their results with innate responses could be mapped onto other experimental results obtained with learned responses. This also allowed the replicable testing of drugs on the behaviour—the start of ethopharmacology (Blanchard and Blanchard, 1990a).

Innate reactions are not always 'functional' or 'adaptive'. Survival systems produce responses that were advantageous in the phylogenetic past, on average, but not always then and perhaps not at all now. This will help us explain psychological dysfunction in the absence of overt neuropathology; and why anxiety disorders are now a major health problem. Further, anxiety that is adaptive in some can be maladaptive in those with lower intelligence; and usual precursors of anxiety, such as rumination, may be adaptive when coupled with high intelligence (Perkins and Corr, 2014). We have argued that this phylogenetically-viewed adaptive functionality ('teleonomy') should be used to define specific emotions (McNaughton, 1989b). But we simplify here with two *working* assumptions: 1) the function of behaviour in a threatening situation will be intuitively obvious to us; and, 2) this function will be currently relevant to the animal. Both derive from the expectation that threat-related systems will be highly conserved in evolution (see, e.g. LeDoux and Daw, 2018) as will the trait control of their hierarchical neural organization (McNaughton, 2020).

For a proper functional analysis of behaviour, we must compare across species. Patterns of defensive behaviour vary depending on the specific situation, the type of threat, the animal's past history, and many other factors. However, ethologists have managed to categorize this amazing variety of behaviour into a number of fairly simple *functional classes*. Thus, 'avoidance, flight and defensive responses are found in all animal Phyla' (Eibl-Eibesfeldt and Sutterlin, 1990, p. 381) and the functional relationship between these responses is also predictable although the responses may not be.

Animals avoid when they can, flee if avoidance has not been successful, and defend themselves, usually aggressively, when flight is impossible or difficult. 'The basic principles... for birds and non-human mammals hold true for [humans] except that [humans have] many cultural expressions of agonal behaviour including elaborations of group aggression in war' (*op. cit.*, p. 388). These cultural refinements, however, do not require any major theoretical changes. They are founded on innate reactions, many of which are not only homologous to the reactions of other mammals but also surprisingly similar to them in phenomenological detail. Further, culturally transmitted behaviour patterns are themselves subject to the same adaptive constraints and requirements as genetically transmitted patterns.

The similarities between humans and other primates are particularly obvious; culture has also been attributed to whales (Rendell and Whitehead, 2001); and human cultural refinements, while extensive, are in any case no different in principle from the learned modifications to agonal (defensive and aggressive) behaviour that occur in other mammals. Similarly, we have argued that even human cognition, at the process level, is no different in principle to non-human cognition except in so far as non-human species also differ from each other (McNaughton and Corr, 2008).

2.2 Ethoexperimental analysis

Classical ethology, operating in the wild, cannot control events. This limits deductions about the underlying control of behaviour. To solve this problem, the Blanchards created an

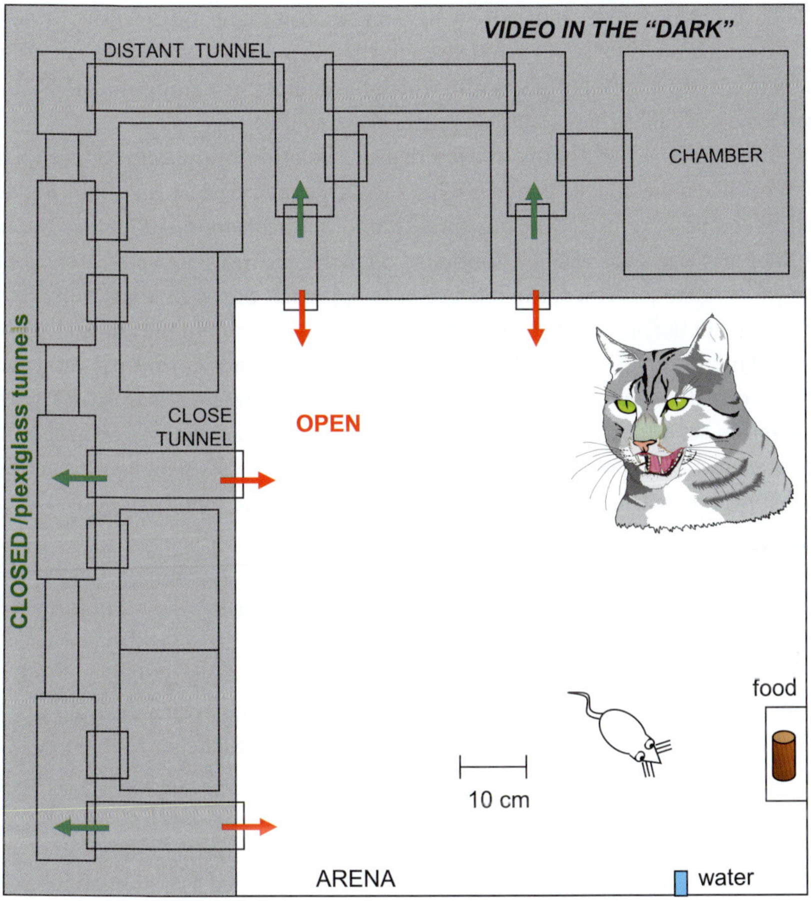

Fig. 2.1 The Visible Burrow System. For explanation, see text. Redrawn and adapted from Blanchard, R. J. & Blanchard, D. C., 'An ethoexperimental analysis of defense, fear and anxiety'. In: McNaughton, N. & Andrews, G., eds., Anxiety, p. 130, Figure 2. Copyright © 1990, University of Otago Press.

apparatus that provided an environment half-way between a natural ecology and an artificial experiment: the 'Visible Burrow System' (VBS; Fig. 2.1, Blanchard and Blanchard, 1989; see also Blanchard et al., 1995 for a mouse version of this test). The VBS had two main parts: an arena where rats could obtain food and water and where experimenters could introduce a cat; and a permanently dark artificial burrow system made of plexiglass tubes where the rats could live and where they could escape from the arena. Critically, the burrow system was illuminated with red or infrared light, which the rats treated as darkness but which allowed video recording. The rats lived permanently in colonies in this apparatus, with a cat occasionally presented. So, the experimenters could categorize many different types of behaviour and determine their contexts through ethoexperimental analysis.

The VBS allowed, in particular, comparison of the immediate responses to a cat (when it was placed in the arena with the rats) with the pattern of responses after removal of the cat when, from the rat's point of view, the cat was potentially rather than actually present. The important difference, here, is that 'while such potential threat situations necessarily elicit some defensive behaviours,... defensive behaviours such as flight and defensive threat/defensive attack, which work well to present, discrete, threat stimuli, may be useless or even counterproductive in threatening situations in which the actual threatening animal or object has not been localized' (Blanchard and Blanchard, 1990c, p. 128).

Using the VBS, the Blanchards showed that presentation of the cat produced a characteristic sequence of behaviour patterns. First, was the expected defensive fight/flight. Flight resulted, of course, in return to the burrows. Second was behavioural inhibition and freezing within the burrow system—which continued after the cat was removed. Later, as the duration of cat absence increased, the rats began to approach the open arena, initially poking their heads out of the burrow. Even once the rats were active, and in the arena, there was still behavioural inhibition of non-defensive behaviours, such as eating. The post-cat pattern also occurred to cat odour, but with a shorter initial immobility phase. The similarity of responses post-cat and to cat odour, and their clear common functions, mean we can group them together as reactions to a 'potential cat'; characterized by 'risk assessment behaviour' (periodic tentative approach, rearing and scanning, defensive quiescence, and thigmotaxis), eventually replaced by the return of pre-cat behaviours.

To allow parametric and pharmacological analysis of this plethora of defensive behaviours, the Blanchards constructed an ethoexperimental test battery: a set of limited laboratory situations that allowed a high degree of control over stimuli; but which also used 'a wide enough range of conditions to make it possible for a variety of defensive behaviours to appear and be recognized, and moreover, to suggest by the conditions in which they appeared something of their specific functional significance' (Blanchard and Blanchard, 1990d, p. 125). This battery consisted of two separate sets of tests: the 'Fear/Defence Test Battery', which tested immediate reactions to an actual, proximal predator; and the 'Anxiety/Defence Test Battery', which tested reactions to a potential predator.

Critically, the Fear/Defence Test Battery used wild rats, which treat humans as predators. (This reaction has been largely bred out of laboratory rats.) The behaviour of the predator (i.e. the experimenter) could then be controlled in a way that is impossible with wild predators (e.g. Blanchard et al., 1986).

The experimenters manipulated both the distance of the human predator from the rat and also whether escape was available or not (for details see Blanchard and Blanchard, 1990d), with results summarized in Fig. 2.2A. At near-zero predator-prey distances, defensive attack (including vocalization, jumping and biting) is elicited. At larger distances flight is elicited, if this is possible, or freezing if flight is not possible. The intensity of both flight and freezing decreases with increasing defensive distance. Note that, except for freezing, the behaviour that the Blanchards observed would be inappropriate if the predator were not clearly present and, in many cases, close.

The 'Anxiety/Defence Test Battery' employed the odour of a cat or brief presentations of a non-contacting cat as the eliciting stimulus in a battery of tests that allowed measurement of defensive quiescence, risk assessment, suppression of eating, and other behaviour previously characterized as occurring after exposure to the cat in the VBS (Fig. 2.2B).

The Blanchards summarize their overall conclusions as follows:

> natural defensive behaviours of nonhuman mammals are very different in situations involving potential danger as opposed to present danger, and... specific behaviours seen in

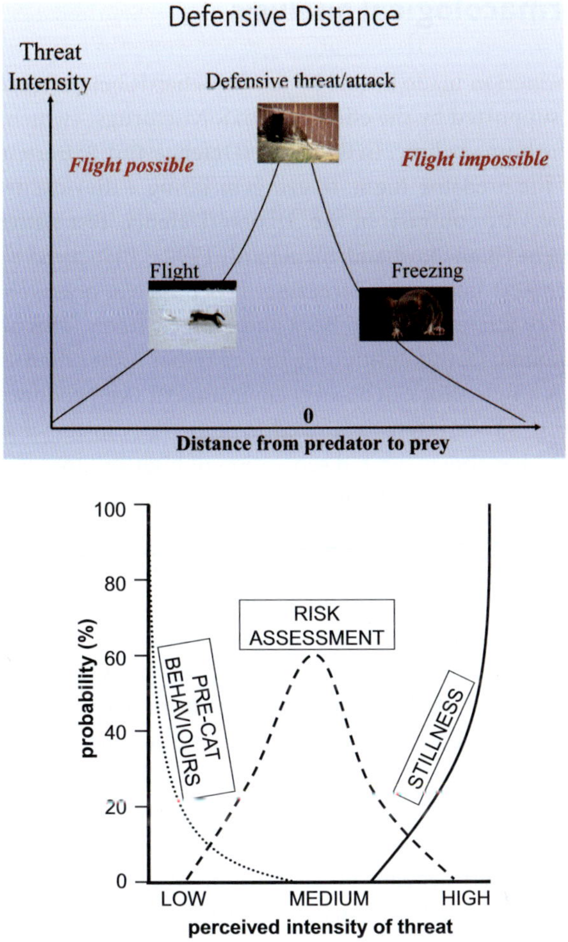

Fig. 2.2 Defensive distance. For an individual this can equate to actual physical distance—but across individuals is better seen as perceived intensity of threat. (A). As distance from a predator decreases, the intensity of fear is held to increase in an accelerating fashion. This intensity controls very tightly a progression from flight or freezing (depending on whether flight is available or not) through defensive threat to defensive attack. Image provided by and © D. C. Blanchard. (B). Effects of equivalent variation in defensive distance (perceived intensity of threat) for a potential predator. Stillness (including defensive quiescence rather than freezing) gives way to risk assessment, and then pre-cat behaviours.

the former situation may be especially relevant to an analysis of anxiety. These behaviours centre around a 'risk assessment' pattern *which includes approach and scanning of potentially dangerous stimuli or situations*, accompanied by changes in posture and movement characteristics. In contrast, reactions to specific, present, threat stimuli involve flight, freezing, and defensive threat and attack. We suggest that *risk assessment is the central component of an anxiety pattern*, while the reactions to present threat are best characterized as indicating fear.

Blanchard and Blanchard (1990d, p. 124, our italics)

2.3 Ethopharmacological analysis

The ethological distinction made in rats by the Blanchards between actual and potential threat is generally supported by the effects of anxiolytic drugs—which were quite separately classified in the human clinic. In their Fear/Defence Test Battery, anxiolytics did not affect avoidance of the predator, flight, freezing, or biting. (They did reduce vocalization and defensive threat.) By contrast, in the Anxiety/Defence Test Battery, anxiolytics reduced risk assessment (Blanchard and Blanchard, 1990a; Blanchard et al., 1993) but, as in the Fear/Defence Test Battery, not freezing. It is possible, however, that conditioned freezing is sensitive to anxiolytics (e.g. Beck and Fibiger, 1995). This is particularly clear with so-called contextual fear (conditioning to a chamber rather than a discrete stimulus, see section 4.6.2). A single shock in a novel environment can produce freezing 24 hours later that is related to shock intensity, linked to static cues in the chamber, reduced by anxiolytic drugs, and has shown a rapid separation of high and low conditioned freezing strains (i.e. those with anxious of non-anxious personalities) with selective breeding (León et al., 2017).

There is a possible parallel of innate freezing and other fear-related reactions with human clinical phobic reactions. If simple phobia is viewed as a type of anxiety, the failure of anxiolytics to reduce avoidance of, for example, snakes (Sartory et al., 1990) is difficult to understand. However, on the Blanchards' analysis, simple object (e.g. snake) phobia is better viewed as the result of fear rather than anxiety, since it involves active avoidance of a present, distinctly localized, predator. Given the Blanchards' results with anxiolytic drugs, we would predict that simple phobic avoidance should not be affected, as indeed it was not in the Sartory et al. (1990) experiment. The sensitivity to anxiolytics of verbal report (as opposed to physical avoidance) in human snake phobics (Sartory et al., 1990) might be accounted for, *post hoc*, if verbal report depends on anticipation of the requirement to approach the snake and, therefore, reflects risk assessment rather than avoidance of the snake itself. The therapeutic situation is clearly one where the distinction between fear and anxiety is difficult to make. For example, the presentation of the snake by the experimenter (unlike the sudden appearance of a snake in the wild) could result in its being perceived as a potential rather than actual threat, since the patient might be aware that the possibility of being bitten during therapy should have been excluded by the ethics committee before they approved the therapy! Furthermore, presentation of the snake by the experimenter could well create pressure for the patient to approach the snake, and approach to a potential source of danger is a prime characteristic of the Anxiety/Defence Test Battery. These issues would repay further experimental attention (the experiment by Sartory et al. has not, so far as we know, been followed up by others) but should be easy to implement with novel computer-based methods (Robillard et al., 2003).

The specific nature of the drug effects on risk assessment measures that the Blanchards observed is also interesting; and emphasizes that care must be taken with parametric aspects of tasks if they are to be properly interpreted. Across different components of their anxiety/defence battery, the Blanchards found that anxiolytic drugs both increased and decreased risk assessment measures. As the time since presentation of an actual cat increased, the control rats in the VBS went from freezing to high levels of risk assessment and then, finally, to low levels of risk assessment and a return of normal daily routines. In specific tests of the anxiety battery in which an actual cat was used to generate anxiety, risk assessment was low in controls and was *increased* by an anxiolytic drug. In tests where cat odour rather than an actual cat was used, risk assessment was high in controls and was *reduced* by the drug. Thus, in all cases the drug-induced change in risk assessment could be interpreted as an increase in effective defensive distance and hence a decrease in anxiety (this is discussed further in section 4.6.4).

2.4 The ethology and ethopharmacology of anxiety and fear

It is clear from the ethological analysis we have summarized that defensive responses to threat take many specific behavioural forms, each finely tuned to the precise circumstances of the threat. However, there are at least two global functional categories that the Blanchards (e.g. Blanchard and Blanchard, 1990d; Blanchard and Blanchard, 1994) identify with fear and anxiety respectively.

Confrontation with an inescapable predator elicits an explosive attack (the precise details of which vary with the species and situation). This attack can be intermixed with undirected escape attempts (flight). A more distal/escapable predator also elicits escape (now directed rather than undirected) or, if escape is not available, a complete absence of movement (freezing). A critical point, to which we shall return, is that all of these forms of behaviour can be seen as outputs from a system that controls behaviour when the animal is moving, or intends to move, *away from* a dangerous situation, i.e. when the goal is a repulsor and simply requires some form of withdrawal.

Where a predator is potential rather than actual (e.g. it has just gone out of view, or its smell is present), this elicits behavioural inhibition as the predominant response when the perceived risk is high. Behavioural inhibition (in the sense of inhibition of pre-predator behaviours) persists, but is accompanied by risk assessment behaviour when the perceived risk is moderate. Finally, risk assessment decreases when non-threat behaviour patterns are released from behavioural inhibition as the perceived risk becomes negligible. Risk assessment functions to reduce the level of perceived potential threat, while behavioural inhibition both prevents competition between risk assessment and non-defensive behaviour and reduces risk should threat prove actual.

Crucial to our theory is that both risk assessment and behavioural inhibition are part of a behavioural program that restrains the animal when it has positive reasons to move, *towards* a dangerous situation. They must operate only when the animal is faced with two incompatible goals—an attractor and a repulsor (e.g. approach to food versus avoidance of a predator). As we shall see, however, when we come to the full version of our theory, behavioural inhibition in the absence of observable external (behavioural) risk assessment can nonetheless be viewed as involving internal risk assessment (comprising, e.g. attentional shifts and the scanning of memory stores rather than the environment). Accompanying these changes in risk assessment are changes in heart rate and in the sensitivity to startling stimuli. Not only are these latter reactions sensitive to anxiolytic drugs in a way that predator-avoidance reactions are not, they also appear to be quite distinct ontogenetically (Hunt et al., 1994). As to the anxiolytic drugs, their central action is not on withdrawal (escape/active avoidance) but rather on the capacity of signals of danger to reduce approach to the appetitive goal (passive avoidance). This distinction is discussed further in Chapter 4.

2.5 Some terminological problems

We can now make a preliminary assessment of some of the problems involved in analysing anxiety. Anxiety can be viewed, to some extent as DSM-III-R (American Psychiatric Association, 1987) suggests, as a set of responses to threat. But theoretically, and ethologically, there are at least two quite separate types of threat. On the one hand there is a definite, localizable, actual threat such as a predator, from which one must withdraw to a safe distance; and, on the other, there is indefinite, diffuse, potential threat, which (for other reasons, e.g. loss of food resources) should often be cautiously approached. Both the functionally desirable and the observed skeletal responses are quite different depending on which of these two situations is present. This distinction is more or less captured by DSM-5[2] with fear seen as a response to imminent threat and anxiety as a response to anticipated future threat (American Psychiatric Association, 2013, p826; see also American Psychiatric Association, 2022).

The Blanchards' analysis links 'fear' and 'anxiety' with actual and potential threat, respectively. However, actual/potential as a categorical distinction between fear and anxiety does not fit with the everyday tendency to conflate the two terms; nor with other ethologically-based usage (e.g Ursin, 1980). There are also specific functional reasons for treating the actual/potential distinction with caution.

First, neither the form nor the function of the behaviour is driven solely by the actual versus potential nature of the threat. For example, a potential threat which *need not be approached* requires only withdrawal (in the form of unurgent active avoidance or escape), and so is functionally equivalent to a paradigmatic case of actual threat. Similarly, a localized actual *mild* threat (e.g. a competing conspecific) which *has to be approached* (if some appetitive goal is to be obtained) will require behavioural inhibition and risk assessment, and so is functionally equivalent to a paradigmatic case of potential threat.[3]

Second, and of particular relevance to our analysis of learning in the next chapter, even when there is an approach-avoidance conflict, escape responses are regularly observed. For example, in the Blanchards' paradigm case there are frequent rapid returns of the animal to its burrow. This escape from a potential predator is not only functionally equivalent to escape from an actual predator but is similarly insensitive to anxiolytic drugs (Appendix 1).

Thus, instead of focusing on the paradigmatic eliciting stimuli, use of which allowed the Blanchards to characterize the separate classes of behaviour and their functional consequences, we shall focus in the remainder of this book on the behaviour patterns themselves and, most importantly, their *adaptive functions.*

Rather than refer (except in the loosest way) to fear, therefore, we shall refer to the Goal Repulsion System (GRS) the function of which is to remove the animal from negative goals and the lower levels of which incorporate the classical fight/flight/freezing system. We hold that this system in animals such as rats is homologous to the systems that control panic and simple phobia in human beings; and that are insensitive to anxiolytic drugs but sensitive to panicolytic drugs. It is important to note here that fight (defensive aggression) involves, at

[2] As already noted in Chapter 1.

[3] The threat must be only mild if approach is to be a viable option. The importance of this point will become clearer in the next chapter. But it is implicit in the Blanchards' emphasis on risk assessment (see also section 2.6) that the reactions to the potential predator involve a major *conflict* between achieving the goal of food (and engaging in other survival-oriented behaviour outside the burrow), on the one hand, and achieving the goal of safety, on the other. Risk assessment involves active attempts to gather sufficient information to resolve the approach-avoidance conflict either with avoidance (if a cat is detected) or approach (if a cat is proved to be absent).

the observational level, approach to the threatening stimulus; but has the *adaptive function* of achieving withdrawal from it—it only occurs when flight is not available (Fig. 2.2); and, critically, it is either unaffected or may be increased by anxiolytics (see Gray, 1977, p 451). We discuss this meaning of fight in the context of personality questionnaires in §12.14.

Similarly, rather than refer (except in the loosest way) to anxiety, we shall refer to the GIS: a system presumed to control not only inhibition of pre-potent responses to positive and negative goals but also risk analysis; to be homologous to the systems that control anxiety (as opposed to fear) in human beings; and to be sensitive to anxiolytic drugs. As justified in Chapter 1, the GIS is essentially identical to what was previously labelled as the BIS with its renaming being an solely an attempt to avoid confusion with systems controlling action stopping and with lexically derived questionnaires that have not been neurally validated.

Thus, the GIS (originally BIS) is a system that not only inhibits pre-potent behaviour, but also generates risk assessment behaviour. In addition, in preparation for the sudden appearance of a predator, we would expect increased negative bias, vigilance, faster reactions and a variety of more general autonomic changes (Fig. 1.2). One of these preparatory reactions may well be the basis for the phenomenon of 'fear-potentiated startle'. This consists of an enhanced startle response to an intense stimulus if this is presented in a threatening context (most commonly provided in animal experiments by a fear CS previously associated with a source of pain). Fear-potentiated startle has been much studied in the laboratory but is simple enough to have superficial ecological validity even there. In human beings, potentiated startle has been shown to occur in the context of fear provoking images, but not with affectively positive (sexual) images that produced similar levels of arousal (Jansen and Frijda, 1994) or even with affectively negative (disgusting) images of a non-threatening type (Balaban and Taussig, 1994; Kaviani et al., 1999).

This is not to say that we can always unambiguously distinguish the output of the GRS from that of the GIS. Freezing occurs very clearly in response to a fairly close, inescapable predator, but something very like it can occur as the initial stage of the response pattern to a potential predator. The latter could be a high intensity form of behavioural inhibition that is neurally distinct from freezing, but behaviourally difficult to distinguish from it because both involve cessation of movement. (Remember that 'behavioural inhibition', as we have defined it, is of pre-potent responses. It does not imply loss of all behaviour and can be accompanied by active risk assessment.) It is unclear, therefore, whether stillness as such should be classified as purely a response to actual threat or also as a response to extreme potential threat.[4] There are some indications of differential pharmacological sensitivity relating to the two (putative) types of response; and it may also be possible to distinguish them in operant paradigms (e.g. Kim et al., 1996) or via the specific body postures used to achieve stillness (Blanchard et al., 1996). This issue is impossible to resolve on purely functional grounds and will, therefore, be set aside until a detailed analysis of neural mechanisms is available (Chapter 6), where we will argue that the lower levels of approach, withdrawal, and conflict control can all involve stillness that involves different precise body postures and different functions (Silva and McNaughton, 2019).

[4] Lordosis could be viewed as a positive form of stillness, with all three forms controlled by the periaqueductal grey (Silva and McNaughton, 2019).

2.6 Confirmation in human studies

The power of the ethoexperimental approach to clarify the functions of behaviours is most easily harnessed in rodent studies: where presentation of an innate predator can be achieved fairly easily. Recently the practical and ethical objections to equivalent work in humans have been largely bypassed by studies using scenarios or computer gaming and have essentially obtained similar results to the original rodent studies (as reviewed by Blanchard, 2017).

The scenario studies use descriptions of threatening situations that allow variation of defensive direction/ambiguity of threat, defensive distance, and avoidability of threat. Participants then provided open-ended descriptions of their likely defensive behaviours for each of the scenarios (Blanchard et al., 2001). Note that while presentation of the stimuli and recording of the response use the verbal channel, the paradigm matches the original VBS paradigm much closer than the lexical derivation and factor analytic extraction of items in a conventional questionnaire. Where the scenarios and the described defensive responses were non-linguistic the patterns of results showed good cross-species homology (rats versus mice versus people) but 'human language – both as a component of threatening situations and as a response to them – provides substantial complexity to these patterns' (Blanchard, 2017, p 24). This is as we would expect given the varying meanings assigned by different people to threat-related words (McNaughton, 2018; Davitz, 1969) and the relative lack of ambiguity in words referring to more concrete situations and specific behaviours. The resultant scenario measures also generally show the expected relationships to questionnaire measures of neuroticism, fear, and anxiety (Perkins et al., 2010).

The computer game studies take advantage of modern technology to allow a virtual participant (i.e. a controlled avatar) to be faced with a virtual predator (e.g. Fung et al., 2019; Qi et al., 2018; Korn and Bach, 2019; Bach et al., 2020). A key feature of the virtual predator is that contact with the participant's avatar generates a very real painful consequence to the participant, either via electric shock or via loud white noise. In these experiments the verbal channel is not used and the results with defensive distance and direction are essentially as would be expected from the rodent work, including (e.g. Lippold et al., 2020) the effects of anxiolytic drugs (as reviewed by Blanchard, 2017, who also describes studies of facial expression and stabilometry that require a range of assumptions for their interpretation). The brain activations involved are also as would be expected from prior rodent work (see McNaughton, 2019). Computer delivery of stimuli can also tap, fairly realistically, into existing specific phobic reactions (Robillard et al., 2003) and can expand on the rodent work by demonstrating, for example, that defensive helping in humans is elicited more by immediate than distal threat—linking it to escape reactions (Vieira et al., 2020).

Blanchard (2017) makes the important point that, in the human studies, the link between ambiguous threat and risk assessment behaviour is particularly strong and most clearly homologous to the rodent work (Fig. 2.2B). In the context of outputs from the GIS, this is noteworthy as risk assessment is a distinctive behaviour *generated* when pre-potent approach or withdrawal behaviours are *inhibited*. However, this behaviour is also an external sign of an internal form of processing that stands at 'the interface of cognition and emotion... [with] a more extensive cortical representation than other specific defenses' (Blanchard, 2018, p. 69). Risk assessment, on this view, is equivalent to 'affective cognition' (Blanchard and Meyza,

2017), and so would 'encompass processing of emotionally salient information in contexts requiring cognitive evaluation to generate an appropriate response' (Elliott et al., 2011, p. 153). Risk assessment more generally, then, would normally function to reduced goal conflict by reducing the uncertainties related to action outcomes. That is, uncertainty or ambiguity may be essential to anxiety as defined by anxiolytic drugs—a point we will return to in the next chapter.

2.7 Conclusion

In this chapter, we have depended on the ethological study of *unlearned* defensive responses. This has given us a reasonable basis for the categorical distinctions we have tried to make in terms of the presumed *functions* of the behaviour concerned. A preliminary functional categorization of different emotional terms, derived from this analysis and including the distinction between avoidable and unavoidable threats (which require different responses, see Fig. 2.2A), is provided in Fig. 2.3. With the addition of ethoexperimental and ethopharmacological analysis, this approach has also given us some idea of the control of the relevant forms of behaviour. From this we have concluded that anxiety represents activity in the GIS: a system that is active when the animal is faced with a threat that it has some reason to approach, and the major outputs of which are inhibition of pre-potent responses to the conflicting positive and negative goals, risk assessment, and increased arousal or vigilance.

The emphasis in this chapter has been on our evolutionary past. However, while many would accept that human emotion has evolutionary roots, most would argue that a key feature of both normal and pathological human fear and anxiety lies in the specificity of the eliciting stimuli. This specificity owes little to genetics and much to learning and cognition. We therefore turn to this issue in the next chapter.

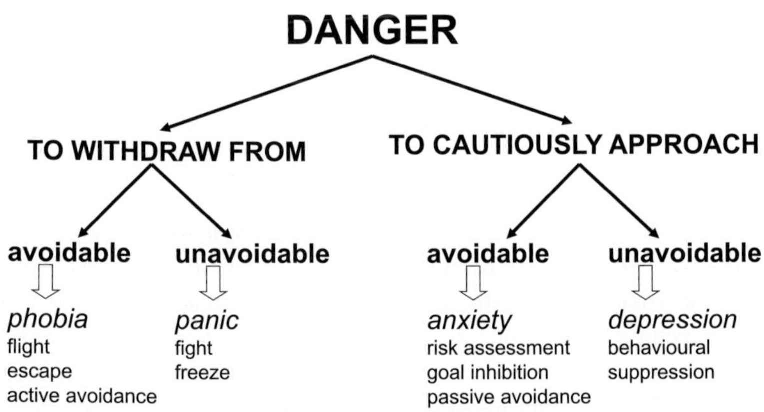

Fig. 2.3 A functional classification of different types of clinical disorder and normal response in terms of different classes of danger. Adapted from McNaughton (1993).

2.8 Caveat—rumination and worry

Even with its discussion of the human data, this chapter has not discussed rumination, obsession, or worry. There are those who would see these as central to anxiety, or at least anxiety disorder, in humans (e.g. LeDoux, 2015). But we have three reasons for excluding them.

First, this chapter focuses on basic approach-avoidance conflict and its parallels in rats and humans. Especially with acute state anxiety we do not see rumination about the past, obsession about the present, or worry about the future as having a place; and, of course, it is hard to tell when a rat is engaging in these activities.

Second, we see rumination and worry as linked to causes of anxiety rather than being part of anxiety itself. We take rumination to include both reflective pondering and brooding (Treynor et al., 2003). In one sense rumination pure and simple need not be negative but, in practice, is often 'a repetitive and passive focus on one's negative emotions' (Treynor et al., 2003, p 247). It is in this form that it contributes to and provides some coincident context for anxiety disorder; but without being part of anxiety proper (in our terms) itself. Crucially, we see rumination/worry as part of, or strongly linked to, the effects of neuroticism (see Chapter 12, 13). We follow Gavin Andrews in seeing neuroticism as a risk factor for the range of neurotic disorders including phobia, obsession, and depression as well as anxiety (Andrews et al., 1990). Importantly, in this context, Nolen-Hoeksema would see rumination as a key factor in the *generation* of depression (Treynor et al., 2003) with at least part of its role (in e.g. gender differences) being a predisposing one rather than a symptomatic one (Nolen-Hoeksema, 2001).

Thirdly, and importantly, rumination tends to block external sources of problem-solving information and may even 'inhibit instrumental behavior by increasing uncertainty, resulting in further rumination and behavioral paralysis' (Ward et al., 2003, p 96). This paralysis seems to us to be a direct precursor of the 'failure to cope' at the core of depression (including cases, of e.g. incarceration, where there is no obvious threat and little comorbid anxiety). So, this paralysis would exacerbate ongoing anxiety/depression and thus increase the probability of clinical manifestation but, like life events, would not be inherent to anxiety/depression proper. Critically, from a functional point of view, the internal focus of rumination/worry has the exact opposite results of risk assessment. Rather than resolving conflict, it can be seen to enhance it.

For pharmacological and ethological reasons, we would want to distinguish anxiety *per se* from depression. We would also want to strongly distinguish neuroticism/rumination (whether they are separate or one is part of the other) from anxiety and depression—since a risk factor (e.g. high blood pressure) for something (e.g. stroke) clearly cannot be the something that it is a risk factor for however clinically coincident it tends to look.

Importantly, in relation to worry, we should note that, while worriers are more likely to experience anxiety, depression, and hostility than non-worriers (Borkovec et al., 1983), when assessed within a group of GAD patients worry 'does not correlate with other measures of anxiety or depression indicating that it is tapping an independent construct' (Meyer et al., 1990, p. 487).

Elicited rumination also appears to generate 'effects of negative cognition on health [that] go far beyond the recovery periods usually measured in the laboratory, thus playing a pathogenic role' (Ottaviani et al., 2011, p453). Thus a tendency (i.e. a trait) to rumination/worry would act as a mediator of the general effects of stress (bodily and mental) and 'what differentiates individuals with greater worry is their personal tendency to worry rather than having more stressors to worry about' (Cristina, 2018, p 3).

So, stress can generate anxiety/depression/PTSD in anyone if it is strong enough or chronic enough. Worriers are more likely to have anxiety/depression/PTSD because their background tendency to worry amplifies and multiplies the effects of stressors to which others would be resilient. Here it is worth noting that 'stress' is to a large extent the internal, particularly cognitive, response and is not the external stimulus that elicits it (for which we prefer stressor). So, rumination (pure cognitive recycling) would be a bad thing if the contents of cognition are negative because that would generate, in effect, chronic stress from what would otherwise be acute stress.

We have a recent model that focuses on neuroticism but that could also fit with rumination/worry. In our view high trait neuroticism/worry is one of two necessary conditions for clinical disorder and some specific trait (anxiety, depression, obsession, etc.) is a second (McNaughton and Glue, 2020, for more detail see Chapter 13). In this context, rumination/worry can be viewed as linked to high levels of obssessionality, which we would link to fear of threats for which there is no safety signal, not to anxiety (Rapoport, 1989).

However, if one wants to *define* anxiety in terms of worry these arguments fail at the linguistic level. But, if you do so, you must then explain what it is that anxiolytics are acting on, and rename their target to match your theory.

3
Learning theory and anxiety

3.1 Why learning?

With cognitive accounts rampant in psychology and neuroscience, why discuss learning theory—an archaic child of extreme behaviourism? Our answer is that starting with a learning theory approach grounded in behaviour analysis not only provides a rigorous evidential ground for our key theoretical constructs but also reduces our temptation to employ complex ones, when simple ones are sufficient to account for the data. As we will see particularly in relation to personality (Chapter 12) complex linguistic constructs often add only ambiguity and confusion not explanation. In particular, we will argue that 'reward' and 'punishment' are such confused constructs.

A focus on behavioural evidence, and learning, is compatible with a cognitive approach. Critically, behaviour provides a solid (and we would argue necessary) foundation for cognitive theorizing and, in particular, translational work. On this view 'the conditioning experiment is primarily an analytically tractable tool for studying the *cognitive changes* that take place during learning' (Dickinson, 1980, p. xi, our emphasis). That is, rigorously recorded behaviour then requires a complex internal explanation. Paradoxically, such apparently artificial and restricted conditioning experiments provide the clearest objective evidence that what changes during learning is not the strength of an internal connection between a stimulus and a response, but rather knowledge of a situation and its motivational values, i.e. a goal (see §1.12.4; McNaughton, 1989b, pp. 22–24; McNaughton et al., 2016). In this chapter, therefore, we will draw on the experimental rigour and concrete data of the behaviour analyst to arrive at conclusions about the internal (i.e. *cognitive*), processes that resolve goal conflict and that generate anxiety. Importantly, these methods also are a species-general tool that can easily deliver homologies.

Ethoexperimental analysis (Chapter 2) clearly separated stimuli that indicate a present, localizable, proximal danger from stimuli that warn of the possibility of (often non-localizable and distal) danger. The former stimuli require only escape but the latter often require cautious approach if suitable appetitive goals are to be achieved; and only the effects of the latter are sensitive to anxiolytic drugs—whether testing rats or humans.

The related distinction between a primary aversive event and a signal that warns of the primary event has received considerable attention within learning theory; with *purely behavioural evidence* supporting a view of emotions as 'central' states, i.e. in the brain or *in the mind* (e.g. Mowrer, 1960; Plutchik, 1962; Millenson, 1967). This view is typical of 'two-process' theories of learning, which we will summarize briefly next (for further detail see Gray, 1972; Gray, 1975; McNaughton, 1989b, Chapter 9).

The Neuropsychology of Anxiety, Third Edition. Neil McNaughton and Jeffrey A. Gray, Oxford University Press.
 DOI: 10.1093/oso/9780198843313.003.0003

3.2 ReinforceMENT versus ReinforCER

In earlier editions, we focussed on 'reinforcement' and freely used the terms 'reward' and 'punishment'. However, particularly with the development of Reinforcement Sensitivity Theory (Corr, 2008b), it has become clear that reward/punishment are ambiguous. Indeed, we discovered that one of us had previously (Gray, 1970a) used the word 'punishment' with three different meanings within a single sentence (McNaughton and Corr, 2019b, p. 129).

We have recently argued, therefore, for an approach that splits valuation from motivation, taking into account contingencies, and so separates a 'reinforCER' view of systems controlling goal-oriented behaviour from a 'reinforceMENT' view of learning (Corr and McNaughton, 2012; see also Chapter 12, where we will also revive the idea of reinforceMENT sensitivity).

To our original focus on motivation, then, we have added an emphasis on valuation that links our theory to analysis of decision making in neuroeconomics (Glimcher and Rustichini, 2004; Zak, 2004; Sanfey et al., 2006; Glimcher et al., 2009) and its implications for psychiatry (Hasler, 2012). We summarize this in the second half of this chapter.

Nonetheless, 'reinforCER' remains an appropriate term; since, whether it generates an innate response, or changes the course of current of future behaviour, we are talking about goals and the motivated control of changes in behaviour not habitual behaviour. However, further consideration of the role of dopamine in reinforcement §12.8 will eventually return us to a view that the simple early form of RST focussing on processes of positive and negative *reinforceMENT* (referred to later as RST2) can be *retained in parallel* with a more nuanced and complex view of three hierarchically organized *reinforCER*-oriented motivational systems depending on two forms of evaluation (RST5; see also §12.10).

3.3 Reinforcer versus goal—the role of contingency

> The capacity of a single class of motivational stimuli to give rise to opposite goals in different circumstances is most obvious with consummatory stimuli (like food and water) and in economic experiments. The presentation of a positive stimulus produces positive goals but the omission of expected food, omission of expected water, loss of money, and any other negative contingencies of positive events generate the aversive state of frustration (Amsel, 1962; Amsel, 1992; Amsel and Roussel, 1952). The situation linked to omission or loss will therefore be associated with negative motivation and so their compound will be a negative goal. When the same situation occurs in the future, it will then generate avoidance, thereby reducing exposure to frustration. An important point, here, is that the immediate experience of frustration produces escape (Adelman and Maatsch, 1956), fighting (Amsel, 1962), learned avoidance and many other responses that are also typical of the immediate experience of pain (Gray, 1987b). In general, then, the omission of negative and positive events can be treated as having the same effects as the presentation of positive and negative events, respectively.
>
> The idea that omission of a positive event creates a negative goal in exactly the same way as presentation of a negative event requires one caveat – the two

outcomes do not have the same value. For an event to affect behaviour, it must first be valued. This value, for any given object, will vary with both time and the particular individual. Gorgonzola cheese will have a high positive value for many hungry adults but will usually have a high negative value for young children. Likewise, a rat that is not hungry will not value food highly (i.e. will not work hard to obtain it), and a rat that has undergone taste aversion conditioning for a particular flavour will not value a food with that flavour but will value other food. You might think that a specific object (like a dollar) will have the same value, whether it is being gained or lost – after all, it is the most fungible of all stimuli. But it turns out that, in a wide range of situations, a lost dollar is treated as having greater value than a gained dollar. That is, someone will work harder to avoid a dollar loss than they will to make a dollar gain. This important and very general phenomenon, discovered in behavioural economics (Kahneman and Tversky, 1979; Novemsky and Kahneman, 2005; Tversky and Kahneman, 1991), is termed loss aversion...

Individual differences in valuation are often not important for means obtained in experiments in which some manipulation affects approach or avoidance. For example, individual variation in hunger drive among a group of rats will simply increase variation in speed of running within a group and will not, in the absence of sampling biases, change the difference between the means of the groups. However, there are times when we may want a full understanding of the effects of individual variations in approach and avoidance tendencies. There are often times, in particular, when we want to assess the long-term sensitivities of approach and avoidance systems—i.e. individual personality traits. If so, we will want to take account of both the valuation of specific objects (via their specific exchange rates in relation to the single internal currency on which choices are based) and whether the situation involves a positive or negative contingency with the occurrence of the object [Fig. 3.1]. If we use only positive objects to assess trait approach our measures will be confounded by variation in trait positive valuation. It should also be noted that valuation, as we have used it here, involves an essential interaction between 'wanting' and 'liking' components of a positively valued object that have different neural correlates (Berridge, 2004; Berridge, 1996).

(McNaughton et al., 2016, pp. 28–29)

3.4 Two-process theories of learning (or maybe three)

The preceding discussion of approach and avoidance links directly to detailed learning theory analysis of reinforcement. Here, the central argument has been whether there is only one process of 'learning' or whether there are two learning processes. Our theory is a two-process one and this section covers the formal details for those who find these useful.

The two processes of two-process learning theory are those of classical ('Pavlovian', 'respondent', Stimulus–Stimulus, Sign–Significate, S–S) and instrumental ('Thorndikian', 'operant', Stimulus–Response, S–R) conditioning. Initially, the fundamental separateness of

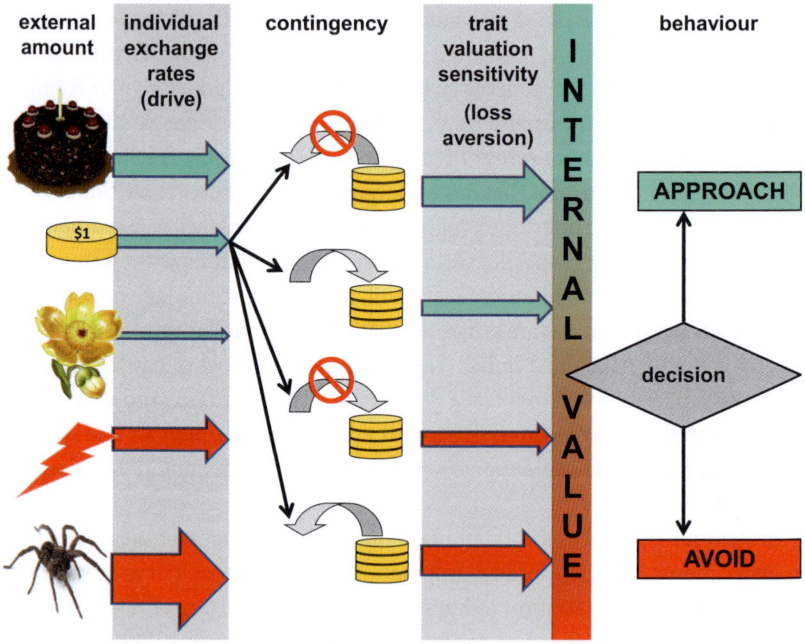

Fig. 3.1 Relations between external amount, contingency and value. An external item will have a specific amount (e.g., 1 entire cake) that, together with the current level of drive (which acts like a currency exchange rate) for that kind of item for that person, determines its primary internal value (thickness of arrows in first column). As shown for the case of $1, this interacts with whether the item will be gained or lost to determine the direction *and* size of its internal value as ultimately measured by the effect on behaviour. The direction of this effect is reversed if the gain or loss is omitted. Loss (removal from a store of items) is most easily controlled with money but will also occur when, for example, one rat steals the food from another rat. Figure and legend from McNaughton et al. (2016) with permission.

these process was controversial (e.g. Mackintosh, 1974) but since then there has been behavioural evidence that they are distinct (Gray, 1975; McNaughton, 1989b). Critically, there is now good neural evidence for quite separate purely associative and reinforcement forms of classical plasticity dependent on long-term potentiation (Bliss and Lomo, 1973) and activity-dependent facilitation (e.g. Kandel and Hawkins, 1992), respectively; and recent evidence for a third distinct dopaminergic instrumental process that can be viewed as combination of activity-dependent and long-term potentiation (Wickens et al., 2003; Reynolds et al., 2001). However, in any particular situation, the acquired behaviour normally involves an interaction between these three learning processes.[1] Critically, across different species or experimental conditions, this can reflect one process more than the other despite the formal contingencies that the experimenter believes they have imposed.

[1] More complex processes can also become involved with, e.g. trace conditioning (Lindquist, 2020).

3.4.1 Classical conditioning

Classical conditioning is the process whereby the subject learns the associative relationships between discrete stimulus events. Suppose a stimulus (S1) can be followed by a second stimulus (S2). Also suppose that S2 has a fixed probability (pS2) of occurring on occasions when it is *not* preceded by S1. There are now three possibilities for the conditional probability of S2 occurring given that it does follow S1 (pS2/S1): pS2/S1 may be greater than, equal to, or less than pS2. In classical conditioning experiments animals are sensitive to all three of these relationships (Dickinson, 1980). Even in the case where (pS2/S1)=pS2, and S1 apparently has no signalling value, this lack of signalling value is itself learned, producing 'learned irrelevance' (Mackintosh, 1973).

In experiments using Pavlov's (1927) paradigm with (pS2/S1)>pS2, it often seems that S1 (the conditioned stimulus, in this positive case conventionally designated CS+) comes to elicit a conditioned response (CR) by gaining control of responses that originally occurred to S2 (the unconditioned stimulus or UCS). However, it can be demonstrated (Dickinson, 1980) that the CS-UCS association is formed independently of whether the UCS elicits any observable response (but see Blackman, 1983 for a contrary view), as would be expected from the properties of associativity underlying long-term potentiation (see, e.g. Abraham, 1988). It is also generally better (see next) to view the CR as being elicited by the anticipation of the UCS rather than necessarily consisting of any component of the UCR. This is also the case when (pS2/S1)<pS2. Here S1 (designated CS-) may often seem to have little effect other than to reduce responses to a CS+ ; however, in a number of cases the animal produces a completely new response appropriate to the anticipated *omission* of the UCS.

Thus, we can conclude that the animal learns the relationship (positive, neutral or negative) between the stimuli and then, quite separately, produces a response that is generally adaptive given the anticipated situation. That is, the animal learns about a particular *goal* and may well use either an innate or a previously learned response to achieve that goal. It should be noted that the experimenter has no control, in such a straightforward Pavlovian conditioning experiment, over the nature of the CR, once the specific UCS has been chosen.

3.4.2 Instrumental conditioning

Instrumental conditioning is the process whereby the subject acquires new behaviour patterns that have the capacity to alter the frequency of its exposure to stimulus events; it can therefore be viewed as response-stimulus or R-S learning (although we shall qualify this view somewhat next). As with classical conditioning, there are three possible cases for the occurrence of S when it is preceded by the response, R. The experimenter can arrange that pS/R is greater than, equal to, or less than pS. However, since the subject rather than the experimenter controls the occurrence of R, we also need to consider the subsequent probability of occurrence of R, conditional on the R-S relationship: pR/(R:S). For each of the pS/R:pS cases we must consider whether the animal produces R so that pR/(R:S) is greater than, equal to, or less than pR (pR is usually referred to as the baseline response rate). The 9 combinations that result from the 3 × 3 cases we have discussed (Table 3.1) can be simplified in a number of ways.

First, while the subject can learn that pS/R = pS (i.e. that the occurrence of the stimulus is completely independent of the occurrence of responding), this learning does not usually change pR/(R:S) or pR, and any effects of the conditioning procedure can probably be viewed as a special case of classically conditioned learned irrelevance. Where S is an aversive stimulus, as defined next, it has been claimed to produce a special type of learned irrelevance called 'learned helplessness', which Seligman (1975) has related to the emotional state of depression.

Second, if pR/(R:S)=pR (that is, there is no change in the probability of responding when S is made a consequence of responding) for either of pS/R>pS or pS/R<pS, it will be found that pR/(R:S)=pR also for the other (S would be what is usually termed a motivationally neutral stimulus). Taken together with our first simplification we have now dealt with the middle row and middle column of the 3 × 3 cases with which we started (Table 3.1).

Third, an important feature of the particular version of two-process theory that we prefer is that it takes the remaining 2 × 2 cases and treats their instrumentally conditioned effects as arising from changes in only two systems, one concerned with maximizing GAIN ('rewards' as objects) and the other with minimizing LOSS ('punishments' as objects).

Table 3.1 Instrumental reinforcing procedures with unconditioned reinforcing events (S). The items within the table and their abbreviations are defined by the intersection of the columns, which categorize the change in probability of a specific operant response (R) given the prevailing R-S contingencies (i.e. a relationship determined by the learner); and of the rows, which categorize the change in probability of S given the occurrence of R (i.e. a relationship determined by the experimenter). 'GAIN' and 'LOSS' indicate two specific classes of stimuli—previously identified as a reward or a punishment (in the sense of objects), respectively. LOSS includes both removal from a positive store of a value and presentation of an affectively negative stimulus; '+' and '–' indicate the presentation or omission, respectively, of GAIN or LOSS consequent on a particular response

			pR/(R:S)	
		> pR	= pR	< pR
	> pS	GAIN+ (approach)	Neutral	LOSS+ (passive avoidance)
pS/R	= pS	Learned irrelevance	Neutral	learned helplessness
	< pS	LOSS– (active avoidance)	Neutral	GAIN– (extinction)

3.4.3 Two systems from four conditions—the effects of omission

Consider the diagonals of Table 3.1. In the top left-hand corner, we have the situation where a stimulus increases response probability when it is presented contingently upon that response. Empirically, it is usually the case that the same stimulus will also decrease response probability when its omission (or termination) is contingent on the response. In Skinner's (1938) terminology such a stimulus is a 'positive reinforcer', or more colloquially a 'gain' ('reward'). Thus, the top left-hand corner and bottom right-hand corner of Table 3.1 may be logically independent but they are not independent in practice—the same physical stimulus can be used in the two cases. We indicate this similarity by using the same descriptor, GAIN, for each and then adding + to indicate an increase in probability of occurrence of the stimulus or — to indicate a decrease in its probability, consequent on the response.

Similarly, any stimulus that will decrease response probability when it is presented contingently upon that response (top right-hand corner of Table 3.1) will also usually increase response probability when its omission (or termination) is contingent on the response. Such a stimulus can be called a 'negative reinforcer' or 'LOSS' ('punishment'). In general, any specific type of stimulus, within certain limits of intensity, duration, etc., will be regularly classifiable as GAIN, neutral, or LOSS.

We have (tacitly) supposed so far that, for a given animal species, there exist stimuli that may act without prior learning as GAIN and others that may similarly act as LOSS. However, these stimuli ('primary reinforcers') can also act as UCSs in a classical conditioning paradigm, as a result of which, in addition to any UCRs and CRs that ensue, they confer on CSs, which are initially neutral, 'secondary' or 'conditioned' GAIN or LOSS properties. It is a convenient fact for the simplifications we have been attempting that the reinforcer property of the secondary stimulus is the same (i.e. GAIN or LOSS) as that of the UCS with which it was paired as a CS.

3.4.4 Conditioning, central motivational states, and emotions

The central states elicited by such secondary reinforcers have played a key role in theories of emotion. Thus Mowrer (1960) treats 'hope' as the state elicited by secondary GAIN ('rewarding stimuli'); and 'fear' similarly as the state elicited by secondary LOSS ('punishing stimuli'). It should be noted that these states—which anticipate GAIN (primary reward) and LOSS (primary punishment), respectively—form a necessary background for the bottom row of Table 3.1. For it is only when an animal anticipates GAIN (hopes) that the omission of GAIN ('frustrative non reward'; Amsel, 1962; Amsel, 1992) can affect its behaviour; and only when it anticipates LOSS (fears) that it can be affected by the omission of LOSS ('relief'). (For a recent detailed analysis of omission, inhibitory learning, safety and frustration, and their neural substrates, see Cassaday et al., 2023.)

For any particular imposed contingency between response and stimulus, Table 3.1 provides two different ways of parcelling out behavioural outcomes. We can focus on the specific direction of change in response (the columns) or on the specific class of stimulus (GAIN or LOSS), the increase (+) or decrease (–) in the probability of which gives rise to the changes in response. It is, of course, an empirical question as to which, if either, of these classifications reflects real distinctions in the way the nervous system processes information in different learning situations. However, the parsimony of Table 3.1 (and learning theories in general) depends on there being general mechanisms for increasing or decreasing response rate, respectively (via positive and negative *reinforcement*), which are each common to all *reinforcers* of that class (i.e. positive or negative). In the absence of specific contrary evidence, then, consistency requires us to parcel together GAIN+ with LOSS—, and GAIN— with LOSS+, on the basis of their effects on response probability, in just the same way and for just the same reasons that we parcel one GAIN+ (e.g. food for a hungry rat) together with another qualitatively different GAIN+ (e.g. water for a thirsty rat). It will be recalled that we placed the same emphasis on functional consequences as opposed to physical stimuli in the ethological analysis of the previous chapter.

Since we will often distinguish between LOSS+ and LOSS—, it is worth re-stating the distinction in a slightly different manner. 'LOSS+' means that, if a specified response is made, then it will be punished; 'LOSS—', that, if the response is made, impending LOSS will be omitted. In still other words, successful avoidance of LOSS requires a *passive* avoidance response in the former case, but *active* avoidance in the latter. Similarly, 'GAIN+' means that, if a response is made, then it will be followed by GAIN (rewarded); 'GAIN—' that, if the response is made, GAIN will be omitted.

3.5 Elicited reactions in learning experiments

Data also favour this particular parcellation—most obviously in two-process analyses of frustrative non-reward. The omission of an expected GAIN not only suppresses subsequent responding (so that GAIN— is located in the right-hand column of Table 3.1 and generates negative *reinforcement*), but also elicits behaviours like those elicited by LOSS+ (Wagner, 1966; Gray, 1967; Gray, 1975) and so is an innate negative *reinforcer*. Likewise, a stimulus paired with frustrative non-reward (CS-GAIN—) becomes secondarily punishing in the same way as a stimulus paired with punishment (CS-LOSS+).

We have until now ignored the eliciting properties of stimuli on which the previous chapter focussed. The similarities between the eliciting properties of LOSS+ and the eliciting properties of GAIN—, especially since they are not complete, may not seem as surprising as they should. Pause for a moment and consider the hungry and sexually receptive female rat who will work to obtain both food and a male rat (Bermant, 1961b). She clearly treats both a piece of food and a male rat as GAIN+. However, the elicited responses supported by these different stimuli are quite different. The female rat will present herself for copulation to the male rat but will eat the food. She never attempts to eat her mate as he approaches her, nor adopt a sexually receptive posture to the food. Given the different eliciting properties of these stimuli that have in common the reinforcing property of being GAIN+, the fact that the *eliciting* properties of LOSS+ and GAIN— are similar is surprising.

The similarity between the eliciting properties of LOSS+ and GAIN— is even more remarkable when we consider that this is not a general property of negatively reinforcing stimuli. Primary and secondary aversive stimuli (LOSS+ and CS-LOSS+), respectively, elicit responses through quite different systems. For example, in the rat, an electric shock elicits as a UCR a great deal of activity (running, jumping, etc.) and noise (squealing); but a CS that predicts such a UCS actually elicits the reverse—immobility (freezing) and silence (Myers, 1971). Similarly, a shock may elicit aggressive behaviour if a suitable object of aggression is present, but a CS paired with shock inhibits aggressive behaviour (Baenninger, 1967; Myers, 1971). There are less specific elicited responses. 'From the functional perspective, skin conductance, pupil size, and respiratory amplitude are valence-unspecific measures that do not directly relate to active defensive or escape behaviors' (Ojala and Bach, 2020, p. 103).

In this respect, aversive stimuli provide a clear contradiction to the idea that properties acquired by a CS as a result of classical conditioning are properties also possessed by the UCS employed to establish the CR. Thus aversive stimuli do not conform to Pavlov's (1927) stimulus substitution hypothesis. This is a particularly powerful demonstration of the fact that the CS alerts the animal to a particular goal rather than simply eliciting the UCR. These results should surprise only the hardline S-R theorist, as opposed to the cognitive learning theorist (e.g. Dickinson, 1980). They might, in contrast, be *predicted*, and to some degree in specific behavioural detail, by the ethologist. For, as we saw in Chapter 2, the functional requirements for responses elicited by a predator, or a warning of a predator, change markedly depending on whether the source of danger can simply be avoided or must be approached. These distinctions were made on the basis of ecologically valid reinforcers. Nonetheless, on the reasonable assumption that a shock can be equated with contact with a predator, then a CS-shock should be equated with a potential or close predator, depending on whether it must be approached or avoided, respectively. In the former case, following the logic developed in the previous chapter, we expect anxiety to be elicited.

The key conclusions from the aforementioned considerations, then, are that: (a) we can to some extent equate LOSS+ with GAIN—, as well as CS-LOSS+ with CS-GAIN—; but that (b) we need to distinguish carefully between the primary events (LOSS+, GAIN—), on the one hand, and CSs for those primary events, on the other, since they can have quite opposite eliciting properties and functional requirements. Nonetheless all produce the same basic effect of positive reinforcement when they are presented conditionally.

3.6 The GIS revisited

We now have the main distinctions that will allow the goal inhibition system (GIS), introduced in the previous two chapters, to provide the core of our theory.

Originally, Gray (1975) proposed a behavioural inhibition system that mediated certain responses to secondary punishing and secondary frustrative stimuli (CS-LOSS+, CS-GAIN—; Table 3.1). He attributed the similar responses elicited by these two classes of stimuli (Wagner, 1966; Wagner, 1969; see also the aforementioned) to their acting on the same central system. This system—the GIS—governs approach to, coupled with passive avoidance of, stimuli that warn of danger, either innately (e.g. cat odour) or as a result of the conditioning process that gives rise to CS-LOSS+ or CS-GAIN—. Gray also held that primary punishing and primary frustrative stimuli (LOSS+, GAIN—) act on the same system as each other, the fight–flight system (Gray, 1971; Gray, 1975; extended to fight–flight freeze system by Gray and McNaughton, 2000), which we located in the lower levels of the Goal Repulsion System (GRS; §2.5).

The GRS, as we have seen, is quite distinct from, and to some extent has opposite properties to, the GIS. These two systems have in common, however, the property that neither is activated by primary GAIN stimuli (each subclass of which acts on its own specific appetitive system) or by secondary GAIN stimuli and safety signals (CS-GAIN+; CS-LOSS—), which all act on the separate GAS, which has been linked to approach (Gray, 1972; Gray et al., 1991) and behavioural activation (Fowles, 1980).

As noted already, the distinction we have made here between LOSS+ and CS-LOSS+ can be mapped directly onto the one made in Chapter 2 between actual and potential threat. Here, we take this argument one step further to claim that the parallel between these two distinctions is not mere analogy, but reflects an identity. This is justified on both functional and ethological grounds.

From the functional point of view, a CS-LOSS+ is a potential threat stimulus, since it involves an explicit conflict between a goal that would normally elicit a prepotent approach response and stimuli that warn of LOSS should that goal be approached. (If there is no prepotent approach tendency then there will be no occasion when the LOSS+ contingency can be demonstrated.) This is true despite the fact that the animal depends on conditioning rather than evolution for both the nature of the prepotent response and for the nature of the warning stimulus. From the ethological point of view, a CS-LOSS+ normally releases the same behaviour patterns as does an innate potential threat stimulus such as cat odour. To complete the terminology developed in the present chapter, we can therefore code such an innate potential threat stimulus as 'IS-LOSS+' (IS standing for 'innate stimulus').

It follows from this argument that the GIS should react to both conditioned aversive stimuli (CS-LOSS+, CS-GAIN—) and innate ones (IS-LOSS+, IS-GAIN—). For human beings, darkness could be one IS-LOSS+; in our phylogenetic past it often contained (and in many modern cityscapes still does) a plenitude of potential dangers. Whether there are any true IS-GAIN— is not clear. Care must in all cases be taken in the classification of innate stimuli, unless their functional status is very obvious. In a conditioning paradigm, we have experimental control over the functional status of any particular stimulus and so can usually determine whether it is LOSS+ or CS-LOSS+. In contrast, with innate stimuli, all we can determine from conditioning experiments is that they are aversive. It is clear enough, however, that a bite from a predator can be equated with LOSS+. A close approach from the predator (involving no pain but requiring avoidance) should probably, then, be treated as functionally equivalent to a CS-LOSS—, i.e. it is an 'innate fear stimulus' (Gray, 1971, Chapter 2; Gray, 1976), for example, snakes for primates (Hebb, 1946 see also §13.6). The odour of the predator (involving no pain, warning of danger, but often occurring in a context that requires approach) should in many cases, therefore, be equated with CS-LOSS+. But careful functional analysis (as in the Blanchards' work on cat odour, discussed in Chapter 2) is required to be sure that any particular stimulus is an innate anxiety stimulus (IS-LOSS+) rather than an innate punishing stimulus (LOSS+). To repeat: the key issue in all cases will not be simply whether the stimulus signals actual or potential danger but rather the extent to which other aspects of the situation require approach or avoidance.

In addition to innate signals of potential threat such as cat odour, which will retain their warning value even after many presentations, the same functional considerations lead to the view that the GIS should react to at least certain forms of novelty. On first encounter, stimuli such as unexplored environments should be treated as sources of potential danger and should be dealt with in the same manner as a CS-LOSS+, CS-GAIN—, or IS-LOSS+. There are two critical distinctions between such novel stimuli and true innate anxiety stimuli. The first is that after a period of habituation they become neutral stimuli. Thus the phenomena described by Sokolov (1963) as the 'orienting reflex' and by Pavlov (1927) under the rubric of 'external inhibition' should be closely related to the activities of the GIS. The second is that novelty has the approach and avoidance components of conflict both instantiated in the same stimulus. A novel object or environment should be treated, not only as a potential source of LOSS, but simultaneously as a potential source of GAIN. Unlike other aversive stimuli, therefore, it does not require any concurrent appetitive stimulus to generate the required conflict.

At this point in the development of the model, then, we view the GIS as being activated in any approach-avoidance conflict; we equate anxiety with activity in the GIS; and we view anxiolytic drugs as having a selective effect on the GIS. In Chapter 10, the full theory will slightly expand on the specification of adequate inputs to the GIS. In the interim, until we have considered the pharmacology and neurology of anxiety, we can take anxiety-provoking stimuli to be: CS-LOSS+ ('conditioned fear stimuli'), CS-GAIN— ('conditioned frustrative stimuli'), IS-LOSS+ such as cat odour ('innate anxiety stimuli'), and some but not necessarily all novel stimuli. With all of these stimuli, their definition implies that they activate the GIS, not because they are aversive as such, but because the animal has some additional tendency to approach rather than simply avoid them. *Given an innate or learned requirement to approach the source of potential danger*, the animal would normally be advised to inhibit non-defensive behaviours (including the prepotent approach response) as well as the GRS/FFFS (provided this is not extremely highly activated). Then, while maintaining this behavioural inhibition, it should actively assess the degree of threat while at all times actively scanning/assessing its environment. All of these responses also imply increased arousal and attention in the sense of heightened readiness to convert cautious approach (requiring activity in the GIS) to avoidance (mediated by the GRS/FFFS) as fast as possible should conditions require this (see Kim and Anderson, 2020 for evidence that threat-induced activation of gain representations is linked to blocking of attention to them).

This analysis suggests the system of Fig. 3.2. There are a number of key points to be borne in mind when interpreting this figure.

First, while we have included CS-LOSS+ within the class of anxiety-provoking stimuli, we have explicitly excluded LOSS+. For some, it is CS-LOSS+ that elicits 'fear' and we have

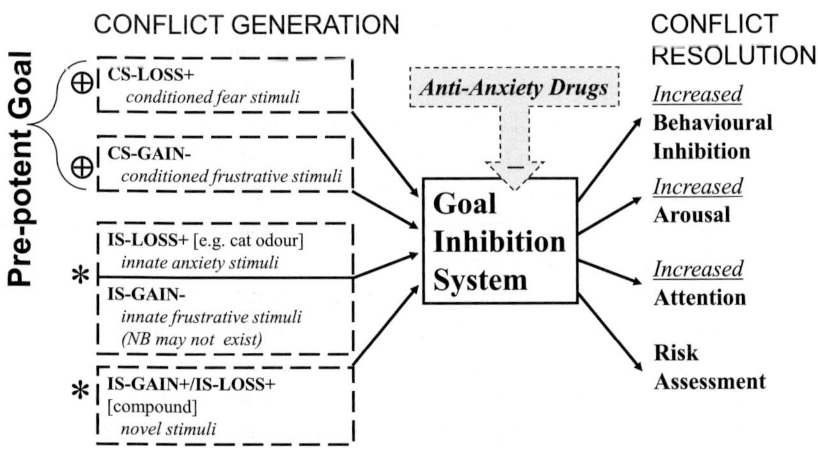

Fig. 3.2 The Goal Inhibition System (GIS)—expanded. Re-specification of the inputs of Fig. 1.2 in terms of the learning theoretic analysis of the current chapter.

explicitly recognized this by referring to these stimuli as 'conditioned fear stimuli' in Fig. 3.2. However, for others such as the Blanchards (Chapter 2), fear is a state elicited by LOSS+. We can acknowledge this usage by referring to these stimuli as 'unconditioned fear stimuli'. As just noted, however, conditioned and unconditioned fear stimuli usually have quite different eliciting properties, resulting in behavioural inhibition and escape respectively; and, as we shall see later, they have quite different pharmacologies. It follows that conditioned and unconditioned fear are often significantly different emotions, and it may therefore seem problematic to label them both 'fear'. We shall attempt to avoid using the term as far as possible (replacing it with, e.g. activity in the GRS or GIS as appropriate); and, when we are forced to use it, we shall preface it with 'conditioned' or 'unconditioned'. However, conceptually and at the level of neural analysis, there is no real problem. By our current definition, anxiety involves an approach-avoidance conflict. This necessarily implies that fear systems could be activated; but pure fear can be contrasted with anxiety because, in the latter case, the tendency to avoid (based on fear) is combined with a tendency to approach. As we shall see, this leads naturally to the idea of levels of control of the defence system; anxiety then reflects activity in a higher order system that modulates the output of a more fundamental pure fear system.

Second, while we have included CS-LOSS+ (i.e. stimuli that generate an approach-avoidance conflict) within the class of anxiety-provoking stimuli, we have explicitly excluded CS-LOSS— (i.e. safety signals). A stimulus that predicts that a particular response will escape or avoid an aversive stimulus would be presumed to activate the GAS and therefore to generate conditioned relief. However, precisely the same stimulus can, and often will, predict that some other (usually many other) responses will produce, or fail to avoid, the aversive stimulus. In many situations, therefore, particularly during the initial phases of active avoidance conditioning, conditioned fear (elicited by CSs paired with the primary aversive UCS) is likely to participate in the processes leading to both anxiety (engendered by CS-LOSS+) and relief (dependent on CS-LOSS—). That is, both the GIS and the GAS will be activated concurrently, with some patterns of behaviour being produced by the one system and some by the other.

Third, at the stimulus level, we have mapped a distinction derived from learning theory (the difference between, on the one hand, LOSS+ and GAIN— and, on the other, CS-LOSS+ and CS-GAIN—) onto a distinction derived from ethology (the difference between actual and potential threat). However, the reverse mapping is not possible. The experimental difference between LOSS+ and CS-LOSS+ is simply one of conditioning. However, the ethological point of view contradicts the idea that anxiety can be defined uniquely in terms of this conditioning. In particular, the odour of a cat, as used in the experiments by the Blanchards discussed in the previous chapter, is an *innate anxiety* stimulus. Thus, the commonly perceived relationship between fear and innate stimuli, on the one hand, and anxiety and conditioned stimuli on the other (as emphasized by Gray, 1982), is an artefact of conventional laboratory methodology rather than a logical necessity.

Fourth, this same ethological analysis resolves an apparent problem with the categorization of stimuli provided by Gray (1982). There, anxiety-provoking stimuli were defined as the aggregation of: signals of punishment, signals of reward omission, novel stimuli and innate fear (the term then used) stimuli. In this set, if the definition of anxiety and the GIS *requires* the involvement of conditioning, both novel and innate fear stimuli constitute *ad hoc* additions to signals of LOSS and GAIN omission. However, given that we have already distinguished ethologically between threat avoidance (depending upon the GRS) and threat approach (producing conflict and hence risk analysis and behavioural inhibition, mediated by the GIS), there is no problem in identifying CS-LOSS+ and CS-GAIN— as anxiety-provoking stimuli and adding them to the novelty and innate anxiety stimuli already identified in the ethological analysis.

From an ethological point of view, CS-GAIN— is not so easy to classify, although such stimuli can be readily identified within the experimental tradition of learning theory. The strongest reasons for including them with the other anxiety eliciting stimuli lie in the similarity of their reinforcing and eliciting properties to those of CS-LOSS+. However, *post hoc* it can be suggested that, under normal ecological circumstances, LOSS of food can be just as life-threatening as predation, and that anticipated LOSS of food requires behavioural inhibition and risk analysis in the same way as potential predation.

Fifth, while the ethological analysis corrected some inappropriate inferences from the learning theory analysis, the latter in turn highlights an important point about the coactivation of anxiety and relief mechanisms in the ethological situation. In the situation studied by the Blanchards (Chapter 2), after prior experience of a cat, rats inhibit their exit from the burrow system and, when they exit, engage in scanning, this behaviour being motivated by anxiety. However, when the rat has entered the arena and then chooses to escape back into the burrow system, this is escape from the same source of fear, but now motivated by anticipatory relief or hope (i.e. by the response to the equivalent of a CS-LOSS—, namely, the burrow). Thus (as we have already argued for the case of avoidance conditioning), in the arena responses will be activated (or primed) that are appropriate to both an actual and a potential predator, and the animal can rapidly switch between these repertoires by releasing one or the other system (see McNaughton, 1989b, Chapter 2).

Sixth, not all *stimuli* that technically fit the specific labels of Fig. 3.2 will always be anxiety-provoking. A novel stimulus that the animal has no innate basis for perceiving as potentially threatening (e.g. a smell of roses) will be different from one for which there may be such a basis (e.g. a loud noise). Similarly, what is formally a CS-LOSS+ from the experimenter's point of view will be anxiety-provoking only if the rat truly anticipates LOSS, as would be the case in a conditioned suppression paradigm where the shock is unavoidable, for example. However, in a *well-learned* avoidance task, habitual suppression of responding in the presence of the CS means that the shock is seldom or never obtained. In this case the CS should no longer produce anxiety.

Seventh, not all individuals will respond in the same way. Sex, daring, intelligence, and cognitive complexity all affect caution in humans in a risky foraging task with a virtual predator with, in this particular case, greater risk-taking being linked to higher success in obtaining gains (Bach et al., 2020). We will have much more to say about the role of personality in Chapters 12 and 13.

Eighth, while we have covered considerable complexity in the effects of reinforcers on observed behaviour, it remains the case that positive reinforcers, when used in conditioning paradigms, activate a common positive *reinforcement* system to change *future* behaviour, however different the behaviours they may currently elicit.

As was the case with the ethological distinctions made in Chapter 2, experiments with anxiolytic drugs (McNaughton, 1985a) support the distinction just made in relation to conditioning paradigms. Anxiolytic drugs given before every training session impair the *acquisition* of both successive negative discrimination (a paradigm in which behavioural inhibition to a CS-LOSS+ results in shock avoidance) and conditioned suppression (which is similar except for the fact that shock cannot be avoided). However, if the drug is administered after suppression has been acquired and the dose is increased progressively rather than suddenly, then anxiolytics impair performance of conditioned suppression but not successive negative discrimination. This supports the inference that, provided a CS-LOSS+ warns that a shock is likely to occur, it will generate anxiety; but that, once behavioural suppression is well developed and shocks no longer likely, then such a stimulus no longer generates anxiety. Similar conclusions have been drawn for changes in fear after prolonged training with CS-LOSS— (Kamin et al., 1963; see McNaughton, 1989b, p. 125). Indeed, it seems generally to be the case that, once a consistent pattern of active or passive responding to an aversive *or* appetitive reinforcer is established, not only do the eliciting properties of the CS disappear, but the response itself may become a simple habit unrelated to the value of the original reinforcer even if, as in the case of positive reinforcers, the reinforcer continues to be delivered (see McNaughton, 1989b, pp. 124–128). Interestingly, in such cases, goal-relatedness can be reinstated by unexpected reinforcer delivery of a range of different types (Trask et al., 2020; Bouton et al., 2020).

3.7 Conclusions

We believe that Blanchard and Blanchard (1990d) are right that functional analysis is required if we are to understand the unity of the various different forms of behaviour labelled 'anxious'. However, the methodologies of the two-process theorists, with which the Blanchards contrast their 'ethoexperimental' methodology, provide an independent basis for categorizing and, in particular, generalizing. While ethology may tend to overcategorize, learning theory tends to overgeneralize. The combination of the two provides a better balanced and potentially deeper perspective. We apply this perspective to the symptoms and syndromes of anxiety and anxiety-related disorders in Chapter 13.

Whether we consider the learning theory analysis of the present chapter or the ethological analysis of the previous one, the anxiety we have defined has proved specifically sensitive to anxiolytic drugs. Indeed, in a number of cases, we have seen that the effects, or lack of effects, of anxiolytic drugs in specific tests have clarified psychological analysis. In particular, we have found that variations in apparently trivial parametric aspects of experimental procedure (e.g. the extent of training) that do not change the superficial behavioural results, nonetheless often dramatically change the underlying psychological processes involved. In the chapters that follow then, we shall use the anxiolytic drugs as a probe, or marker, for activity in the GIS and hence for its neural location. Our immediate next step, therefore, will be to review the behavioural effects of these drugs. We will later relate this profile of behavioural effects to that of damage to specific parts of the defence systems of the brain.

4

The anxiolytic drugs—our key tool

4.1 What is an 'anxiolytic'?

4.1.1 'Anxiolytics' as a key integrative tool

In the more than half a century since the core of the GIS theory was proposed psychology and psychiatry have changed their use of words such as 'fear' and 'anxiety'. Even with this apparent evolution, there is still little agreement as to their meaning (§1.4; McNaughton, 2018) and, at the next level up, the complexities of 'emotion' (McNaughton, 1989b) mean that the age-old question 'What is an emotion?' (James, 1884) remains not only unanswered but seldom asked.

Although scientific semantics have changed, the effects of drugs and the systems on which they act have not. The barbiturate that killed Marilyn Monroe in 1962 is still the same chemical, would treat anxiety similarly now, and acts through the same fundamental $GABA_A$ system as do the less lethal benzodiazepines still used in clinical practice (§4.3.1). It is certain, then, that the behaviours affected by any specific 'anxiolytic' drug (however labelled) remained the same—as do the neural systems on which it acts.

We have already used anxiolytics and panicolytics to dissect classes of behaviour (Chapter 2, Chapter 3) and to link those classes to the clinical targets of the drugs. In later chapters we will use the drugs to identify key neural systems and validate a biomarker.

Here, we take a close look at the selective anxiolytic drugs (that are not also panicolytic). We will look at their actions, and at a means of separating their main anxiolytic effect from their extremely various other effects. We will call this method 'triangulation' in analogy to how surveyors both locate positions and assess the accuracy of that location. In relation to psychology and psychiatry, an important methodological point is that we will look across *batteries* of symptoms, or behavioural tests, and deduce from the *pattern* of positive, null, and negative drug-induced changes the functional nature of the main common effect of the drugs as a class.

In the process, we will find that the GIS inhibits goals (and so certain actions indirectly) but does not stop actions either directly or in general (generating, e.g. risk assessment behaviour). We will also find that goal inhibition has important effects in tasks that are often seen as testing spatial memory (see also Chapter 7).

The Neuropsychology of Anxiety, Third Edition. Neil McNaughton and Jeffrey A. Gray, Oxford University Press.
 DOI: 10.1093/oso/9780198843313.003.0004

4.1.2 'Anxiolytic' action in the laboratory

In Chapters 2 and 3 we used the selective actions of 'anxiolytic' drugs to validate distinct pre-defined 'fear' and 'anxiety' classes of behaviour. The classes were based on either (a) ethoexperimental or (b) learning theoretic analysis. That any *pharmacologically* defined type of drug consistently affects all items within only one class strongly supports the class definition. The parallel drug effects also strongly link the separately derived and superficially distinct ethological and learning-theory constructs of 'fear' and 'anxiety'.

In principle, class-specific action of any type of drug would be a cross-check on our behaviour-based categories. However, importantly, we argued that the drugs were reducing the construct of anxiety itself rather than always reducing specific anxiety-related behaviours. (For example, an anxiolytic can increase rearing if a rat is so anxious that it is freezing; or decrease rearing if mild anxiety is eliminated allowing the return of non-defensive behaviour; see also §4.6.4). So, the quite independent definition of anxiety-related behaviour by ethology and learning theory means that each, in return, provides evidence that the clinical labelling of the drugs as 'anxiolytic' is correct. This three-way interlocking pharmacological consensus (see also §1.5 and 1.6) provides our unique, bootstrapped, answer to the question 'What is "anxiety"?' (§1.4).

Here, we take it as a matter of definition that anxiolytic drugs do in fact reduce anxiety as opposed to fear in the clinic. But we must emphasize that what we term 'anxiolytic action' is only that *subset* of effects that are *common to all* classes of clinically effective anxiolytics. $GABA_A$ anxiolytics are also muscle relaxant, anticonvulsant, euphoriant, and addictive. $5HT_{1A}$ anxiolytics, if anything, increase tension and convulsion and can be unpleasant enough that the clinician may need skill to make their patient willing to keep taking the drug.

For this reason, also, we will generally distinguish panicolytic drugs from anxiolytic despite their also having anxiolytic action. This is important since, with current definitions, what we call anxiolytic drugs are not effective in some of what DSM or ICD would call 'anxiety disorders' but that we would classify as 'fear disorders' (see §4.1.2); whereas panicolytics do affect the latter (and usually depression as well). The *common* actions of the specifically anxiolytic drugs thus tag the psychological processes that contribute specifically to anxiety (as opposed to the fear on which panicolytics would act). Similarly, a common action across different classes of anxiolytic drug will identify the specific neural systems that underly anxiety-related processes.

4.1.3 What does a psychiatrist mean by 'anxiolytic'?

It is important for our approach that anxiolytics not only can treat anxiety but also do so specifically. Concurrent actions on joy, anger, and the sex drive would confound any deduction about anxiety. Similarly, if the benzodiazepines, for example, were as effective in controlling schizophrenic thought disorder as anxiety, they would be much more useful to the clinician but of little value as scientific tools. Fortunately for us, the relative specificity of anxiolytic drugs as a class is clear. They are of little use in schizophrenia. Nor are they effective in the control of anger or aggression; indeed, they can facilitate aggression (Lynch et al., 1975). But we need some caution when distinguishing the specifically anxiolytic drugs from other drugs with anxiolytic action that would be classified as panicolytic or antidepressant rather than anxiolytic.

In the ideal case, an anxiolytic drug should act to reduce anxiety as defined by, e.g. DSM-5 (American Psychiatric Association, 2013), while affecting no other psychological state or syndrome. As we shall see, pooling all classes that have some anxiolytic action together we can treat this as being essentially the case, but this pooling extends beyond what psychiatrists specifically term 'anxiolytics'. One complication is drugs, particularly panicolytic antidepressants, that not only have anxiolytic action but also reduce panic and/or obsession and/or depression. A second complication is the regular need to update psychiatric diagnostic criteria, with DSM already having undergone five major revisions of the original (as well as interim more minor revisions)—so what DSM calls 'anxiety disorder' has changed while the drugs have not.

We argued in Chapter 1 (and will again in more detail in Chapter 10 and 13) that panic and obsession proper are neurally quite distinct from the anxiety that can accompany them; and DSM-5 (unlike previous DSM editions) does not include obsession or depression with anxiety disorders. Conversely, DSM-5 sees simple phobia as anxiety whereas we see it as fear (and so like simple avoidance in animal experiments, not sensitive to anxiolytics). The ethology of Chapter 2 sees fear of a spider or snake as quite distinct from anxiety (§13.6; Fig. 13.10), which is consistent with the failure of anxiolytic drugs to prevent a patient's *avoidance* of a phobic object such as a snake (see Sartory et al., 1990, p. 273, for a brief review). Further, simple phobia does not activate the areas of the brain that we shall associate with anxiety, nor are changes in the pattern of brain activity produced by a phobic stimulus altered by anxiolytic drugs (Fredrikson et al., 1995). Conversely, we would agree with the more recent term 'social anxiety' rather than the older 'social phobia'.

Given these caveats, we shall discuss anxiolytic drugs on the working assumptions that they all treat anxiety (as opposed to phobia, panic, obsession, etc.), and do so equally well (or poorly given the high levels of treatment resistance) if there is proper adjustment of dose. While this is consistent with the normal classification of certain drugs as anxiolytic, the set of target disorders is more restricted than the set of DSM anxiety disorders or ICD-10 neurotic, stress-related and somatoform disorders (World Health Organization, 1992; World Health Organization, 2021). A specific action on anxiety also allows validation of biomarkers that could provide a basis for quite novel biologically based diagnoses that cut across the current symptom-based schemes. We discuss one such possible biomarker in later chapters.

4.1.4 Using anxiolytics to re-define 'anxiety'

How can we draw a line between primary defence systems and systems mainly involved in anxiety? Our principal tool will be a careful comparison (Appendix 1; §4.6.2; Table 4.2) of the profile of behavioural effects of the anxiolytic drugs with those of specific lesions of potentially relevant structures.

Drugs may seem a tricky a tool for the dissection of specific psychological processes: any drug has a wide range of disparate effects. Is the specific behavioural action of a drug due to its main effect, in which we are interested, or to some side effect or additional un-interesting main effect? In answering this question, we are now on a much sounder footing than previously. The theory was founded on classical anxiolytics (initially sodium amylobarbitone), which shared common side effects of muscle relaxation, addiction, anticonvulsant action, etc. The second edition could add 'novel' monoaminergic anxiolytic drugs, with none of these particular side effects; allowing us to compare the behavioural effects of the two classes. We now have available a third specific anxiolytic class operating via calcium channels (e.g. pregabalin); and a fourth entirely novel neurotic-disorder-general class: dissociative drugs the primary action of which is unknown (§14.4; Table 14.1), exemplified by ketamine.

Where the effects of these classes overlap, we can be almost certain that the effects reflect their anxiolytic action. Where they differ, we can ignore the separate effects as being unrelated to anxiety—but to keep analysis simple we will focus most on drugs that are anxiolytic but not panicolytic (i.e. the drugs clinically labelled as anxiolytics not the ones clinically labelled as panicolytics or antidepressants). In its most basic form, this strategy assumes that when drugs that are not also panicolytic have an anxiolytic action this will be similar to the effect of a lesion of those neural structures most involved in anxiety. But before proceeding we must survey the drugs concerned and their clinical and behavioural effects.

There has long been a vast literature on anxiolytic drugs (see Nutt, 1996 for a review of earlier data on human subjects) with recent meta-analysis (Slee et al., 2019) providing clear evidence of efficacy in generalized anxiety disorder of drugs that reduce panic and depression (e.g. sertraline, fluoxetine, ketamine), depression but not panic (buspirone), and neither panic nor depression (but are anticonvulsant and with abuse potential, e.g. pregabalin, low dose benzodiazepines).

We will gain maximum scientific specificity by taking a surveyor's triangulation approach. Each chemical class of anxiolytic has its own non-specificities, described in detail next. But, as a larger therapeutic class taken together, the selective anxiolytic drugs can be treated as specific to anxiety. Here we summarize conclusions originally justified in detail in Appendix 1 and in its secondary sources, particularly Gray (1977) for the classical anxiolytics, and Griebel (1995) and Handley (1995) for compounds acting selectively at the 5-hydroxytryptamine (5HT) 1A receptor and for imipramine. We update these where necessary with more novel serotonergic compounds and with discussion of ketamine, the most recent and effective current anxiolytic known to act on the SHS in the same fashion as specific anxiolytics. We include compounds validated with human patients and exclude those that have only been tested in animal models, some of which are of dubious validity (McNaughton and Zangrossi, 2008; Luyten et al., 2011).

We first look briefly at the clinical use of drugs that treat anxiety in human beings to define our target 'anxiolytic' compounds, and then consider their effects in animals. Critically, we first use the clinical data to provide an ostensive definition of anxiolytic drugs, then use the animal data to discover the psychopharmacology, and in later chapters the neuropharmacology, common to these drugs, treated as a single functional class. A key assumption of this cross-species approach (justified in more detail in §1.5) is that the drugs concerned act on fundamental, ancient, systems that have been highly conserved in evolution (McNaughton, 2020), allowing fish to provide neurobehavioral models of a range of human psychiatric disorders (Soares et al., 2018) and neurodevelopmental disorders (de Abreu et al., 2020). Given this essentially neurohormonal approach, we have excluded non-drug treatments such as non-invasive brain stimulation (Vicario et al., 2019) and ECT.

4.2 Clinical anxiolytic usage

It has been said that all drugs go through an essentially similar clinical life cycle. On intro duction to medical practice, they are hailed as wonder drugs, able to cure 100% of cases of the target disorder (as well as, sometimes, everything else). Next, it is reported that they are totally without effect on the original target disorder and, far from curing other disorders, produce a range of life-threatening side effects. Finally, it becomes accepted that in a subset of cases of the target disorder the drug can be helpful, at least in controlling symptoms, but doses must be controlled with care and precautions taken.

The drugs generally classified as anxiolytic have followed this pattern, inasmuch as the classical anxiolytics have fallen out of favour because of their side effects. But it is interesting to note that they have not been replaced by drugs with any greater or more general therapeutic main effect; indeed, somewhat the reverse appears to be the case for the novel anxiolytics. As a result, pharmaceutical companies have been driven to produce many chemically unrelated compounds, all of which share the same essential main effects. In this respect ketamine (as other, similarly effective, dissociative/psychedelic drugs) appears to be genuinely novel—likely because it was not developed as an anxiolytic and, even now, is used off-label.

4.2.1 Drugs generally used in the clinic

There have been six major drug types of interest in the clinical treatment of anxiety in general and generalized anxiety disorder in particular. First, the oldest anti-anxiety drug of all is alcohol. Clinically this is unattractive because of its depressant, toxic, addictive, and intoxicant effects. Second, came the barbiturate family. These were the earliest drugs used regularly for the specific treatment of anxiety. Third, for a brief period came 'Miltown' (meprobamate, a carbamate that binds to a barbiturate site). However, each of these successors had, albeit to a lesser extent, the same problems as alcohol—and none is used now. Fourth, sweeping the other classical anxiolytics into the dustbin of history, came the benzodiazepines: with much less pronounced sedative effects; a wide margin of safety between the clinically effective dose and the dose at which you can kill yourself; and, it was wrongly thought, little potential for producing dependence and withdrawal symptoms. Fifth, about 30 years ago, the benzodiazepines themselves were challenged by novel classes of compound such as the azapirodecanediones, buspirone, and ipsapirone; and by novel uses of older drugs, particularly the tricyclic antidepressant, imipramine. Sixth, developed from the tricyclics and now the first line drugs for anxiety treatment, are the more specific serotonergic and noradrenergic reuptake inhibitors (such as fluoxetine/Prozac and venlafaxine/Effexor).

For as long as different classes of drug have been available there has been debate as to which is best for the treatment of anxiety in general (see e.g. Goldberg, 1990; Marks, 1990; and their accompanying commentaries on each other). The most important differences are side-effect variations that affect tolerability between drugs and of the same drug between individuals. Surprisingly, the benzodiazepines are still grossly overprescribed as their addictive properties keep the drug companies, patients, and many physicians happy. While very brief use of benzodiazepines for acute sleep problems may be indicated,

> anxiety disorders should be treated with psychological therapy, pharmacotherapy, or a combination of both. Cognitive behavioral therapy can be regarded as the psychotherapy with the highest level of evidence. First-line drugs are the selective serotonin reuptake inhibitors and serotonin-norepinephrine reuptake inhibitors. Benzodiazepines are not recommended for routine use. Other treatment options include pregabalin, tricyclic antidepressants, buspirone, moclobemide, and others.
>
> (Bandelow et al., 2017, p. 93; see also Slee et al., 2019; added emphasis)

The second generation of apparently more specifically anxiolytic benzodiazepines are partial agonists (this seems more important than the type of benzodiazepine receptor to which they bind) that retain the anxiolytic effect of benzodiazepine receptor activation, but essentially act as their own antagonists with respect to the sedative and addictive effects (Facklam et al., 1992; Doble and Martin, 1992; Haefely, 1990c; Haefely, 1991; Sanger et al., 1994). At higher doses they are antidepressant and panicolytic; but this also seems to be true of older benzodiazepines if given at high enough dose (Noyes et al., 1996; van Marwijk et al., 2012)—so the new benzodiazepines are not that different from the old (see §4.3).

Similarly, the $5HT_{1A}$ agonist ipsapirone is like buspirone in being effective in treating generalized anxiety disorder while lacking the effect of buspirone on dopaminergic systems (Cutler et al., 1993). Interestingly, it is buspirone rather than ipsapirone that continues to be increasingly used clinically, rising to 10 million prescriptions in the USA in 2017 (Kane, 2020). SSRIs are, as noted earlier, the first-line drugs for anxiolytic treatment clinically. However, their broad (panic, depression, obsession) spectrum of action reduces their usefulness for our academic triangulation, especially since like buspirone their specific anxiolytic and antidepressant actions appear to be $5HT_{1A}$ mediated (Vahid-Ansari et al., 2017). So, in relation to anxiety, there is good reason to group buspirone, imipramine, and specific serotonin reuptake inhibitors (SSRIs) like fluoxetine together in terms of their agonist actions on $5HT_{1A}$ receptor systems and to use the most psychologically specific, buspirone, as the paradigm case.

Newer variants on either the benzodiazepine or the $5HT_{1A}$ theme, represent an attempt to retain the main effect of the parent compound while eliminating unpleasant side effects. Since the more recent, and apparently more specific, drugs all appear to share the key actions common to the older classical (e.g. benzodiazepines) and novel (e.g. buspirone) anxiolytics, we have largely excluded them from the academic focus of our discussion later.

One new drug of note is pregabalin. This has actions somewhat like classical anxiolytics but acts presynaptically on voltage-dependent calcium channels (Field et al., 2001) to reduce transmitter release, rather than on the $GABA_A$ receptor to increase inhibition (see §4.3.1). It is anticonvulsant, sedative, and has at least some abuse potential (Baldwin et al., 2013) and has a clear effect on social anxiety disorder (Pande et al., 2004). Its tolerability makes it clinically attractive and its quite distinct mechanism of action, bypassing $GABA_A$ makes it particularly useful for our triangulation exercise as it has no effect on panic or depression.

4.2.2 Ketamine, the new kid not quite on the block

As we have noted, conventional drugs are often ineffective and they can take weeks to have their full therapeutic effect. It has come as something of a shock, therefore, that ketamine (commonly used as a dissociative anaesthetic) has been found to be effective, within hours

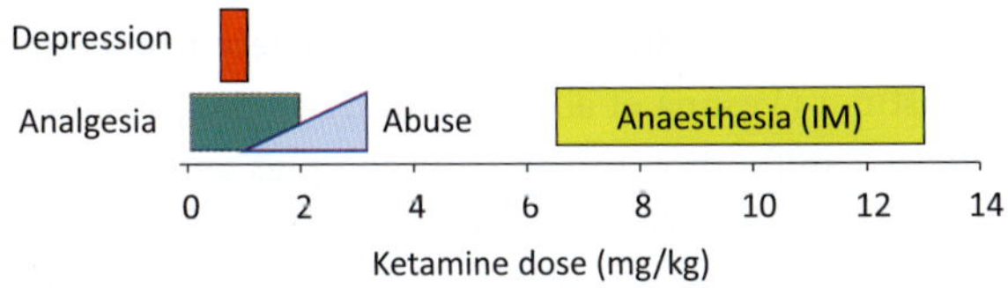

Fig. 4.1 Dose-indication relationships for different uses of ketamine clinically. Redrawn with permission from Biological Psychiatry, 70 (4), Paul Glue, Abhishek Gulati, Martin Le Nedelec, and Stephen Duffull, Dose—and Exposure-Response to Ketamine in Depression, pp. e9-e10, Figure 1c, https://doi.org/10.1016/j.biopsych.2010.11.031, Copyright © 2011 Society of Biological Psychiatry. Published by Elsevier Inc. All rights reserved.

of a single dose, in cases of depression, anxiety, and related internalizing disorders that are resistant to psychological treatment, SSRIs, and related conventional drugs (Rodriguez et al., 2013; Zarate Jr et al., 2006; Feder et al., 2014b; Glue et al., 2017; Loo et al., 2016; Zhang and Hashimoto, 2018). This has already led to 'a paradigm shift for depression research and treatment' (Krystal et al., 2019) and at least proof-of-concept for anxiety (Glue et al., 2017; Banov et al., 2019; Glue et al., 2018; Glue et al., 2019; Glue et al., 2020). So, ketamine appears equally effective across the span of mood and neurotic, stress-related, and somatoform disorders as classified by ICD-10 (World Health Organization, 1992; World Health Organization, 2021) and across different classes of DSM-5 anxiety disorder.

But the neural effects of ketamine (Table 14.1) are complex (see also Vollenweider and Preller, 2020). At a very high dose (>6 mg/kg) it is anaesthetic (and is approved for paediatric use). At lower doses (1–3 mg/kg) it is used as a drug of abuse (and so is scheduled) and at somewhat lower doses still is used as pain relief. But its effects on neurotic disorders occur in a much lower and very narrow dose range (0.5–1.0 mg/kg, see Fig. 4.1; Glue et al., 2011). Notably, high versus low doses of ketamine can have opposite effects on both behaviour and protein expression (Wu et al., 2020). The shared fast response of neurotic disorders to ketamine suggests dysfunction of a single common neural system distinct from those acted on separately by the conventional drugs (McNaughton and Glue, 2020).

Ketamine arrived in the 1960s as an anaesthetic (see Domino, 2010). But, while it has a clear action at N-methyl-D-aspartate (NMDA) receptors 'clinical trials indicate that … alternative NMDAR antagonists lack the rapid, robust and/or long-lasting antidepressant actions of ketamine in humans' (Zanos and Gould, 2018, p. 804; see also Matveychuk et al., 2020). So, the therapeutic effect of ketamine might not involve NMDA antagonism at all. However, it appears that

> the mechanism of ketamine's antidepressant action involves the following cascade of sequential events. Ketamine has a greater affinity for NDMA receptors on γ-aminobutyric acid (GABA) interneurons, which are inhibitory neurons and act to suppress excitation of downstream glutamatergic neurons. As a result of NMDA receptor antagonism, ketamine prevents activation of GABA interneurons and causes downstream disinhibition of glutamatergic neurons and a consequential glutamate surge.
>
> (Matveychuk et al., 2020, p. 5)

As we noted at the start of this section, compounds touted as wonder drugs must be approached with caution. Ketamine is old enough for its problems to be known. It is scheduled because it is addictive. Its normal administration for anxiety results in dissociation that is likely to be neurally distinct (Vesuna et al., 2020) and has the potential for dangerous systemic effects that require careful monitoring. This complex administration needs to be repeated once a week. Its R-isomer may be more tolerable (Leal et al., 2021) but it and any similarly improved compounds will be very expensive and likely have undiscovered problems once they are in general use.

Current drug development includes a range of other compounds that may share some form of glutamate-related action including riluzole and xenon (Sartori and Singewald, 2019)—with glutamate and glutamine *levels* likely being a key factor for therapeutic action (Milak et al., 2020). We will discuss how this widespread action (both neurally and therapeutically) can fit with the quite different actions of our other drugs of interest when discuss the effects of drugs on the hippocampal theta rhythm. We will also discuss ketamine's relationship to them when we cover personality in Chapter 12 and its relationship to disorder in Chapter 13 and treatment in Chapter 14 (for a summary of the take-home message, see McNaughton and Glue, 2020). However, like the SSRIs, ketamine's very broad spectrum of action means that we will largely exclude it from our triangulation.

4.2.3 Various other exclusions

We shall briefly discuss next the use of anti-adrenergic drugs (e.g. those that that block β-adrenergic receptors, aka 'beta-blockers') in the control of anxiety; but we conclude that their action is primarily peripheral and so do not group them with the other anxiolytics in our search for the neuropsychology of anxiety.

There are indications that the neuropeptide cholecystokinin (CCK) may be panicogenic (Harro et al., 1993); that CCK antagonists may have anti-panic activity (see Crawley and Corwin, 1994); and that the effects of certain benzodiazepines may be through direct or indirect interaction with CCK receptors rather than through benzodiazepine receptors (Boden and Woodruff, 1994). But, while hope is still maintained for CCK-related compounds (Crespi, 2019) there are no data at present on successful clinical trials of CCK antagonists on either panic disorder or, more importantly for our present analysis, generalized anxiety.

There were indications that $5HT_2$ antagonists may be anxiolytic (e.g. Hensman et al., 1991; Katz et al., 1993). Their effects appear to be like those of buspirone. However, 2B receptors appear to be important for SSRI action and specific $5HT_2$ antagonists are still unavailable (Quesseveur et al., 2012). We have therefore excluded them from our triangulation exercise.

Other drugs with efficacy in anxiety disorders (Bandelow et al., 2017) but where there is insufficient data for our use include: moclobemide (a selective monoamine oxidase-A inhibitor); agomelatine (a melatonin agonist and $5HT_{2C}$ antagonist); and quetiapine (an atypical anti-psychotic).

4.3 The different pharmacologies of drugs used for anxiety disorders

This section discusses the pharmacology specific to each class of selective anxiolytic drug. The key point is that there is essentially no overlap among them in terms of their direct targets.

Those in search of an anxiolytic-specific pharmacology can ignore these details; while those interested in our triangulation method for assessing behaviour and neural action should see the details as strong evidence for its lack of confounds.

4.3.1 The classical anxiolytics and the $GABA_A$ receptor

Ethanol, barbiturates, meprobamate, and benzodiazepines can be grouped together as the classical anxiolytics, which we shall contrast as a group with the (relatively) novel anxiolytics. But first we must note some of the similarities and differences within the group of classical anxiolytics themselves. Chemically they are very different from each other and, rather than acting on a single binding site, simply share a final common pharmacological path—a chloride channel—so their similarities far outweigh their differences.

The benzodiazepines include a number of drugs in exceptionally wide past or present use: both older low-potency ones such as Librium (chlordiazepoxide) and Valium (diazepam); and more recent high-potency ones like Xanax (alprazolam). More than 60 million benzodiazepine tablets were prescribed annually in the United States alone in the 1970s (Tallman et al., 1980). This was

> the decade of peak usage, [but] alarm was expressed about the 'relentless march of the psychotropic drug juggernaut' and the benzodiazepines were stigmatized ... as 'the opium of the masses' ... In the [1980s], 'a dark shadow has been cast over the benzodiazepines by the spectre of dependence'.
>
> (Lader, 1990, p. 3)

So, even at the time of our second edition, it was generally agreed that benzodiazepines should be restricted to only short-term treatment and as an adjunct to other therapies (see Ashton, 1994). However, 20 years later, physicians remain as addicted to benzodiazepine use as their patients.

> Alprazolam is not only the most commonly prescribed benzodiazepine, but it is the most commonly prescribed psychotropic medication in the United States, accounting for more than 48 million prescriptions dispensed in 2013 [with] high misuse liability and ... a more severe withdrawal syndrome than other benzodiazepines, even when tapered according to manufacturer guidelines.
>
> (Ait-Daoud et al., 2018, p. 4)

The classical anxiolytics as a group all enhance the effects of the inhibitory neurotransmitter, GABA, but through quite different primary actions. Each type of classical anxiolytic alters the functioning of the $GABA_A$ receptor complex (Fig. 4.2A) through a quite different binding site (Fig. 4.2B). It should be noted that 'the' $GABA_A$ receptor has five subunits (usually two α, two β, and one of γ, δ, ε, π, ρ) with 19 possibilities (α1-6, β1-3, γ1-3, δ, ε, π, ρ1-3). Since binding sites can involve more than one subunit and different $GABA_A$ variants occur on different neurons, these 'provide the opportunity for possible subtype-selective pharmacological ligand specificity and clinical therapeutics with minimal side effects' (Olsen, 2018, p 11), including with neurosteroids (Hosie et al., 2006). There has been detailed analysis of $GABA_A$

function via mice with mutated subunits (Rudolph and Mohler, 2004). As a result, there is continued pharmaceutical development but, so far, with no truly anxiolysis-specific $GABA_A$ candidate. In what follows we will provide a simplified view of binding sites (Fig. 4.2B) that nonetheless provides a model for understanding the actions of all the relevant ligands sufficient for our triangulation approach.

GABA itself binds to a site that opens the channel as do, each with their own sites: the barbiturates with actions linked to the picrotoxin receptor (Olsen et al., 1978a; Olsen et al., 1978b; Ticku and Olsen, 1978; Braestrup and Nielsen, 1980; Olsen, 2018); and ethanol (Suzdak et al., 1986; see also Coop et al., 1990). Ethanol also binds to receptors for the excitatory amino acid transmitter, NMDA but this does not appear to contribute to its anxiolytic effects (Criswell et al., 1994).

In contrast, the benzodiazepines do not affect the chloride channel directly. They bind to a site linked to the GABA site, with anxiolytic benzodiazepines increasing the affinity of the latter for GABA (Fig. 4.2B; Guidotti et al., 1978; for early detailed reviews see Haefely, 1990c; Haefely, 1990a; Haefely, 1990b; Haefely et al., 1990; Richards et al., 1991). The low toxicity of the benzodiazepines, relative to the other classical anxiolytics, appears to be due to their modulation of GABA action only when it is released endogenously; unlike the direct effects on the chloride channel of other classical anxiolytics (Fig. 4.2B). But note that some $GABA_A$ receptors react to GABA in the extracellular space rather than in the synapse and can generate a 'tonic' inhibition (Glykys and Mody, 2007).

Benzodiazepine modulation of the GABA site generates a pharmacological peculiarity. While benzodiazepine agonists increase the affinity of the GABA receptor and so enhance GABA action, benzodiazepine antagonists such as flumazenil block only endogenous or exogenous benzodiazepine receptor ligands and do not block GABA. In most behavioural tests, the antagonists have little or no effect until a benzodiazepine is administered and have little clinical action (Haefely et al., 1992) except on performance-induced anxiety, possibly by antagonizing the effects of an endogenously released (anxiogenic) benzodiazepine receptor ligand (Kapczinski et al., 1994). However, some benzodiazepines are 'inverse agonists' that reduce the affinity of the GABA receptor and so decrease the effects of GABA, with effects opposite to the anxiolytic benzodiazepines.

Two additional points should be noted about benzodiazepines. First is that the classification of a compound as agonist, antagonist or inverse agonist depends to some degree on the behavioural test used (File and Cooper, 1985). This is consistent with the more selective effects on anxiety of partial agonists. These are presumed to act as full agonists in some parts of the nervous system and as antagonists or even inverse agonists in other parts. The second point is that there is now considerable evidence for endogenous benzodiazepines, which may be the natural ligands of the receptors (Medina et al., 1993). In this context, it should be noted that neurosteroids also potentiate GABA responses at $GABA_A$ receptors and their dysregulation has been linked to a range of mental disorders (Hosie et al., 2006; Gravielle, 2018). We will not discuss neurosteroids further but, at the moment, have no reason to see their actions and varying specificities as any different from endogenous benzodiazepines.

If classical anxiolytics (and some neurosteroids) share a final common path of direct or indirect $GABA_A$ agonist action, this suggests that the necessary common denominator of anxiolytic action is enhanced GABAergic transmission. But, this 'GABA' hypothesis of anxiolytic action has long been known to have problems. GABA receptors, *per se*, are far too widely distributed in the brain. Even if we convert the 'GABA' hypothesis to an 'endogenous

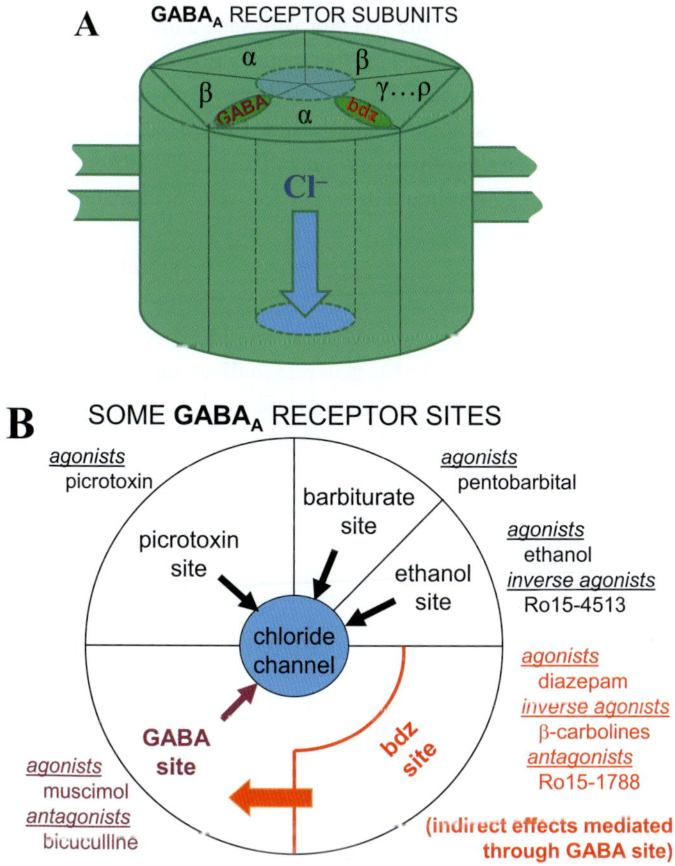

Fig. 4.2 The GABA$_A$ receptor. **A.** A set of 5 transmembrane subunits forms a ligand-gated chloride ion channel. There are usually two α and two β sub-units, with the 5th subunit being from γ, δ, ε, π, or ρ family, allowing 19 variants altogether (see text). There are binding sites, often between the subunits, that can cause conformational changes, e.g., GABA and benzodiazepine (bdz). Binding of GABA to its site (purple) causes the channel to open (blue shading) and chloride (Cl-) to pass through and so hyperpolarize the cell (Haefely, 1990c). **B.** There are distinct sites (Teicher, 1988; see also Gravielle, 2018) that bind picrotoxin, barbiturates and ethanol—all of which can affect the chloride channel directly without the need for endogenous GABA (for elaboration see Olsen, 2018; Rudolph and Mohler, 2004). The benzodiazepine (bdz) site by contrast alters the GABA site rather than the channel itself. It can thus increase (agonists) or decrease (inverse agonists) the effects of GABA. Benzodiazepines, therefore, only have effects if GABA is released and benzodiazepine antagonists are not GABA antagonists. Adapted from Medical Clinics of North America, 72 (4), Martin H. Teicher, Biology of Anxiety, p. 793, Figure 1, https://doi.org/10.1016/S0025-7125(16)30745-3 Copyright © 1988 Elsevier Inc. All rights reserved.

benzodiazepine' one, benzodiazepine sites are rich in many regions of the central nervous system that are unlikely to play a role in anxiety (e.g. the cerebellum and spinal cord, Braestrup and Squires, 1977; Williamson et al., 1978; Möhler and Okada, 1977; Robertson et al., 1978; Young and Kuhar, 1980). Furthermore, drugs that enhance GABAergic transmission do not generally appear to be anxiolytic (Sanger, 1985). Indeed,

> it is surprising that a neurotransmitter receptor with such a ubiquitous distribution as the $GABA_A$ receptor can serve as the target for therapeutically useful anxiolytic drugs with excellent tolerability. The explanation is that the mechanism of allosteric modulation by the benzodiazepine receptor does not profoundly alter the spatial and temporal pattern of GABAergic synaptic activity. Furthermore, potentiation of GABAergic transmission by benzodiazepine receptor ligands should be most effective in neuronal networks engaged in pathological overactivity.
>
> (Haefely, 1992, pp. 165–166)

Given the widespread inhibitory role of GABA, we would expect drugs that facilitate its action to act not as specific anxiolytics but as general sedatives and anticonvulsants (Meldrum, 1975). This is, indeed, the case for the benzodiazepines, barbiturates, and ethanol (Simon and Soubrié, 1979; Schallek et al., 1972; Randall and Kappell, 1973; Browne and Perry, 1973; Olsen, 2018; Nutt and Lister, 1987). So is classical anxiolytic action secondary to sedative, muscle relaxant, and anticonvulsant properties? We will argue that this may be true of the drugs' immediate but not their long-term effects.

4.3.2 Buspirone and the $5HT_{1A}$ receptor

The treatment of anxiety with buspirone started only after our first edition and revolutionized GABA-centric views of anxiolytic action. For our second edition, it provided the basis for our triangulation approach, which then greatly strengthened our understanding of the neural mechanisms underlying anxiolytic action. It provided predictive confirmation of the role of the SHS. Survival of similar challenges from other more recent drugs is described later. The original theory can be viewed as having, since 1982, predicted all the relevant neural and behavioural effects of the full chemical range of anxiolytics without prior knowledge of any anxiolytic drug that did not have a classical (Fig. 4.2) mode of action.

Except for its anxiolytic effects (Goldberg and Finnerty, 1979), buspirone is so unlike the classical anxiolytics that it was touted as 'anxio-selective' (e.g. Goldberg, 1990). This overstatement ignored a variety of side effects. Unwanted ones include: dizziness; nervousness; headache; nausea; insomnia; somnolence; and a range of less common symptoms (Schwob et al., 1989). Some of these unwanted effects may result from an increase in corticosterone levels (Urban et al., 1986; see also §4.6.2). A wanted side effect, unlike the majority of benzodiazepines at anxiolytic doses, is an antidepressant action.

Buspirone is notable in not having an anti-panic or anti-obsession action (see Deakin, 1993; Ravindran and Stein, 2010). This differs from reuptake blockers, despite their common action on generalized anxiety and unipolar depression and their common interaction with $5HT1_A$ systems. This lack of additional effects may be why buspirone has a lower efficacy compared to other anxiolytics on anxiety scale scores on meta-analysis (Bandelow et al., 2017). In head-to-head trials with GAD it appears equivalent to a benzodiazepine but suffers from limited efficacy in other anxiety and mood disorders that are often comorbid with GAD (Ravindran and Stein, 2010). Critically for our triangulation strategy, it (like other $5HT_{1A}$ agonists we will discuss next) does not share with classical anxiolytics their sedative, hypnotic, euphoriant, anticonvulsant, muscle relaxant, or addictive properties. Paradoxically, then, the various lacks of action that make buspirone a second-line choice for the clinician make it particularly useful for our academic purposes.

Inconveniently (like other $5HT_{1A}$ agonists), buspirone must be taken for at least 10 days to achieve a therapeutic effect (Feighner, 1987; see also §4.6.2). But, with clinical measures such as the Hamilton Anxiety Scale, there appears to be 'no overall significant difference between buspirone and the benzodiazepines in treating patients with anxiety symptoms, with a maximum effect for both medications between the 2nd and 4th week of study' (Schuckit, 1984, p.64).

Buspirone is thought to owe its clinical efficacy to being a partial agonist at the $5HT_{1A}$ receptor (Ravindran and Stein, 2010), with which the classical anxiolytics do not interact. Its antidepressant action is likely to be the result of a consequential down-regulation of $5HT_2$ receptors (Robinson, 1993). It also interacts with dopamine D_2 receptors and indirectly affects noradrenergic systems (Jann, 1988), something we return to later in the book. The fact that ipsapirone appears equally anxiolytic (see Glaser, 1994) is consistent with the hypothesis that it is the $5HT_{1A}$ rather than dopamine D_2 actions of buspirone that are critical for its anxiolytic effects, since ipsapirone lacks the latter.

However, the most important property of buspirone for our triangulation approach is that it does not increase the effects of GABA nor interact directly with the $GABA_A$ receptor. It has been reported to increase benzodiazepine binding *in vivo* (Goeders et al., 1988), but its behavioural effects cannot be blocked by benzodiazepine receptor antagonists (see Jann, 1988). Thus, the reason that buspirone does not share the common side effects of the classical anxiolytics is buspirone's lack of interaction with GABAergic transmission. Conversely, that buspirone and classical anxiolytics are both clinically effective in treating the symptoms of anxiety suggests they act indirectly on the same final common path within the brain; but do so through quite distinct primary mechanisms. A major task of later chapters is to identify this final common path.

4.3.3 Panicolytic antidepressants

Drugs that change the levels of the monoamines serotonin and noradrenaline in the synaptic cleft usually reduce not only anxiety but also panic, depression, and in some cases obsession. In many cases, their action on anxiety cannot be taken at face value and could be secondary to a primary effect on panic attacks, obsessions or compulsions that generate anxiety as a consequence (see Chapter 13). However, the tricyclic antidepressants (and related SNRIs and SSRIs) are at least as effective as benzodiazepines in the treatment of generalized anxiety disorder.

This might appear to make the distinction between anxiety and depression difficult to maintain, especially when we remember that buspirone is also an effective antidepressant. However, there are two reasons for believing that there are distinct neural systems that are involved in anxiety and depression to different extents. First, most benzodiazepines are much more effective in treating anxiety than depression. The specific exceptions, like alprazolam (see, e.g. Dellemijn and Fields, 1994, Table III), merely remind us that different drugs of the same chemical family can have different effect profiles. Second, there is no evidence that monoamine oxidase inhibitor antidepressants are effective in controlling generalized anxiety disorder. Where there are reports of apparently anxiolytic effects of the monoamine oxidase inhibitors, these appear to be in cases of atypical depression or anxiolytic-resistant anxiety with phobia (Sheehan et al., 1981), in which they are much more effective than tricyclics (Klein, 1993; Sheehan et al., 1981).

As with buspirone, a task of later chapters will be to show how far the anxiolytic effects of antidepressants can be attributed to effects on final common paths in the nervous system. Given the assumption that buspirone reduces anxiety in virtue of its action as a partial agonist at $5HT_{1A}$ receptors, it is possible that both tricyclic and monoamine oxidase inhibitor antidepressants may vary in the ratio of their relative anxiolytic:antidepressant potency depending on the extent to which their effects on serotonin reuptake are greater at $5HT_{1A}$ than other 5HT sites. An insufficient range of antidepressants has been tested on generalized anxiety disorder to assess this possibility.

4.3.4 Drugs effective in obsessive-compulsive disorder

Clomipramine is structurally very similar to standard tricyclic antidepressants, differing from imipramine in the addition of a single chlorine atom. As you would expect from §4.3.3, it is antidepressant and panicolytic. However, it is also particularly effective in the treatment of obsessive-compulsive disorder (see Rapoport, 1989; Modigh, 1990). This specificity is consistent with the removal by DSM-5 of obsessive-compulsive disorder from the general class of anxiety disorders. Comparison with imipramine also supports a separation of obsession from depression and, indeed, 'the majority of investigators have come to the conclusion that the effect of clomipramine in obsessive-compulsive disorder is unrelated to its antidepressant effect' (Modigh, 1990, p. 94). We will argue in later chapters that, in obsessive-compulsive disorder, clomipramine has no direct effect on anxiety *per se*. We follow Rapoport (1989) in seeing it as a disorder primarily of obsessions (anterior cingulate cortex) interacting with compulsions (basal ganglia), and anxiety arising only when compulsive safety rituals conflict with other goals. Clomipramine would differ from imipramine by targeting reuptake in the cingulate and basal ganglia; but, like imipramine, may also be at least partially effective in treating anxiety by blocking reuptake at $5HT_{1A}$ sites (Akimova et al., 2009) in other areas. A similar broad neural action would account for the SSRIs now being the primary 'on label' drugs for OCD (Sartori and Singewald, 2019).

4.3.5 Anti-adrenergics

The 'beta-blockers' act at the ß subclass of adrenergic receptor and affect both central and peripheral adrenergic transmission. Our focus is central anxiolytic action, and yet the beta-blockers appear to act largely in the periphery; although one of the most commonly used, propranolol, is also a non-selective 5HT antagonist (see Griebel, 1995, Table 1). However, propranolol too appears to have its greatest effect on somatic rather than psychic symptoms of anxiety, and to be as effective as benzodiazepines only in those patients whose predominant anxiety symptoms are somatic (Noyes et al., 1981). Clinically, beta-blockers are used most commonly for performance anxiety. Given these complications and the paucity of data on the behavioural effects of these drugs in animals, we have left them out of our triangulation strategy.

Other, centrally acting, anti-adrenergics like clonidine and prazosin can be useful in 'anxiety disorder' and post-traumatic stress treatment. But they have complex effects (e.g. Hoehn-Saric et al., 1981) and appear to be most useful in treating symptoms linked to non-specific sympathetic arousal.

4.4 Clinical actions of the anxiolytics—a summary

All drugs have multiple effects. Where therapeutically undesirable or irrelevant (in any particular context), they are termed 'side effects'. But, from a physiological point of view, side effects can be as closely related to the principal mode of action as a drug's official therapeutic effect. Drugs acting on the $GABA_A$ receptor reduce not only anxiety but also, whatever their binding site, muscle tension, and seizures. For our first edition, therefore, muscle relaxant or anticonvulsant action could have been necessary properties for an effective anxiolytic. But then came incontrovertible evidence that an anxiolytic need not be sedative or anticonvulsant: buspirone, ipsapirone, and imipramine are anxiolytic but shared none of the $GABA_A$ side effects. This remains true for what are now the first line drugs (SSRIs).

This parallel clinical effectiveness is subject to one apparent caveat. The novel anxiolytics require at least 10 days' administration to produce their therapeutic effect; so are generally seen to differ markedly from the apparently immediate benzodiazepines. This apparent immediacy likely explains the preference for benzodiazepines (Trimble, 1990) that remains among some clinicians to this day (Ait-Daoud et al., 2018). But on the Hamilton Anxiety Rating Scale, benzodiazepines take as long as novel anxiolytics to produce their effects (e.g. Wheatley, 1990, Fig. 14.2) and even with preoperative anxiety, which might have been expected to be especially susceptible to acute anxiolytic effects, the benzodiazepines do not act immediately (Wikinski et al., 1994). The benzodiazepines appear to have two separate effects: 1) immediate euphoria and muscle relaxation (which show rapid tolerance); and 2) a slower truly anxiolytic effect (which does not show tolerance) that appears as the muscle relaxation and euphoria fade. For example, patients treated with long-term alprazolam for panic disorder show apparently normal baselines, but greatly depressed responsiveness to diazepam in tests of saccadic eye movements, growth hormone secretion, memory, and self-rated levels of sedation. By contrast they show no differences in diazepam-induced changes in measures of anxiety or cortisol levels (Cowley et al., 1995). In later chapters, we will link this delayed truly anxiolytic clinical action of all drugs to anterograde reductions of emotional memory and to interactions with sleep.

The data we have briefly reviewed so far suggest that there could be a single neural system that mediates the common effects of all the anxiolytic drugs. However, the anxiety affected by these drugs must be distinguished from atypical depression and simple phobia, and from anxiety that is consequent on panic or obsession. For, in the case of each of these conditions, there are drugs which are ineffective in treating them but effective in treating generalized anxiety (Table 4.1). For example, while atypical depression can be treated with the monoamine oxidase inhibitor (MAOI) anti-depressant phenelzine, it does not respond

Table 4.1 Comparison of the effects of different drug classes on internalizing disorders. Drugs are ordered in approximate relation to general effectiveness from most effective to least effective (or least available data). Disorder abbreviations: GAD = generalized anxiety disorder; MDD = major depressive episode; OCD = obsessive-compulsive disorder; PD = panic disorder; PTSD = post-traumatic stress disorder; SAD = social anxiety disorder (previously termed 'social phobia'); SP = simple phobia. Activity codes: blank = no data; 0 = inactive; (0) equivocal inactivity; (+) = equivocal or high dose activity; + = active; ++ = more strongly active than related drugs

	GAD	SAD	MDD	PD	PTSD	OCD	SP
Ketamine	+	+	+	+	+	+	
Mirtazapine	+	+	+	+	+	+	
SSRI	+	+	+	+	+	++	(+)
SNRI	+	+	+	+	+	+	
TCA_2 (≈CMI)	+	(+)	+	++	(+)	++	
TCA_1 (≈IMI)	+	(+)	+	+	+	(+)	0
MAOIs		+	+	+	(+)	(+)	(+)
NRI		(+)	+	(+)	(+)		
Buspirone	+	(+)	+	0	0	(+)	
BDZ_2	+	(+)	(+)	(+)	0	0	0
BDZ_1	+	(+)	0	0	0	0	0
Pregabalin	+	+	0*	(0)			

* PG unpublished results, Hauser et al. (2010), but see also discussion in Strawn and Geracioti (2007)

BDZ_1 early benzodiazepines, e.g. chlordiazepoxide and diazepam administered at typical (i.e. low) antianxiety doses. Other sedative antianxiety drugs (barbiturates, meprobamate) have similar effects.

BDZ_2 Later high-potency benzodiazepines, e.g. alprazolam. The antipanic effect is achieved at higher doses and this has also been reported with equivalent high doses for BDZ1 (Noyes et al., 1996). See also van Marwijk et al. (2012).

CMI clomipramine.

IMI imipramine.

MAOI MonoAmine oxidase inhibitors, e.g. phenelzine.

NRI selective noradrenaline reuptake inhibitors, e.g. reboxetine.

SNRI selective serotonin/noradrenaline reuptake inhibitors, e.g. duloxetine, venlafaxine.

SSRI selective serotonin reuptake inhibitors, e.g. fluoxetine, citalopram.

TCA_2 high effect tricyclics, e.g. clomipramine.

TCA_1 imipramine and related tricyclic antidepressants, but excluding clomipramine.

Table and legend taken from McNaughton and Glue (2020), some abbreviations and font changes added. Updated from McNaughton and Zangrossi (2008) data from or as reviewed in (Gray and McNaughton, 2000; McNaughton, 2002; Stein et al., 2004; Stevens and Pollack, 2005; Westenberg, 1999; Stein et al., 1992; Rickels and Rynn, 2002; den Boer and Westenberg, 1988; Spivak et al., 2006; Albucher and Liberzon, 2002; Pande et al., 2004; Feltner et al., 2011; Ravindran and Stein, 2010; Ravindran et al., 2009; Atmaca et al., 2003).

to benzodiazepines. MAOIs offer a particularly useful point of comparison in Table 4.1, since atypical depression shares many symptoms, particularly autonomic, with those of the anxiety disorders, which complicates differential diagnosis on the basis of symptoms. (Note that there is a 'a lack of randomized double-blind placebo-controlled trials for anxiety disorders and few studies comparing novel treatments to existing anxiolytic agents', Garakani et al., 2020, p. 1.)

The lack of clear specificity to any one DSM-5 type of anxiety (e.g. GAD versus SAD) of this wide range of anxiolytic drugs is consistent with the unitary view of the GIS presented in Chapter 3. The fact that, taken as a class, the drugs do not affect simple object phobia or panic (see Chapter 13) is consistent with the separation of the GIS from the GRS/FFFS. Critically, the consistency of anxiolytic but not other effects across novel and classical anxiolytics forms the basis for the triangulation that generates the neuropsychology of anxiety presented in this book. However, a complete neuropsychology must also account for the differences between the subclassifications of anxiety (a topic dealt with in Chapter 13), as well as for the clinical experience that nonetheless leads to their being grouped together (a major theme of Chapters 12 and 14), as for example, in the DSM system.

4.5 Bridging the species gap

Psychiatrists are seldom clear as to exactly what anxiety is; but have agreed for decades as to which drugs are anxiolytic. This allowed us to use the drugs to clarify some details of diagnostic classification (see Table 4.1; Chapter 13). We will now use them, in a similar fashion, to cross the species barrier.

As we briefly noted in §4.1.4, anxiolytics act on fundamental, ancient, chemical receptor systems that have been highly conserved in evolution (McNaughton, 2020). The key idea (Fig. 4.3) is that benzodiazepine receptors in the dorso-lateral nuclei of the primordial periaqueductal grey allowed a degree of control of a primitive goal inhibition system by circulating endogenous ligands (Silva and McNaughton, 2019; (gis) in the figure). Phylogenetic expansion resulted in the budding-off and progressive functional freezing of lower-level structures with a hierarchical rostral expansion producing a GIS with ever-more sophisticated conflict processing. This splitting of enlarged structures generally retained benzodiazepine receptors and so benzodiazepine control. This conserving of key ligands and receptors across a range of control system allows us to use fish to provide neurobehavioral models of a range of human psychiatric disorders (Soares et al., 2018).

Critically for our analysis, classical and novel drugs share anxiolytic action despite quite different primary actions on the brain. This gives us two reasons for reviewing the effects of the anxiolytic drugs in animals. First, the profile of behavioural effects <u>common</u> to both classical and novel anxiolytic drugs will represent truly anxiolytic, as opposed to other, action: providing insight into the psychological nature of the anxiolytic action. Second, the neural effects common to anxiolytics should map the neurology of anxiety. By comparing the behavioural profile obtained in the present chapter with the effects of lesions of the nervous system we shall, in the following chapters, narrow the search for the neuropsychology of anxiety.

However, here we must make explicit an assumption that has until now been largely implicit: that anxiety exists in other animals as well as human beings, and that all respond in much the same way to anti-anxiety drugs. This assumption is critical, not only for our arguments, but also for the whole research endeavour on which they are based. With drug effects, as we will see, the match in terms of changes in the control of behaviour is a matter of observation.

Yet many people will find the assumption of homology of what <u>they</u> may mean by anxiety (McNaughton, 2018) hard to accept. Anxiety is commonly believed to be a uniquely human

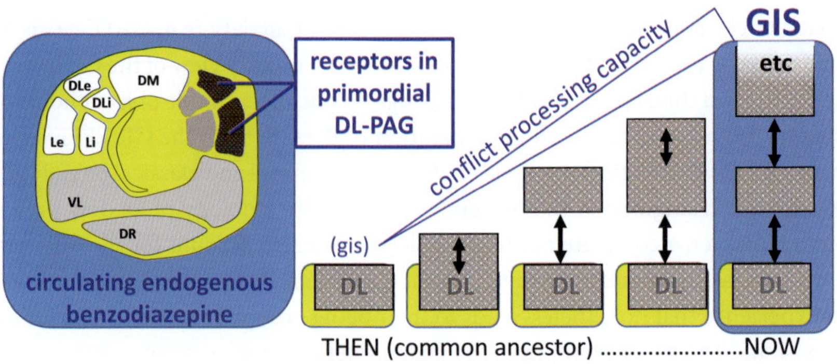

Fig. 4.3 Conservation of the primordial PAG with expansion of motivational controls systems such as the GIS. The primitive core is retained during phylogenetic expansion as higher levels of control are added. During expansion, receptors for endogenous benzodiazepines are conserved in those structures for which benzodiazepine modulation is not maladaptive. **Abbreviations:** DL = dorsolateral; DR = dorsal raphe; e = external; GIS = goal inhibition system; I = internal L = lateral; VL = ventrolateral. **Source:** Adapted from *Personality Neuroscience*, 3 (e4), Neil McNaughton, 'Personality neuroscience and psychopathology: should we start with biology and look for neural-level factors?', p. 11, Figure 2, DOI: https://doi.org/10.1017/pen.2020.5 Copyright © McNaughton, 2020. Published by Cambridge University Press. Licensed under CC-BY 4.0. With elements from *Progress in Neurobiology*, 177, Carlos Silva and Neil McNaughton, 'Are periaqueductal gray and dorsal raphe the foundation of appetitive and aversive control? A comprehensive review', p. 63, Figure 19, https://doi.org/10.1016/j.pneurobio.2019.02.001 Copyright © 2019 Elsevier Ltd. All rights reserved.

state, dependent on such complex cognitive capacities as the ability to foresee the future, to form a self-image, or to imagine one's own mortality. If this were true our present approach would be misconceived. But we believe that the reflexive separation of cognition from biology is driven by a range of common fallacies that particularly afflict the analysis of personality and emotion (McNaughton and Corr, 2009). That said, we accept that 'science has not yet reached a point where it can be shown that cognitive and biological explanations of emotion and personality must always be intertwined' (McNaughton and Corr, 2009, p. 111). Critically, the belief that cognition sets 'us' apart from 'them' cannot be lightly brushed aside. The general continuity of human and animal behaviour is not open to serious dispute on biological grounds. But this does not avoid the need to demonstrate that there is sufficient continuity in each specific case.

Indeed, a criticism (Eysenck, 1992b, p. 166) of our first edition was that:

> Gray may well be right that there are important similarities between rat and man in terms of the brain structures which mediate anxiety, but it is much less likely that the cognitive processes associated with anxiety are the same in the two species.... Even if the layman or clinician were to accept that perceiving events as, say, signals of punishment or non reward called forth biological responses that we have in common with other species, they might still argue that the cause of complaints of anxiety was in perceiving events in this way, and not in possessing the biological mechanisms of these responses.

Eysenck argued, in particular, that the book failed to capture some specifically cognitive components of human anxiety because of its foundations in animal work. We discuss these cognitive components in some detail in Chapter 14.

Likewise, Joe Ledoux, despite a lifetime's focus on animal work, says of the second edition that 'in my opinion, it still gives the septum and hippocampus too prominent a role, at the expense of the amygdala and prefrontal cortex' (LeDoux, 2002, p. 288). More recently, he has promoted the view that 'anxiety, in short, is a conscious feeling... Anxiety (worry, dread, apprehension, trepidation, angst, and worry*[sic]*) involves a particular kind of conscious thought. It is all about self' (LeDoux, 2015, p. 257). Linking anxiety to working memory and conscious worry places it, for Ledoux, primarily in the prefrontal cortex, the area of the brain in humans that is least like that of other animals. We will discuss this further in Chapters 11 and 14 (see also McNaughton and Corr, 2009) but our view is that a key difference is semantic. We define 'anxiety' differently and in a way that would make worry distinct—and indeed common to neurotic disorders not specific to anxiety (§12.8.4). It is also our view that making consciousness the key construct not only puts analysis out of the range of animal work but also puts it out of the range of science, since I have no means of directly accessing your consciousness or even of being able tell, in the hard sense, if you are conscious at all.[1]

In one sense, of course, human anxiety cannot be like that of any other species. We have our own unique sensory and cognitive systems and this must affect the way we perceive stimuli able to elicit anxiety. Yet, taken to the extreme, this is a counsel of despair that would imply that we cannot generalize even from one human being to another, since everyone has their own unique concerns and perceptions (and neurology). (People who agree as to what is turquoise will often disagree as to whether it's a blue or a green; some people are completely blind to specific smells; and we have no way of knowing if someone else experiences anxiety the way we do.)

However, anxiety and other emotions can be viewed as resulting from particular *functional classes* of situation that are species-general (McNaughton, 1989b). While these may produce certain species-specific adaptations, the similarities between species and individuals would be expected vastly to outweigh the differences and to be driven by common general factors. To take a physiological example, human beings neither eat grass nor ruminate, and cows do not eat meat. Nonetheless there are virtually no differences in the basic physiological principles of digestion and metabolism (e.g. the Kreb's cycle) between the two species, and surprisingly few detailed practical differences. So, we accept Eysenck's point that the specific stimuli that give rise to a specific occasion of human anxiety are unique, and that their anxiogenic potential depends on individual interpretation. Nonetheless, the cognitive processes that give rise to such interpretations share with those of other animal species a reliance upon such universal principles of learning as those of classical conditioning. Our cognitions depend upon some processes that cannot occur in a non-linguistic species; but they also depend on developmental processes that can differ markedly between individual humans. However, once formed <u>as</u> anxiogenic stimuli, their action in eliciting the *conserved* emotion of anxiety is essentially similar in humans and other mammalian species. Thus, a full analysis of anxiety requires an understanding of <u>both</u> the specifically human cognitive processes (Dalgleish and Power, 1999) that lead to a particular individual's construing a particular

[1] The week this sentence was written, the Guardian Weekly published an article completely written by a self-trained machine learning algorithm. Can you be sure that 'my' sentence was not generated by a machine?

event as a threat, e.g. to self-esteem (the kind of process emphasized by Eysenck), <u>and</u> the processes that convert that construal into the emotion of anxiety, which are common to the human and other species—leading Dalgleish among others to currently analyse human anxiety reactions via exposure to virtual predators (Mobbs et al., 2015; Rigoli et al., 2016). We also need to allow for cognitive processes in non-humans that may be similar to those that in humans support sex differences in anxious responding (Blanchard, 2023).

As we shall now see, the observed effects of anxiolytic drugs in animals suggest that they act on an anxiety that is very similar to the human type. The final crucial steps will be taken in Chapters 12–14. There we take our theory of anxiety based largely on animal experiments and apply it to the phenomena of anxiety in humans. In particular, we describe an anxiety biomarker derived from rat neuropharmacology that is measured in human prefrontal cortex and that we have shown is high in some (new) type of human anxiety disorder. In the last analysis, this is the touchstone of the theory's success: the understanding it brings of human anxiety and fear, and their disorders, and their treatment.

4.6 The behavioural effects of anxiolytic drugs in animals

4.6.1 General approach

In the previous chapters we focussed on specific views of anxiety and so specific related effects of anxiolytics. In what follows, we progress to an increasingly general view of anxiolytic drug action, and hence, given our triangulation approach, of anxiety.

In Chapter 2, we took as our paradigmatic case the innate behaviour that is likely to occur in the context of potential threat. But we concluded that the critical feature for such behaviour is the approach-avoidance conflict inherent in a situation of potential threat, rather than the potentiality of the threat as such (see also §4.6.4). In the present chapter, we deal with explicit cases of approach-avoidance and find that, as with the case of predatory defence, the anxiolytic drugs shift the balance of the conflict from avoidance towards approach. Nonetheless uncertainty or unexpectedness of events will remain as <u>one</u> important means of generating conflict—linking back to one feature of potential threat.

In Chapter 3, moving from innate to learned behaviour, we found reason to broaden the notion of approach-avoidance conflict and to treat as potentially threatening: novel stimuli of certain kinds, signals of loss, and signals of gain omission, in addition to the (ethologically speaking) paradigmatic innate anxiety stimuli. In what follows, we shall deal with all of these cases, and find reason to emphasize both the role in anxiety of passive (inhibitory) avoidance and the necessity for true conflict between highly primed (activated) incompatible goals. This leads naturally to the fact that anxiolytic drugs also shift an active avoidance-passive avoidance conflict away from inhibitory avoidance.

Importantly, and underpinning the renaming of the key inhibitory system from BIS to GIS, described in Chapter 1, we will distinguish between action stopping and goal inhibition. The former is not sensitive to anxiolytic drugs and (Chapter 11) depends on structures outside the limbic system.

The end of the chapter generalizes still further. Anxiolytics affect tasks that, at first sight, have no aversive component at all, but instead appear to involve memory. However, the tasks do involve conflict—but between approach to one stimulus and approach to another. The common thread here is that choice of correct action requires inhibition of competing goals that are currently inappropriate.

4.6.2 Interpretation, dose-response, and conventional screening

A careful description of the effects of the anxiolytic drugs on the behaviour of experimental animals, and where possible of human beings, is essential, then, for the arguments pursued in this book. There have been many hundreds of experiments on these effects, starting with the pioneering work of Jules Masserman on alcohol and Neal Miller on sodium amylobarbitone (Masserman and Yum, 1946; Miller, 1951). Appendix 1 provides details for the overall summary of anxiolytic effects presented in Table 4.2, which are mostly independent of the drug used or the species investigated, and annotations in the table indicate where new data have been added. Note that, to avoid duplication and allow easy comparison, this table also includes lesion data that will be covered in later chapters.

Table 4.2 has been organized into blocks of paradigms that appear related conceptually and in terms of what treatments (including lesions) are effective or ineffective. In the text that follows, however, we will often compare pairs, or sets, of tests where an unaffected test (e.g. simultaneous discrimination, elevated T-maze escape) provides a form of control for an affected test (e.g. successive discrimination, elevated T-maze inhibition, respectively) and so allows us a clearer picture of the psychological processes that the drug is affecting. We will also attempt in §4.7 to treat the entire Table in the same way and see how far we can account for all the drug effects in terms of some single process or single set of processes.

Our key triangulation question is how far novel anxiolytics such as buspirone are like the classical anxiolytics. We will see that, where buspirone has been investigated, the similarities are surprisingly good, extending to some tasks that are superficially unexpected (such as the Morris water maze). However, it should be remembered that the data on buspirone and similar compounds (labelled $5HT_{1A}$) seldom include more than one test with any particular experimental regime (with the exception of the classic 'screening' tests for anxiolytic action), and its entries in Table 4.2 usually reflect only one experimental regime for each major class of behavioural test with a number of key classes still empty.

Where null results are encountered in the literature on buspirone, it should also be borne in mind that in many, but not all, animal tests buspirone has an inverted-U dose-response curve. There is some indication (Johnston and File, 1988) that this is because, at higher doses (above 1 mg/kg in rats), it releases corticosterone (Urban et al., 1986). This corticosterone acts, effectively, as an anxiolytic antagonist (McNaughton et al., 1996b) but then develops tolerance at about the same rate as buspirone's development of effectiveness in the clinic. Benzodiazepines have an opposite interaction with corticosterone with opposite effects of their tolerance (McNaughton et al., 1996b). The inverted-U dose-response curve may arise also because buspirone is only a partial rather than a full agonist at $5HT_{1A}$ receptors. In either case, it can have more convincing anxiolytic effects with chronic pretreatment (e.g. Zhu and McNaughton, 1995b), possibly because of tolerance of dopaminergic action or tolerance of corticosterone-based antagonism (see Matheson et al., 1996; and §4.3.2).

Table 4.2 Comparison of the common behavioural effects (ANX) of novel ($5HT_{1A}$) and classical ($GABA_A$) anxiolytics with the com effects (S/H) of septal (SEP) and hippocampal (HIP) lesions and lesions of the amygdala (AMYG) dorsal ascending noradrenergic b (NA), ascending serotonergic system (5HT), and (usually systemic) blockade of the cholinergic system (ACh). For details of the literature, please see the Appendices. Changes based on later publications are marked and cited below. Variable effects of $5HT_{1A}$ drugs are likely due to higher doses (>1 mg/kg) releasing corticosterone

	$5H_{T1A}$	GAB_{AA}	ANX	S/H	SEP	HIP	AMYG	NA	5HT	ACh
Defecation, emotional	+	0	0	0	–	0		0		
Drinking	0	+	0	0	+	0	0	0	0	
Simple rewarded learning	0/–	0	0	0	0	0	0	0	0	–
Simultaneous spatial discrimination		0	0	0	0	0		0		
Simple stopping		0[r0r0r]	0[r0r0r]	0	0?		0?[u0?u0?u]		–?[s–?s–?s]	0[t0t0t]
Elevated T – escape	0[b0b0b]	0[b0b0b]	0	0		0[c0c0c]	0[e0e0e]	0[g0g0g]	–/0[d–/0d–/0d]	
Frustration		0	0	0	0	0	–	0		
Classical aversive conditioning	0[o0o0o]	0	0	0	0	0	–			
Escape	0	0	0	0	0	0	–	0	0	
One-way avoidance	0/–	0	0	0	–	0	–	0		0
Response to aversive stimulation	–	0	0	(+)	+	+/0	–	0	0/+	
Latent inhibition	0[n0n0n]	0[n0n0n]	0	–	–	–	0	0	–[p–p–p]	
Eating	+	+	+	0	0/+	0	0	0	+	
Defensive burying	–	–	–	0	–	0	0		–[b–b–b]	
Conditional/delayed discrimination	(–)	(–)	(–)	0?		–/0	0		+	–
Single alternation		–	–	?	+?	+/0/–	–	–		

Conditioned suppression on baseline	–	–	–	0	(–)	0	–	–	–	
Social interaction	–/0	–	–	–?	–?	–/0[j]–/0[j]	–	0	–	
Fear-potentiated startle	–	–	–	0		0	–		+	
Extinction		–	–	–	–	–	0	–	–/0	–
Reversal		(–)	(–)	–	–	–	0/–	0		
Water maze	–	–	–	–	–	–	0	0		–
Elevated + maze	–/0	–	–	–	–	–[k]–[k]	0	+[h]+[h]	–	–[v]–[v]
PREE		–	–	–	–	(–)	0	–		
Fixed interval	–/0	–	–	–	–	(–)	0	0/–		0
Successive discrimination	–/0	–	–	–	–/0	–	–	–	0	–
Conditioned freezing to context	–[a]–[a]	–	–	–	–	–[c]–[c]	–	+/0		–[v]–[v]
Passive avoidance	–/0	–	–	–	–	–	–	+[h]0/–+[h]0/–	–	–
Elevated T – inhibition	–[b]–[b]	–[b]–[b]	–	–	(–)[f](–)[f]	–[c]–[c]	–[e]–[e]	+[g]+[g]	–[d]–[d]	
DRL	–/0	–	–	–	–	–	–	0	–	–
Aggression (no shock)	–[i]–[i]	–[i]/+–[i]/+	–	–	–	–	–	0		–
Radial arm		0/–*	0/–	–	–	–	–			–
Spontaneous alternation	–?[m]	–	–	–	–	–	–	–		–
Rearing (low threat)	–	–	–	–	–	–	+	–	–	–
Two-way avoidance**	+/–[l]	+	+	+	+	+	–	0/+	+	+
Non-spatial Avoidance		+	+	+	+	+		0		+

(continued)

Table 4.2 Continued

[a] Tandospirone (Nishikawa et al., 2007), flesinoxan (Li et al., 2001) fluvoxamine (Li et al., 2001).

[b] (Graeff and Zangrossi, 2002).

[c] Effects on inhibition with hippocampus (Trivedi and Coover).

[d] Median raphe lesion (Andrade et al., 2004) electrolytic lesion also affected escape.

[e] (Strauss et al., 2003).

[f] Clear effect but with successive alleys task not conventional T maze (Bannerman et al., 2004).

[g] NA in PAG *decreased* inhibition (Estrada et al., 2016).

[h] (Pelosi et al., 2009).

[i] (Ferreira et al., 2000).

[j] (Becker et al., 1999; Deacon et al., 2002).

[k] (Kjelstrup et al., 2002).

[l] Buspirone anxiolytic at 0.05 (Fernández-Teruel and Tobeña, 2020) and anxiogenic at 10 mg/kg! (Alhaider et al., 1993).

[m] Baited arms used (Rhoads et al., 2012).

[n] (Moser et al., 2000).

[o] (Hellewell et al., 1999).

[p] Effect with median raphe lesions that deplete hippocampal serotonin but not dorsal raphe lesions that did not deplete (Solomon et al., 1980).

[q] (Treit et al., 1993) but see also (Pobbe et al., 2011).

[r] (McNaughton et al., 2013, Shadli et al., 2015).

[sI] Inferred from cortical noradrenaline infusion (Bari et al., 2011).

[t] (Eagle et al., 2009).

[u] Hippocampal lack of involvement inferred from magnetic resonance spectroscopy (Schmitz et al., 2017).

[v] Chen et al., 2021.

* Effect of drug with high dose or complex non-spatial radial maze.

**For review, see Fernánde-Teruel & Tobeña (2020).

For this, and similar reasons with the benzodiazepines, throughout what follows, we consider only the effects of low doses of the drugs. In the case of the classical anxiolytics, these are doses that do not produce sedative, motor, or anaesthetic effects (e.g. 5 mg/kg of chlordiazepoxide in the rat). In the case of buspirone, they are doses (usually less than 1 mg/kg) that, across a range of tasks, produce effects quantitatively similar to those of low doses of benzodiazepines, and are below those which show diminished or reversed acute effects.

In looking at the behavioural effects of the anxiolytic drugs, we shall take the opposite approach to that adopted by most modern screening tests such as

> the social interaction test, light–dark exploration, the anxiety/defense test battery, the open field test, the elevated-plus maze, shock-probe burying, fear-potentiated startle after cued fear conditioning, and conflict tests... Systematic examination of the validation criteria in these models is largely lacking in the literature, and although there is often (some) pharmacological similarity between these models and GAD, behavioral or etiological resemblances are mostly absent.
>
> (Luyten et al., 2011, p. 229)

Most screening tests are designed for speedy automated testing of many compounds, but allow minimal theoretical analysis (McNaughton and Zangrossi, 2008) and appear each to be measuring a somewhat different behavioural trait with no common factor of anxiety uniting them (File, 1992; see also Broekkamp et al., 1989; Davies et al., 1994; Dawson et al., 1995). Resultant replication problems (which remain, Rosso et al., 2022) led to more ethological analyses (e.g. Cole and Rodgers, 1993; Rodgers and Cole, 1994; Miczek et al., 1995), but not usually to the parametric analysis that, in the Blanchards' hands, showed the U-shaped relationship of many behavioural measures to the underlying construct of anxiety (Chapter 2; for more detail see §4.6.4 and Fig. 4.4; see also Rodgers and Cole, 1993). As noted by Dawson and Tricklebank (1995), the increased labour of ethological analysis removed the time-saving that is perhaps the sole attraction of the conventional screening tests (see e.g. Griebel, 1995).

Before looking at the list of measures in Table 4.2 we should distinguish between an animal screen for anxiolytic *action* (or, e.g. the human startle model, Grillon and Ernst, 2020) and an animal model of anxiety *disorder*. For example, Luyten et al. (2011, p. 231, our emphasis) propose, as 'an animal model of [generalized anxiety disorder], contextual conditioning in rats, with one or more training and testing sessions, using freezing *and/or* startle amplitude as measures of anxiety'. Luyten et al. justify such 'contextual conditioning'[2] as a model of GAD in terms of face (e.g. symptom patterns) and construct (aetiology, neural circuitry) validity. Importantly for us, they also provide some evidence of predictive validity—with positive effects of $5HT_{1A}$ agonists and benzodiazepines on freezing to 'context'. But they do not seem to cite any contextual conditioning study with $5HT_{1A}$ agonists on fear-potentiated startle. That said, $5HT_{1A}$ agonists are effective in conventional (somewhat 'contextual') startle paradigms. Nonetheless, we think that their model would be safer with a requirement to use freezing and startle amplitude as measures. Notably, we have not included a simple category 'contextual conditioning' in Table 4.2 but have retained our original separate 'conditioned freezing to context' and 'fear-potentiated startle' items, especially since the former but not the latter is sensitive to hippocampal lesions. This means that a positive result with freezing does

[2] In the second edition, we included 'conditioned freezing to context' as a drug- and lesion-sensitive category and focused on cases where there is both foreground (tone-shock) and background (apparatus shock/context-shock)

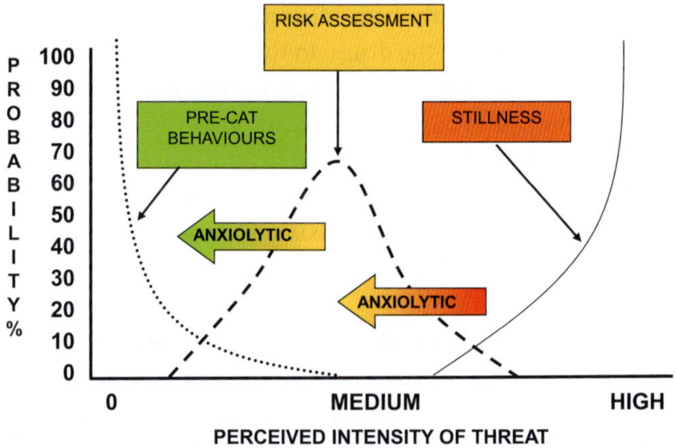

Fig. 4.4 Ethopharmacological analysis revisited. As threat intensity decreases, risk assessment behaviours such as rearing appear at a low level then increase to a maximum and then decrease and vanish. Anxiolytics given on a high threat/low rearing baseline increase rearing (right hand arrow); given on a medium threat/high rearing baseline they decrease rearing (left hand arrow). In both cases the effect of the drug is the same as a reduction in perceived intensity of threat—the anxiolytics consistently reduce anxiety and so have variable effects on observed behaviour.

not guarantee a positive result with startle. It would also seem necessary for the test to be a more complete model of GAD that, in addition to contextual freezing and potentiated startle, measures should also be taken of defecation, ACTH, corticosterone (c.f. human cortisol), and heart rate (see Luyten et al., 2011, Table 1, p. 232). Otherwise, the result is no different from previous separate freezing and startle studies. The use of selected strains seems promising here (e.g. for GAD, León et al., 2017; Cruz et al., 2023).

One honourable exception to the atheoretical screening approach is the elevated T-maze test developed by Graeff's group (Viana et al., 1994; Graeff et al., 1998; Jardim et al., 1999; Pinheiro et al., 2008; Zangrossi and Graeff, 1997; Roncon et al., 2012). This uses the same innate tendencies as the + maze but harnesses them to discrete types of learning that, as we shall see, distinguish anxiolytic and panicolytic drugs (for a theoretical analysis of the T versus + difference, see McNaughton and Zangrossi, 2008; for positive comparison with other screening tests see Luyten et al., 2011).

> Benzodiazepine anxiolytics such as diazepam and midazolam, but also 5HT-related drugs such as buspirone, ipsapirone and ritanserin impair inhibitory avoidance in the T maze while leaving one-way escape unchanged (Graeff and Zangrossi, 2002). This selective effect in favour of defensive approach correlates with the clinical effectiveness of these drugs on generalized anxiety, as opposed to their lack of efficacy (at least at anxiolytic doses) on panic disorder. Similarly, one-way escape is impaired by chronic (but not acute) administration of the tricyclic antidepressants such as imipramine (Teixeira et al., 2000) and clomipramine as

conditioning possible. Since then, 'context' has come to be generally used to describe conditioning to a large apparatus *even if there is no foreground conditioning*. We object to this use in detail in Chapter 7, in particular noting that the key thing is not context *per se* but use of 'a complex, spatially and temporally extended CS' (second edition, p. 169). But we fear this is a lost cause.

> well as by the selective 5HT reuptake blocker fluoxetine (Poltronieri et al., 2003)—all drugs that are used to treat panic disorder.
>
> (McNaughton and Zangrossi, 2008, p. 21)

That said, 'although animal models of anxiety have relatively good validity, anxiolytic drugs with novel mechanisms have been slow to emerge' (Cryan and Sweeney, 2011), so we largely ignore the screening tradition (but include the + and T-maze in Table 4.2) and, in contrast, our approach is to treat the entire literature as one massive test battery; and to interpret the results in terms of our prior ethological and learning-theory analysis. Thus, as we have done in miniature already in the last two chapters, we shall use a lack of effect in one test to rule out the various psychological processes involved in that test from any contribution to the effect of the drugs obtained in some other test.

4.6.3 Simple appetitive and aversive stimuli

Since many experiments require the use of appetitive or aversive stimuli to control behaviour, we start our review with the simplest effects of these stimuli. Our immediate focus will be on ruling out effects of the drugs on active approach and active avoidance so as to allow a clear interpretation of the effects, described later, on the inhibitory avoidance inherent in approach-avoidance conflict.

In Chapter 2 we concluded that the paradigmatic case of pure fear, the response to an immediately present predator, is unaffected by anxiolytic drugs. This result encompassed each of fight, flight and freezing (and contrasts with the conditioned 'contextual' freezing discussed in §4.6.2). Consistent with this conclusion, in more artificial laboratory situations this form of behaviour is again not affected. A key finding here is that, with simple active avoidance (as opposed to two-way avoidance, which we consider shortly), there is no effect of the drugs, matching their lack of effect on the Blanchards' Fear Defence Battery. It can also be seen from Table 4.2 that anxiolytic drugs do not affect any responses related to simple appetitive motivation, nor to the learning of active responses to avoid noxious stimuli or approach appetitive ones. These results immediately rule out any general actions of the anxiolytics on simple motivation (including pure fear), on sensory discrimination, on motor control, or on learning and memory in general.

4.6.4 Simple conflict, e.g. approach-avoidance, successive discriminations

As can be seen from Table 4.2, in tests in which there is explicit approach-avoidance conflict (Miller, 1951) involving a painful stimulus, such as foot-shock, the anxiolytic drugs shift the balance of the conflict from avoidance towards approach (as was the case with predatory defence, Chapter 2). As previously noted in Chapter 2, the effect of the drugs on risk assessment behaviour is a complex function of defensive distance (hence the ethological approach to screening tests mentioned in the previous section). This function explains, for example, the opposite effects of anxiolytics on rearing in open field tests depending on whether loud noise and bright lights are used or not. In a high stress version of the open field test, which includes loud white noise and bright light, anxiolytics increase rearing (McNaughton et al., 1984), whereas, in a low stress version of the test, anxiolytics decrease rearing (McNaughton, 1985b). This result is explicable if rearing in this test reflects risk assessment in the same way that it does in the Blanchards' paradigms.

Note that the effects of the drugs in these cases cannot be attributed to an action on fear since they did not change the crucial behaviours in the Fear/Defence Test Battery (see also §4.6.3). Nor can they be attributed to a direct effect on the motor systems which control risk assessment, or risk assessment would be uniformly decreased.

Rather (Fig. 4.4), they must be interpreted as a reduction in the underlying construct of anxiety. This is, by hypothesis, linearly related to defensive distance; which is in turn, by observation, non-linearly related to risk assessment behaviour in undrugged animals. This non-linearity of the relationship between risk assessment and anxiety demonstrated by the drugs is a reason for preferring goal inhibition as the primary measure of this emotional state. With goal (and so behaviour) inhibition we see a simple progression from no threat, where there is no inhibition; to moderate threat, where there is inhibition of non-defensive but not defensive (risk assessment) behaviour; to high threat where there is inhibition of both non-defensive and defensive behaviour. Effects on risk assessment appear the same for conflicts with both innate and conditioned stimuli (Illescas-Huerta et al., 2021).

A selective action of anxiolytics against goal inhibition is seen in tasks in which the conflict is with an active avoidance response, as in the well-studied two-way active avoidance task in the shuttlebox. The superficially paradoxical effect of the drugs is to improve two-way active avoidance. This reduction follows from unaffected one-way active avoidance (§4.6.3) coupled to reduced passive avoidance of the part of the apparatus from which the animal had to escape on the previous trial (for a recent review, see Fernández-Teruel and Tobeña, 2020).

The same selective reduction in passive avoidance is seen when the avoidance component of the approach-avoidance conflict is based, not upon a painful stimulus, but upon omission of expected gain. Perhaps the clearest cases of this are extinction and successive discrimination. Anxiolytic drugs have no effect, in the rat, on learning to run down a runway, but they greatly impair learning *not to run* when the food the rat wants is no longer available. Note, here, the similar complexity and similar uncertainty involved in the two pharmacologically distinct cases. Similarly, when responding is reinforced by food in the presence of one stimulus (S+) and a second stimulus (S–) explicitly indicates that food is not available (or that shock will be presented), the animals can learn the required response if the S+ and S– are presented as a concurrent choice (simultaneous discrimination) but not if they are presented successively (go/no go), so that the S– requires the animal to inhibit the responding that obtained gain in the immediately preceding S+ period.

Particularly interesting in this context is the stop signal task (SST). Here, an S+ is presented but, before the rat or person has made a response, a 'stop' signal (essentially an S–) is presented. If the S– were presented before the S+ the task would become a successive discrimination and be anxiolytic-sensitive. However, in the SST the capacity to stop (which even in controls is only marginal) is not affected by anxiolytic drugs—we will discuss in §11.5.4 electrophysiological and lesion evidence that anxiolytic-sensitive limbic goal inhibition circuits are activated during the SST but are too slow to control the fast action stopping, which instead depends on prefrontal circuits (see also Neo et al., 2011).

4.6.5 Operant schedules, including delayed matching

The actions of the anxiolytics on the bulk of operant schedules (fixed interval, FI, differential reinforcement of responding, DRL, etc.) are again consistent with the notion that they reduce inhibition of responses that are followed by both gain and omission of gain. In all cases, the way in which responding has changed indicates that the animal retains knowledge of the task to be performed, but that its capacity to inhibit prepotent responding is reduced.

The data on anxiolytic drug action in Table 4.2 thus licence the generalization, from behaviour that occurs in the context of approach to potential predators, to behaviour that involves approach to a wide array of conditioned and unconditioned aversive stimuli. Additional data in the table show that we must generalize still further. The drugs are effective in a number of tasks that appear to have no aversive component at all, involving instead memory. However, this generalization does not involve as big a step as might at first appear: the tasks do involve conflict, but conflict between approach and approach. In delayed matching to sample with trial non-unique stimuli, for example, in order to approach the correct goal on any particular trial, the animal must inhibit responding to a goal that would have been correct previously (often on the immediately preceding trial). Thus, correct performance of the task requires inhibition of competing responses that are currently inappropriate.

4.6.6 The Morris water maze

Probably the most theoretically significant of the 'memory' tasks is the Morris water maze (Morris, 1981; Morris, 1984). This is the quintessential test of spatial navigation, and nowadays the most commonly used test of temporal lobe dysfunction in non-human subjects. It consists of a circular featureless swimming pool containing a submerged, and hence invisible, platform that is always located in the same spatial position. The rat is placed in the pool at different positions on different trials. Control rats quickly learn to find the platform and to swim almost directly to it. The invisibility of the platform also allows the use of transfer tests to determine what the rat has learned. In such tests, at the end of acquisition, the rat is placed in the water as usual, but there is no platform to swim to. Control rats show that they know the precise position at which the platform should have been located. They swim to this position and then swim in very tight circles on the spot where the platform would have been before eventually searching in other areas (Fig. 4.5 bottom right). Chlordiazepoxide, buspirone, the $5HT_{1A}$ agonist 8OH-DPAT, ethanol and other anxiolytic drugs eliminate acquisition of spatial navigation in the water maze (McNaughton and Morris, 1987; Devenport et al., 1989;; Rowan et al., 1990; McNamara and Skelton, 1991; McNamara and Skelton, 1992; McNaughton and Morris, 1992; Carli and Samanin, 1992), while leaving intact non-spatial (or less accurate) strategies for finding the platform. It is of note that in this task, unlike many of the standard screening tests for anxiolytics, buspirone has a purely linear dose-response curve (McNaughton and Morris, 1992).

There are two features of the effects of anxiolytics in the water maze that are particularly important for the analysis of behavioural inhibition. These are discussed more fully in Chapter 7, but will be mentioned here.

First, it is clear that the drugged rats are motivated to learn the task and are capable of at least some learning. On successive trials in the apparatus, they reduce the distance they swim

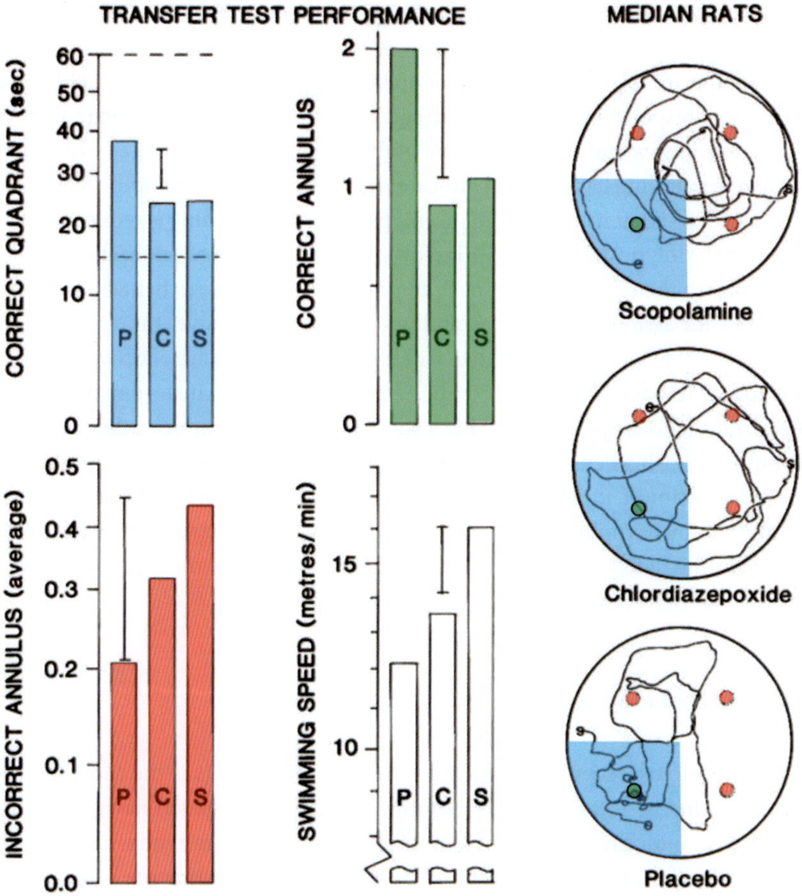

Fig. 4.5 Effects of the benzodiazepine chlordiazepoxide and the anticholinergic scopolamine in a transfer test after spatial learning in the water maze. Both drugs impair the capacity of the rats to find the location at which a platform had been during learning. Note that the paths taken by the median rats of each group show that control rats tend to swim with a zig-zag path to where the platform was and then circle on the spot; that scopolamine rats tend to swim in circles and that chlordiazepoxide rats show no consistent pattern. **Source:** Adapted from *Behavioural Brain Research*, 24 (1), N. McNaughton and R.G.M. Morris, 'Chlordiazepoxide, an anxiolytic benzodiazepine, impairs place navigation in rats', p. 43, Figure 2, https://doi.org/10.1016/0166-4328(87)90034-9 Copyright © 1987 Published by Elsevier B.V.

and towards the end of acquisition appear, on the basis of path length, to be solving the task nearly as well as controls. However, in the transfer test, they swim straight through the position at which the platform would have been (Fig. 4.5 middle right) and show little indication that they know where it is. This suggests that they have a simple non-spatial rule that allows them to bump into the platform when it is there.

Second, while this task involves aversive motivation (deriving from immersion in water), it is formally an escape task, not one of passive avoidance. However, we concluded earlier that it is only passive avoidance, not escape or active avoidance, which anxiolytic drugs normally impair. The deficit produced by anxiolytic drugs in this task cannot therefore be attributed to the use of a negative reinforcer. Nor can it be attributed to a general failure of memory, since respectable learning occurs, but accuracy is reduced by a failure to determine the position of (or at least to correctly approach) the platform. Finally, the deficit cannot be attributed, except *ad hoc*, to a loss of specifically spatial capacities, since many of the other tasks we have considered (FI, DRL etc.) are not distinguished by specifically spatial requirements. Further, administration of buspirone only during the probe trial at the end of acquisition has no effect (Rowan et al., 1990) and diazepam has no effect on performance (McNamara and Skelton, 1991; Kant et al., 1996) or even on acquisition if the rats have first been habituated to swimming in the maze (Zanotti et al., 1994, see also §4.6.8).

4.6.7 Other spatial tasks

In a radial arm maze task, the rat is placed into the centre of a maze in the shape of a star burst (*) with, typically, 8 or 16 arms. In the simplest version of this task all arms contain a piece of food at the beginning of any one trial, and the most efficient performance is for the rat to visit each arm only once. This might seem very simple in that this outcome can be achieved by a rule such as 'turn sharp left as you come out of each arm'. In practice rats do not solve the task in this way, tending rather to choose arms roughly opposite to that which they have just visited. They must, therefore, maintain in working memory information (presumably, spatial information) about the arms they have visited.

We discuss different types of memory more in Chapter 8. Suffice it to say here that a normally anxiolytic dose of chlordiazepoxide (5 mg/kg) is without effect in the simplest form of this task (data from J. N. P. Rawlins, cited by McNaughton et al., 1980b, p. 188), but a high dose (20 mg/kg) is effective (Rawlins personal communication). The $5HT_{1A}$ agonists also impair performance in the radial arm maze (Winter and Petti, 1987).

The importance of task complexity, as opposed to space, is underscored by the fact that, if the radial arm maze is modified to be more complex but less spatial, anxiolytics become effective even at low doses. Instead of putting food in all eight arms of the maze, one can place food in only four, and signal which four by placing non-spatial cues (e.g. a sandpaper floor), in each baited arm. The arms containing the food are changed from trial to trial. Chlordiazepoxide significantly impairs acquisition of this task at a dose of only 5 mg/kg (Hodges and Green, 1986; Olaman and McNaughton, 2001) by impairing non-spatial reference memory while, perhaps, leaving spatial reference memory intact (Olaman and McNaughton, 2001).

4.6.8 Anxiolytics, space, and hippocampal lesions

When we view nominally spatial tasks as a whole, we see a progression from simple to complex tasks. In the simplest—position learning in a T maze—there is little effect of the drugs; in more complex tests (spontaneous alternation and radial arm maze), there is a clear effect only at high doses; finally, in the most complex (spatial navigation as opposed to other solutions of the water maze), there appeared to be total abolition of the capacity for spatial learning. However, there are also anxiolytic effects in complex non-spatial tasks (most obviously the cued radial arm maze we have just discussed but also operant tasks requiring response inhibition). We can ask, therefore, if 'spatial' effects are in fact due to spatial processing or due to the fact that many spatial tasks generate complexity (and particularly interference). It will be useful, here, to preview our analysis of the supposedly spatial effects of hippocampal lesions.

'Complexity' is an elastic term; it may well relate, however, to the concept of conflict that has been at the root of our analysis so far. In the case of the water maze, we can make some progress in drawing these ideas closer together. As we discuss later (Chapter 7; Appendix 7), septo-hippocampal lesions produce an even larger deficit in spatial navigation in the water maze than do anxiolytic drugs. However, there are a number of data that suggest that space *qua* space is not the critical factor in determining the lesion deficit. For example, Eichenbaum et al. (1990) found that rats with fimbria/fornix lesions (which disconnect the septum from the hippocampus) could perform the task nearly as well as controls, but only if they started from the same position on every trial; yet a probe trial showed that they were solving the problem using spatial cues and not some simpler rule (see also Whishaw and Tomie, 1997). The main cause of the drug-induced deficit in the standard form of the water maze may, therefore, be due to an inability to inhibit conflicting response tendencies (particularly thigmotaxis) when starting from different positions on each trial. This seems particularly likely, given the findings of Zanotti et al. (1994) that prior experience of the maze (which would be expected to eliminate initial exploratory tendencies) eliminates the effects of anxiolytics on spatial navigation. The concept of complexity may perhaps, therefore, be made more precise along these lines.

4.7 Anxiolytic action—some conclusions

We have now completed a general overview of the behavioural profile of the anxiolytic drugs. We find little evidence that the drugs affect basic motivational, perceptual, or simple memorial processes. With only a few exceptions (for some of which we have been able to provide possible, albeit *ad hoc*, explanations), the effects of the drugs have been seen in tests that involve approach-avoidance conflict (with which we started our analysis in Chapters 2 and 3), or avoidance-avoidance conflict (as in two-way active avoidance), or approach-approach conflict (as in delayed matching to sample). In all these cases, whether because of reinforcement of specific responses or of the nature of the stimuli presented, the animal is faced with conflicting goals of similar strengths. This is particularly a feature of the standard spatial tasks. The effect of the drugs is to reduce the power of the inhibitory component of the conflict (i.e. with approach-avoidance, they reduce avoidance and hence increase approach).

The extent to which this pattern is generally applicable to all of the chemically different anxiolytic drugs is remarkable, especially so in the case of buspirone (at least with low doses, lengthy administration, or blockade of corticosterone release). As noted earlier, buspirone shares none of the side effects of the classical anxiolytics. It might have been expected, therefore, that a large part of the common behavioural profile of the classical anxiolytics would not be reproduced by this compound.

The clearest effects of buspirone and the clearest similarity to the effects of classical anxiolytic drugs are in what might be viewed as the least emotional, most stimulus-oriented measures: spatial navigation in the water maze and rearing in the low stress open field. The least clear effects and the greatest departure from those of classical anxiolytics are seen, paradoxically, in tasks supposedly designed as screens for anxiolytic drugs: the elevated plus maze and social interaction. It may be that these latter tests suffer from being more tests of action at benzodiazepine sites on GABA-A receptors than of anxiety. But, as we have noted, another possibility is that the anxiolytic effect of buspirone is masked by an antagonist action of corticosterone, released both by the drug and in consequence of the inherently stressful nature of this type of test, which may be lost with repeated administration (as first suggested by Johnston and File, 1988; see also Zhu and McNaughton, 1995b; McNaughton et al., 1996b; Matheson et al., 1996). For our present purposes, this issue is not critical, since in the great majority of cases benzodiazepine-like effects of buspirone can be obtained if suitable dosing regimens are used. In Chapter 8, and in Appendix 10, we discuss the complex involvement of 5HT systems in both the regulation of the GIS and the control of other aversive behaviour. As summarized by Handley et al. (1993, p. 203), the evidence 'that decreasing serotonergic function is anxiolytic and increasing it is anxiogenic, is most consistent in models of behavioural inhibition where the stimulus inhibits an approach response (conflict models). However, paradoxical drug effects are also frequent, especially where the aversive stimulus evokes an active response'.

The similarities between the anxiolytic drugs, classical and novel, strongly imply that they act upon a common neural system (or systems). Central to our understanding of the effects of the drugs is that they do not affect either the eliciting effects of gain or loss, nor the learning of simple responses, nor the learning of discriminations reinforced by such stimuli. They also appear not to affect the simple eliciting properties of novel stimuli. Thus, they do <u>not</u> act on systems mediating perception, motivation, action, or any general kind of reinforcement or memory. By far the widest range of their effects, and the most easily understood, are found in tasks where behavioural inhibition of some prepotent response is central to correct acquisition: passive avoidance, extinction, successive discrimination, etc. It appears, then, that anxiolytic drugs may be characterized as producing a specific interference with the GIS (largely as defined by Gray, 1975); the key properties of which were detailed in Chapter 3 and Fig. 3.1.

Note that the GIS, so defined, does not mediate all cases where behaviour occurs at a low level and so might in some sense be described as inhibited. We have already seen this in the case of innate predator-induced freezing. The stimuli that activate the GIS are taken to be conditioned fear stimuli, conditioned frustrative stimuli and other stimuli which have been paired with primary negative reinforcers, and also novelty and other innate anxiety stimuli. As argued in Chapter 3, the common function of all such stimuli is to signal potential threat, and they activate the GIS only when they do in fact signal potential threat in such a way as to generate conflict. It follows that there can be both cases in which the frequency of behaviour is reduced by some process other than goal inhibition, and cases in which stimuli that initially produced their behavioural effects through the GIS subsequently cease to do so. An example of the former case is positive conditioned suppression, in which an animal can obtain food by holding still; this is not affected by anxiolytic drug treatment (Miczek, 1973). An example of the latter case is over-learned successive discrimination (S– signalling shock for responding); once the habit is learned to the point that shocks are no longer received, anxiolytics no longer disinhibit responding (McNaughton, 1985a). Similarly, action stopping in the SST (§4.6.4) must occur too fast to allow goal inhibition circuits to control behaviour.

Nor is the GIS, as we define it, solely concerned to produce goal inhibition. As described in Chapters 2 and 3, its outputs include increased risk assessment behaviour and increased levels of arousal and attention. Descriptively, these outputs involve behavioural activation rather than inhibition, yet they are sensitive to anxiolytic drugs (although the U-shaped relationship of risk assessment measures to level of anxiety discussed in Chapter 2 creates great problems for interpretation unless anxiety is parametrically varied within a single experimental paradigm).

The overt exploratory behaviour that forms part of risk assessment results in increased attention to environmental stimuli. The effects of anxiolytic drugs on this attentional output of the GIS have been studied in connection only with novelty as the input to the system. A lone experiment by McGonigle et al. (1967) has taken this type of analysis furthest, by measuring the degree to which a drugged animal learns about a novel element in its environment. These workers trained rats on a random 50% partial reinforcement schedule of gain for choosing the positive cue (black or white) in a choice box, choice of the negative cue never obtaining gain. The rats were then shifted to a combined-cue discrimination (black vs. white and horizontal vs. vertical stripes, both cues being presented together) in which the old positive cue remained positive. During this stage of the experiment half the animals received a barbiturate and half placebo. Finally, transfer tests were conducted with only horizontal vs. vertical stripes and no drug. Controls chose correctly on the transfer trials, but the drugged animals did not. Since the task was a simultaneous discrimination, not normally affected by anxiolytic drugs, it is likely that the critical element that made it sensitive to these agents was the requirement to attend, and transfer control, to a novel environmental cue. However, the problem of attention requires much more research before we can be sure whether anxiolytic drugs decrease this output from the GIS.

There are several examples of a blockade by the anxiolytic drugs of the increment in level of arousal that is postulated to result from activity in the GIS. This too remains a neglected problem. In part this is because the concept of arousal is much less firmly embedded in animal learning theory than in human experimental psychology (e.g. Gray, 1964; Eysenck and Eysenck, 1967; Broadbent, 1971), so that there are few experimental paradigms that unambiguously address this issue. One paradigm which comes close to this ideal is the partial reinforcement acquisition effect. This consists in an increase in running speed, relative to animals receiving food on every trial, in animals receiving food on a 50% random partial reinforcement schedule for traversing a straight alley. The partial reinforcement acquisition effect has been explicitly treated as reflecting an increased level of arousal arising from exposure to secondary frustrative stimuli (Amsel, 1962; Amsel, 1992; Gray and Smith, 1969), and it is blocked by anxiolytic drugs. A second experimental demonstration of the increased arousal output of the GIS is the potentiated startle response, produced by preceding the startle stimulus by either a conditioned fear (Brown, 1961) or conditioned frustrative (Wagner, 1963) stimulus. Fear-potentiated startle is blocked by benzodiazepines, barbiturates, and buspirone (Chi, 1965; Davis et al., 1993) when these are given during the test as opposed to acquisition phase.

In general, then, we can make the case that the anxiolytic drugs impair the functioning of the GIS as this was defined in the previous chapters (Fig. 3.1). The drugged animals care less about threats of loss, omens of failure, or the uncertainties of a novel environment. In caring less, they inhibit behaviour less, they are less attentive to threatening stimuli, and they are less aroused. This description is surely one that applies to people who are being treated with anxiolytic drugs. Thus, it is reasonable to conclude that *these drugs reduce anxiety in non-humans as in humans.*

Our description of anxiolytic drug effects has emphasized a change in mood or disposition. However, we have also seen data that suggest that, related to this alteration in mood, there is a cognitive factor. It is the cognitively complex tasks that demonstrate the clearest drug effects. Rather than discuss the issue of cognition in the present chapter, we leave it until we present the full theory (Chapter 10), by which time we shall have taken a detailed look at brain mechanisms of memory (Chapter 9). We also leave, until Chapter 7, discussion of the effects of the anxiolytics on memory. For the moment, we merely note the possibility that anxiolytic drugs produce indirect effects on the expression of anxiety by interfering with cognitive mechanisms that impact on emotional bias.

The behavioural effects of the anxiolytic drugs, then, provide a reasonably coherent pattern, which we can seek to see replicated by dysfunction of specific neural systems. It will be the business of later chapters, then, to attempt to match these drug effects to some part or parts of the neurology of defence (see Appendices 2 and 3 for additional details).

5
A conceptual theory of the goal inhibition system

5.1 GIS versus BIS—a terminological difference

This chapter integrates the picture of the Goal Inhibition System (GIS) that arises from the previous four chapters. Before proceeding, it is important to provide a reminder (see §1.7; Table 1.1) that the GIS, as defined in this edition, is in pharmacological, neural, and behavioural terms *fundamentally* the same as the Behavioural Inhibition System (BIS) of previous editions. Likewise, Goal Attraction System (GAS) and Goal Repulsion System (GRS) largely map to what were previously the Behavioural Approach System (BAS) and Fight, Flight, Freeze, System (FFFS).

Some *newly emphasized* issues are that the GIS deals with goal inhibition *but not* action stopping (McNaughton et al., 2013; Shadli et al., 2015), and that attraction can be produced both by GAIN and by omission of expected LOSS; and repulsion by both LOSS and omission of expected GAIN (Chapter 3). Thus, loss aversion (Tversky and Kahneman, 1991; Novemsky and Kahneman, 2005; Tom et al., 2007) can affect both attraction and repulsion (Fig. 3.1). Importantly, also, it must be emphasized that these systems respond to reinfor<u>cers</u> and are impacted by reinforce<u>ment</u> with its own sensitivities (§12.7.2) with resultant care needed in the use (or, better, avoidance) of 'reward' and 'punishment'. A related adjustment is that the lowest levels of the GRS (i.e., those activated by a close predator) have retained the label !FFFS as a subsystem since they control special predator-specific forms (hence!) of fight, flight, and freezing—with, e.g., !FIGHT meant to be limited to explosive attack and not confused with the various forms of aggression that have been termed 'fight' in the development of RST scales. Although not labelled as subsystems, the lowest levels of the GIS and GAS also control specific proximal patterns, including ones involving complete stillness (stretch attend, lordosis), rather than general conflict or approach behaviour. Note that the stationary behaviours can be distinguished by body posture but are most clearly different in terms of their function in the situations in which they appear.

A final point to note (see Chapter 12) is that all future personality measures intended to assess the GIS should be pharmacologically or neurally validated and, ideally, derived. Most importantly, it should be noted that the most-used *BIS* scale (Carver and White, 1994) contains no items assessing goal inhibition (or behavioural inhibition) and is, in practice, a worry scale (§12.8.4) that will be linked to neurotic disorders in general and not disorders of anxiety (as we define it) in particular. Indeed, this is the main reason for a new nomenclature. A number of more recent RST scales share the problem of lacking biological derivation or validation and have a lack of consensus on the matter of the constructs nominally being measured (§12.12.3, §12.12.4).

So, in this chapter, we provide a high-level picture of the GIS as defined by anxiolytic drugs. We account for the ethology, learning theory, and behavioural pharmacology we have

The Neuropsychology of Anxiety, Third Edition. Neil McNaughton and Jeffrey A. Gray, Oxford University Press.
 DOI: 10.1093/oso/9780198843313.003.0005

discussed so far via a single conceptual system that we think is central to anxiety. This conceptual outline will guide our search, in subsequent chapters, for the neural basis of the GIS, and therefore of anxiety.

5.2 System inputs—an ethoexperimental perspective

Let us first deal with the eliciting stimuli that activate the GIS. The Blanchards' analysis of the ethology of threat systems (Chapter 2) distinguished responses to immediate present threat from responses to a potential threat. In theory, their paradigm predator-based cases (present and potential threat) pose different functional requirements; and, in practice, give rise to quite different types of behaviour. Active responses (including attack) to a *present* threat implement simple repulsion from danger. Active responses (including risk assessment) to a *potential* threat implement cautious approach to danger (driven by attraction to gain, which can include the termination/omission of threat).

Defensive distance is a key concept within the Blanchards' analysis; and will have a major impact on our analysis of neural systems. In the specific case of the *potential* threat paradigm (i.e., producing anxiety not fear), a small defensive distance (high expectation of potential danger) produces goal inhibition so great that there is no active behaviour; with a larger defensive distance, goal inhibition (i.e., inhibition of prepotent behaviour) is present, but is accompanied by active risk analysis and distinctive conflict-related behaviours such as the 'stretched-attend' posture; with very large defensive distance (no expectation of potential danger), both goal inhibition and active threat-related behaviour disappear and pre-threat behaviour returns. An important point was that active threat-related behaviour (risk assessment) showed an inverted U relationship to defensive distance, and anxiolytic drugs had effects consistent with an increase in defensive distance (Fig. 4.4). That is, the drugs increase or decrease active threat-related behaviour, depending on whether the defensive distance is smaller or larger, respectively.

Despite the apparent clarity of the Blanchards' analysis, there is a problem with viewing the categories of behaviour in terms solely of their nominal eliciting stimuli. Certainly, the response pattern to a potential cat includes risk analysis and goal inhibition (that is inhibition of pre-threat behaviours) as the rat enters the threatening situation; and both of these are sensitive to anxiolytic drugs. However, even a potential cat can produce active escape from the threatening situation and this escape is anxiolytic-insensitive. The key here is the generation of repulsion, not whether the threat is actual or potential. Conversely, the very certain presence of an immoveable shock prod can elicit *cautious approach* and defensive burying, which is also sensitive to anxiolytic drugs. Further, the animal's response to a discrete, non-moving, source of shock appears to depend markedly on how distinctive the source of shock is. A poorly localized source elicits similar behaviour to that which would be normally be elicited by a potential predator.

Our perspective replaces a classical behaviourist stimulus-bound position with a more contemporary cognitive and functional view of the situation. We proposed that, on the one hand, we have a GRS that controls behaviour whenever the animal's primary purpose is to move *away* from a source of danger (or, more generally, loss)—that is, when there is a negative goal creating repulsion. On the other hand, we have a GIS that controls behaviour whenever the animal's primary purpose is to achieve some goal that requires it to move *towards* a source of danger—that is, when it has *concurrent conflicting goals*: attraction and repulsion. The Blanchards distinguish, at the stimulus level, an actual from a potential predator but we see this as highly correlated with, but not a necessary condition for, activation of the GRS and GIS, respectively. Instead, we see the fundamental distinction as being a conflict between the goals of entering (GIS) or leaving (GRS) a dangerous situation—a matter of 'defensive direction'. This distinction is an extension of, and enriched by, the Blanchards' ethological analysis of responses to a potential predator, which we have attempted to incorporate in more detail in the new version of Fig. 5.1.

Note that GIS activation (and hence anxiety) not only necessitates activation of the GRS (or there would be no threat to approach) but also necessitates activation of the GAS or there would be no reason to approach the danger. Activation of the GIS can be most simply thought of as resulting from concurrent similar substantial activation of the GAS and GRS.

5.3 Presentation/omission of gain/loss—a learning theory perspective

The ethological perspective on the GIS has the advantage of functional clarity in its dependence on innate responses in ecologically reasonable circumstances. However, it is at a disadvantage if we want to gain greater insight into the cognitive processes that can give rise to the animal's decision to enter or leave a dangerous situation. In Chapter 3, therefore, we looked at a learning-theory analysis of the capacity of threatening stimuli to support new learning.

As with the ethological analysis, but for different reasons, our learning analysis found it necessary to categorically differentiate repulsion (active avoidance) from goal conflict and inhibition (passive avoidance). The results of learning experiments also led us to expand the concept of the GIS from that of a system specifically activated by the requirement to approach danger to a system generally activated by any approach–avoidance conflict. We concluded that such conflicts could be produced, not only by the innate fear stimuli analysed by the ethologists and not only by learned signals of impending pain, but also by signals of impending frustrative non-reward and by novelty. Crucially, it is not the presence of the aversive stimuli themselves that activates the GIS, but their conjunction with appetitive stimuli or other conditions that result in the animal having to choose between conflicting, incompatible goals. Novelty as a stimulus is special in this respect in that the same stimulus can be presumed often to give rise to both the approach and the avoidance tendencies constituting the conflict.

At this stage of the analysis, then, the GIS was viewed as a system that is engaged by a need to approach aversive stimuli. From this point of view, we can derive both its normal adequate stimuli (signals of pain, signals of frustration, novelty, and innate anxiety stimuli—all *when they must be approached*) and its normal outputs (inhibition of prepotent behaviour, arousal, attention and, where appropriate, risk assessment).

5.4 System outputs—the pharmacological perspective

In both Chapters 2 and 3, we used the effects of selective anxiolytic drugs to validate the categorical distinctions between anxiety and fear that we had made on ethological and learning theory grounds. These compounds appear to leave the functioning of the GRS and GAS intact while quite generally impairing that of the GIS in a manner consistent with an increase in perceived defensive distance. Since the drugs concerned were defined by human clinical work, and the behavioural categories by two quite independent analyses of the behaviour of un-drugged non-humans, this matching up of anxiolytic drug effects with anxiety-related behaviour is not tautological. (Indeed, in a few minor cases, like the anxiolytic reduction of vocalization in the presence of a predator, discussed in Appendix 1, the match is not perfect.)

Chapters 2 and 3 suggested that the common actions of the different classes of anxiolytic drugs could be used as a probe for anxiety itself. So, Chapter 4 reviewed the effects of the anxiolytic drugs on both clinical and animal behaviour. Importantly, there was high congruence between the effects of classical and novel anxiolytics, despite their different mechanisms of action, and profiles of side effects. The picture was of anxiety involving, and anxiolytics reducing, goal inhibition, risk analysis, and a variety of other responses resulting not only from approach–avoidance conflict, but also approach–approach and avoidance–avoidance conflicts. That is, anxiolytics affected all situations that required goal inhibition (or produced it in practice), including a number of effects in what would normally be considered tests of memory. Full analysis of the memory tests is postponed until Chapter 7; but these 'amnesic' effects of anxiolytics suggest that their actions in non-memory tasks may be exerted on the cognitive processes that ultimately lead to emotional responses, as much as directly on the emotional responses themselves.

Chapter 4 also substantiated the distinction between the GRS/FFFS and the GIS. The anxiolytic drugs are ineffective in reducing innate or conditioned escape or active avoidance responses. We were in addition able to distinguish the GIS from the GAS/BAS, since anxiolytics do not affect appetitive learning or a wide variety of other responses that are uncontaminated by the presence of conflicting goals. The only potential exceptions to this rule were a subset of memory tests (which, as argued in Chapter 7, must involve at least one of a number of types of goal conflict if they are to be sensitive to the drugs). There was also confusion surrounding the results obtained in a number of the more recent screening tests for anxiolytic drugs. This could be due to the fact that these tests are not firmly grounded in classical learning theory and, as a result, often contain elements that could activate both the GRS and GISs concurrently with clearer results when these elements are separated (Graeff et al., 1998; McNaughton and Zangrossi, 2008). In the case of the novel anxiolytics, a further potential confound is the interaction between these compounds and the activity of the pituitary–adrenal system (§4.6.2).

5.5 The conceptual GIS updated

Putting Chapters 1–4 together, then, we have an updated view of the basic psychological (Conceptual Nervous System) components of the GIS (Fig. 5.1; c.f. Fig. 1.1). The GIS is most characteristically involved in, and may have originally evolved to cope with, the requirement to enter threatening situations. However, potential predatory threat is not the only situation that engenders approach–avoidance conflict, and all approach–avoidance conflicts have many functional features in common. Either originally, or subsequent to its initial evolution, the GIS broadened its scope from potential predators to all the aversive stimuli that we can at present envisage as requiring resolution of approach–avoidance conflict: innate and acquired signals of punishment, innate and acquired signals of frustration, and initially threatening

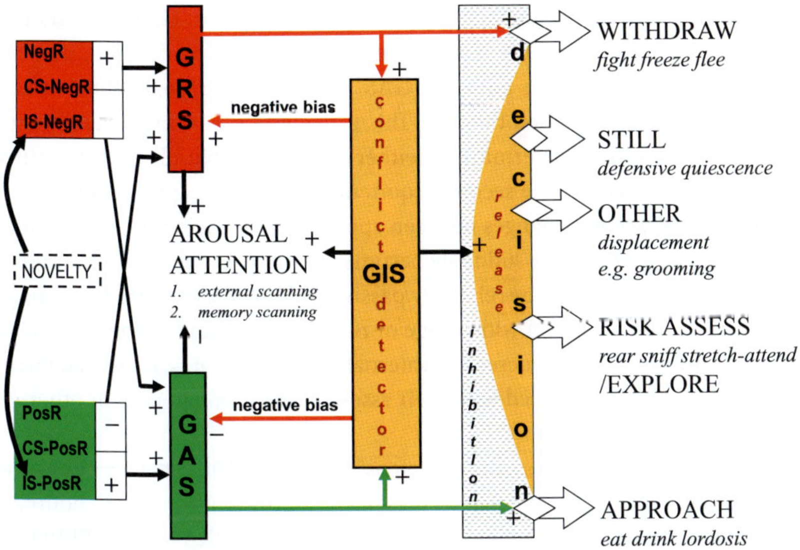

Fig. 5.1 An expanded view of the GIS (c.f. Figures 1.1 and 3.1) showing its relation to the GRS and GAS. The inputs to the system are primary positive (PosR) or negative (NegR) reinforcers that can be delivered [+] or omitted [-] (see Chapter 3); or conditional (CS) or innate (IS) stimuli that predict the primary reinforcers. General system outputs are in capitals (e.g., APPROACH, WITHDRAW); reinforcer-specific proximal rodent behaviours are shown in italics (*freeze, stretch-attend, eat*). The simplest way to activate the GIS is to concurrently activate the GRS and the GAS, i.e., face the animal with an approach-avoidance conflict. In this case both simple approach and simple avoidance will be inhibited and replaced with environmental scanning (in the form of altered attention), external scanning (risk assessment behaviour) and internal scanning of memory. Note that all of these scanning operations are aimed at confirming/ denying the presence of affectively negative information and involve an increase in the salience of such information. As a result, a secondary consequence of activation of the system, is a shift of the balance between approach and avoidance tendencies to a negative bias in the direction of avoidance by opposite return inputs to the GAS and GRS. The coloured areas indicate zones in which distinct traits (e.g. loss aversion, see Kim and Anderson, 2020) operate.

Source: Figure and legend are modified from Gray and McNaughton (2000), Corr and McNaughton (2012), and McNaughton and Corr (2014).

novel stimuli. In sum, the GIS functions to resolve conflicts between approximately equally activated and incompatible goals.

In Fig. 5.1 we have made explicit the requirements for approach–avoidance conflict for each of the different classes of stimuli. That is, the presence of stimuli or contingencies *per se* is not sufficient to activate the GIS. The animal's knowledge of those stimuli and contingencies must be such as to engender within it a genuine conflict between mutually incompatible goals (e.g., danger and food). As noted already, once an animal has learned to avoid shock, its behaviour is controlled by habit and the GIS is no longer involved. Thus, the operation of the GIS is fundamentally concerned with the 'hesitation and doubt' of Simonov's quotation at the head of Chapter 1.

Not only the inputs, but also the outputs of the GIS can be derived from the requirement to correctly resolve conflicting goals. Given an approximately equal balance between appetitive and defensive drive, neither should control behaviour. Gluttony may turn you into someone else's lunch; timidity may starve you to death. The first requirement then is inhibition of the output from both the GAS and GRS—the 'goal/behavioural inhibition' from which we have named the GIS. This provides a preliminary resolution to the appetitive–aversive conflict by permitting neither of the incompatible goals to gain immediate control over behaviour. The second requirement is an increase in arousal: one must be prepared for split-second changes between approach to the appetitive goal and escape from a potential danger that may suddenly become manifest. The third requirement is that of increased attention. This may be relatively passive and involve increased scanning of the environment, or it may involve a wide range of risk assessment behaviours. To anticipate somewhat, it could also involve increased 'internal scanning', that is, increased retrieval of associations from memory coupled with their assessment for threatening or otherwise adverse implications.

Fig. 5.1 also contains elements of both defensive distance and defensive direction. The relative balance between GRS and GAS is represented by position from top to bottom on the right-hand side. With balanced conflict (in the middle), WITHDRAW and APPROACH are both inhibited and, e.g., RISK ASSESS occurs. An effect of defensive (and appetitive) distance is indicated in reinforcer/species-specific behaviours that occur with a proximal reinforcer (indicated in italics, e.g., *displacement grooming*) and reinforcer/species general tendencies that occur with a distal reinforcer, e.g., WITHDRAW, APPROACH. Note the reciprocal relation of inhibition of prepotent behaviours and release of GIS-specific ones indicated in the **decision** box. Note also that while the systems affect decision antagonistically, they summate to affect arousal and so the intensity of whatever behaviour is decided on (Gray and Smith, 1969). Paradoxically, increased GAS arousal may even decrease attention to its stimuli through arousal-biased competition (Kim and Anderson, 2020).

5.6 The search for the brain's GIS—evolution, anxiety, and rules of thumb

Given this behaviour-based sketch of the GIS, our next step will be to try and find its neural substrate. We have already deployed the basic principles that will guide us to the neurology of anxiety: where both classical and novel anxiolytics affect behaviour in the same way, that behaviour is likely to involve elements of anxiety. Similarly, where both classical and novel anxiolytics produce a common change in neural function, that change is likely to involve the neural substrate of anxiety. In Chapter 6, then, we use the effects of the anxiolytic drugs as a marker for the neural systems involved in anxiety.

For clarity, we need first to take a close look at the implications of the functional analysis just carried out—and the core idea that the GIS is specifically adapted to one aspect of threat processing. Threat is phylogenetically universal and its physiological and behavioural requirements (e.g., for successful escape) are similar across species. The species with similar responses to anxiolytic drugs include fish, birds, mice, cats, dogs, pigs, monkeys, and people. It is striking (Gray, 1977) there is virtually no need to qualify any of the resulting conclusions with respect to species. Where there is such a need, this is because of the intrusion of a species-specific complicating factor superimposed on the basic effect of interest, not because of an inherent lack of replication of the effect in that species. Further, there is no sign of any change, qualitative or quantitative, in the effects of the anxiolytic drugs as one approaches, phylogenetically speaking, our own species.

This implies that the substrate upon which the anxiolytic drugs act includes components that are phylogenetically old—old enough to be present (so far as we know) in all contemporary mammalian species and to have homologues in all vertebrates. Anxiolytics affect the behaviour of birds and fish much the same as of rats and monkeys. Classical anxiolytics act on a benzodiazepine receptor present in the brains of all vertebrates, including fish, quite generally (Nielsen et al., 1978). These data give us good reason to treat human beings as fundamentally similar to other mammalian species in the specific case of anxiety, as do other data for other emotions (LeDoux, 1996) and mental functions generally (Chapter 11; McNaughton, 1989b; Thomas, 1996; Macphail, 1996; Steckler and Muir, 1996; Zinbarg and Mineka, 1991).

If the action of the anxiolytic drugs in so many diverse species is to reduce anxiety (and that is what the data suggest), it follows that anxiety itself is phylogenetically old. This greatly weakens any attempt to explain the fundamental mechanisms of human anxiety in terms that are specific to human beings, by recourse, say to consciousness as a key element (LeDoux, 2015), let alone specific to the pressures of modern life. Second, we now have an important clue as to at least some of the brain areas that must mediate human anxiety and on which the anxiolytic drugs act. These are likely to include, as major components, systems that are common at least to most mammals—with origins as primitive as the periaqueductal grey (Silva and McNaughton, 2019)—and likely, therefore, to have important elements outside the cerebral cortex, which has achieved most prominence in ourselves and other primates.

Of course, this does not mean that phylogenetically recent structures do not play a major role in anxiety among the creatures that possess them. Even in the simpler organisms, conditioning and expectation play major roles in the production of anxiety. It follows that the range of stimuli that can elicit anxiety must depend on the perceptual and cognitive equipment available to the species in question. (To take a trivial case, the rat, being colour blind, cannot respond differentially to a red as opposed to a green stimulus that predicts a shock, while a pigeon can.) Nonetheless, given the evidence from studies of the anxiolytic drugs, it is virtually certain that the core mechanisms involved share much in common between human anxiety and the anxiety experienced by a rat or mouse, enough at any rate for it to be reasonable to search in the brains of these small creatures for the neural mechanisms that mediate the clinically important aspects of human anxiety. In fact, in our final theory the phylogenetically oldest mechanisms are assigned a general modulatory function that is, if anything, more important for more highly encephalized species, while being chemically and functionally the same across all species. By studying these mechanisms in less encephalized species we can get a clearer picture of their function than we could in people (and indeed in other primates).

Perhaps because of their phylogenetic ubiquity, benzodiazepine receptors are remarkably widely distributed in the brain. Despite this, there is no evidence that the putative endogenous ligands of these receptors are released as neurotransmitters or even neuromodulators. An alternative possibility is that these ligands consist of a family of hormones or neurohormones able to affect multiple spatially separated targets in the brain (and possibly the rest of the body as well). Evolution often proceeds through phylogenetic conservation of simple mechanisms combined with elaboration of function by the progressive addition of further simple mechanisms; these are then able to extend the range of circumstances to which the animal is adapted or otherwise to modify the operation of the existing mechanisms. A process of this kind might give rise to multiple sites of action of the anxiolytic drugs, sensitivity at each site arising from its own combination of random mutation and selective advantage. This possibility is consistent with our ethological analysis. This has shown that, even when we restrict ourselves to the GIS in particular as opposed to defensive reactions in general, we are dealing with a complex system with multiple effector components, each of which has been subject to somewhat different adaptive pressures (see Marks and Nesse, 1994; McNaughton, 1989b; McNaughton, 2020).

We have previously argued (McNaughton, 1989b; McNaughton, 2020) that each emotion is best defined as a set of reactions to its own unique historical functional class of situation (see also LeDoux, 1996). In the case of at least the 'basic' emotions (Ekman, 1982; Ekman and Friesen, 1986), there are two points to note. First, a large part of the form of the emotional reaction is the result of evolution (although this does not mean that it is rigidly fixed). Second, most emotions (and certainly anxiety) involve action tendencies, autonomic responses, hormonal responses, and probably immune responses. Thus, all the effector systems of the brain are likely to be involved simultaneously. However, it does not follow that this plethora of activity, which we call 'an emotion', must be produced via the activation by a single environmental stimulus or a single central state that then triggers all the responses of all the effector systems. If that were the case, we would probably have had a generally agreed theory of the emotions a century ago. Rather, there are good evolutionary reasons for believing that most, if not all, emotions give only the appearance of a single source of central control. The pattern of effector output to which we assign a specific emotion label, such as 'anxiety', could result more from consistencies in the functional characteristics of the external eliciting stimuli than from the presence of some single locus in the animal's brain controlling all the outputs of all the co-activated effector systems.

Let us illustrate this point with the example used by William James (1884). You are faced with a lion (or any animal is faced with a predator). Your capacity to recognize that the lion is dangerous may be the result of learning, and the precise form of your fear reaction may have been modified by experience, but to a large extent your 'motor tension, autonomic hyperactivity, apprehensive expectation, and vigilance and scanning' (e.g., DSM-III-R, American Psychiatric Association, 1987) are determined by the fact that your ancestors have frequently been faced with predators (if not lions) and that in the presence of any predator certain responses will increase the chances of survival. Your responses, therefore, are in part due to the prior meeting of random mutation with selective advantage. The necessary involvement of random mutation, here, has some interesting consequences for emotion. In particular, the response of each effector system will be subject to its own evolutionary equation; and, to the extent that the response of any effector system is genetically determined, it will be the result of a mutation that in many cases will be specific to that system. We have detailed the consequences of this state of affairs elsewhere (McNaughton, 1989a), but they can be understood by brief inspection of Fig. 5.2.

Fig. 5.2 shows, at the top, the logical situation to which we are referring. A range of stimuli S1-S9 can occur in the environment and, with the exception of S8 and S9, usually occur together. These could be, for example, the smell of the lion, the sight of its teeth, its outline and so on. Each of these stimuli, alone, is a good predictor of threat, i.e., the presence of a predator or some other situation requiring the same general classes of response. Given that a threat *is* detected, each of the responses in Fig. 5.2 will, in general, be advantageous (though not necessarily for the same reasons; e.g., if escape is successful, there is no need for an increase in

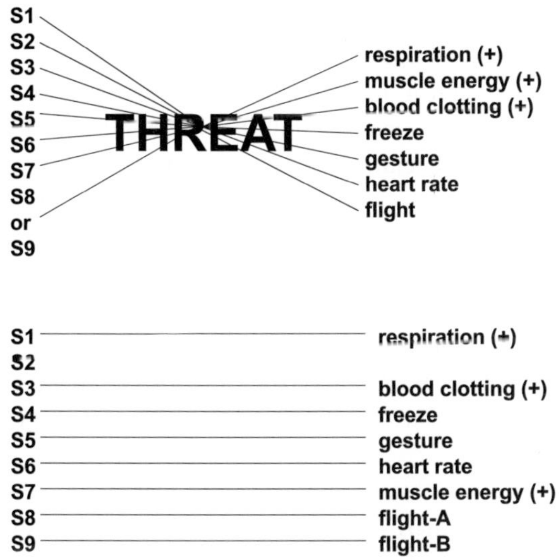

Fig. 5.2 The extremes of the possible neural relations which could have evolved to control responses to threat. The top half of the figure shows the functional relations linking stimuli (S1-S9) to responses where the stimuli may be regular predictors of threat (S1-S7) or where different stimuli are predictive of threat at different times (S8, S9). It can also be viewed as a representation of the simplest view of emotional states, namely that all stimuli activate a single neural representation of threat and this in turn activates the separate response systems. The bottom half of the figure shows, in its most extreme form, the opposite type of neural organization suggested by Hofer's experiments (see text). Here, each response system is under its own private stimulus control.

Source: Reproduced from *New Zealand Journal of Psychology*, 18 (2), Neil McNaughton, 'Anxiety: One label for many processes', p. 53, Figure 1, © Copyright New Zealand Psychological Society, 1989.

blood clotting factor). What is the probability that the neural (or mental) control situation will parallel the logical one represented by the top half of the figure? Is there a single central node which detects all forms of threat and triggers all effector systems? Given the normal workings of mutation and selection, an equally likely scenario will be that shown in the lower part of the figure, each effector system, and each response of each class of effector system, now being under separate control.

William of Occam would not be pleased with this suggestion, and evolutionary arguments are notoriously slippery, so what evidence do we have that such a complicated view might be necessary? One example should suffice to show that we must at least take the possibility seriously.

Separation anxiety occurs in both children and the young of other mammals such as rats, dogs, and primates. When the 'reaction is beyond that expected for the child's developmental level', it becomes[1] Separation Anxiety Disorder (DSM-III-R American Psychiatric Association, 1987, p. 58). In the case of rats, separation anxiety is manifest in both behavioural and autonomic responses. These occur in concert when the mother is removed and

[1] Adult separation anxiety has a higher prevalence with >75% of cases with adult onset (Katherine Shear et al., 2006). We emphasize childhood onset here and quote DSM-III-R as that matches the available non-human data. DSM-5 uses different criteria.

appear, therefore, to be different effector outputs of a single, unified central state. Certainly, one could argue that, if either output were missing, the result would not be separation anxiety. However, it has been shown that the behavioural reactions can be eliminated by the presence of a non-lactating foster mother, while the autonomic reactions can be eliminated by feeding with milk, but not in either case *vice versa* (Hofer, 1972). Thus, the two effector aspects of the 'one emotion' can be doubly dissociated in the laboratory. This does not make the label 'separation anxiety' any less useful, but it does mean that we must view the term as referring only to a particular class of evolutionarily recurring situation (loss of parents) that gives rise to a regular effector pattern (behavioural and autonomic) and hence a consistent central state, but not as referring to, or in any way implying a single central control mechanism. The source of the apparent unity in ecologically normal circumstances is that removal of the mother necessarily eliminates simultaneously both her behavioural and her nutritional support of the pups.

Thus, both for the individual pattern of reactions making up a 'single emotion' on a single occasion and for the patterns making up 'the same emotion' on separate occasions, we must be prepared for apparent coherent, integrated activity to result from the activation of a number of what have been termed 'rules of thumb' (see Krebs et al., 1983). In the current edition the fragments are numerous but, with neural hierarchies mirroring motivational distance, present a coherent two-dimensional picture (McNaughton and Corr, 2004; Silva and McNaughton, 2019) for decision-making. However, new to this edition, is inclusion of the circuitry controlling arousal that, as we have noticed, involves additive rather than subtractive logic and so additional areas (Fig. 11.15) that have been subject to somewhat different selection pressure.

The potential complexity of the neural systems involved in mediating anxiety does not mean, however, that a search for them must be for the proverbial needle in a haystack. On the contrary, our search will be highly focused by the actions of the anxiolytic drugs. Specifically, we shall look for neural systems: a) activity in which is altered by the anxiolytic drugs; and b) dysfunction in which produces behavioural effects similar to anxiolytics (Table 4.1). Nor need we search at random for structures fulfilling these criteria. Given our phylogenetic arguments, the logical place to start our search will be in the limbic system. This is complex enough to subserve the functions we have delineated and phylogenetically old enough to be a realistic common substrate across many organisms. However, in our ethological, learning-theory and pharmacological analyses we have also found it useful to link the operations of the GIS with those of the GRS/FFFS, acting, as they do, to control different modes of response to similar classes of situation. In the next chapter, therefore, we approach the deeper aspects of the limbic system from the direction of the periaqueductal grey, hypothalamus and amygdala, subcortical structures known to be involved in the integration of primary defensive reactions.

6
The neurology of anxiety—survival circuits

6.1 Overview

Here we review the neurology of what we term anxiety in the context of what have recently come to be called 'survival circuits'. Survival circuits 'instantiate functions that allow organisms to survive and thrive by detecting and responding to challenges and opportunities . . . [e.g.] defense, maintenance of energy and nutritional supplies . . . [they] and their adaptive functions *are conserved to a significant degree* across mammalian species, including humans' (LeDoux, 2012, p. 654, our emphasis). We include, in this chapter, a preliminary view of the cingulate cortex; but keep for Chapter 11 prefrontal areas that have undergone a greater degree of phylogenetic differentiation and, we argue in §6.8, involve a different class of processing.

The neural control of defence can appear complex. Even simple classical conditioning of fear to so-called contextual cues (see also §4.6.2) produces noticeable reactions in the allocortex, isocortex, subcortical telencephalon, thalamus, hypothalamus, and many areas of the brainstem; and many of these reactions are reduced (but not eliminated) by peripheral administration of anxiolytics (e.g. Beck and Fibiger, 1995). So, a detailed analysis would require a book at least as large as the present one.

We provide three solutions to this complexity problem: (a) this chapter is largely a summary, with more detail in Appendix 2; (b) in the key area of the amygdala, even at the time of the previous edition, we could depend on excellent reviews (Davis, 1992c; Aggleton, 1993; LeDoux, 1994; LeDoux, 1995; see also Aggleton, 1992; and, for an amygdalo-centric view of emotions in general, LeDoux, 1996; but see also, LeDoux, 2015; Li and Kirouac, 2012; Krout et al., 1998)—and we can now cite similar reviews for other areas; and (c) there is broad agreement about the general organization of the Goal Repulsion System (GRS) and developing consensus for the Goal Inhibition System (GIS).

We present, therefore, a brief largely-consensus view of systems organized hierarchically in terms of both motor control and stimulus analysis; which comprises structures that represent an interface between stimulus and response; and which essentially code for goals. The neural hierarchies we describe (Table 6.1, see also Table 1.1 and Fig. 1.8) build primarily on Graeff (1994) but have other venerable origins that include the opposing of hypothalamic activation by hippocampal inhibition (see McNaughton, 2011, for review). We start with Graeff's view because, even now, the simple picture it presents is one that many would share. We will then show how our own picture diverges from his. We omit discussion of the likely role of the cerebellum in assessing prediction errors and so provide high-speed regulation of integrated cardiac and behavioural responses in defence (da Silva et al., 2023).

The Neuropsychology of Anxiety, Third Edition. Neil McNaughton and Jeffrey A. Gray, Oxford University Press.
 DOI: 10.1093/oso/9780198843313.003.0006

6.1.1 From behavioural hierarchy to neural hierarchy

In terms of behaviour and functions (Table 6.1A), Graeff (1994) starts with the hierarchical primary defence organization of the Blanchards (Chapter 2). Fight (explosive defensive attack, !FIGHT), flight (undirected escape, !FLIGHT), and proximal freezing (!FREEZE) are at the lowest level; and result from a contacting or proximal danger, when there is little time for analysis—which behaviour is observed will depend on freedom of action. Directed escape is at the next level and results from a more distal but clearly present danger (with more time for analysis, more possible responses and outcomes, and more room for learning). We would then include active avoidance of an imminent danger that need not be approached (a category omitted by Graeff). With active avoidance, analysis and motor programming will often have high levels of abstraction and often involve learning. However, it should be noted that the simplest learned avoidance may be supported by tegmental systems (Hormigo et al., 2021; but see also Hormigo et al., 2016).

Above and beyond primary defence, Graeff places risk assessment resulting from a potential predator that must be approached. We would add to this goal inhibition resulting from the high level of conflict generated; and note that, absent a need to approach, simple avoidance is all that is required. This highest level requires not only processing of information by the structures that mediate the competing avoidance and approach, but also additional distinct information processing and priming of action tendencies so as to resolve the discrepancy between the outputs of the approach and avoidance systems.

We would agree with Graeff (1994) that this logical hierarchy at the psychological level maps essentially directly onto the largely hierarchical anatomical and functional organization of the neural systems involved. At the lowest level is the periaqueductal grey (PAG), above that the medial hypothalamus, the amygdala, and septo-hippocampal system (SHS); to which we would add the anterior and posterior cingulate cortices (Table 6.1B).

6.1.2 Adding defensive direction

We diverge from Graeff most importantly by adding to his dimension of defensive *distance* (proximal-distal-uncertain, Table 1A) a quite separate dimension of defensive *direction* (repulsion-conflict resulting from simple avoidance of versus approach to danger; McNaughton and Corr, 2004). In Chapters 2 and 3, we distinguished fear and anxiety as two classes of defence (although others use both these terms differently; McNaughton, 2018). The simplest defence requires only escape or attack controlled by the Goal Repulsion System (GRS) at the base of which is the traditional fight/flight/freeze system (!FFFS[1]). In parallel with this simple defence system is the similarly simple Goal Attraction System (GAS; not included in Table 6.1) at the base of which are the traditional neural modules controlling feeding, drinking, and copulation. Defence becomes more complicated when GRS outputs conflict with GAS outputs. With such goal conflict, control passes to the Goal Inhibition System (GIS). Here, we will paint a picture of the GAS, GIS, and GRS as three parallel

[1] The ! is included to differentiate this label from the earlier FFFS which included all of the current GRS. See also §12.14.

Table 6.1A Levels of defence processing, related behaviours, proposed emotions, and proposed neural substrates. A) as B) key features of an updated two-dimensional (defensive distance/defensive direction) model (McNaughton and Corr, 200 are not included (see Chapter 11). Note that responses to proximal dangers (below the dashed line) are object-specific; reflect both our mapping to components of Table 6.1A and the tendency in the real world for proximal stimuli to be m and GRS—and so, in consequence, the GIS *Abbreviations:* ACC = anterior cingulate cortex; Amyg = amygdala; bl centromedial; dm = dorsomedial; dl = dorsolateral; MH = medial hypothalamus; MR = median raphe; PAG = PeriA hippocampal system.

A. One dimensional model—defensive distance				B. Two-dimensional model defensive distance and defensive direction					
				Repulsion (fear/panic)			Conflict (anxiety)		
Danger	Behaviour	Emotion	CNS	Danger	Behaviour	CNS	Danger	Behaviour	CNS
Uncertain	Risk Assessment	Anxiety	Amyg/SHS	Future (to avoid)	Avoidance (complex)	ACC	Future (to approach)	Avoidance (complex)	PCC
				Imminent (to avoid)	Avoidance (simple)	Amyg (bl)	Imminent (to approach)	Goal Inhibition	SHS
				Imminent (to avoid)	Arousal	Amyg (cm)	Imminent (to approach)	Potentiated Startle	Amyg (bl/cm/BNST)
Distal	Freezing/escape	Fear	PAG-MR-SHS/MH	Distal (to avoid)	Escape Flight (directed)	MH	Distal (to approach)	Risk Assessment	MH
Proximal	Fight/flight	Rage/ panic	PAG	Proximal (to avoid)	!FREEZE !FIGHT !FLIGHT (undirected)	PAG (dm)	Proximal (to approach)	Defensive Quiescence (Conditioned freezing)	PAG (dl)

Table 6.1B Levels of threat processing and related levels of neural integration (largely drawn from Graeff (1994); see text for modifications). See also Fig. 1.8

Level of processing	Behaviour risk assessment and behavioural inhibition	Neural substrate
Potential danger (to approach)		Posterior cingulate Septo-hippocampal system
Potential danger (to avoid)	Avoidance	Anterior cingulate amygdala
Distal danger	Escape Inhibition of aggression	Medial hypothalamus
Proximal danger	Freezing flight fight	Periaqueductal grey

hierarchical systems (see Fig. 6.5B), with the hierarchies of each deriving from defensive or appetitive distance and the GIS interacting with both the GAS and GRS.

The key active output of the GIS, as a survival circuit, is risk assessment (McNaughton and Corr, 2018). For risk assessment to occur, or even for internal memory scanning of possible risks, the active *outputs* of the GAS and GRS must be blocked by inhibitory control from the GIS. Further, even if the cause of risk assessment is conflict detected at a very low neural level such as the PAG (§6.2), the generation of appropriate risk assessment behaviour will usually engage much higher-level circuits (Fig. 6.2B; Motta et al., 2017). So, the neurologies of the GAS and GRS are not only parallel to but also intertwined with the neurology of the GIS. A further complication is that goal conflict need not involve fear proper. We concluded that anxiety can also result from frustrative non-reward. However, fear is the clearest precursor of anxiety (and many of its key proximal behaviours, such as aggression, are shared with frustrative non-reward); so, we will focus on fear for the neurology of the GRS and GIS discussed next.

Our first specific point of divergence from Graeff is that, as discussed earlier, we do not equate !FREEZE with behavioural/goal inhibition, and so we do not see the SHS as mediating freezing, in this most basic sense of the word. The highest intensity of freezing occurs in response to a proximal predator, and usually precedes explosive attack or flight. Like Graeff, we believe that both high intensity freezing and explosive attack are mediated by the PAG. This !FREEZE response forms an integral part of a set of behaviour patterns that remove the animal from the dangerous situation.

As noted earlier (Chapter 2), the problem with any distinction between high intensity behavioural inhibition and at least low intensity freezing is that both are most easily characterized by an absence of behaviour. This, no doubt, is the basis for Graeff's amalgamation of the two. Our own analysis bears a greater burden of theory. We use the term 'behavioural/goal inhibition' to indicate that there is indeed a form of behaviour that is being inhibited, in particular, a form of approach behaviour. In the theoretically simplest case, this is approach to an appetitive goal (e.g. food, water, or merely a part of the environment that might contain these valuable commodities). In a more complex case, the approach behaviour that is inhibited is approach to safety, as in a learned escape or active avoidance response, which (like approach to an appetitive goal) we see as mediated by the GAS. Thus, in our usage, 'behavioural inhibition' does not necessarily imply a cessation of all behaviour. Indeed, it can, and often does, occur concurrently with *active* risk assessment. It is only at the shorter defensive distances (e.g. when close to contact with a predator) that complete behavioural inhibition occurs. As we have seen, behavioural inhibition, in this sense, appears distinguishable from !FREEZE by being sensitive to anxiolytics (Chapter 2) and, less tautologically, by the body postures adopted, e.g. the 'stretched attend' posture which would not be seen in true freezing. Blanchard and Blanchard (1996) have suggested the term 'defensive quiescence' to refer to this type of behaviour. It should be noted that freezing (GRS), quiescence (GIS), and lordosis (GAS) are all proximally-elicited forms of stillness that may only be distinguishable in terms of posture at high intensities.

Our second specific point of divergence from Graeff's scheme results from defensive direction (Table 6.1B). We agree that the SHS is neurally and logically above the amygdala. However, as far as active avoidance (repulsion) tendencies are concerned, the linear sequence with increasing defensive distance is: dorsomedial PAG →medial hypothalamus →cortico-medial amygdala →anterior cingulate. In contrast, with passive avoidance (conflict/goal inhibition) the linear sequence with increasing defensive distance is: dorsolateral and ventrolateral PAG (Silva and McNaughton, 2019) →medial hypothalamus[2] →basolateral amygdala [arousal]/SHS[decision][3] →posterior cingulate.

6.1.3 Hierarchical (quick and dirty versus slow and sophisticated) stimulus inputs

The separate, but also hierarchical, organization we describe for stimulus processing is largely that proposed by LeDoux (LeDoux, 1992; LeDoux, 1994; LeDoux, 1995; LeDoux, 1996). On this view, several levels of sensory processing are connected, independently, to each single structure such as the amygdala.

For example, the amygdala receives input from both the visual thalamus and from the highest levels of visual cortex. The central underlying principle of this type of organization is illustrated in Fig. 6.1. The lowest levels of stimulus processing provide the amygdala with only partially digested information, but they do so with greater speed than the higher levels.

Having parallel inputs to the amygdala results in a number of useful properties. It allows extremely fast processing of the simplest and most discriminable danger stimuli. In the case of complex or poorly discriminable stimuli, it allows for priming (rather than full blown activation) of defence circuits by lower levels of processing to speed up the subsequent response to input from higher levels of processing. Finally, it allows for receipt by the defence system of information about danger from the very highest levels of cognitive analysis, even if such danger has not been detected by any of the lower levels.

> Animals, and humans, need a quick-and-dirty reaction mechanism.... Failing to respond to danger is more costly than responding inappropriately to a benign stimulus.... Details are irrelevant and, in fact, detrimental to an efficient, speedy and potentially lifesaving reaction.

[2] This will be a different part of the medial hypothalamus for the GIS as compared to GRS, with the lateral hypothalamus for the GAS.

[3] Note that arousal summates across the motivational systems, while decision is competitive.

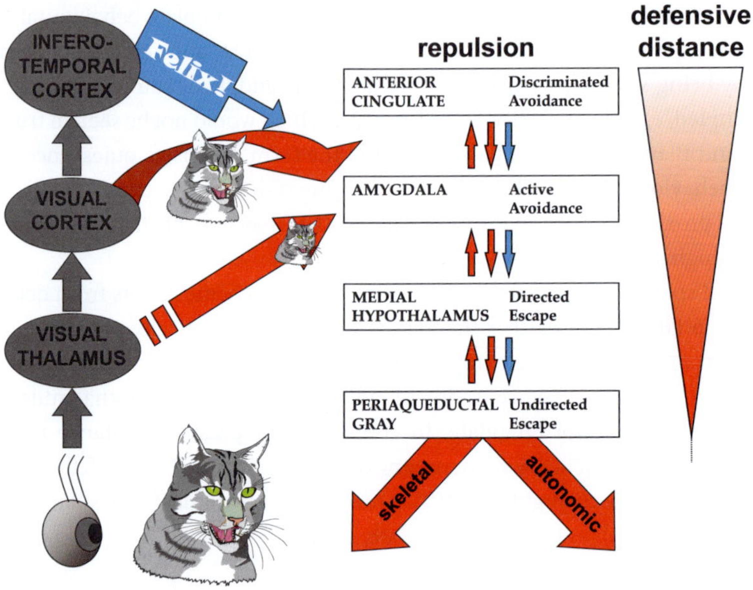

Fig. 6.1 'Quick and dirty' versus 'slow and sophisticated' processing of threat stimuli. The cat in the external world creates impulses at the retina which proceed to the visual areas of the thalamus and then quickly via a direct pathway to the amygdala. The representation in the thalamus will be very sketchy but will allow either priming, or generation, of escape responses with the minimum of delay. Slower processing, via the various levels of primary visual and inferotemporal cortex will ultimately produce a more detailed and exact classification of the stimulus, which will then also be sent to the amygdala—allowing either completion of escape or, if the quick and dirty system produced a false alarm (as when the cat is identified as a friend called 'Felix'), cancellation of the escape response. (See LeDoux 1995, Fig. 2 for the snake/human original on which this cat/rat Fig. is based.) Note that similar parallel inputs will go to all levels of the defence system and the reciprocal connections shown will allow transfer of excitation (red arrows) from lower to higher areas and transfer of excitation and inhibition (blue arrows) of unwanted outputs from higher to lower areas. **Source:** Fig. and legend are modified from Gray and McNaughton (2000, Fig. 6.1 and 1.8).

> The brain simply needs to be able to store primitive cues and detect them. Later, coordination of this basic information with the cortex permits verification... or brings the reaction to a stop.
>
> LeDoux (1994, p. 38)

6.1.4 Warp and weft in 'The Enchanted Loom'

As we describe next, this parallel organization of perceptual inputs, coupled with the capacity for plasticity of synapses in the amygdala, provides a simple basis for the learned association of a wide variety of stimuli with output from that part of the defence system. It also provides a basis for the evolution of innate threat stimuli. However, essentially the same inputs interact as a weft with the warp of the hierarchical defence system in The Enchanted Loom[4] of the brain to produce the magic cloak that defends us from threat (see also §6.7).

The parallel inputs can activate all levels of the hierarchy and, when quick and dirty is incorrect, slow and sophisticated must take over. In Fig. 6.1 (and elsewhere) therefore we have inserted bi-directional arrows to flag the passage of threat information both from lower levels to activate higher levels and from higher levels to activate lower levels. Importantly, the downward flow also includes control signals that block inappropriate aspects of quick-and-dirty responses (e.g. undirected escape) while retaining useful aspects (e.g. autonomic) and allowing higher centres to control behaviour (e.g. directed escape, simple avoidance) without interference from more primitive responses.

When we compare the schemes of Graeff and LeDoux, we see that the SHS figures in both but differently. Graeff sees it as the top level of the hierarchical defence control system for both fear and anxiety. LeDoux sees the SHS as one of the highest levels of the threat analysis system, essentially a stage *beyond* polysensory neocortex (despite its greater phylogenetic age and simple architectonics). The picture we shall paint of the SHS to some extent combines these points of view but, as discussed in Appendix 3, sees the anterior cingulate cortex, not SHS as the 'top' of the active defence survival circuits, providing a transition to the planning circuits of prefrontal cortex.

However, as will become clear when we consider the SHS in detail in the following chapters, we agree

> that limbic circuits are loops, rather than one-way streams of information flow. Anxiety arises from activity in these circuits when ambiguous environmental stimuli are interpreted as threatening.... The highly interconnected circuits... 'interpret' the meaning of those stimuli and determine whether they portend danger.... Additional circuits including the PFC and nuclei at the intersection of the limbic system and motor effectors must evaluate whether the external events reflect expectations and whether they meet or contradict the animal's needs in order to engage the appropriate... downstream motor pathways, brainstem nuclei in control of autonomic responses, and the neuroendocrine system.
>
> (Calhoon and Tye, 2015, p. 1400)

A final point to note about Table 6.1B is that, while we have provided a completely symmetrical two-dimensional scheme at the *qualitative* level, a less symmetric view is possible at the *quantitative* level. In particular, because we have removed 'uncertainty' as a key defining construct (used by both Graeff and the Blanchards), we allow for quite distant and uncertain pure fears (see §6.7 on the anterior cingulate). Note here, that the extended amygdala (unlike frontal cortex) does not appear to respond differently to uncertainty versus certainty (Hur et al., 2020). However, at the quantitative level and in practice, uncertainty is likely to generate goal conflict; and, further, the perception of uncertainty can be aversive. Similarly, while a proximal threat may generate anxiety (if it is balanced by a similarly strong appetitive input), it is much more likely to generate fear; whereas a future one is more likely to generate anxiety. So, our shaded areas in Table 6.1B reflect not only our mapping to components of Table 6.1A but also the tendency in the real world for proximal stimuli to be *more likely* to

[4] Originally coined by Sherrington, according to Wikipedia (https://en.wikipedia.org/wiki/Enchanted_loom).

activate the GRS and distal ones to activate both the GAS and GRS—and so, in consequence, the GIS (for a human fMRI example, see Hur et al., 2020).

Having briefly described the defence survival circuits as a whole, we now provide more detail on each element, starting with the lowest and proceeding to the highest. We will take much of the neurology of the lower levels of the defence system as given.[5] As noted in the previous chapter, the key tool we shall use to draw a line between the GRS and GIS lies in the behavioural effects of the anti-anxiety drugs (Chapter 4 and Appendix 1). We shall compare the resulting 'behavioural profile' of these compounds with that of specific lesions of the key candidate structures (Table 4.2), in the belief that anxiolytics are likely to act like a lesion of those neural structures most involved in the control of anxiety. Where data are available, we also take particular note of the effects produced by injecting anxiolytics directly into the structures of interest. (Detailed consideration of the advantages and problems of this strategy of drug-lesion comparison is provided in Appendix 8.)

6.2 The periaqueductal grey (PAG)

Note: This section draws heavily on a major review by Carlos Silva, in which appropriate citations will be found (Silva and McNaughton, 2019).

The PAG appears to be the lowest command level of the GRS, GIS, and GAS (Fig. 6.2; see also Motta et al., 2017; Reis et al., 2021a).

> Many see the PAG as a region responsible for the downstream control of defensive reactions. Here we [include] the dorsal raphe, which completes the circle of periaqueductal nuclei.... We provide a comprehensive functional view of the PAG, going beyond simple panic and escape to integrate data on fear, anxiety, and depression. Importantly, we conclude that this periaqueductal cluster of nuclei is broadly involved in motivated behavior controlling not only aversive but also appetitive behavior and with some involvement in more complex motivational processes such as approach-avoidance conflict resolution. In sum, these highly conserved nuclei surrounding the aqueduct appear to be the simplest, foundational, elements of integrated motivated goal-directed control of all types.
>
> Silva and McNaughton (2019, p. 33).

Stimulation of the PAG can elicit a range of environmentally dependent integrated defence responses; and it also appears to *mediate* the control of such responses by higher-level systems (see also §6.1.4) with, in rodents and humans, 'a prominent role... in more complex processes, including representing behavioral states and influencing fear learning and memory' (Reis et al., 2023, p. 1). With strong stimulation, and an appropriate nearby object, 'all of the behavioural signs of defence, including directed attack, are found within the periaqueductal grey' (Bandler and Carrive, 1988)—including, from posterior dorsal PAG, the explosive, undirected escape typical of an animal in close proximity to a predator. It should be noted that its function organization is not completely columnar, the sparse, distinct, cholecystokinin

[5] Detailed reviews are provided for the periaqueductal grey (Appendix 2; (Silva and McNaughton, 2019)), medial hypothalamus and amygdala (Appendix 2); the SHS (Chapters 7–10, Appendices 4–9, McNaughton and Bannerman, 2024); and the cingulate and prefrontal cortices (Appendix 3).

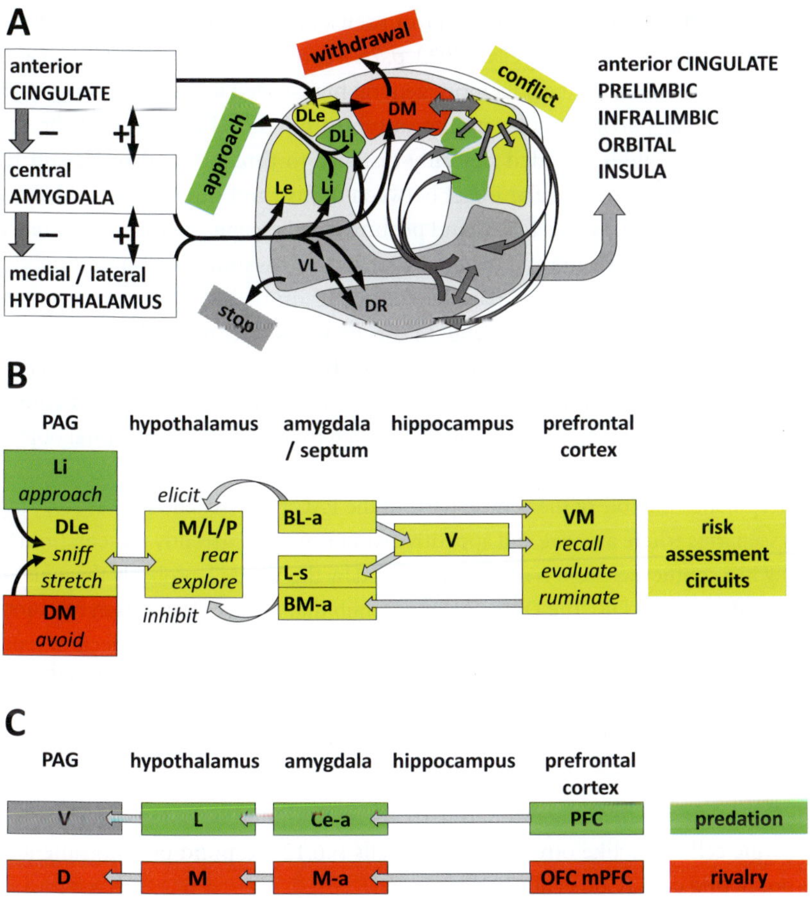

Fig. 6.2 A. Diagrammatic representation of the organisation of GAS (approach), GRS (withdrawal), and GIS (conflict) within the PAG. The VL PAG and DR are treated as related serotonergic areas. The internal and external parts of the L and DL PAG are functionally distinct; as is DM PAG. Note that approach (e.g., lordosis, prey pursuit) is somewhat more associated with rostral PAG and avoidance with caudal. Other important rostro-caudal distinctions that we have ignored in this figure are detailed in Silva and McNaughton (2019). **B.** Simplified picture of risk assessment circuits. **C.** simplified circuits for predatory and defensive aggression. *Abbreviations:* a = amygdala; Ce = central; D = dorsal; e = external; i = internal; L = lateral; M/m = medial; OFC = orbital frontal cortex; P = posterior; PFC = prefrontal cortex; R = raphe; V = ventral.

Sources: A—modified from Figure 16 of Silva and McNaughton (2019). **B—Fig.** modified from graphical abstract for McNaughton and Corr (2018) for greater detail see Motta et al. (2017); (Ennis et al., 1997). **C—modified** from Haller (2018).

(CCK) expressing cells appear to drive flight to safe regions (but not other reactions) and do so even within the lateral and dorso-lateral PAG that are more associated with freezing (La-Vu et al., 2022).

Interestingly, input to the cuneiform nucleus from the dPAG can elicit *goal-directed* flight, which 'suggests that critical spatial information required for remembering, orienting to, and actively tracking shelter position reaches the defensive escape pathway downstream of dPAG, possibly as a result of converging afferents from sensory-receptive areas in superior and inferior colliculus and cortex' (Tsang et al., 2023, p. 7). At present it appears that direct activation of the cuneiform nucleus itself elicits more general high-speed locomotion; and so, it seems likely that additional, particularly ascending, outputs from dPAG support goal-directedness.

Dorsal PAG 'ensembles encoded not only distance to threat, but also relevant features, such as predator speed and angular offset between mouse and threat.... [and] defensive behaviours, including freezing, stretch-attend postures, and escape... with a shared representation to encode these behaviours and distance to threat across innate and conditioned threats' (Reis et al., 2021b, p. 5399). It has parallel control of immediate defensive responses and aversive learning via nitric oxide-dependent mechanisms (Acuna et al., 2023). Graeff (e.g. 1994) views the PAG as being the principal locus for generating panic in human beings.

Especially with the inclusion of the dorsal raphe (DR) within the circle of structures round the aqueduct; and seeing the PAG generally as limited to proximal motivational objects,

> we conceptualize the role of the ventral parts of the PAG (VLPAG and DR) as stopping action in scenarios where aversive and appetitive stimuli are concurrently present. Immediate stopping in a conflict scenario is mostly conducted by the VLPAG, probably through inputs from the DLPAG and DR. The DLPAG acts as a hub that receives input from relevant cortical and subcortical regions that aid in resolving these goal conflicts. The effects of repeated conflicts generate a more systemic reduction in drive, which is mediated by the DR sending inhibitory inputs to the motivational regions of the PAG and the forebrain.
>
> Silva and McNaughton (2019, p. 57)

While DR is often seen as a serotonergic structure, it should be noted that it also contains dopaminergic cells that, like other dopamine cells (§6.12) respond both to salience and to reward-predicting cues (Cho et al., 2021).

While we will next emphasize connections between adjacent levels of the defence system (with the hypothalamus being particularly strongly connected to PAG) it should be noted (Fig. 6.2A) that PAG both receives input from midline frontal cortical areas and (particularly in the case of DR) sends output to them. Indeed, in the case of proximal risk assessment, conflict detected in PAG may elicit responses in higher-level circuits (Fig. 6.2B). There are, then, direct connections between the top and the bottom of the hierarchy as well indirect. In contrast to higher levels of the defence system, the PAG/DR complex has no direct *input from* the SHS; while ventral aspects of PAG/DR do send *output to* the hippocampal formation.

6.3 The hypothalamus

The medial hypothalamus is in many ways functionally similar to PAG. Matching Graeff's suggestion for the PAG, Shekhar (1994) has suggested that activation of the dorso-medial hypothalamic 'cardiostimulatory' area can give rise to panic; likely due to spill over of activation to the PAG (see also Esteban Masferrer et al., 2020).

However, escape responses elicited from the medial hypothalamus lack upright jumping and are interspersed with rearing, suggesting a greater defensive distance and possibly some shift in defensive direction. Notably, escape elicited from the medial hypothalamus is blocked by lesions of the PAG (and not *vice versa*); and medial hypothalamic lesions increase aggression, whereas PAG lesions decrease it. With other data (Appendix 2), these suggest that the medial hypothalamus represents the next level up in the GRS. Increased aggression would result from loss of hypothalamic inhibition of the quicker, dirtier PAG when controlling aggressive behaviour (see also Yamaguchi and Lin, 2018); and with 'distributed encoding of sensory and motor features in the medial hypothalamic-brainstem instinctive network' (Esteban Masferrer et al., 2020, p. 9283). In particular, the medial hypothalamic defence area acts as a way station for both ascending and descending circuits between the amygdala and PAG (see Fig. 2 in Canteras, 2002), with ascending and descending collaterals producing distinct results via their different targets (e.g. avoidance and immobility, respectively, Wang et al., 2015; or spatially versatile and panic-related flight, respectively, Wang et al., 2021). Effects of ascending activation of the thalamus by a predator provide a basis for 'contextual' fear conditioning.

While activation of the medial hypothalamus can increase experimental anxiety in various animal tests, it also increases escape and avoidance. In particular, it appears to be a locus at which social defeat can enable social avoidance (Krzywkowski et al., 2020). Thus, the increases in, e.g. rearing produced by activation could be due to a simple increase in fear under conditions where this can conflict with prepotent responses. However, there is some indication of effects of anxiolytics on the medial hypothalamus (Appendix 2; Talalaenko et al., 2003; Jardim and Guimaraes, 2001; Milani and Graeff, 1987; Shekhar, 1993; Shekhar et al., 1993; Silveira and Graeff, 1992; but see also Woodnorth and McNaughton, 2005), and particularly the supramammillary area (Woodnorth and McNaughton, 2002b; Pan and McNaughton, 1997). There are also good reasons to see the medial hypothalamus—and particularly the perifornical area (Horii et al., 2020)—as part of an anxiety/risk assessment system originating in the PAG (Fig. 6.2B; Motta et al., 2017) and so contributing to the GIS. There is topographic output from the SHS to the hypothalamus, which we will consider in detail in Chapter 9, especially Fig. 9.7.

While our focus is on the GRS and GIS here, it is worth noting that the *lateral* hypothalamus can be viewed as being part of the GAS (McNaughton et al., 2016), with the hypothalamus as a whole acting 'as a central gateway modulating homeostatic and nonhomeostatic drives' (De Silva et al., 2012, p. 1). Conversely there is evidence that avoidance of a predator-odour-paired context (likely mediated by the GRS, see Chapter 2) is controlled by output from the central amygdala to the lateral hypothalamus (Weera et al., 2021).

6.4 The amygdala

6.4.1 A general role in emotion

As with the PAG and hypothalamus (medial + lateral) we will argue that distinct parts of the amygdala contains components of the GAS, GIS, and GRS. Lesions of the amygdala produce much wider emotional deficits (the Klüver-Bucy syndrome) than would be expected if it were a purely defensive structure (see, e.g. LeDoux, 1992). It is a locus at which, quite generally,

> sensory stimuli are endowed with emotional and motivational significance... Thus, when the amygdala is damaged, monkeys act tame in the presence of humans because the sight of a

> human is no longer coded as a threatening stimulus. Similarly, *dietary and sexual preferences change since environmental stimuli no longer elicit their normal affective responses.*
>
> (LeDoux, 1992, p. 340, our emphasis).

> The amygdala is a 'polymath',... a nodal point in the control of several emotions and behaviors, including anxiety, depression, drug dependence and addiction, learning and memory, sexual behavior, pain, etc. It also plays important roles in aggression control. General theories of human aggression place the amygdala somewhere between cortical decision making centers and hypothalamic and/or brainstem centers of execution.
>
> (Haller, 2018, p. 34)

Indeed, even if we limit our observations to aggression of different types (rivalry/defensive; predatory/appetitive), we get a picture of separate streams passing through different parts of the same hierarchy of structures (Fig. 6.2C) and even food-liking and consumption decisions appear to involve distributed representations within the amygdala (Tiedemann et al., 2020).

Given the anatomical and functional complexity of the amygdala, we shall follow a strategy that we apply later, on a much larger scale, to the SHS. We attempt to combine the anatomical, lesion and physiological data into a coherent picture, in the hope that each discipline will correct the faults inherent in the others. We concentrate on the role of the amygdala in anxiety and omit, for example, any discussion of its possible role in the symptomatology of depression (e.g. Schulkin, 1994; Schulkin et al., 1994; ; Abler et al., 2007; Holmes et al., 2012; Ludwig et al., 2015). We start with the anatomy of the amygdala because its details provide a solid foundation for findings in the other disciplines.

6.4.2 The amygdala: anatomy

Note: We take much of this section without detailed attribution, and much simplified, from Sah et al. (2003); (see also Appendix 2, and Amaral et al., 1992).

The amygdala is extremely complex (~13 nuclei, differing in cellular composition and connections, and with some variation across species), with even human fMRI studies differentiating as many as 10 areas (Boccardi et al., 2011). Its nuclei can be grouped into four clusters (Table 6.2).

A straightforward, simplified view sees the main information flow as essentially unidirectional: from lateral to basal to centromedial (Fig. 6.3A). The amygdala appears to receive, in the lateral nucleus, information that can be used to identify affective situations (e.g. threat). This information is sent directly (i.e. without influence from additional information received by the basal and central amygdala) from the lateral nucleus to the hippocampal formation (particularly the entorhinal cortex) and to the dorsomedial thalamus.

The basal nucleus has an unusually reciprocal (and unusually restricted) connection with the hippocampal formation and also has extensive reciprocal connections with the frontal and cingulate cortices. In the latter case, we suggest that the projection to the cortex provides information about affect, with the return projection providing information about current plans (essentially read out from working memory). This reciprocity between the basal

Table 6.2 Grouping of amygdala nuclei into related clusters based on Sah et al. (2003); (see also the stria terminalis is normally treated as part of the extended amygdala rather than amygdala pro

Cluster	Basolateral	Cortical-like	Centromedial	Other
Nuclei	Accessory Basal/ basomedial	Nucleus of the lateral olfactory tract	Central nucleus	Anterior nucleus
	Basal/basolateral	Bed nucleus of the accessory Olfactory tract	Medial nucleus	amygdalo-hippocampal area
	Lateral	Periamygdaloid cortex	(bed nucleus of the stria terminalis)	intercalated cell masses
		Anterior cortical nucleus		
		Posterior cortical nucleus		

amygdala and the neocortex could allow a recursive updating of current plans in the context of the predicted affective consequences. When we discuss the SHS in detail, we shall argue for a roughly similar, but more hippocampopetal, organization. The basal nucleus also provides output to all levels of visual processing in the cortex. We suggest that this could provide an affective bias to the processing of incoming information. The main clearly unidirectional output of the basal nucleus is to the striatum; this could provide affective bias to ongoing motor programmes and their modification.

The centromedial complex receives information from both the lateral and basal areas. This organization raises the possibility that the centromedial complex takes into account, not only the primary affective information being determined in the lateral nucleus, but also the interaction between that information and concurrent processing in the frontal cortex, cingulate cortex, and hippocampal formation relayed via the basal nucleus. The primary output of the centromedial complex, in contrast to that of the basal nucleus, is subcortical and appears to involve interaction with a range of detailed 'lower' level units of affective control for which the amygdala represents a higher-level of integrated control, the hierarchical organization of which terminates in PAG (see Fig. 6.4). The central amygdala also sends output more rostrally, e.g. to the globus pallidus, that is likely to be involved in fear conditioning (Giovanniello et al., 2020).

> Each portion of the prefrontal cortex has a distinctive projection to the amygdala. The ventral areas of the lateral and medial prefrontal cortices, which receive olfactory projections, are the only prefrontal cortical areas with projections to the olfactory-related superficial amygdaloid nuclei. The more dorsally situated prefrontal areas, the dorsal agranular insular area and prelimbic cortex, have complementary projections to the basal nucleus.
>
> McDonald et al. (1996)

Similarly, 'The perirhinal area, along with other areas in the frontal cortex that project to the amygdala, receive reciprocal connections from the LA, B, AB, M, and periamygdaloid cortex. The cortical nuclei that receive olfactory projections all send substantial reciprocal

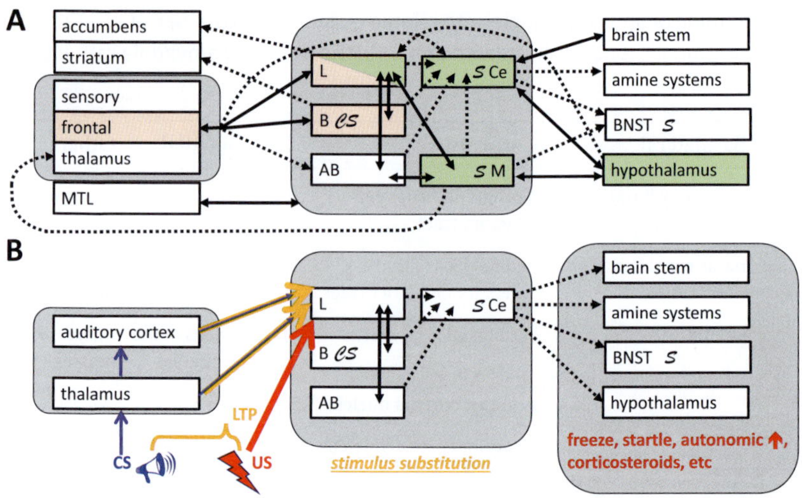

Fig. 6.3 Greatly simplified picture of amygdala anatomy and involvement in learning. **A.** Complex sensory (particularly olfactory) and memory information arrives in the basolateral area (primary input stages shaded pink). There are substantial reciprocal connections with the frontal cortex to the lateral area (L) and basal area (B). The basal, accessory basal (AB), and medial (M) areas supply increasing processing steps within the amygdala that finish (primary output stages shaded green) in unidirectional connections converging on the central amygdala (Ce). Central and medial output is via reciprocal connection to the hypothalamus and brainstem; and via unidirectional connections to the ascending amine systems (cholinergic, serotonergic, and noradrenergic) and to the bed nucleus of the stria terminalis (BNST). There are reciprocal connections between various parts of the medial temporal lobe 'memory' system (MTL) and the amygdala as a whole. There are limited specific inputs from hippocampal area CA1 (C) to the basal area; and from the subiculum (S) to the basal, central and medial areas. For a more complex picture and evidence for the connections in the Fig., see Sah et al. (2003); (see also Appendix 2, and Amaral et al., 1992; Cullinan et al., 1993). **B.** Slow and fast stimulus inputs (c.f. Fig. 6.1) of 'weak' stimuli (e.g., a tone/CS) converge on the L area, but normally have no effect (blue arrows). If paired in time with an input that <u>does</u> have an effect (e.g., shock/UCS) the simple association causes LTP and so stimulus substitution; and the tone now elicits at least some of those effects elicited by the shock. Note the parallels with innate responses (Fig. 6.1).

projections back to the olfactory cortex' (Sah et al., 2003, p. 809). The amygdala, then, may share the organization into a dorsal and ventral trend that we shall discuss in more detail for the frontal cortex (see next and Appendix 3) and SHS.

6.4.3 The amygdala: effects of lesions

The amygdala is clearly involved in a wide range of motivations. It may be the most important structure for fear. However, in human patients with amygdala lesions, CO_2 inhalation induces not only panic but also fear suggesting that the amygdala is required only for the triggering of fear by external rather than internal threats (Feinstein et al., 2013). Further, even in simple Pavlovian fear conditioning (Fig. 6.3B) 'a simple model involving plasticity of synapses made by a given input in one structure cannot entirely account for the complexity of the

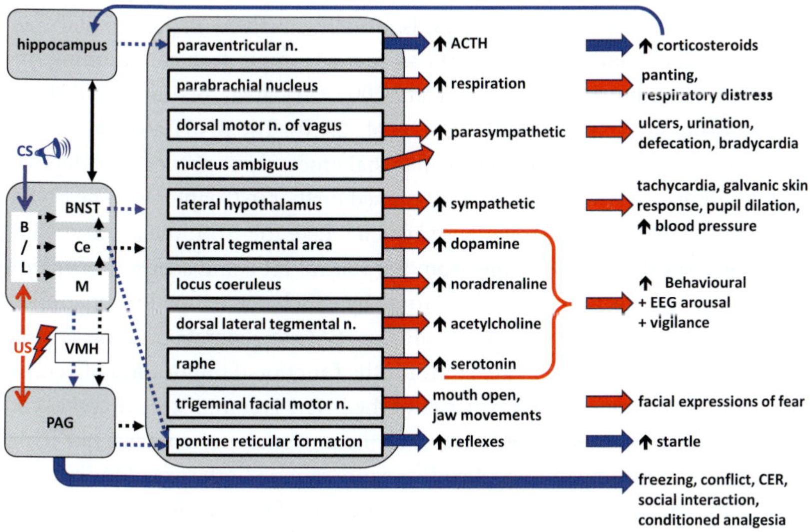

Fig. 6.4 Outputs from the amygdala produced by either an unconditioned stimulus (US) such as a shock, or a conditioned stimulus (CS) such as a tone previously paired with a US. 'CS' can also be read as a Complex Stimulus that is diffuse and/or unpredictable. In both cases, the amygdala can be viewed as the final stage where 'fear' (red arrows) or 'anxiety' (blue arrows) is encoded in its full form before signals are sent to separate areas that deal with specific desired outputs. Thus, a total amygdala lesion blocks all of the outputs listed while stimulation or lesions of the anatomical targets of the amygdala (other than the PAG) produce or block only the indicated subsets of effects (based on Davis et al., 1994) (Davis, 2006). Importantly for our hierarchical model, the PAG has parallel outputs to all the same nuclei as the amygdala and so can produce the same reactions in response to an unconditional stimulus but with much less nuanced stimulus control (Silva and McNaughton, 2019; Krout et al., 1998; Li and Kirouac, 2012; Ennis et al., 1997; Farkas et al., 1997). PAG is thus the true end of the line for integrated innate responses, but the amygdala (coupled with the PAG) is the key area for conditioned, and more complex, reactions. Anticipatory stimuli can release ACTH (and so then corticosteroids) via the paraventricular nucleus and it is noteworthy that the negative feedback control of this release is via corticosteroid receptors in the hippocampus.

phenomenon of learning' (Sah et al., 2003, p. 827). The key question, here, is 'how far is the amygdala the central structure for anxiety?'.

We previously reviewed the effects of amygdala lesions (Appendix 2). These are compared with the effects of anxiolytics, septal lesions, and hippocampal lesions in Table 4.2. The list of behavioural effects of amygdala lesions is both positively and negatively discrepant from the anxiolytic drug syndrome. Lesions of the amygdala decrease one-way active avoidance, decrease two-way active avoidance (in the basolateral but increase in the central, see also §6.8, Fig. 6.5C, D), increase rearing, and decrease the double-runway frustration effect. In all of these cases anxiolytics (and, as discussed further next, septal and hippocampal lesions) are without effect or have the opposite effect. Conversely, lesions of the amygdala are without effect on most delayed matching to sample tasks and on behaviour reinforced on fixed interval schedules. Both of these are affected by anxiolytics (and, again, by SHS lesions). It follows that, if anxiolytic drug effects are a good (inverse) guide to the nature of anxiety, anxiety does not easily map onto enhanced amygdala function.

Further, while the basolateral complex is usually involved in 'contextual' (as is the basomedial area, Rajbhandari et al., 2021) as well as simple fear conditioning, it can be bypassed by overtraining (Ponnusamy et al., 2007) via areas of the BNST that receive hippocampal formation (HPF) input (Poulos et al., 2010). The BNST also appears to be one of the key targets of inhibitory paraventricular thalamic output needed for adaptive choice between competing goals (McNally, 2021, discussed further in Chapter 9). 'The BNST is capable of undergoing experience-dependent plasticity. Like the BLA, the anteromedial group of the BNST receives direct projections from the ventral HPF and sends information to the vPAG. Such neural connectivity provides a route by which contextual information encoded by the HPF could bypass the BLA and activate the vPAG to generate freezing' (Poulos et al., 2010, p. 14881; see also Oleksiak et al., 2021, for the functional importance of ventral as opposed to dorsal hippocampal input). The role of the BNST is complex since context fear conditioning activates anterolateral BNST input to the amygdala in male but not female rats; while large BNST lesions impaired context fear expression in both sexes. Similarly, while the caudal part of the BLA appears to mediate some aspects of response suppression by punishment, it does not appear to mediate choice between an unpunished and a punished alternative (Jean-Richard-dit-Bressel and McNally, 2015).

6.4.4 The amygdala: single cell responses

The complexity of cellular responding in the amygdala is considered in some detail in Appendix 2. Many single cells respond, each relatively selectively, to a wide range of stimuli: visual, auditory, objects, faces, novelty, reward, punishment—even heights (Liu et al., 2021). There appears to be a progression from relatively high stimulus selectivity in the lateral amygdala to relatively low selectivity in the centro-medial amygdala (with the basolateral nucleus intermediate). Changing the affective associations of a stimulus frequently changes the response of the amygdala to that stimulus. Interestingly, *extinction* of fear is encoded in BLA 'reward' neurons that then inhibit the BLA neurons encoding the fear (Zhang et al., 2020b). The extent of response often seems tied to what could be termed the 'importance' of the stimulus and in the central amygdala appears to encode a 'salience' signal (see also §6.12) biased to unconditioned stimuli that is necessary for both appetitive and aversive learning (Steinberg et al., 2020). The coding of importance is also true of the coding of responses. With BLA principal neurons during benzodiazepine-sensitive punishment learning

> excitatory activity transients to the footshock punisher and inhibitory transients to lever-presses... activity around the punished response transformed from inhibitory to excitatory and similarity analyses showed that these punished lever-press transients resembled BLA transients to the punisher itself.... the degree to which [benzodiazepine] alleviated punishment was associated with how much punished response-related BLA transients reverted to their prepunishment state. Together, these findings show that punishment learning is supported by aversion-coding of instrumental responses in the BLA and that the anti-punishment effects of benzodiazepines are associated with a reversion of this aversion coding.
>
> (Jean-Richard-dit-Bressel et al., 2021, p. 1)

So, stimulus processing *per se* appears to depend on other parts of the brain; and amygdala firing appears to signal affective value and to precede autonomic changes and freezing. Thus, the firing of amygdala cells may relate more to the programming of output than to the detection of particular complex events. Importantly, with conditioned stimuli, distinct groups of cells in the BLA are activated by appetitive (R) and aversive (S) stimuli, respectively (and inhibited by the opposite valence stimulus).

> When the CS-S was presented in the safe context, rats entered a long-lasting, anxiety-like state characterized by increased inter-CS freezing and impaired reward seeking. During this state, a subset of BL cells ('state cells') showed sustained shifts in baseline activity whose time course matched that of the behavioral changes. Many state cells with increased firing rates were S cells, whereas R cells only included state cells with reduced firing rates. Thus, anxiety involves persistent activity changes that are differentially expressed by subsets of valence-specific BL neurons.
>
> (Lee et al., 2017, p. 81)

The long-lasting nature of the freezing elicited when a signal of danger was presented in a previously safe place could be the basis for the persistence of anxiety and, in an extreme form, be a substrate for anxiety disorders (Sah, 2017). Here, we should note that such second-order conditioning creates a CS_2–CS_1 link within the BLA that allows the context (CS_2) to track (via the CS_1-US link) the threat level of the US (Lingawi et al., 2021).

6.4.5 The amygdala: effects of anxiolytics

The discrepancies between the effects of anxiolytics and those of amygdala lesions (Table 4.2) suggest that the amygdala is not a 'single anxiety centre'. But, as with PAG and the medial hypothalamus, it appears have at least some involvement in anxiolytic action.

> The amygdala has a high density of benzodiazepine receptors... Local infusion of benzodiazepines into the amygdala (for review see Davis, 1992a) has anxiolytic effects in the operant conflict test, social interaction test, measures of conditioned freezing and hypoalgesia [and] the light-dark box test in mice... However, benzodiazepines can still have anxiolytic effects in animals with lesions of the amygdala.
>
> (Davis et al., 1994, pp. 212–213)

Intra-amygdaloid benzodiazepine injection has also been reported to impair step-down passive avoidance (Tomaz et al., 1993; Harris and Westbrook, 1995), shock-probe avoidance (Pesold and Treit, 1994), conditioned suppression of drinking (Shibata et al., 1989), measures of anxiety and memory in the elevated T maze (Tomaz et al., 1993), and thigmotaxis in an open field (McNamara and Skelton, 1993). Despite the effect of amygdala lesions on conditioned suppression of drinking, they do not appear to interact with the effects of benzodiazepines on this test (Kopchia et al., 1992); and may even increase the effects of anxiolytics (Yadin et al., 1991).

In contrast, injection of benzodiazepines into the amygdala normally has no effect on water maze learning (McNamara and Skelton, 1993), on behaviour in the elevated plus-maze or on defensive burying (Treit et al., 1993a; Pesold and Treit, 1994). The lack of involvement of the amygdala in the latter two cases is also shown by the fact that amygdala lesions neither affect behaviour by themselves, nor interact with the effects of systemic benzodiazepines on these measures (Treit et al., 1993a). More detailed analysis of parts of the amygdala may be required, however, since it appears that effects in the plus-maze and in passive avoidance can be obtained with injections into the basolateral but not central amygdala, while the reverse appears to be the case with shock-probe avoidance (Pesold and Treit, 1995; De Souza Silva and Tomaz, 1995).

We consider the relationship between amygdala lesions and anxiolytic action again below. However, we note here that such lesions affect fear responses even when these are uncontaminated with conflicting approach tendencies, while anxiolytics do not. Conversely, infusion of benzodiazepines into the amygdala impairs response suppression resulting from shock but not from reward omission (Hodges et al., 1987). Overall, anxiolytics seem to produce only some of their effects via the amygdala and, conversely, only some amygdala processes are affected by anxiolytics.

6.4.6 Fear-potentiated startle

The phenomenon of fear-potentiated startle requires special consideration in relation to the hierarchical organization of defence that we have been describing. It is one of the few cases where amygdala lesions act like anxiolytics, but hippocampal lesions do not. It is also more than an academic curiosity since: (a) it has received extensive psychological analysis; (b) the neural systems involved are known in extensive detail; (c) as is its pharmacology; and, most importantly, (d) it is clearly affected by state anxiety in human beings and in their anxiety disorders (e.g. Grillon et al., 1993), and (e) it may be useful as an anxiolytic screen in healthy humans (Grillon and Ernst, 2020). The key facts are reviewed by Davis (Davis, 1992c; Davis et al., 1993; Davis, 2006); where references are not given for statements in the rest of this section, they will be found in his reviews.

The paradigm itself is simple. A rat is first exposed to pairings of a light with a shock in a conventional classical conditioning arrangement. Then, in the dark, a loud noise is presented that results in a startle response. Finally, the loud noise is presented but now with the light and at about the time that the shock would have been delivered. A much larger (potentiated) startle response is produced as a result of the prior fear conditioning compared to the lesser response that might have been expected if habituation to the tone stimulus had occurred. A range of tests suggest that potentiation results from true fear conditioning and not from postural adjustments nor other secondary effects (Davis, 1992a, p. 257). An essentially identical result can be obtained using the eyeblink to measure startle in human subjects (see Grillon and Ernst, 2020 for recent review of human potentiated startle).

The neural pathways involved have been worked out in considerable detail (Fig. 6.4) and conform tightly to the general plan described earlier. The light CS is received by the retina and sent to the lateral and basolateral nuclei of the amygdala usually via the perirhinal cortex. Interestingly, 'complete removal of all primary and secondary visual cortices does not block the expression of fear-potentiated startle using a visual conditioned stimulus' (Davis, 1992a, p. 274). So, 'quick and dirty' thalamic input can support conditioning in the absence of a clear cortical signal. The unconditioned stimulus (shock) is detected by the footpads and relayed in the spinal cord and then in parallel through the parabrachial area (which relays to the intralaminar thalamus not the amygdala, Deng et al., 2020), intralaminar thalamus, and insula before arriving in the basolateral complex. Here the conditioning of the CS by the UCS depends on an NMDA receptor dependent process (see Davis et al., 1993, p. 190), presumably long-term potentiation. The information from the lateral and basal nuclei is then transferred to the central nucleus, which may also engage in long-term potentiation (Samson and Pare, 2005); this makes a monosynaptic connection with the nucleus reticularis pontis caudalis, which constitutes 'an obligatory part of the acoustic startle pathway' (Davis, 1992a, p.263; Hitchcock and Davis, 1991). The central nucleus also relays in the superior colliculus; while the medial nucleus relays via the ventromedial hypothalamus and PAG. The full details of the startle pathway are given by Davis (2006); (see also Davis, 1992a; Frankland and Yeomans, 1995).

While the paradigm is universally referred to as *fear*-potentiated startle, Davis links it with anxiety in a number of ways. First, he notes that potentiated startle indicates *anticipation* of the shock. Second, he links the increased startle response with equivalent changes in heart rate, salivation, ulceration, respiration, scanning and vigilance, urination, defecation, grooming, and freezing—all of which have corresponding features in generalized anxiety disorder. Third, and most critically (as we noted earlier), fear-potentiated startle is blocked by the majority of anxiolytics (ethanol, barbiturates, benzodiazepines, buspirone, propranolol); so we, with others (Grillon and Ernst, 2020), see fear potentiated startle as a valid animal model of anxiety that is paradigmatic for the 'increased arousal+attention' output of the behavioural inhibition system (Fig. 5.1; see also, e.g. Gray, 1987b).

Given the emphasis on goal conflict in Chapter 5, we must then ask: what is the source of conflict in fear-potentiated startle? A light that threatens shock is followed by the startle-eliciting auditory stimulus and there is no explicit goal with which startle can come into conflict. But the light produces potentiation of the startle response later elicited by the loud noise. At the time of the light-increased arousal, and before the noise, the animal is usually immobile. Since the shock was inescapable, the light predicting it is likely to produce defensive quiescence as a result of the conflict between a variety of different (equally useless) potential escape responses. Leaton and Borszcz (1985, p. 421) found that 'startle amplitude was positively correlated with freezing [during the CS] under all conditions [although there was]... a non-monotonic relation between potentiated startle and shock intensity'. Since conditioned freezing is sensitive to anxiolytics, these data suggest, then, that potentiated startle is linked to anxiolytic-sensitive behavioural inhibition. On this view, the paradigm is one of anxiety-potentiated startle, not fear-potentiated startle. Crucially, the fact that anxiolytics do not affect one-way active avoidance, and actually improve two-way active avoidance and Sidman avoidance (Chapter 4), shows that their reduction of fear-potentiated startle cannot be the result of a reduction in fear itself; and, conversely, that the potentiated startle phenomenon does not contribute to learned avoidance.

6.4.7 Autonomic activity as a special case

Autonomic symptoms of anxiety include, for example, raised skin conductance, increased spontaneous fluctuations in skin conductance, raised heart rate, increased forearm blood flow; (Lader, 1975). As summarized in Fig. 6.4 (and see Davis, 2006), the central nucleus of the amygdala provides outputs to a whole range of lower structures that collaborate to organize the entire spectrum of autonomic responses that occur during anxiety.

These autonomic changes are not specific to anxiety: they occur during other types of defensive behaviour as well and in some cases also with some types of appetitive behaviour. Autonomic changes function to increase the body's readiness for, and ability to sustain, vigorous action in general (Gray, 1987b; McNaughton, 1989b, pp. 8–9). The patterns of autonomic change are more general than specific to particular states of emotion (Gray, 1987b, Chapter 5).

As with other emotions (McNaughton, 1989b) it is useful to look at the relation of the GRS and GIS adaptively. With potential threat processed by the GRS, the need to increment arousal arises from the possibility that vigorous fight or flight may suddenly be required. Using potentiated startle as an explicit model, we can see the part of GIS output that consists in heightened arousal and increased activity in the autonomic nervous system as shared with (and on occasion amplifying) GRS output—and correspondingly in human states of both panic and anxiety (Lader and Mathews, 1970). In contrast, the behaviour-related outputs of the GIS would, among other things, block the fight and flight *outputs* of the GRS.

Anticipation of a negative goal will in any case activate the GRS and conflict can increase that activation as a precaution—provided the output of fight/flight behaviour is blocked. Such (continuously pre-programmed) behaviour can then occur by simple release from inhibition. Indeed, there can be very sudden (milliseconds) switching between them because of their essentially complementary but opposing roles in directing the animal's behaviour under what are likely to be rapidly changing circumstances. Autonomic changes, by contrast, are relatively slow and required to a similar extent whichever system is at any given time in control of behaviour. This slow speed also accounts for the greater involvement of the amygdala (often dealing with conditioned or complex stimuli and anticipation) than the PAG (often dealing with instantaneous requirements that must precede any autonomic reaction).

At this point in the hierarchical picture that we are painting of the defence systems, we can see fear-potentiated startle as largely dependent on the amygdala. Critically for our next step, it is *not* dependent on the SHS nor are other aspects of *increased* arousal that are a feature of anxiety (Gray, 1982, p. 182; and see §6.5, next). So, we will now proceed from lower levels of the GIS that deal with immediate consequences of goal conflict (such as attention, arousal, and simple inhibition) to higher levels that deal with resolution of conflicts between the goals or less immediate threats. But first we will briefly recap the story so far.

6.5 Interim summary 1—2D lower-level survival circuits

We have now covered the lower levels of Table 6.1, presenting a strongly hierarchical view of the defence control system, based on Graeff (1994) and extended to two dimensions (McNaughton and Corr, 2004; Silva and McNaughton, 2019) and so mapping to the Blanchard's ethopharmacological analysis (Chapter 2). Table 6.1 is, of course, too categorical, too 'cut and dried', given the extensive reciprocal connections between adjacent levels (e.g. Fig. 6.2B, C). However, we believe it to be correct in general principle and so leave it as it is for the sake of simplicity.

As detailed in Table 6.1B, defensive systems are organized hierarchically—and in parallel. We have also noted, in passing, that appetitive systems are similarly organized. The PAG appears to be at the lowest level at which integrated control occurs (Fig. 6.4; Blanchard et al., 1981). It releases a suite of motor programmes with the minimum of analytical finesse. For defence, these include freezing, *undirected* escape, and aggression; removing the animal from harm as quickly as possible.

Next is the hypothalamus; which performs essentially the same functions but with greater finesse given more time, more flexible options, and allowing the influence on responding of conditioning. Defence (controlled by the medial hypothalamus) includes risk assessment and *directed* or learned escape, coupled with the *inhibition* of aggression that would otherwise be generated by the PAG and interfere with successful responding. The hypothalamus produces many effects via connections with the PAG region. Excitatory outputs achieve effects such as escape (but with control of direction) and inhibitory ones prevent unwanted more proximally-appropriate actions such as attack or freezing.

Above the hypothalamus is the amygdala. Here complex conditioning is possible with, e.g. active anticipatory avoidance replacing (and inhibiting) directed escape. Critically, the amygdala mediates the GIS outputs of increased arousal (e.g. potentiated startle) and, via outputs from the basal nucleus to cortical areas, attention (LeDoux, 2015, his Fig. 8.6, p. 218). The amygdala also mediates frustrative non-reward (Henke, 1977). The combination of excitatory and inhibitory connections with the hypothalamus and PAG allows a nuanced and guided subset of reactions to be released (Blanchard et al., 1981) by those structures (as originally suggested by Fanselow, 1991, his Fig. 12).

A particularly pleasing picture of the contribution of the amygdala to defence is provided by combining the ideas of Davis (2006) with those of LeDoux (LeDoux, 1994; LeDoux, 1996). The amygdala receives relatively low grade, but affectively labelled, information about sensory inputs from the thalamus. It receives (with somewhat greater delay) extremely highly processed, cognitive more than affective, information about the same sensory inputs from the highest levels of unimodal and polymodal cortex. Novel sensory stimuli are sent to the lateral nucleus of the amygdala but, unless they are associated with affective input, they rapidly habituate. Learned avoidance depends on the pairing of a CS (arriving in the lateral nucleus) with a UCS, arriving in the basal nucleus, and on the resultant long-term potentiation of the connection between the CS and the UCR. This is the paradigm case of Pavlovian stimulus substitution. In principle, specific biologically prepared stimuli (§13.6.5) could operate in a similar fashion with their initial input being sufficient, even in the absence of long-term potentiation, to produce a UCR. The various outputs of the central nucleus of the amygdala then control the different components of different UCRs and CRs. Fear would, on this view, result from activity in the basal nucleus of the amygdala and this could lead to: (a) defensive reactions including arousal via the subcortical outflow from the central nucleus; (b) the adjustment of learned avoidance via the outflow from the basal nucleus to the striatum; (c) anxiety via the outflow to the SHS; and (d) focussing of attention and increased negative cognitive bias via the recursive outflow from the basal nucleus to all levels of the visual cortex and other sensory systems both directly and via the basal forebrain cholinergic system (see Appendix 2; LeDoux, 2015). Some elements of anxiety-related activation would be encoded in the basal nucleus and others in the central nucleus.

So far, then, we have dealt with brain defence systems that provide, e.g. activating responses to goal conflict but that are not involved in conflict resolution. For this, we will move on to the SHS. Like Graeff (1994), we view the SHS as one of the higher levels of the defence control system; and, like LeDoux (1994), we view it as one of the higher levels of the threat analysis system. On either view, the SHS is likely to have a major role to play in the elaboration of anxiety. However, in distinction to both Graeff and LeDoux we view the SHS as having an antithetical, or at least doubly dissociable (Selden et al., 1991), role in comparison to much of the amygdala, since fear and anxiety have, in many cases, opposite outputs and, in many other cases, do not overlap (see also Bechara et al., 1995). Even with anxiolytic drug effects, as we have noted, the amygdala and SHS appear to dissociate in terms of arousal versus goal inhibition, respectively. A particularly important point to note in terms of Table 6.1 is that, for the GRS, we can view some parts of the amygdala as generating the necessary changes in arousal and attention; and other parts controlling specific avoidance behaviour and its conditioning. In contrast, with the GIS, we see GIS-specific aspects of the amygdala as controlling arousal but the SHS as controlling goal conflict processing and so decisions. Indeed, the basolateral amygdala and SHS may exert opposite effects on anxiety-related behaviour (Vo et al., 2021). We have, therefore, reached a point at which the separation between the GIS and GRS (already present in PAG, Fig. 6.2) becomes clear and structurally distinct.

6.6 The septo-hippocampal system (SHS)

This section focuses on the position of the SHS within the defence hierarchy. It asks whether the hippocampus: (1) supplies highly processed, essentially non-emotional, cortical information that is used by the amygdala to generate anxiety only in cognitively complex situations such as 'contextual' conditioning; *or* (2) itself generates anxiety, interacting with the amygdala when the level of anxiety is such that autonomic activation is required (see §6.4.7). We will conclude that neither of these 'single anxiety centre' approaches captures hierarchical reality.

We cover the detailed operation and functions of the SHS in Chapters 7–10 and Appendices 4–9. We will note here only that anxiolytics produce subtle impairment of SHS processes; and that these, when produced selectively, change behaviour in ways that match both systemic administration of anxiolytics and SHS lesions (see §1.3.3, §1.7). We also, here, treat the SHS as a single functional entity. Later we will take account of its essentially two-dimensional topographic organization and the retention of that topography in terms of the areas from which it receives inputs and those to which it sends outputs.

Table 4.2 summarizes the septal and hippocampal syndromes described in detail in Appendix 8 and Gray and McNaughton (1983). It should be noted that: (a) it is based on large lesions of the septum and relatively large lesions of the (often dorsal) hippocampus, both of which are likely to have interfered with fibres of passage involving the whole SHS; (b) our major concern here is to define a 'septo-hippocampal syndrome' based on the overall points of agreement between the two types of lesion; and (c) we have excluded the literature on the involvement of the hippocampus in memory (which is discussed in detail in Chapter 8), because there are few equivalent data on anxiolytics.

We talk of a *septo*-hippocampal *system* because there are extensive interconnections between the septum and hippocampus (Appendix 4; see Figs. 1.4, 9.3, 9.5, 9.7), and the septum controls hippocampal RSA/'theta' rhythm, through which we postulate that anxiolytics produce critical behavioural effects. Nonetheless, you may be surprised how closely the effects of septal and hippocampal lesions resemble each other (Table 4.2). The cases where septal and hippocampal lesions have different effects from each other are discussed in detail in Gray (1982, his §6.24). Here we focus on the concordance of the two kinds of lesion.

The anatomical interconnections between the septal area and hippocampus provide strong *a priori* grounds for expecting the septal and hippocampal syndromes to resemble each other, irrespective of any particular theory of their behavioural functions. However, there are no a priori grounds, other than those derived from our theory, for expecting any similarity between the septo-hippocampal syndrome and the effects of anxiolytics. But it is clear when we compare the third and fourth columns of Table 4.2 that the concordance here is also remarkably strong. Since the value of science is often seen as its predictive power, note that the overwhelming majority of the data that support the concordance in Table 4.2 were collected in the 50 years *after* the original proposal of the links between anxiolytic drug effects and septal and hippocampal lesions (Gray, 1970b).

The degree of concordance between the anxiolytic and septo-hippocampal syndromes is particularly surprising in the case of benzodiazepines, because their receptors are widely distributed throughout the brain. Their muscle relaxant effect, at least, might have been expected to produce many effects that would decrease the concordance with the septo-hippocampal syndrome. However, where it has been tested in the tasks we have considered, buspirone (and the less specific SSRIs) almost invariably shares the effects of the benzodiazepines and hence of septal and hippocampal lesions. This suggests that the battery of tests we have reviewed are not, by and large, sensitive to the muscle relaxant, anticonvulsant, hypnotic, depressant, and addictive properties of the benzodiazepines—since buspirone's side effects do not include any of these properties. The striking feature of Table 4.2 is that, with few exceptions, *wherever* the effects of septal and hippocampal lesions are the same as each other, the effects of the anxiolytics are the same (although there are many cases where relevant data are not available). The size of the drug effect, however, is usually smaller than that of the lesions.

An exception to the rule of anxiolytic/SHS similarity is found in aggressive behaviour. Although the effects of the drugs on aggression are very variable (Gray, 1977), there is reason to suppose that there is a real divergence on this measure between their effects and those of septal and hippocampal lesions. Both septal and hippocampal lesions usually reduce aggression if this is induced by means other than shock (usually by isolating animals). When shock is not used, all the anxiolytics have been reported to increase aggression, particularly at low doses—with the likely exception of decreased maternal aggression (Ferreira et al., 2000).

There are also few discrepancies in the reverse direction. Those that exist can be attributed to one effect of anxiolytics which, as noted in §6.4.6 and §6.4.7, appears to be missing from the septo-hippocampal syndrome, and which is of particular importance for the psychological theory developed in Chapter 5. The drugs impair all three postulated outputs of the GIS: goal inhibition itself, increased attention to novel stimuli, and increased level of arousal. However, SHS lesions do not lower the level of arousal and, particularly, do not reduce fear-potentiated startle whereas all types of anxiolytic drug do (§6.4.6).

Overall, then, Table 4.2 shows a very wide range of similarities between the effects (and lacks of effect) of SHS damage and of anxiolytics. The pattern seems to rule out any general effects on memory as opposed to emotion with, e.g. passive avoidance impaired, and one-way active avoidance unchanged. But, also, includes effects of anxiolytics in tasks that seem to involve memory more than emotion (water maze, delayed conditional discrimination). This pattern offers strong support for the hypothesis that the anxiolytics produce their effects on goal inhibition via the SHS, but on arousal via the amygdala.

At the start of this section, we suggest two ways the SHS and the amygdala could be related if only one of them were 'the anxiety centre': 1) that the SHS is a source of special (perhaps spatial or contextual) information to which the amygdala adds affect to construct anxiety; 2) that the SHS generates anxiety, involving the amygdala only when fear stimuli or high levels of autonomic activation are involved. It is clear that neither of these simple alternatives is correct and the data force us to the more complex position that both the SHS and amygdala, as well as hypothalamus and PAG, must be included if we are to account for the full anxiolytic profile.

6.7 The cingulate cortex

> Above the amygdala, we place the anterior cingulate and assign to it more complex active avoidance that will require a greater degree of anticipation and a less tight temporal linkage of warning stimuli with actual threat than the amygdala. Higher level processing, here, does not imply less involvement in fundamental features of defense. Anterior cingulate is involved in the perception of pain, the production of anger, Pavlovian fear conditioning and avoidance learning. Likewise, anterior cingulate lesions impair avoidance of the CS– in discriminated autoshaping, as well as 'lick suppression during the presentation of a CS+ that had previously been paired with shock...; and active avoidance learning'.
>
> (McNaughton and Corr, 2004, pp. 292–293)

For these reasons, we include here a preliminary view of cingulate cortex. Since the focus of the chapter is on survival circuits, we will cover other aspects of cingulate cortex function together with prefrontal cortex in Chapter 11.

Papez saw the *gyrus cinguli*, plus hypothalamus, and hippocampus, 'as representing theoretically the anatomic basis of the emotions' (Papez, 1937; reprinted in Arnold, 1968, p. 302). It receives major input from the mammillary bodies of the hypothalamus via the anterior thalamic nuclei and so 'may be looked on as the receptive region for the experiencing of emotion as a result of impulses coming from the hypothalamic region, in the same way as the area striata is considered the receptive cortex for photic excitations coming from the retina' (*op cit.*, pp. 305–306). Input from anterior and mediodorsal thalamus distinguishes frontal from posterior cortex, respectively; so, the cingulate appears more frontal than sensory. Indeed, anterior cingulate is contiguous with motor, premotor, and frontal cortex proper. However, we argue (Appendix 3) that the perception of emotion has a much tighter relationship to action than it does to perception of the external world—with anterior cingulate computing: a) the expected values of goals (Yee et al., 2021); b) whether to switch strategy; and c) whether to commit to a particular alternative (Tervo et al., 2021). So, we can still view the cingulate as 'the receptive region for the experiencing of emotion', which is also consistent with the contiguity of posterior cingulate to somatosensory cortex.

While the cingulate cortex as a whole receives input, relayed by the thalamus, from the mammillary bodies, and while posterior cingulate receives direct input from the lateral hypothalamus and the ventral tegmental area, there are many reasons why we can neither treat the cingulate as a homogeneous area nor solely as primary receiving cortex for hypothalamic information (Vogt, 1985). We must divide cingulate cortex into a number of discrete areas, exactly as with frontal cortex, on the basis of parallel 'dorsal' and 'ventral' trends, each subdivided into architectonically progressive levels (Fig. 11.2).

For this chapter we will treat cingulate cortex as consisting of two separate (but reciprocally connected) modules that are anterior and posterior to the central sulcus, respectively. Posterior cingulate is related to posterior cortex, with its thalamic input somewhat like (e.g. the geniculate and collicular input to striate cortex). Anterior cingulate is related to frontal cortex, with its thalamic input equivalent to that of the anterior and dorsomedial thalamic input to frontal cortex. However, the thalamic inputs to the posterior cingulate include ones that send collaterals to frontal cortex. Conversely, given its input from pain pathways, anterior cingulate acts in part as a form of primary sensory cortex. So, both anterior and posterior cingulate differently combine both frontal 'action' and posterior 'perception'. We (see also Appendix 3) link cingulate cortex with the *anticipatory* control of motor programmes, the steps of which are controlled largely by internal events coded as somatosensory input (e.g. nociception) or as hypothalamic input. In this sense cingulate cortex is quite distinct from both frontal and posterior cortex, and we shall treat it (together with the SHS) as a third major 'mesial' division of the cortical mantle with posterior and anterior cingulate cortex representing parallel 'dorsal' and 'ventral' trends (discussed in detail in Chapter 11). We discuss the division of the SHS into dorsal and ventral trend components in Chapters 7–10.

On a small scale, some aspects of the cingulate appear to mirror prefrontal cortex (Chapter 11). The cingulate undertakes the same general tasks but with sequences of motor output that are largely 'innate' as opposed to 'acquired'. (The stimuli that elicit the innate plans can be learned.) Anterior cingulate can add greater range and anticipatory character to the initiation of, e.g. the simple (UCS-UCR) active avoidance reactions of the amygdala—adding greater anticipation in the same way that the amygdala converts hypothalamic escape into simple avoidance. The anterior cingulate is likely to be anticipatory, particularly when there is no explicitly observable UCS (e.g. viruses) to elicit the UCR (hand washing). Similarly, posterior cingulate may add greater range and anticipatory character to the inhibition of ongoing behaviour and the elicitation of risk analysis that can be generated via the SHS.

An important point when we consider clinical conditions later (§13.7; see also §9.6) is that obsessions can be viewed as the activation (pathological or non-pathological) of largely innate affective motor plans within the cingulate cortex that could then place items into the working/active memory areas of prefrontal cortex. Compulsions can be viewed as originating in the basal ganglia, which 'contains a series of modules each controlling a given pattern of behaviour including locomotion, eye-movements, posture, and chewing that contain both the direct pathway to release a motor programme and the indirect pathway to inhibit competing behaviours... the net effect of the direct pathway is to disinhibit brainstem motor centres and release motor programmes' (Grillner and Robertson, 2016, p. R1088).' Critically, hand washing and similar compulsive actions (Rapoport, 1989) involve anticipatory avoidance of very real danger (e.g. viral disease); but unlike the conditioned avoidance controlled by the amygdala has no external stimuli that signal either danger or safety. At least one source of *pathological* obsessions could then be a failure to provide to the cingulate a 'task completed' feedback signal from the motor system analogous to that which, according to Goldman-Rakic (1992), terminates the delay firing of prefrontal neurones (Fig. 11.5); a second source could be a failure of the anterior cingulate itself to determine that strategy-switching is needed (Tervo et al., 2021).

> Using the idea of defensive distance as the basis for speculation, we suggest that the anterior cingulate deals with relatively simple 'surface' expectations of nebulous threat (with prefrontal cortex dealing with deeper aspects). Likewise, using the idea of defensive direction, we suggest that it deals only with obsessional active avoidance with posterior cingulate dealing with obsessional passive avoidance.... Fear of the dark can be viewed as assigning threat to a set of locations and posterior cingulate cortex appears to be involved in spatial analysis particularly in the dark although its exact involvement and the contribution of fibres of passage remains to be determined. A related form of anxiety is agoraphobia (which, in the theory would be better named as agoranxiety). This and other equivalent possible higher order anxieties are classified by a lack of any simple avoidance strategy for the danger (which requires a high level of the defense system for their processing) and the fact that what is required, for normal function, is the capacity to approach and deal with the source of threat (which engages the defensive approach, anxiety, system rather than the pure fear system).
>
> McNaughton and Corr (2004, p. 293, 295)

Posterior cingulate, then, has functions related to the GIS and so could be involved in anxiety.

6.8 Interim summary 2—2D higher-level survival circuits

We have now covered all the levels of the GRS and GIS that could normally be considered to control *conserved* defensive reactions with the highest order of these being motor programmes such as grooming driven by the cingulate cortex. Our basic picture of the GRS follows the conventional picture of 'fear' systems, starting with the PAG, then medial hypothalamus, amygdala, and anterior cingulate cortex. However, particularly with the PAG, we have placed a new emphasis on particular subregions as being involved in the GRS and other subregions being involved in the GIS (and GAS).

Our parallel hierarchical view of the GIS in comparison to the GRS is novel in its detail for the PAG and amygdala and in the extent to which anterior cingulate has been excluded. Areas such as the septum and nucleus accumbens are important, but will be dealt with later as their role is less modular. When we reach frontal cortex (Chapter 11) we will also want to include in the GIS at least some aspects of the orbital frontal cortex and of the insular cortex—but these do not have such a clear role in the control of goal inhibition by aversive stimuli. We will also want to consider the role of the dorsomedial prefrontal cortex in 'teaching signal processing during fear conditioning' via prediction errors (see Fig. 2 in McNally et al., 2011, p. 288). The details of the rostral parts of the GRS (and their reasons for partially excluding anterior cingulate, infralimbic and prelimbic cortex) are reviewed in Jean-Richard-dit-Bressel et al. (2018) and are shown positionally in Fig. 6.5A. Note the relatively consistent ventrolateral location of the structures along the rostro-caudal axis. The systems (with inclusion of the GAS) are represented diagrammatically in Fig. 6.5B; and some ways in which the GRS and GIS interact in Fig. 6.5D, E.

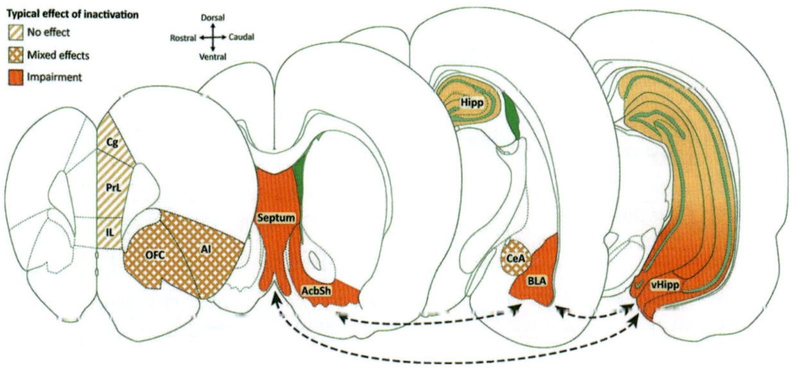

Fig. 6.5A The hierarchical 2D survival circuits. Forebrain regions implicated in punishment. Regions are shaded according to the typical effects of inactivations or lesions of that region on response suppression within punishment protocols. Arrows show regional connectivity implicated in punishment. *Abbreviations:* AcbSh nucleus accumbens shell (ventral striatum), AI anterior insular cortex, BLA basolateral amygdala, CeA central amygdala, Cg cingulate cortex, Hipp hippocampus, IL infralimbic cortex, OFC orbitofrontal cortex, PrL prelimbic cortex, vHipp ventral hippocampus. Fig. panel and legend from Jean-Richard-dit-Bressel et al. (2018).

A key point to note here is that our survival circuits (including the aspects of cingulate function that we have covered here) involve, by and large, the production of phylogenetically old responses that are adapted to specific defensive distances. The prefrontal cortex, in contrast, is more concerned with the organization of novel complex learned response sequences that involve the encoding not just of a goal but specific ordered series of subgoals that may conflict (Morris et al., 1997; Rushe et al., 1999). To this we should add

> the concept of 'subgoal scaffolding', to which Corr (2008a) drew attention.... Subgoal scaffolding relates to the fact that although the primary function of attractor motivation is to move the animal up the temporo-spatial gradient, from a start state toward the final biological reinforcer, this primary function must be subserved by a number of subprocesses:
>
> 1. Identifying the biological reinforcer.
> 2. Planning behavior.
> 3. Executing the plan (i.e., 'problem solving') at each stage of the temporo-spatial gradient.
>
> (McNaughton and Corr, 2019a, p. 162)

Prefrontal subgoal scaffolding goes far beyond the output of basic survival circuits. Likewise, the prefrontal cortex contains areas that carry out quite complex learning-based valuation of situations and endpoints, whereas survival circuits (absent direct frontal input) respond to stimuli the valence of which is easy to detect and often genetically wired-in.

We have paused at this point partly because further upward travel takes us into new goal/subgoal control territory (see Chapter 11) that, while obviously important for survival, does not fall under the rubric of 'survival circuits'. But this pause also allows us to take a step back and consider modulatory systems that not only impact on defence but also on appetitive

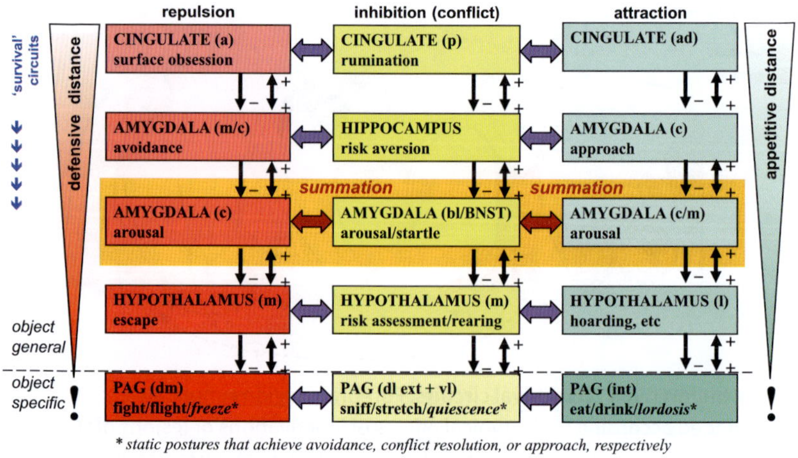

Fig. 6.5B *2D GRS and GIS survival circuits shown diagrammatically, together with parallel GAS circuits*. The lowest levels release proximal object-specific behaviours that in all three cases can include stillness but with different body postures (freezing, quiescence, lordosis). Higher levels release higher order behaviour, while supressing inappropriate output from lower levels. Orange box: components of the amygdala that control arousal. Note that these interact to summate their activities (dark orange arrows), whereas the other components of the amygdala and other areas compete (blue arrows) for goal control. *Abbreviations:* a = anterior; b = basal; BNST = bed nucleus of the stria terminalis; c = central; d = dorsal; ext = external; int = internal; l = lateral; m = medial; p = posterior; v = ventral. Adapted from Silva and McNaughton (2019).

responses. The key point is that our hierarchical parallel systems, while containing lateral and rostro-caudal connections, also *all* receive diffuse neuromodulatory inputs at *all* levels. This modulation, as does a hormone, tunes the systems as a whole (including prefrontal and cingulate cortex); and provides a major source for personality, psychopathology, and the connection between them (covered in the final chapters).

6.9 Neuromodulatory systems—a common anatomical plan

To a first approximation, we can treat all the monoamine systems (Fig. 6.6) and, to a lesser extent, the acetylcholine systems (§6.14), and the relaxin-3 system arising in nucleus incertus (§6.15) as projecting diffusely to much of the forebrain and so acting more like hormones than computational machines. Importantly, their projections have expanded through phylogeny so that they reach the bulk of the neocortex and therefore have effects well beyond the survival circuits. They are best viewed as neuromodulators rather than neurotransmitters as they originate in small caudal nuclei and have massive branching of collaterals to reach their rostral (and more caudal) targets. They also have strong links with hormonal stress systems (Hale and Lowry, 2015).

In our view much the same is true, in reverse, of systems that run through the habenula (§6.16)—although these cannot be characterized by a single chemical. These are also phylogenetically very ancient (e.g. present in the lamprey, which has only the beginnings

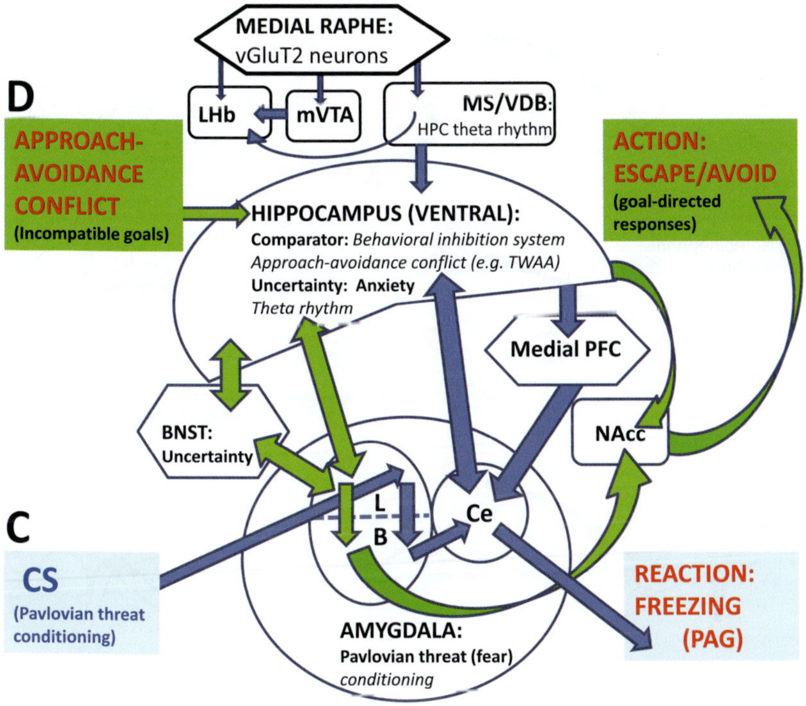

Fig. 6.5C,D *The proposed circuitry for amygdala-centred CS-elicited responses* (**C**; pavlovian threat—fear- conditioning; blue colour) and for the involvement of the hippocampal (E; green colour) system when the situation constitutes an approach-avoidance conflict and involves uncertainty/ anxiety. (**C**) The amygdala is proposed to be responsible for CS-elicited reactions (Pavlovian conditioned freezing) and to be involved in active avoidance actions through its connections with NAcc, hippocampus and medial PFC. (**D**) The hippocampus is proposed to be a crucial node in monitoring and behavioural control under conditions of approach-avoidance conflict (see also Fernandez-Teruel and McNaughton, 2023), thus having a critical role for the selection of appropriate responses to conflict (i.e. initial phases of acquisition of the two-way active avoidance task) through its connections with amygdala nuclei, with BNST, with medial PFC and directly with NAcc. Moreover, medial raphe vGLUT2 neurons modulate aversive experiences and establish synapses on LHb, mVTA and MS/VDB neurons. The latter project to the hippocampus and control RSA/'theta' rhythm, which is also coordinated with firing of LHb neurons. The MS/VDB, through its projections to hippocampus and LHb may coordinate the activity of both structures (see text for further details). Symbols: BNST, Bed nucleus of the stria terminalis; PFC, prefrontal cortex; NAcc, nucleus accumbens; L, B, Ce, lateral, basal and central amygdala. HPC, hippocampus; PAG, periaqueductal grey; vGLUT2 neurons, "vesicular glutamate transporter 2" neurons; mVTA, medial ventral tegmental area; LHb, lateral habenula; MS/VDB, medial septum and vertical limbs of the diagonal bands of Broca. Fig. panel and legend modified from Fernández-Teruel and Tobeña (2020) with permission.

of a telencephalon), have expanded (at least somewhat, with the lateral habenula) to match changes in the telencephalon, and have as their ultimate targets the ascending modulatory systems—essentially completing feedback loops.

Finally, we will ask about the role of the ascending systems that control RSA/'theta' rhythmicity—particularly of hippocampal-cortical interactions. These are not yet will

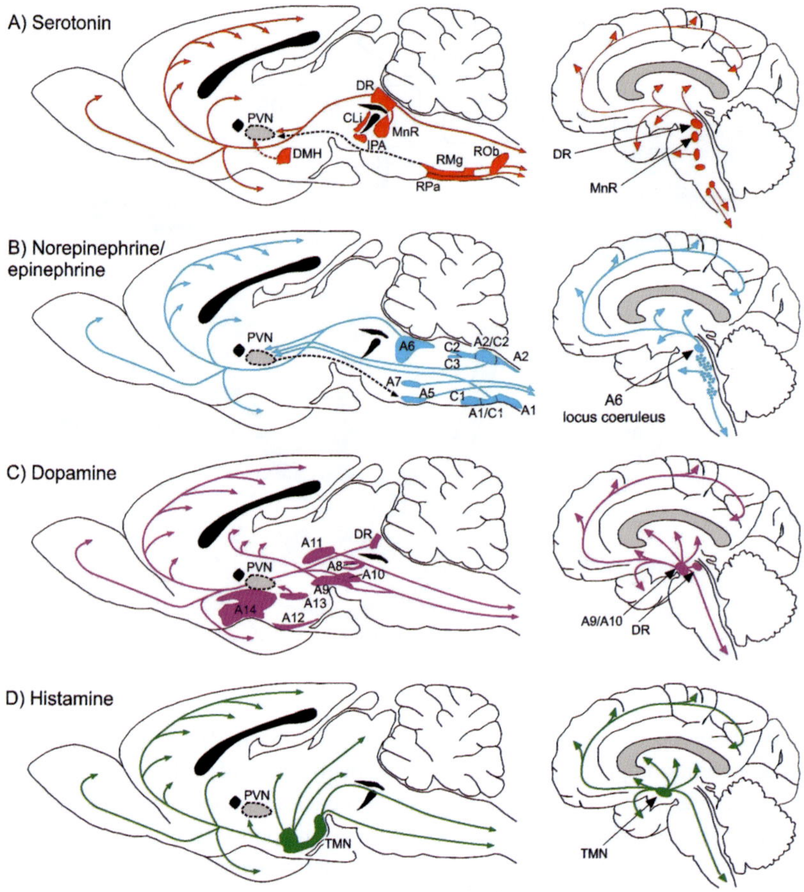

Fig. 6.6 Monoamine innervation of the brain: left, rat; right, human. Systems originate in small caudal nuclei and send collaterals rostrally and caudally to the bulk of the forebrain. *Abbreviations:* CLi = caudal linear nucleus; DMH = dorsomedial hypothalamus; DR = dorsal raphe; IPA = inter-peduncular nucleus, apical; MnR = median raphe; PVN = paraventricular nucleus of the hypothalamus; RPa = raphe pallidus; RMg = raphe magnus; ROb = raphe obscurus; TMN = tuberomammillary nucleus. Figure supplied by Mathew Hale (see also Hale and Lowry, 2015).

mapped and so we will focus (§6.17) on the supramammillary area (which remains active under urethan anaesthesia) while recognizing that it is just part of a distributed control system. The role of RSA/'theta' can be viewed as modulatory and so not unlike the amine systems. The connectional anatomy of the supramammillary area (ignoring any particular neurotransmitters involved) is very similar to the chemically-defined modulatory systems. Importantly, like them, it appears to receive feedback-like input from the habenula.

While in the past there has been a tendency to link specific monoamines with specific goal systems (serotonin with approach, dopamine with avoidance), their projections are more diffuse, essentially innervating all levels of the GAS, GIS, and GRS. As we will see they do not affect all levels equally, and their input to one system may be used for a different purpose than another—but, in terms of Fig. 6.5B, we can see them all innervating all parts of the diagram.

6.10 The serotonin systems

With such broad-ranging targets (Fig. 6.6A; Fig. 6.7A) it is not surprising that the simple modulatory role of collateral output from the serotonin (5HT) system can occasionally seem unexpected. There are also important differences between activation of, e.g. DR neurons that is short-term ('anxiogenic' and 'antidepressant') versus long-term ('antidepressant only') with impact on different neural networks in the two cases (Urban et al., 2015).

> Serotonergic systems play important roles in a number of physiologic and behavioral states, including sleep/wake cycles, locomotor activity and emotional states. In mammals, serotonin is synthesized by neurons in the midbrain, pontine and medullary raphe nuclei (Fig. [6.6A]). The vast majority of forebrain-projecting serotonergic neurons are located in the dorsal raphe nucleus (DR) and median raphe nucleus (MnR). The DR can be further divided into subregions based on anatomical, hodological and functional properties. For example, serotonergic neurons in the ventrolateral part of the DR and adjacent ventrolateral part of the periaqueductal gray contain presympathetic-premotor neurons that innervate the adrenal gland via multisynaptic pathways and are implicated in autonomic control and panic-like behavior, whereas serotonergic neurons located in the dorsal and caudal parts of the DR contain limbic system projections and are implicated in the control of anxiety-like behavior. Serotonergic neurons in the median raphe nucleus send dense projections to the septohippocampal system and may play a role in the suppression of hippocampal RSA/'theta' rhythm and disruption of long-term potentiation and memory formation. Additionally, it has been suggested that serotonergic neurons in the MnR may be important in resilience and an organism's ability to cope with stressors.
>
> Hale and Lowry (2015, p. 23)

> Both facilitatory and inhibitory functions have been ascribed to 5HT. The... view that 5HT enhances anxiety is mainly based on the observed effects of drugs and neurotoxic lesions in animals submitted to conflict tests. In general, operations that decrease 5HT activity in the brain release behaviour suppressed by punishment in the rat. A likely site for this facilitatory action of 5HT is the amygdala, since it has been shown that microinjection of 5HT receptor antagonists inside the basolateral amygdala has anxiolytic effects, whereas 5HT receptor agonists enhance behavioural suppression determined by punishment. [*Added:* Another likely site, particularly with $5HT_{1A}$ agonists is the ventral hippocampus' (Hernandes et al., 2021).]
>
> In contrast, the results of studies using escape from electrical stimulation of the dorsal midbrain of the rat led to the view that 5HT inhibits defensive behavior in the dorsal PAG. For example, it has been shown that systemically administered drugs that enhance 5HT activity have anti-aversive effects while those that impair 5HT transmission have pro-aversive effects....
>
> Taken together, the evidence reviewed above suggests that 5HT facilitates defensive behavior integrated in the amygdala, while inhibiting the defence reaction organized in the PAG. In order to make sense of this seemingly paradoxical situation, Deakin and Graeff (1991) hypothesized that the PAG would be responsible for proximal defence, commanding fixed action patterns that are only adaptive under conditions of extreme danger. Conversely, if the same behaviors were performed in response to potential or distal danger they would

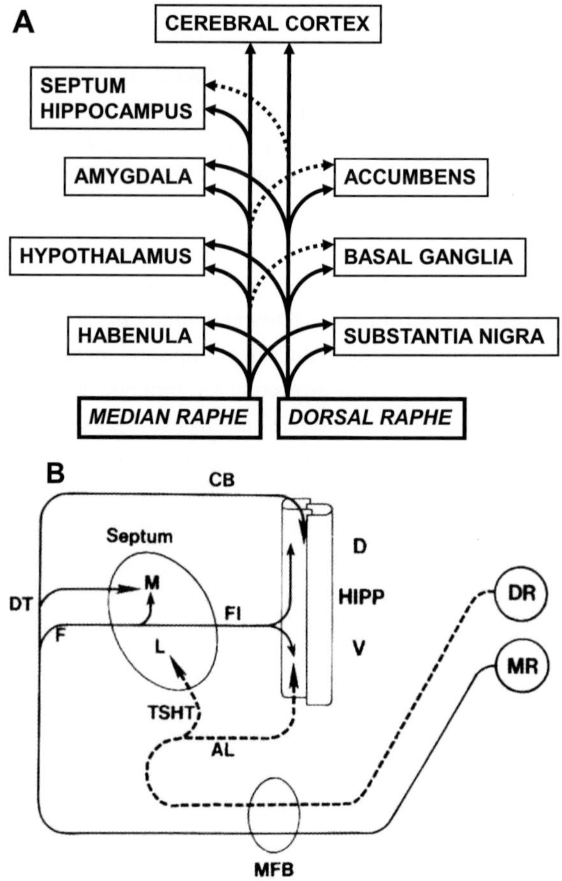

Fig. 6.7 Ascending serotonergic projections. **A.** Schematic diagram of the major projection areas of the dorsal and median raphe. Dashed lines (- - -) represent relatively weak connections. (Figure modified from Soubrié, 1986) **B.** Diagrammatic representation of the main projections to the septo-hippocampal complex. AL, ansa lenticularis; CB cingulum bundle; D, dorsal and V, ventral hippocampus; DR dorsal raphe; DT diagonal tract; F; columns of the fornix; FI fimbria; L, lateral and M medial septal area; MFB medial forebrain bundle; MR median raphe; TSHT, septo-hypothalamic tract. (From Azmitia, in Elliott and Whelan, 1978, with permission)

> enhance the probability of detection by an aggressor. Instead, *more flexible, largely learned behavioral strategies are likely to lead to successful escape from or avoidance of danger....* Translating it into emotional terms, it may be said that 5HT enhances anxiety and fear while at the same time inhibiting panic.
>
> Graeff (1994, pp. 820, 821—emphasis added)

The Deakin and Graeff (1991) model is shown, modified, in Fig. 6.8. The 5HT system, essentially in parallel with the hierarchical defence control system, assists coordination of the different levels. For example, it can also 'explain why the $5HT_2$ receptor antagonist, ritanserin, has been shown to ameliorate anxiety in patients with a diagnosis of generalized anxiety

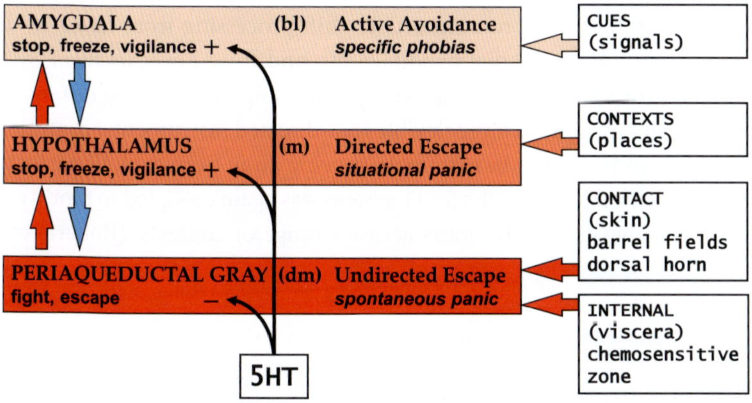

Fig. 6.8 The Deakin and Graeff (1991) model of the role of serotonin (5-HT) in the control of the defense system. A key feature is the opposing regulation (e.g., red and blue arrows) of the PAG compared to more central structures and the specific role of 5HT in this control. The release of 5HT suppresses PAG panic while enhancing hypothalamic directed escape and amygdala avoidance, which accounts for phenomena such as relaxation-induced panic. For further discussion, see text.

disorder, whereas panic disorder patients were found to be either not improved or even worsened by the same drug' (Graeff, 1994, p. 821). Thus, Graeff's view of the raphe 5HT system is that it carries a simple signal that an *avoidable* danger is present. This both activates those areas concerned with avoidance and directed escape and inhibits those areas that would be likely to produce interfering undirected escape responses. The signal of avoidability may also account for a link between serotonin and an increase in risk-taking behaviour under conditions of balanced payoff (Cui et al., 2020a). However, Graeff sees 5HT coordinating activity across multiple levels of the defence system—and with its innervation of GAS and GIS, we would expect a more general influence.

Inhibition of the PAG involves suppression of proximal 'object-specific' outputs (Table 6.1). But the other components of the survival circuits can also be seen as a relatively quick and dirty System 1, relative to the slow and sophisticated System 2, that we will consider in Chapter 11.

We refer to System 1 and System 2 here specifically in relation to the picture presented by Kahneman (2011), who adopted

> terms originally proposed by the psychologists Keith Stanovich and Richard West, and I will refer to two systems *in the mind*, System 1 and System 2.
>
> - *System 1* operates automatically and quickly, with little or no effort and no sense of voluntary control
> - *System 2* allocates attention to the effortful mental activities that demand it, including complex computations. The operations of System 2 are often associated with the subjective experience of agency, choice, and concentration.
>
> op. cit. (pp. 20–21, emphasis added).

It is quite likely, then, that serotonin acts to shift processing from faster to slower circuits including from PAG to medial hypothalamus and from lower levels of System 1 towards higher levels of System 2—thus generally increasing motivational distance. Or, from an evolutionary point of view, 'as more flexible goal-directed instrumental cognition became increasingly viable and complex in mammals, moving away from evolutionarily conserved fixed action and reaction patterns, the 5-HT system was again co-opted to modify the adaptability of several higher-level behaviours across a range of contexts' (Roberts et al., 2020, p. 142). Thus,

> evidence from diverse literatures supports the viewpoint that two modes of self-regulation exist, a lower-order system that responds quickly to associative cues of the moment and a higher-order system that responds more reflectively and planfully; low serotonergic function is linked to relative dominance of the lower-order system; that how dominance of the lower-order system is manifested depends on additional variables; and that low serotonergic function therefore can promote behavioral patterns as divergent as impulsive aggression and lethargic depression. [There is] work on two-mode models; studies of brain function supporting the biological plausibility of the two-mode view and the involvement of serotonergic pathways in functions pertaining to it; and studies relating low serotonergic function to impulsiveness, aggression (including extreme violence), aspects of personality, and depression vulnerability.
>
> Carver et al. (2008, p. 912)

As discussed in Chapter 4, $5HT_{1A}$ agonists (particularly partial agonists) are classified as anxiolytics. Like them, specific disruption of the serotonin systems generally has effects like those of both anxiolytics and SHS lesions (Table 4.2). However, some exceptions for system disruption include: improved conditional/delayed discrimination, increased fear-potentiated startle, increased elevated T inhibition, and a lack of (or weak) effect on context freezing, DRL, aggression, two-way avoidance, and non-spatial avoidance.

6.11 The noradrenaline systems

Noradrenergic systems have in the past been suggested to be crucial for defence in general, aversive learning and arousal, and anxiety in particular (see McNaughton and Mason, 1980). But they also appear to be involved in (e.g. re-organization of 'the cognitive map' in response to novel goal locations; see Király and Hangya, 2020). They innervate all levels of the defence hierarchy (see Fig. 6.6B) and so should be crucial for at least some aspects of anxiety, see Table 4.2, with distinct locus coeruleus efferent targets controlling goal-directed attention and impulsivity (Bari et al., 2020). The pathway most studied (and to which we confine our review) consists of the dorsal ascending noradrenergic bundle, which carries afferents to the whole of the forebrain, including the SHS, from the locus coeruleus.

Briefly, where dorsal bundle lesions have behavioural effects, these usually match the anxiolytic/septo-hippocampal syndrome; but there are a large number of cases where dorsal bundle lesions do not reproduce the effects of anxiolytics (Appendix 10). Interestingly, the effects of serotonergic lesions are often complementary, supplying the missing elements of the anxiolytic/septo-hippocampal syndrome (Table 4.2). This fractionation of the anxiolytic syndrome by the separate monoamine systems shows that neither can uniquely constitute an anxiety 'centre' but appear to contribute in parallel to some common target/s (e.g. amygdala, SHS or both).

Effects of dorsal bundle lesions can become evident only in adrenalectomized animals, suggesting redundancy between it and the hypothalamic–pituitary–adrenal (HPA) axis. Like the SHS,

> a wealth of experimental evidence has implicated serotonergic systems and norepinephrine/epinephrine systems in the control of the HPA axis activity and emerging evidence suggests that dopaminergic and histaminergic systems may also be important in stress neuroendocrinology. Studies continue to support a role for both monoaminergic systems and HPA axis dysfunction in the pathophysiology of anxiety and affective disorders.
>
> Hale and Lowry (2015, pp. 38–39)

It is consistent with this pattern of results that anxiolytics act directly on the locus coeruleus and raphe nuclei (Appendix 10). Both noradrenergic and serotonergic fibres project to the SHS. A direct action of the anxiolytics on the source nuclei should, therefore, have extensive effects on this system and, as a result, reproduce aspects of the septo-hippocampal syndrome. For example, noradrenergic input to the dentate gyrus modulates generalization of contextual fear conditioning (Seo et al., 2021). There is also evidence of synergistic interactions between the monoamine systems, implying that anxiolytics ought to have greater effects than would be predicted from their effects on the noradrenergic and serotonergic systems separately (Appendix 10). This said, we should note that the anxiolytics have important actions on other inputs to the SHS (e.g. the amygdala, §6.4.5, the supramammillary nucleus, §1.9, §6.17). Further, the serotonergic and noradrenergic systems project to many areas other than the SHS (e.g. the amygdala, frontal cortex, and cingulate cortex). On this basis the goodness of fit between the combined noradrenergic plus serotonergic behavioural profiles and the septo-hippocampal profile is surprising. We provide an account of this later, but to some extent it suggests that the SHS is unusually dependent on inputs from its monoaminergic afferents.

6.12 The dopamine systems

Dopamine systems are generally seen as encoding 'reward prediction error' (Schultz, 2002; Schultz, 2016; see also §12.7) or even the formal construct of economic utility (Schultz et al., 2017); and it has been suggested that 'striatal dopamine waves are sculpted by inference about agency and provide a mechanism to direct credit assignment to specialized striatal subregions' (Hamid et al., 2021, p. 2733; see also Mohebi et al., 2019). This is likely to be true, also, of secondary (conditioned) rewarding stimuli (Galaj and Ranaldi, 2021). Note that 'there are functionally distinct dopamine populations in the VTA for promoting motivation and reward association [respectively], which operate on the same timescale to [synergistically] optimize behavioural reinforcement' (Heymann et al., 2020). Importantly, *glutamate* cells in the VTA can reinforce both place aversion and approach without a contribution from dopamine (see Nuno-Perez and Mameli, 2020).

However, fast (<200 ms) dopamine signals (including those in the dorsal raphe, Cho et al., 2021) appear to react more to general salience (independent of valence) and may

> instead have a central role in identifying which aspects of context and behavioural output are crucial in causing unpredicted events[; so] that the reinforcing function of the phasic DA response has more to do with the discovery of new actions than adjusting the relative probabilities of selecting pre-existing actions to maximize anticipated rewards.
>
> Redgrave and Gurney (2006, pp. 967, 973); (see also Redgrave et al., 2011; Bang et al., 2020)

Related to this, dopamine release is a key element of responses to different types of novelty and this links both to novelty seeking and to novelty-induced approach-avoidance conflict (Tapper and Molas, 2020).

Dopamine systems are not generally seen as primarily involved in defence. However, striatal D2 receptor reduction may be linked (Dong et al., 2020) to obsessive compulsive disorder (see discussion of anterior cingulate §6.7). Further, while increased dopamine output can be seen as positive and linked to the GAS, with tonic non-zero levels, decreased output is also possible, contributing to GIS (but not GRS).

> Activity of midbrain dopamine (DA) neurons is necessary and sufficient for reinforcement of behavior. Symmetrically, negative outcomes cause pauses in VTA DA firing. It follows that punishment could be due to inhibition of VTA DA neurons. Certainly, inhibiting VTA DA causes conditioned place aversion and D1 or D2 dopamine receptor manipulations in the ventral striatum, a major target of reward-coding VTA DA neurons, can result in place aversion. However, the role of VTA DA in punishment remains unclear [Fig. 6.9].
>
> Jean-Richard-dit-Bressel et al. (2018, p. 1645)

In particular, the habenula (see Fig. 6.9) detects upcoming aversive events (including both unexpected and expected omission of positive events); and then suppresses VTA dopamine release (Sosa et al., 2021). But this suppression may occur 'only when guided by competing threat and safety memories' (Velazquez-Hernandez and Sotres-Bayon, 2021). Prediction errors as such are likely computed by the cerebellum and so allow it to regulate defensive states (Urrutia Desmaison et al., 2023) and integrate them with cardiac dynamics (da Silva et al., 2023).

On this view *suppressed* dopamine function could contribute to anxiety through punishment (i.e. response supressing not activating) mechanisms and a loss of coping mechanisms (Cui et al., 2020b). This does not seem to be the case for anxiety disorders generally but (combined with suppressed serotonin function) does appear to contribute to social anxiety disorder (for an early review, see Stein, 1998)—where 'separate from fear and arousal systems, the functional neurobiology of central DA systems contribute uniquely to susceptibility and maintenance of [social anhedonia]' (Carlton et al., 2020, p. 1). This suppressed dopamine function appears to result from increased transporter availability and to co-occur with a similar increase in the serotonin transporter (Hjorth et al., 2021). Reduced dopamine has also been linked to trait anxiety in humans (potentially via reduced connectivity between the rostral anterior cingulate and the amygdala, Berry et al., 2019).

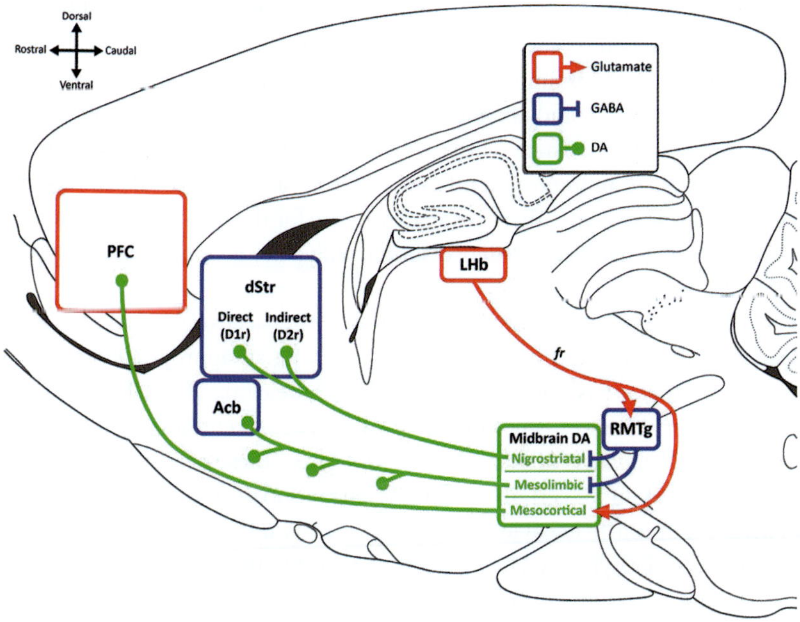

Fig. 6.9 Midbrain dopamine circuits implicated in punishment. Mesolimbic and nigrostriatal projections are generally reward-coding; punishment could be encoded via pauses in DA firing and decreased DA release at projection targets. Mesocortical neurons burst fire to aversive stimuli, ostensibly causing increased DA release within the PFC. Aversion-coding LHb neurons can exert relevant control over each of these pathways, although its role in punishment has been disputed. The role of each of these circuits in punishment remain unclear. Acb nucleus accumbens (ventral striatum), D1r D_1 receptor, D2r D_2 receptor, DA dopamine, dStr dorsal striatum, fr fasciculus retroflexus, LHb lateral habenula, PFC prefrontal cortex, RMTg rostromedial tegmental nucleus. Fig. and legend from Jean-Richard-dit-Bressel et al. (2018) with permission.

6.13 The histamine systems

Histaminergic systems play important roles in a number of physiological processes within and outside the nervous system, including inflammation and immune system function, attention and arousal, and pain perception. In the brain, histamine is stored and released from two cell types, mast cells and neurons. Mast cells are located throughout the body, including in the brain, and contribute to brain histamine concentrations. Histamine-synthesizing neurons are located in the tuberomammillary region of the posterior hypothalamus and project widely to most regions of the central nervous system, including the PVN (Fig. [6.6]D).... [There appears to be] an important role for histamine signalling in HPA axis activity; however, further investigation is required to fully elucidate the role of histaminergic systems in stress neuroendocrinology.

(Hale and Lowry, 2015, pp. 37–38; figure number refers to current chapter)

The histamine systems have not been extensively studied at the behavioural level, and the effects of systemic antagonists can be confounded by anticholinergic action (Masuoka et al., 2007) and interaction with histamine released by Mast cells rather than neurons, particularly during development (Carthy and Ellender, 2021); so we will not try to integrate them into the picture being presented here. There is little evidence to link them directly to fear or anxiety as such; but they may have an important influence on fear- and anxiety-related behaviours via interaction with stress systems. There is some evidence for the use of the H1 receptor antagonist hydroxyzine in generalized anxiety disorder, with a key action being on psychic symptoms (see, Millan, 2003).

The H3 receptor has been linked to arousal and the sleep-wake cycle (Passani et al., 2004; Venner et al., 2019) and has been suggested to be an appropriate target in obesity and cognitive disorders (Passani et al., 2004; Esbenshade et al., 2006). However, the firing of tuberomammillary neurons is not linked to control of wakefulness as such but rather to maintenance of high vigilance (Takahashi et al., 2006). So, these neurons 'may be important for enhancing arousal under certain conditions, such as exposure to a novel environment, but play only a minor role in behavioral and EEG arousal under baseline conditions' (Venner et al., 2019, p. 8939). Presynaptic H3 receptors can modify the input from glutamatergic afferents to the nucleus accumbens from the basolateral amygdala, ventral hippocampus, and prelimbic cortex; and in the latter case appear to reduce anxiety- and obsession-related behaviours generated by restraint stress (Zhang et al., 2020a). Likewise, lateral septal injections of histamine reduce anxiety-related behaviour in the plus-maze and with suppression of feeding by novelty (Chee et al., 2014, which also reported effects on RSA/'theta' that we will discuss in Chapter 9).

6.14 The acetylcholine systems

Compared to monoaminergic systems, the ascending cholinergic system originates more rostrally, has somewhat different general organization, and is linked more often to memory (and its retrieval, Soma et al., 2021) than to emotion. Nonetheless, the distribution of cholinergic afferents to cortex, hippocampus and amygdala is equivalent to those of the monoamine systems (compare Fig. 6.6. with Fig. 6.10) and, like them, is involved in the control of hippocampal RSA/'theta' activity (see Chapter 9). We need to consider, therefore, whether it too may make a contribution to the control of anxiety.

The data in the cholinergic column of Table 4.2 are not entirely satisfactory in that they have largely been provided by systemic injections of anticholinergics rather than specific neurotoxic lesions. However, if they can be taken at face value, they suggest a superficially surprising similarity to the anxiolytics. The similarity with SHS lesions is less surprising, given the extensive cholinergic innervation of the hippocampus and, as we discuss in Appendix 5, the crucial contribution of cholinergic input for the production of one type of hippocampal RSA/'theta' rhythm. Probably because anticholinergics are not used clinically as anxiolytics, drugs of this class have seldom been tested in the conventional anxiolytic screening tests. Where they have, they appear (unlike the data obtained in other types of experiment) *anxiogenic* rather than anxiolytic (Smythe et al., 1996). In contrast, largely because of the links between Alzheimer's disease, hippocampal dysfunction, and cholinergic neurodegeneration, anticholinergics have been extensively tested in memory paradigms (see

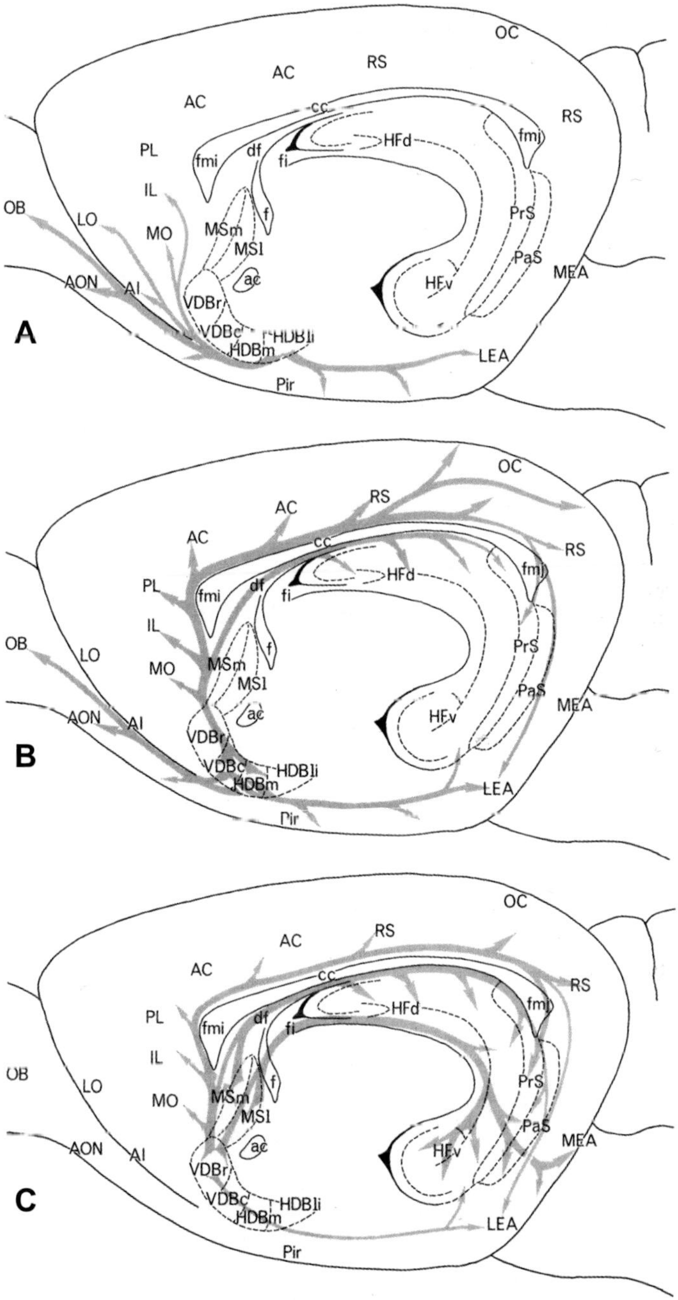

Fig. 6.10 Ascending cholinergic projections from the basal forebrain. These projections are topographically organized with relatively caudal basal forebrain areas projecting to more ventral areas of the forebrain; relatively rostral areas projecting to more dorsal areas of the forebrain; and relatively dorsal areas projecting relatively weakly to more dorsal areas of the forebrain and relatively strongly to the hippocampal formation. Note the tendency of fibres to follow the same routes as, and to have a similar innervation pattern overall to, the noradrenergic and serotonergic inputs to the forebrain. (From Gaykema, 1992).

also Hasselmo, 2006, for a detailed mechanistic picture). Given that anxiolytics have effects similar to hippocampal lesions on many memory tests, the resulting parallels in the table cease to be surprising.

For the present we conclude that such similarity as there is between anticholinergics and anxiolytics is probably in large measure due to the fact that both classes of drug can act through the SHS. However, this overlap should be seen as at least partly accidental, since there are data suggesting that the qualitative nature of the drug effects is different even in tasks where they produce similar quantitative decrements (McNaughton and Morris, 1987), and some types of memory task may be much more sensitive to anticholinergics than to anxiolytics (Kirk et al., 1988b; Tan et al., 1990). Given the quite different patterns of impairment of RSA/'theta' control produced by the different classes of drug (Appendix 5), an incomplete overlap in their 'SHS' behavioural effects is not surprising. Some non-SHS parallels can also be expected, at least with benzodiazepines, since these compounds block release of cortical acetylcholine through an action in the basal forebrain, from which cholinergic neurones project to the neocortex (Moore et al., 1995; Holley et al., 1995; McGaughy et al., 1996).

6.15 The relaxin-3 system (nucleus incertus)

The amine systems that we have just considered have been a strong focus of attention for more than half a century. However, other systems are likely to have similar roles and, in particular, the relaxin-3 system[6] shows strong similarities (Fig. 6.11A, compare Fig. 6.6).

> A major challenge in systems neuroscience is to determine the underlying neural circuitry and associated neurotransmitters and receptors involved in psychiatric disorders, such as anxiety and depression. A focus of many of these studies has been specific brainstem nuclei that modulate levels of arousal via their ascending monoaminergic projections (e.g. the serotonergic dorsal raphé, noradrenergic locus ceruleus and cholinergic laterodorsal tegmental nucleus). After years of relative neglect, the subject of recent studies in this context has been the GABAergic nucleus incertus, which is located in the midline periventricular central gray in the 'prepontine' hindbrain, with broad projections throughout the forebrain. Nucleus incertus neurons express receptors for the stress hormone, corticotropin-releasing factor (CRF), are activated by psychological stressors, and project to key nuclei involved in stress responses and behavioral activation. *The nucleus incertus is also a node in neural circuits capable of modulating hippocampal theta rhythm,* which is related to control of spatial navigation and memory. A significant population of nucleus incertus neurons express the recently discovered, highly conserved neuropeptide, relaxin-3.
>
> Ryan et al. (2011, p. 1327, our emphasis)

Much more work is required to integrate our knowledge of the relaxin-3 systems with that of the main systems. It also seems likely that further non-amine systems will be discovered.

[6] My thanks to Andrew Gundlach for interesting me in this system and explaining many of its details to me. NMcN

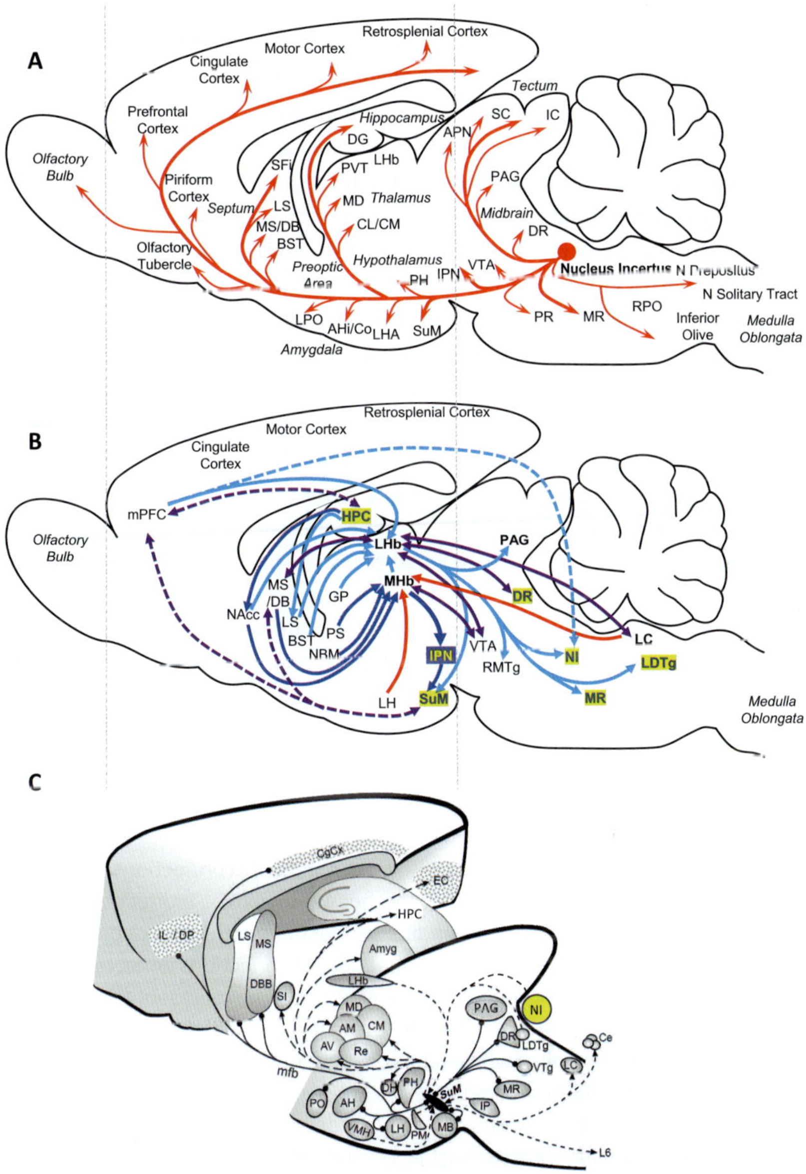

Fig. 6.11 Schematic representations of non-amine systems. A. The major projections of the nucleus incertus in the rat brain, which is characterised by containing relaxin-3 (Figure and legend adapted from Ryan et al., 2011). Note the superficial similarity to the projections of the amine systems. B. The connections of the medial (MHb) and lateral (LHb) habenula. These are phylogenetically very old structures and contrast strongly with the other neuromodulatory systems in having very limited neocortical connections and appearing to be involved in predominantly descending (light blue via LHb, dark blue via MHb) rather than ascending (red, as in A) control. Reciprocal connections in purple; secondary connections via IPN shown as highlights; some additional secondary connections shown dashed (see text). Connections shown based on Batalla et al. (2017); Hones and Mizumori (2022); McLaughlin et al. (2017); Zhao et al. (2015); Loonen and Ivanova (2022). C. The connections of the supramammillary area (SuM)

(Contd.)

6.16 The habenula

The habenular complex consists of two main zones the medial (MHb) and lateral (LHb) habenula[7]; each of which can be further subdivided. The habenula is both phylogenetically old (being well developed in the lamprey, see Loonen and Ivanova, 2016) and highly conserved, particular with response to its outputs (Loonen and Ivanova, 2015). The bulk of its descending inputs are from the 'cholinergic' basal forebrain (an exception is the medial prefrontal cortex) with MHb inputs being from more ventral and posterior nuclei (Loonen and Ivanova, 2022). The bulk of its ascending inputs are from the monoamine systems; with its descending outputs into or close to the pons; and, in complete contrast to the neuromodulatory systems we have just reviewed, no direct ascending outputs.

Both MHb and LHb are reciprocally connected with the ventral tegmental area. The MHb also outputs to the LHB, which connects with a range of ascending systems (dorsal raphe, median raphe, nucleus incertus, latero-dorsal tegmental nucleus, supramammillary area—yellow highlight in Fig. 6.11B) that also receive indirect input from MHb, relayed by the interpeduncular nucleus. Nucleus incertus also receives direct input from medial prefrontal cortex (dashed blue line in Fig. 6.11B). Exceptions to this parallelism for LHb include output to the PAG (which has separate parts devoted to basic appetitive, aversive, and inhibitory goal control, Silva and McNaughton, 2019) and the rostromedial tegmental nucleus (which encodes aversive stimuli and generates goal inhibition while sparing or enhancing active fear responses, Jhou et al., 2009). An exception for MHb is output relayed by the interpeduncular nucleus (yellow highlight in Fig. 6.11B) to the hippocampus (which we see as the primary area controlling more complex forms of goal inhibition). As discussed in the next section

---

Fig. 6.11 *(continued)*

ignoring its division into parts. Dashed lines with arrows indicate connections currently thought to be unidirectional, solid lines with balls indicate those known to be bidirectional. There appears to be a topographic division of ascending connections with bidirectional connections going to more ventral and rostral areas and unidirectional connections going to more dorsal and caudal areas (DH, VMH and PM appear to be exceptions). The representation of LHb has been displaced caudally to achieve clarity and to locate it closer to the superior colliculus (the area above CG), CG and DR with all of which it has connections. Figure and legend adapted from Pan and McNaughton (2004) with permission. Abbreviations: AH, anterior hypothalamic area; AM, anteromedial thalamic nucleus; Amyg, amygdala; AV anteroventral thalamic nucleus; Ce, cerebellar nuclei; CgCx, cingulate cortex; CM, central medial thalamic nucleus; DB/DBB Diagonal Band of Broca; DH, dorsal hypothalamic area; DP, dorsal peduncular cortex; DR, dorsal raphe nucleus; EC, entorhinal cortex; Hip, hippocampus proper; IL, infralimbic cortex; IP/IPN, interpeduncular nucleus; L6, spinal cord, lamina 6; LC, locus coeruleus; LDTg, laterodorsal tegmental nucleus; LH, lateral hypothalamus; LHb, lateral habenula; LS, lateral septal nucleus; MB, mammillary bodies MD, mediodorsal thalamic nucleus; mfb, medial forebrain bundle; MR, median raphe nucleus; MS, medial septal nucleus; PAG, periaqueductal grey; PH, posterior hypothalamic area; PM, premammillary nucleus; PO, preoptic nuclei; PS, posterior septum (including triangular); Re, nucleus reuniens; SI, substantia innominata; SuM, supramammillary area; VMH, ventromedial hypothalamus; VTg, ventral tegmental nucleus.

[7] My thanks to Anton J. M. Loonen for drawing the habenula to my attention and helping me understand it. The key uncited ideas in this section come either from his work or were developed in discussion with him.

(and Chapter 9) the direct (LHb) and indirect (MHb) connections to the supramammillary area could also impact on goal inhibition and, in particular, alter the control of the hippocampus and other areas by RSA/'theta' rhythmicity (purple dashed lines in Fig. 6.11B).

The relative conservation of the habenula, its small size, its relative lack of neocortical connections, and its predominant targeting of ascending neuromodulatory systems all suggest that it is a neuromodulatory (rather than information processing) system. Its primary input from the basal forebrain and general descending control suggest that it represents a feedback control system that keeps the other ascending systems in check. 'The habenula... plays an essential role in regulating the intensity of reward-seeking and adversity-avoiding behavior... by regulating the activity of ascending midbrain monoaminergic tracts' with, for example, input from the GP (Fig. 6.11B) causing it to inhibit unsuccessful reward-seeking (Loonen and Ivanova, 2019, p. 233). It also appears to go beyond inhibition to generating aversion and so avoidance. Like the monoamine systems, it is likely that the habenulae 'play an essential role in the pathogenesis of mood and stress disorders and addiction' (Loonen and Ivanova, 2019, p. 233; see also McLaughlin et al., 2017; Zhao et al., 2015; Loonen and Ivanova, 2018b; Batalla et al., 2017).

A more cognitive perspective of simple actions of the habenulae has been suggested.

> LHb has often been cited as a structure critical for adaptive and flexible responding when environmental contexts and internal state changes. A challenge, however, has been understanding how LHb promotes response flexibility.... We hypothesize that the LHb enables flexible responding following the integration of context memory and internal state information by signaling downstream brainstem structures known to drive hippocampal theta. In this way, animals respond more flexibly in a task situation not because the LHb selects a particular action, but rather because LHb enhances a hippocampal neural state that is often associated with greater attention, arousal, and exploration.
>
> Hones and Mizumori (2022, p. 1)

In addition to its output to the monoamine systems that we emphasized in relation to mood, stress, and addiction (and which influence hippocampal RSA/'theta'), LHb has direct output to the supramammillary area (§6.17, Chapter 9) and nucleus incertus (§6.15) both of which are involved in the control of hippocampal RSA/'theta'. Consistent with this, LHb appears to be involved in context memory. 'LHb inactivation results in disruption of memory retrieval as well as an inability to update the spatial configuration of the environment... [It keeps] track of choice outcomes, implicating it in memory for decisions made during goal-directed tasks... [and] a perhaps more general modulatory role in memory' (Hones and Mizumori, 2022, p. 3).

Despite a cognitive perspective, Hones and Mizumori (2022, p. 11) emphasize the role of LHb in aversion and say 'excessive LHb activity can also lead to impaired motivated behaviour and result in the pathophysiology of depression. In fact, the LHb is the only brain region that exhibits consistent hyperactivity in depression'.

What of the MHb? This has been much less studied. But a superficial inspection of the anatomy (Fig. 6.11B) suggests that it should control more complex processes than LHb. LHb has direct connections to all the ascending neuromodulatory systems as well as to PAG and RMTg, which can be seen as final stages in the generation, or prevention, of proximal stimulus-specific behaviours (consummatory or defensive). Except for VTA, MHb has its output relayed by IPN, which has many of the same targets as LHb (including all of those involved in the control of hippocampal RSA/'theta' rhythm), except that it also projects directly to the hippocampus. These hippocampal connections bring us to consideration of a remaining 'neuromodulatory' system, exemplified by the supramammillary area.

6.17 The supramammillary area (SuM)

We will discuss SuM (and other areas that control hippocampal RSA/'theta' rhythm) in detail in Chapter 9. We have also subjected it to detailed review previously (Pan and McNaughton, 2004, for which see citations for the following statements). It has a complex anatomy with distinct parts each associated with a wide range of neurotransmitters. It is also not the only area involved in RSA/'theta' control. These appear to form an integrated network and so we will take SuM here as an exemplar.

Briefly (see also Chapter 9), SuM controls RSA/'theta' rhythmicity (among other things) but does not appear to process more complex information. Despite its many transmitter systems, it appears to act as a time-based neuromodulatory system. Its basic output connections (Fig. 6.11C) are of the same general form as the relaxin-3 and monoamine systems including connections to medial prefrontal cortex, cingulate cortex, entorhinal cortex, and hippocampus—but omitting more extensive neocortical connections. Although we focus in this book mainly on its connections to the septum and hippocampus, it has similarly intense connections to, e.g. the claustrum that suggest it may coordinate isocortical sensory processing (Barbier and Risold, 2019).

It receives input (which it sometimes reciprocates) from all the targets of LHb except for RMTg and LC (to which it sends output). It also receives input from IPN, which is the main output target of MHb. In the current neuromodulatory context, and given the cognitive perspective discussed in the previous section, SuM could be seen as being an important for habenula feedback to more rostral systems—with its RSA/'theta'-related and other outputs being passed to (and often reciprocated by) the LH, MS/DBB, LS, IL/DP, and HPC; as well as to other areas less closely connected to the habenula: thalamus, amygdala, entorhinal cortex, and hypothalamus. It seems likely, given their ascending projections, that the other neuromodulatory areas are reciprocally connected with SuM to allow some integration of ascending control (e.g. when all the systems are responding to a stressor). SuM has recently been suggested to be particularly involved, together with dopamine systems, in the control of information-seeking behaviour (Kesner et al., 2022).

6.18 Overview—2D survival circuits

We have now ascended to the top of the hierarchy of *survival circuits* supporting defence, with its levels varying in terms of the defensive distance with which they deal. At the bottom, the PAG controls the simplest, undirected, escape responses. The highest of what we can view as a survival circuit is in the cingulate cortex, which controls more complex and anticipatory avoidance responses, including those (like hand washing) that lack safety signals. In Chapter 11, we will renew our journey upwards, treating the cingulate as a transitional zone between lower-level survival circuits and higher-level planning ones. In this context, it should be noted that an apparently complex social reward can activate all levels of the hierarchy, from frontal cortex to brainstem (Martins et al., 2021; see also Noritake et al., 2021).

At all levels of the systems, we have also distinguished defensive direction (GRS versus GIS) and commented in passing on parallel appetitive control (GAS). Thus, all three systems are represented within the PAG (Fig. 6.2), with similar separations at the levels of hypothalamus, amygdala/SHS, and cingulate cortex. In terms of the control of behaviour, as opposed to arousal, the amygdala and anterior cingulate are largely concerned with repulsion; and the SHS and posterior cingulate cortex are largely concerned with goal conflict (and its related risk assessment).

However (§6.9–6.17), there is a complex set of ascending neuromodulatory systems that have the capacity to interact with all three primary systems; are interconnected; and appear to be governed by a descending arm mediated by the habenula. We have not discussed the role of glutamatergic and GABAergic cells in the pontine central grey—these provide general bottom-up attraction and repulsion signals, respectively (acting on the medial septum, hypothalamus, ventral tegmental area, and thalamus; Xiao et al., 2023). All the ascending systems have been implicated in mental disorder—and will be important in future chapters both for specific (gating) control of the SHS and for more general contributions to its function and, particularly, dysfunction.

Our review has shown that the match between the behavioural effects of lesions of a structure and those of injections of anxiolytics (as outlined in the preceding chapter) is greatest in the case of the SHS. To some extent this appears to be because many of the structures on which anxiolytics have their direct actions (locus coeruleus, raphe nuclei, supramammillary nucleus, amygdala) have connections with the SHS, each providing a separate component of the overall anxiolytic/septo-hippocampal syndrome. One important exception to this generalization, however, is that the output of the GIS that increases arousal (Fig. 5.1) is clearly mediated by parts of the amygdala (orange area in Fig. 6.5B) and not by the SHS.

Our overall conclusion, then, is that anxiolytics act on a GIS that is distributed and hierarchical (Fig. 6.5B) but with many key effects achieved directly or indirectly via the SHS. That is, because of its connections, we see the SHS as the core of the GIS and will draw similar conclusions in relation to frontal cortex (Chapter 11). We will later discuss the involvement (or otherwise) of the GIS in the various anxiety disorders as variously categorized by the DSM (American Psychiatric Association, 1987; American Psychiatric Association, 1994; American Psychiatric Association, 2013; American Psychiatric Association, 2022) and ICD (World Health Organisation, 2010; World Health Organization, 2021). But first, in the next part of the book, we provide a more detailed analysis of the SHS itself to clarify its role as the core of anxiety processing and to account for the common view that it is the core of memory processing.

7
What do hippocampal cell fields represent?

Chapters 7–10 will analyse the detailed functions of the septo-hippocampal (SHS). Here, as a guide to those functions, we start with the firing patterns of hippocampal cells in relation to the environment and experimental paradigms. These patterns are most often described as 'place fields' (§7.4) but we argue that, instead, firing is in 'goal fields' (for a detailed argument see McNaughton & Bannerman, 2024, which updates Appendix 6). Such goal fields will often include place as an important aspect. But they do not code for even goals in a strong sense, but rather are efference copies from other goal-encoding areas.

The spatial (cognitive map) theory (O'Keefe and Nadel, 1978) is undoubtedly one of the most important contributions to our understanding of hippocampal function. Strictly speaking, the spatial theory is a theory of memory, with spatial maps stored in the hippocampus (Nadel, 1991). We look at this in detail, with other memory theories, in the next chapter (see particularly §8.13). But, 'place fields' provided the initial impetus for the cognitive map theory, and their properties and the neural basis of their control are still being intensively studied more than 40 years after their discovery (Burke et al., 2011; Gener et al., 2013; Fattahi et al., 2018; Wohlgemuth et al., 2018; McKenzie et al., 2021).

Any essentially non-spatial theory (such as ours) must provide an account of 'place' fields. This chapter does so by first looking at simpler paradigms, where the spatial element is minimal and the nature of the fields easy to demonstrate (for more detail, see McNaughton & Bannerman, 2024). Using this foundation, we then provide a brief survey and reinterpretation of the data from experiments related to behaviour or stimuli in spatial tasks. (We revisit these paradigms in Chapter 10, where they inform mechanisms. Here, they provide only a foundation for our translation of 'place fields' to 'goal fields'.)

7.1 Eyeblink fields: a paradigm example

We will start with hippocampal cell coding of the eyeblink, a simple response with a stereotyped unidimensional trajectory.

An air puff or shock US can elicit an eyeblink without any associated hippocampal response. However, the blink can be conditioned by a tone/light CS, producing a unidimensional CR. Importantly, the hippocampus shows 'eye blink' fields that appear during conditioning (Berger et al., 1983), including in humans (Cheng et al., 2008), and often have the conformation of the CR but not of the CS (Alger and Teyler, 1976; Weiss et al., 1996; but see, Green and Arenos, 2007). Importantly, the primary plasticity underlying eye blink conditioning occurs in the cerebellum not the hippocampus (Thompson, 1986; Knowlton et al., 1988), even with delay conditioning (where the US overlaps the offset of the CS).

The blink and its field may seem very mechanical; but 'neurotic introverts usually condition faster and extinguish slower than other people [consistent with] *susceptibility to fear*

The Neuropsychology of Anxiety, Third Edition. Neil McNaughton and Jeffrey A. Gray, Oxford University Press.
 DOI: 10.1093/oso/9780198843313.003.0007

and particularly its induction by punishment' (McNaughton and Corr, 2019b, pp. 122–123). Consistent with this, as well as cerebellum, blink conditioning involves plasticity in parallel hippocampal and amygdala circuits (Stanton, 2000; Choi et al., 2001).

In contrast to simple and delay conditioning, with trace conditioning (where the CS terminates before the US would have occurred) there is an early 'additive neural response of the combined CS- and US-evoked neural activity similar to reflex facilitation or modification' (McEchron and Disterhoft, 1997, p. 1037), i.e. the hippocampus anticipates the need to act. It is for this reason that the hippocampal response does not always model the CR.

When interpreting the function of these (and other hippocampal cell fields) we should note that trace conditioning is sensitive to hippocampal lesions (Ivkovich and Stanton, 2001) but simple and delayed conditioning are not (Berger et al., 1986a; Logan and Grafton, 1995; Blaxton et al., 1996; Steinmetz, 2000). Similarly, in humans, 'comparable delay and trace activation was measured in the cerebellum, whereas greater hippocampal activity was detected during trace compared with delay conditioning' (Cheng et al., 2008, p. 8108).

The most important general conclusion is that the pattern that we perceive in the field does not match function. More specifically, the hippocampus is not the site at which a model of any stimulus, response, or goal is *stored*. Rather, the hippocampus appears to receive a *copy* of the output from a model constructed elsewhere in the brain. It can then serve as a location at which the requirement for exploration, for example, is indicated by any mismatch between actual and modelled input.

The extra-hippocampal location of the representation of the goal, and the receipt by the hippocampus of an efference copy of its activation, are particularly well illustrated by the data on eyeblink conditioning. During simple conditioning tasks, the firing of hippocampal cells closely tracks the nictitating membrane response (rather than the stimuli that give rise to that response, Berger and Thompson, 1978a; Berger and Thompson, 1978b). Despite this tracking, hippocampal lesions do not affect in any way the production of the nictitating response that has been so tracked (Appendix 6, § A6.2.2). Presumably, a pattern of firing similar to that observed in hippocampal cells must exist in the effector (blink) circuits themselves, so as to produce the observed muscular response. It seems parsimonious to assume, therefore, that these circuits send on to the hippocampus information about their own activation (i.e. an efference copy). In turn the hippocampus sends information on to areas like medial prefrontal cortex (Green and Arenos, 2007) or retrosplenial cortex (Berger et al., 1986b see also §7.5) to control more complex (e.g. trace or reversal) conditioning.

7.2 Habituation of orienting and hippocampus-related circuits

Simple tasks (habituation to a novel stimulus; simple CS-UCS pairing; and simple simultaneous discriminations) have allowed analysis not only of fields but their development along septo-hippocampal-entorhinal circuits, most especially by Olga Vinogradova (1975). Changes within circuits in these simple tasks illuminate fields in more complex tasks.

The medial septum provides short latency multimodal input ('quick and dirty', c.f. thalamic input to the amygdala, Fig. 6.1) that is primarily a flag for a need to cope with a situation (i.e. a goal is present and either orienting or some other subcortical, response mechanism is primed). Absent a suitable pre-programmed reaction (signalled via the entorhinal cortex), hippocampal output elicits exploratory behaviour (c.f. simple avoidance as elicited from the amygdala). With repetition of a novel stimulus, neocortical areas build up a model of the stimulus and of any required responses. These goals are passed to the hippocampus by the entorhinal cortex, with the final step of model building (or at least plasticity) occurring in the dentate gyrus (c.f. Lian and Burkitt, 2021, for a related spatial model). An important point is that separate models of the stimulus must be passed simultaneously for all current potential goals, or inappropriate exploration will be elicited.

Note that overlaid on this simple circuit, there appear to be logical conditions that can operate a series of gates (see §10.3). These gates augment activity in dentate only, or dentate and CA3 only, or dentate and CA3 and CA1 only, or through the entire trisynaptic circuit, or, finally, in the targets of hippocampal output. Importantly, Vinogradova's (1975) data indicate that long-term potentiation (see Chapter 10, §10.3; Appendix 6, § A6.2.1.8) of dentate input *cancels* rather than enhances hippocampal responses. Further, she has shown (Vinogradova, personal communication) that, if long-term potentiation is artificially induced by perforant path stimulation, the hippocampus proper becomes totally unresponsive to natural stimuli that previously elicited a response (see also Miller et al., 1995). As with the eyeblink data of §7.1, these results show that the hippocampus does not code primary goals. If it did, experience would enhance rather than eliminate hippocampal responses, and removal of the hippocampus would eliminate rather than leave intact goal directed behaviour.

Matching the parallel septal and entorhinal inputs to all levels of hippocampus proper (demonstrated anatomically), there is good evidence that (like septal information) quite specific entorhinal information can frequently be passed directly to area CA1 and that the same information can be separately filtered by the dentate gyrus and the septal inputs and then appear, effectively degraded, within area CA3 before being passed on 'to meet itself' in CA1. It is, of course, not 'the same information' and the entire purpose of the linear organization of hippocampal fields[1] may be to provide a hierarchical series of logical gates, with output possible from each level of the system (see Fig. 10.3).

7.3 An initial view of hippocampal cell fields

Sections 7.1 and 7.2 focused on simple stimuli and simple learning paradigms in rats and rabbits, frequently under conditions of restraint; but nonetheless demonstrate quite complicated hippocampal reactions. Further, McNaughton and Bannerman (2024) describe a number of cases where the reaction shows little obvious relation to the apparent stimulus or response involve; and also, cases where there are systematic relations between the different components of the hippocampal formation. We believe these simpler cases are paradigmatic of hippocampal fields, including 'place'.

The picture so far is that that fairly non-specific information, related to the priming of subcortical response systems, is sent from the medial septum to the hippocampal formation; and

[1] While we talk about CA3, CA1 and subiculum as three distinct fields, the mapping may be more spread out than this: area CA2 has long been recognized as potentially distinct (Brown et al., 2020; Middleton and McHugh, 2020; Lehr et al., 2021; Robert et al., 2021); CA4 may be an extension of CA3 (which itself has occasionally been divided into subregions a, b, and c); the CA1/subiculum border appears to have a specific relation to the amygdala; and other sub-regional strips are appearing in the literature. This dimension may then share the complexity of the longitudinal one (Strange et al., 2014).

that such transfer is more likely in the case of conditioned than unconditioned responses. Consistent with non-specific encoding, in a non-spatial working memory task medial septal activity is occasionally correlated with stimulus presentation, but more often correlated with response emission or reward delivery; and 'incorrect responses are not associated with activation, indicating that the medial septal area is only active under conditions in which the appropriate response rule is retrieved for a given stimulus' (Givens, 1996a, p. 425; see also Kita et al., 1995).

Where reinforcement is present, the simpler paradigms suggest that the non-specific septal input and specific entorhinal input are combined to produce CA3 and CA1 responses. Consistent with a combinatory function of this kind, there are hippocampal cells with highly specific, apparently 'relational', fields. This specificity (within any single task) extends even to apparently simple tasks, such as differential reinforcement of low rates of response (DRL), during which each of many cells has a unique firing field linked to task demands that seldom involve any spatial component (Young and McNaughton, 2000). In all these cases, we argue (see Chapter 1) that hippocampal activity reflects relatively simple information about available goals (and hence choices) provided to it by other structures such as the cerebellum or orbital frontal cortex (Wikenheiser et al., 2021; Rolls, 2023), gated by aminergic inputs that indicate importance, and by mismatch (in either direction) between septal and entorhinal inputs (Chapter 9), indicating a need for information gathering. We further suggest (following, e.g. Wiener, 1996) that distinct fields within a single task reflect distinct components of that task (subgoals, if you will) and the cell's firing pattern will change with changing demands within the task (beyond so-called re-mapping, §7.4.9), and between tasks.

With our overview of these data as a foundation, we now turn to observations from more complex tasks; for these, however, there is much less information about the transformations occurring between the different areas of the hippocampus (or other brain areas Conejo et al., 2010; González-Pardo et al., 2012) and so we will focus on field correlates not hippocampal processing.

7.4 'Place fields'

7.4.1 Displace, place, and goal

In our paradigm cases (§7.1; §7.2), the animal was unable to move through space; or (§7.3) the predictors of reinforcement were non-spatial. In a complex environment, where reinforcement can be correlated with space, however, two main firing patterns are observed, both connected to 'place' (if we use the term loosely).

'Displace' units: Some hippocampal units fire principally when the animal is moving from place to place, unrelated to its mode of movement or destination. Their firing has a high rate. It is strongly correlated with movement RSA/'theta' (see next) and the relevant units often fire in bursts phase locked to the rhythm (Ranck, 1973; Feder and Ranck, 1973; O'Keefe and Nadel, 1978). As movement speed increases, previously non-rhythmic units become rhythmic and previously rhythmic units increase their rhythmicity (Rivas et al., 1996), so it is not clear whether units with these characteristics constitute a categorically distinct class of

neurone or a set of neurones temporarily showing a particular mode of responding. O'Keefe and Nadel (1978) term the movement-related cells 'displace' units; they are identical to the 'theta units' in other reports (O'Keefe, 1976) and have received little recent interest.

'Place' units: By contrast, provided there are intrinsic or extrinsic reinforcers linked to space, other hippocampal units appear to fire only when the animal is in a particular place. In common parlance, the unit has a 'place field' and is often called a 'place cell' (see O'Mara, 1995; Wiener, 1996 for early reviews; see Colgin, 2020; Goode et al., 2020, for recent comment). These cells do not show clear individual theta activity; but the individual probability of their firing is linked to the phase of ongoing theta rhythm and their average firing as a population shows theta modulation (e.g. Skaggs et al., 1996, Fig. 2), which can support sequences and reversal of their order (Wang et al., 2020). The description of 'place cells' by O'Keefe and Dostrovsky (1971) was the main impetus for the spatial theory of hippocampal function, supported by lesion experiments (e.g. Olton and Isaacson, 1968; Mahut, 1971), which in one form or another is clearly far from defunct (Sanders et al., 2020; Theves et al., 2020; Bevandić et al., 2021; Dorfman et al., 2021).

'Goal' units: Is how we would prefer to characterize hippocampal cell fields. The basic observation of place-relatedness of fields is not in question. What we must consider here is its generality, the extent to which the name applied to the field matches the functional significance of the firing and, most importantly, the extent to which a cell that occasionally has a place-related field can be called a 'place cell'. We argue that 'place cell' is a misnomer and that 'place field' is only occasionally descriptively appropriate, and never functionally accurate. We will consider many different properties of place fields next. A common feature, important for our theory, is that, other than spatial position *per se*, 'hippocampal neuronal activity may reflect the association of movements with their spatial consequences' (Foster et al., 1989, p. 1580; see also Takamiya et al., 2021), with the hippocampal formation involved in path integration (Wiener and Korshunov, 1996; Wiener, 1996; McNaughton et al., 1996a; Whishaw, 1999; Buzsáki, 2005; Johnsen and Rytter, 2021). Association of a class of movement with a consequence matches the idea of an 'available goal' field (see Chapter 1). Certainly, in everyday speech, a goal is often a place; and firing of about a third of hippocampal cells is related to a specific upcoming choice, even when this is incorrect (Takamiya et al., 2021).

7.4.2 What is a place field?

The *specifically spatial* basis of place fields (O'Keefe and Dostrovsky, 1971; O'Keefe, 1976) was demonstrated by O'Keefe and Conway (1978) with the rats trained inside a specially constructed square enclosure (Fig. 7.1A).

> The walls were formed by floor length black curtains. Within the enclosure, there were four cues by which the rat could locate itself: a dim white light, a white card, a buzzer and a fan. Four male hooded rats were made hungry and trained to go to one of the arms of a T maze to obtain food. From trial to trial, the maze and the cues were randomly rotated by some multiple of 90° relative to the environment, but maintaining the same spatial relationship to each other [(Fig. 7.1B)]. In order to rule out other intra-maze cues as a means of solution, the arms were interchanged from trial to trial. Body turns were ruled out by randomly

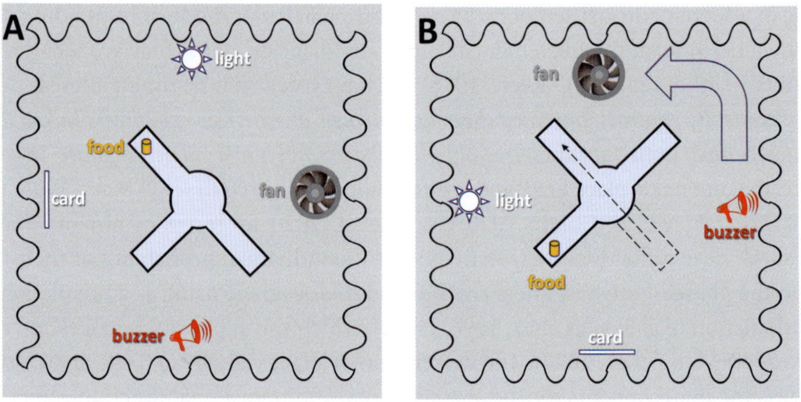

Fig. 7.1 Layout of the cue controlled enclosure used by O'Keefe and Conway (1978) for their single-unit experiment (adapted from their Fig. 1). The curtained-off cue-controlled enclosure (A) was located within a laboratory room and rotated relative to the room (⟲ in B) by multiples of 90° between trials and the start arm was on opposite sides of the maze (dashed arrow and outline) on 50% of trials. For details see O'Keefe and Black (1978, p. 84) quoted in the text.

> rotating the stem of the T maze 180° relative to the cross bar so that on one half of the trials a right turn was required to reach the goal while on the other half, a left turn was required [(Fig. 1B)]. After the rats had learned the task, they were further trained so that after running to the goal arm and consuming the reward they should run to the non-goal arm and thence back to the start arm, where they received a second reward. Thus, on each trial they made a complete circuit of the maze, giving the hippocampal units an equal opportunity to fire on all parts of the maze. The place where the units fired on the maze was recorded by pulsing a light-emitting diode on the rat's head whenever an action potential occurred and photographing these light flashes with an overhead camera.
>
> (O'Keefe and Black, 1978, p. 84)

Using careful transpositions of this paradigm, O'Keefe and Conway showed that a number of cells fired in response to particular relations between the four controlled cues inside the enclosure (light, card, buzzer, and fan). An example of such a place field is shown in Fig. 7.2A–D. On probe trials, one or more of these cues was removed. Some place units responded by increasing their firing field into the entire test environment; others responded by ceasing to fire. In either event, the original place field was lost—as also when the start arm was relocated (Fig. 7.2E, F). When panels A–D were superimposed aligned to the controlled cues, cell firing was located largely in one place (Fig. 7.2G), when aligned with the external world (Fig. 7.2H) or maze components (Fig. 7.2I) firing was distributed.

The increased fields of some cells may be related to the behaviour of the 'misplace' units also described by O'Keefe and Nadel (1978), which fire when the rat goes to a place but *fails* to find a stimulus (e.g. light or food) that has previously been there (O'Keefe, 1976). There were many other descriptions of both place and misplace cells at the time (Ranck, 1973; Olton et al., 1978a; O'Keefe and Nadel, 1978, p. 209); with continuing study, of place cells, since then (see Colgin, 2020, for 50-year overview); and the recent award of a Nobel prize for work that

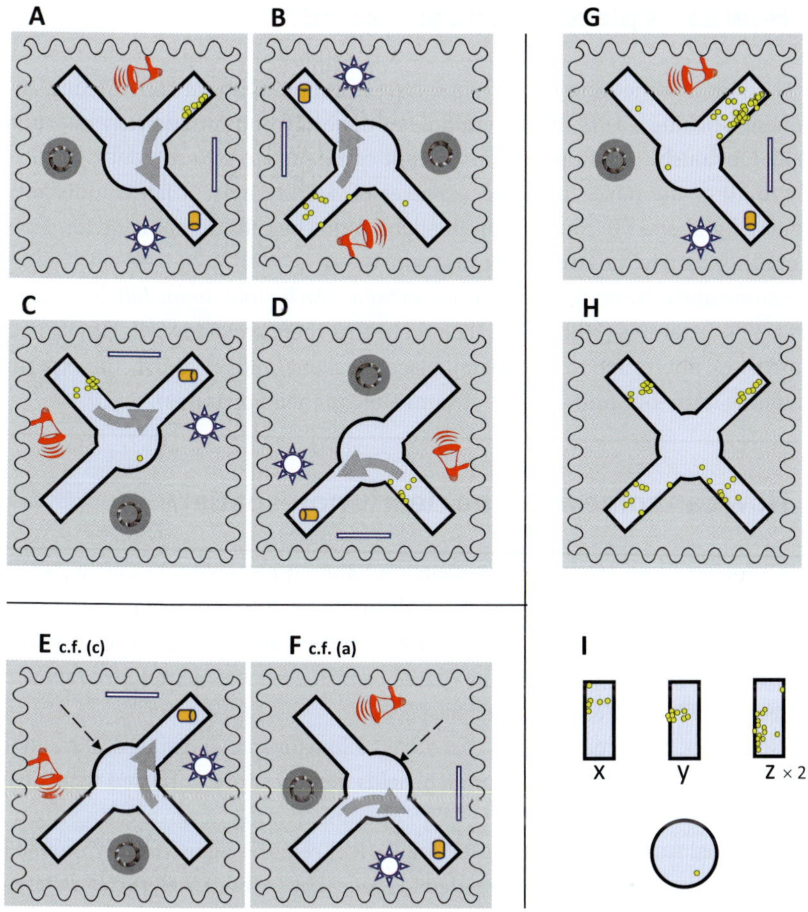

Fig. 7.2 The firing of a place unit when a rat is on the T-maze inside the cued enclosure, adapted from Fig. 3 and 4 of O'Keefe and Conway (1978). Each dot represents one action potential. Four trials are shown in A-D in which the T-maze and the cues on the wall have four different orientations relative to the external world. The orientation of the external world is constant. Note that the unit fires when the rat is in the start arm when it is on the side close to the buzzer, regardless of the orientation relative to the external world (see also G, H). E and F show two trials with the start arm rotated 180° (see Fig. 7.1B) so that it is on the side closer to the light and fan. The unit does not fire on either trial. G, H, I. Cell firing from trials A-D superimposed aligned in relation to: G) the controlled cues on the walls; H) the external world; and I) the individual specific components of the maze. Note that the z-arm was used as the start arm twice while the other arms were used only once each.

sees the hippocampus as a key part of a human 'Global Positioning System' (for overview see Burgess, 2014).

So, if you arrange your task so as to look for 'place fields' (in particular making reward consistently linked to spatial position), you will find them. Let us now look more closely at their specific properties. These do not translate to the coding of a place by the cell in any conventional geographic sense for at least seven reasons.

7.4.3 How can a place field be pre-wired?

Reason 1: There is something more than a little miraculous about constructing an *ad hoc* environment, sticking a wire into the middle of the brain and immediately encountering a place field. Obviously, the hippocampus cannot come prewired to respond specifically and uniquely to all of the novel future occurrences of, for example, 'a fan equidistant from a buzzer and a light, and 90° round from the light' (and the cells do not code for geophysical space since they map to the stimuli not the room).

Yet for some units the place field appears, as far as can be told, *immediately* the animal encounters a new apparatus (Hill, 1978). It could be that there are many cells closely packed together and those not related to the current place are silent (and, of course, the experimenters keep searching until they find cells fire at some time in their apparatus).

7.4.4 How can some fields be clearly non-spatial?

Reason 2: Vinogradova's (1975) experiments on habituation to simple sensory stimuli and Berger and Thompson's (1978a; 1978b) on conditioning of the nictitating membrane response and later developments (§7.1, §7.2, see also Appendix 6 and McNaughton & Bannerman, 2024), demonstrate 'fields' that could be spatial only in a very contemplative rabbit and that correlate better with features not related to space.

Likewise, in rats, task requirements that do not allow for spatial coding still result in many cells with 'cue sampling' and 'goal approach' fields and these are unrelated to available spatial locations (Eichenbaum et al., 1987). With operant chamber lever-pressing there are still small-scale spatial features, but if the schedule (DRL) requires an essentially non-spatial solution, virtually all cells have fields unrelated to space that are nonetheless clearly task-related (Young and McNaughton, 2000).

So, while the firing of a hippocampal unit tells us where a rat is when a task is space-invariant (Wilson and McNaughton, 1993), it cannot tell us where the rat is if the task is space-variant. We believe it was once observed (perhaps by Jim Olds?) that hippocampal cells fire to whatever the experimenter is thinking about (or at least on whatever regularities their paradigm encapsulates).

7.4.5 When is a place not a place?

Reason 3: The same cell has 'place fields' in multiple environments (and often within the same one). This is like London being located both in England and, at the same time, somewhere randomly in France! In the O'Keefe and Conway (1978) study (Fig. 7.1, 7.2) nearly half the cells had one field in the T maze, and a separate field on a platform in the room outside the black curtains. This goes to extremes in an ecologically realistic size of environment, where 'place cells exhibited multiple place subfields of different sizes, akin to those observed along the septo-temporal axis' (Harland et al., 2021, p. 1).

Interestingly, such multiple place fields are 'very different in the different environments ... A single neurone could have a large place field in one situation and a small place field in another situation. [Even in] the same situation a neurone can have single or multiple place fields. This could vary between situations. There was no constancy of the place fields of the same neurone with respect to distal cues [common to the environments]. We have not been able to discover any organizing or over-riding [spatial] principles for the positioning of a single cell's place fields across environments' (Kubie and Ranck, 1983, p. 438; see also Wiener, 1996). Later analysis suggested that time was as important as space (Umbach et al., 2020; Reddy et al., 2021), and that remapping reflected the coding of context (Kubie et al., 2020). Interestingly, odour remains stable when time is remapped (Taxidis et al., 2020).

In monkeys, Cahusac and Miyashita (1988) noted that different cells have spatial correlates in different spatial tasks; and, in rats, the same cell can have one correlate in a clearly spatial task (the radial arm maze), another in a dubiously spatial task (retrieving pups in a nest box), and yet a third in a task that is almost certainly not spatial (bar pressing on a DRL schedule, e.g. Ranck in Elliott and Whelan, 1978, p. 310). This chaos, evident in the early literature where experimenters had less of a spatial focus, goes well beyond the idea of 'remapping' (see *Reason 6, §7.4.8*).

7.4.6 Why is place not sufficient for firing in a place field?

Reason 4: Even when location appears to be a necessary condition for firing, it is not a sufficient one—firing occurs only when a particular organization of the external stimuli is viewed (e.g. McNaughton et al., 1983; Breese et al., 1989; see also Rolls and O'Mara, 1995); and ceases (see also *Reason 6)* if a source of reinforcement is placed within the field (Gothard et al., 1996).

Likewise, the precise details of a field located in a particular place can depend on learning and motivation. 'Hippocampal ensembles encode space at a finer scale following fear memory acquisition. This effect is strongest near the shock grid' (Schuette et al., 2020, p. 8329).

7.4.7 Why does the hippocampus not contain a spatial map?

Reason 5: No-one has ever reported anything approaching a topographic map of spatial fields within the hippocampus. This failure contrasts with the allocentric and body part-related maps found in areas such as the basal ganglia and frontal cortex, and the visual-field-related maps found in visual cortex.

There is enormous variation in the size and shape of spatial fields from cell to cell in the hippocampus (Muller et al., 1987); from time to time, in the same cell; and even of many fields of the same cell within a sufficiently large single environment (Harland et al., 2021). This is inconsistent with a conventional spatial metric.

Notably, pairs of cells with related firing patterns show 'the same interrelations with respect to place field overlap and cross-correlations, irrespective of actual field location' (Hampson et al., 1996), while groups of *neighbouring* cells can show considerable discordance (Tanila et al., 1997).

The true nature of the hippocampal topographic map is discussed further in §7.7.

7.4.8 Why does motivation trump location?

Reason 6: Spatial fields often cluster on important locations ('goals', Hollup et al., 2001; but see also Duvelle et al., 2019) but change radically if the importance changes. Entorhinal grid cells are also attracted to goals (Boccara et al., 2019). Such 'location' change of some cells, relative to adjacent others, continues to be called 'remapping' despite its breaking of all rules to do with conventional maps (Latuske et al., 2018; Grella et al., 2019; Sanders et al., 2020; Schuette et al., 2020; Bevandić et al., 2021; Kubie et al., 2020). (In comparison to *Reason 3*, we now have London jumping from England to France, while Brighton and Lyon remain where they always were.)

In one experiment (Breese et al., 1989), spatial fields clustered on five locations at which water was randomly delivered and tended to omit locations where water was not delivered. Delivering water to only one of the five locations caused most cells (40/47) to shift their field to that location or to change their fields in other ways. The fields appear to relate, then, to task demands; and surprisingly, such remapping, is influenced by the cerebellum (Zeidler et al., 2020).

Direction is also variably important. In a 'foraging task in an open field, . . . hippocampal CA1 pyramidal cells discharge when the rat visits the firing field, regardless of the direction that the animal is facing' (Wiener, 1996, p. 341), whereas 'in tasks involving repeated, stereotyped trajectories between fixed locations, hippocampal place fields are highly directionally sensitive' (McNaughton et al., 1996a; see also Markus et al., 1995). Similarly, O'Keefe and Speakman (1987) rotated a set of spatial cues, which signalled reward location, with respect to the global environment, which did not predict reward location: most cells (33/55) had spatial fields fixed with reference to the cue array, while a more modest number (15/55) had spatial fields fixed with reference to the global environment. Of particular interest is the fact that, if the cues were removed but the spatial field remained the field of the previously cue-related unit predicted the rat's choice—even if this turned out to be an error.

Remarkably, exploration of a range of novel environments can sometimes, after exposure, drastically alter the distribution of place fields in a task and apparatus that is *exactly the same before and after* (McNaughton et al., 1996a); likewise a simple change in running speed 'can cause rapid and reversible transitions between multiple spatial maps *of an unchanging task and environment* . . . synchronized across hundreds of neurons [with] differentially affected navigational cell types' (Low et al., 2021, p. 2967, added emphasis).

In all these cases 'place cells' fire in various places and only given other environmental features of motivational significance for the animal (or its relevance, Allegra et al., 2020). Where there is conflict between the two, motivation trumps location and hippocampal activation in humans is more linked to avoidance than features of threats (Abivardi et al., 2020) and to conceptual dimensions than features of objects (Theves et al., 2020).

7.4.9 Why do people call a failure to correlate with space 'remapping'?

Reason 7: In much of the above, we have seen 'place' fields change as a result of non-geometric factors; or have seen the nature of the immediate distributions of fields inconsistent with a spatial metric. It speaks to the strength of belief in the spatial map concept; that these paradoxical results are often attributed to 're-mapping' even when the result is inconsistent with any spatial metric.

Distortions of the size and shape of the arena in which the animal is placed do not produce equivalent distortions in the spatial fields of all cells, with the single exception of rectangular arenas that vary in side length (O'Keefe and Burgess, 1996). The firing pattern in a rectangular arena could not be predicted from the firing pattern in a circular arena (Muller and Kubie, 1987).

Importantly, if a transparent barrier is placed so that it intersects part of a spatial field, it can destroy the field (or sometimes expand it), whereas the lead base used to hold the barrier does not have this effect when used without the barrier (Muller and Kubie, 1987). So, spatial fields result, not from the rat's being in a place (defined by external detectable sensory cues, see Fig. 7.1), but from the rat knowing what it can do at (or do in the future from) that location (which would be changed by the barrier).

Conversely, a cell will maintain its place field in the dark, if it knows its starting location (see McNaughton et al., 1989; Markus et al., 1994). But, direct placement into a dark environment (eliminating starting location information) can cause a *remapping* that is *maintained* in the light (Quirk et al., 1990). Likewise, conflicting vestibular and visual information can cause 'unpredictable changes in firing characteristics, so that cells either stopped firing, or developed place fields that were altered in overall size, shape, and eccentricity' (Sharp et al., 1995, p. 173).

So, what the experimenter sees as the field and the variable remapping of different fields relative to each other depends on multiple factors, not spatial location alone (or sometimes at all), and can change rapidly. Indeed, 'instantaneous transformation of the spatial context does not change the hippocampal representation all at once but is followed by temporary bistability in the discharge activity of CA3 ensembles. Rather than sliding through a continuum of intermediate activity states, the CA3 network undergoes a short period of competitive flickering between preformed representations of the past and present environment before settling on the latter' (Jezek et al., 2011, p. 246). Likewise, progressive remapping of CA1 place fields with experience is uncoupled from that of place fields in area CA3 (Dong et al., 2021); and medial entorhinal cortex cells remap even more (Cholvin et al., 2021). None of this is consistent with what a surveyor calls space.

7.4.10 So, a 'place' field clearly does not code place

It follows from all of the above (§7.4.1–7.4.9) that 'place field' is a convenient loose descriptive term within specific experimental paradigms at specific (pre-re-mapping) points in time but is not functionally accurate. 'Place cell', in any literal sense, is a misnomer. If a cell has a 'place field' somewhere/sometime, there is no guarantee that the animal will be at that same point in allocentric space when the cell fires again. In two or more shapes of apparatus, there is no obvious allocentric relation between the positions of spatial fields in one as compared to another. There is no topographic mapping in the hippocampus to allow spatial decoding; fields can change dramatically in a spatially unchanged environment; some cells appear to code geographical space and some the cue space, but the majority code whatever multidimensional non-spatial frame of reference predicts reinforcement.

This is not to say that space is unimportant. Spatial fields are not directly related to experimenter-imposed reinforcement, and are usually sufficiently spread to allow (in aggregate) prediction of the animal's position within a specific current space (Wilson and McNaughton, 1993), including when the same space encloses a novel problem (Miller et al., 2023). In monkeys, there is minimal evidence for spatial biases in firing (see O'Mara, 1995) but the monkeys cannot move and spatial position is not a goal correlate. Cahusac et al. (1989) included spatial position as a factor in determining correct responses, and found spatial firing correlates; while, when Rolls and O'Mara (1995) moved a monkey with a robot, cells fired in relation to where the monkey looked, to movement to a place, and to other more complex conditions. The fields appear to relate to what the animal needs to care about—which is often space, for a typical experimental (or ecological) rat—and they lose interest in space if it is not linked to a goal (Hollup et al., 2001).

If 'place fields' do not reflect spatial position, how can we account for them? To answer this, let us first look at the theoretically-simpler head direction fields that have been found in areas that connect to the hippocampal formation.

7.5 From 'head direction' fields to 'place fields'

There is evidence that hippocampal 'place fields' could be constructed from 'head direction' (HD) fields (for an early overview of head direction cells see Taube et al., 1996; and, for more recent perspectives, see Shinder and Taube, 2014; Taube, 2007; Page and Jeffery, 2018; LaChance et al., 2020). HD is in turn derived from landmarks provided by auditory input, visual input (Page and Jeffery, 2018), and optic flow (Arleo et al., 2013); and from idiothetic input from the vestibular (Muir et al., 2009), and proprioceptive systems.

'Motor and proprioceptive information have in particular been shown to be important for updating the HD signal as an animal moves from a familiar environment to a novel one that contains unfamiliar landmarks' (Shinder and Taube, 2014, p. 124; citing Stackman et al., 2003; Yoder et al., 2011). Further, 'the animal's orientation with respect to gravity plays an important role in determining a cell's [preferred firing direction, and] vestibular and proprioceptive cues drive these computations' (LaChance et al., 2020, p. 3035). So, 'head direction' is a fairly subtle concept and as much under internal as external cue control.

The primary visual input to the HD system is most likely to come from 'intermediate/deep layers (IV–VII) of superior colliculus [that] play a special multisensory role in spatially guided behaviour . . . [and] project to the lateral dorsal nucleus of the thalamus (LDN), which also receives direct input from retinal recipient pretectal nuclei. . . . LDN cells . . . in turn project directly to a number of cortical structures, notably the hippocampal formation' (Mizumori and Williams, 1993). These LDN cells 'selectively discharged when an animal's head was aligned along particular directions in space, irrespective of its location in the test room. . . . If the light was . . . turned off, directional firing was maintained briefly . . . [and then] appeared to systematically 'rotate' in either the clockwise or the counterclockwise direction. . . . Maximal directional firing was achieved only when the rat viewed the entire test room, and not just the scene associated with the directional preference of the cell' (Mizumori and Williams, 1993). Up to a minute of exposure to the environment can be needed for the directionality to appear. LDN, therefore, appears to acquire and then retain (like place fields, even in the absence of visual input) preliminary positional information that is head centred. Critically, 'inactivation of the LDN not only impairs spatial performance in rats, but it also disrupts location-specific discharge by hippocampal cells' (Mizumori and Williams, 1993; Mizumori et al., 1994).

Both Mizumori and Williams (1993) and Taube et al. (1996) suggested that the information from the LDN is sent to the post-subiculum (as well as directly to the entorhinal cortex and to the subiculum). The post-subiculum receives a large number of other inputs, but appears to have relatively similar HD cells to those in LDN (Taube et al., 1990a; Taube et al., 1990b). However, LDN lesions do not affect post-subiculum HD fields (see Taube et al., 1996) despite their affecting hippocampal 'place fields'. The LDN information appears to take the direct route to entorhinal cortex to reach the hippocampus (Fig. 7.3, yellow highlighted line) and separate routes, for example, via the anterior dorsal nucleus of the thalamus (ADN), to the post-subiculum. The ADN cells appear to predict *future* HD rather than to indicate current HD (Blair and Sharp, 1995; see also 'drift' in Arleo et al., 2013), and so the post-subiculum likely receives both current and future HD information.

This stimulus-oriented description is easy to follow, but we should note that the source of the original visual information, the superior colliculus, is much more concerned with spatially guided behaviour (and, indeed, affective significance, see Redgrave and Dean, 1997) than visual space itself. For example, when we discuss motor control in frontal cortex, we will make the suggestion that the frontal eye fields are an area of pre-motor processing that, of necessity, engages the eyes via the superior colliculus in order to provide the information required for the upcoming movement (Fig. 11.7). Indeed, Mizumori and Williams (1993, p. 4023, emphasis added) suggested that

> the LDN may be part of a neural system that subserves directed attention to constellations of salient cues in the animal's visual world. In this context it is worth noting that the structurally similar thalamic nucleus in primates, the pulvinar, has been shown to play a significant role in visual spatial attention processes. Specifically, Desimone and colleagues suggest that the pulvinar may *gate extrastriate responses to distracting visual input, thereby focusing one's attention onto a visual target.*

Thus, LDN may be concerned with the inhibition of eye movements to objects of visual attention ('visual goals') that are currently inappropriate.

More detailed landmark information appears to be provided by the extensive connections of the visual cortices with granular (area 29) and agranular (area 30) retrosplenial cortex (Fig. 7.3). As with eyeblink conditioning (§7.1) retrosplenial cortex operates in concert with the hippocampus to achieve control of higher order processes than those that give rise to the observed cell fields (place and HD in this case).

> Area 29 is the primary recipient of hippocampal and parahippocampal spatial and contextual information while area 30 is the primary interactor with current visual information.... Retrosplenial cortex helps to integrate space from different perspectives, e.g., egocentric and allocentric, providing landmark and heading cues for navigation and spatial learning. It provides *a repository of scene information* that, over time, becomes *increasingly independent of the hippocampus*. These processes, reflect the interactive actions between

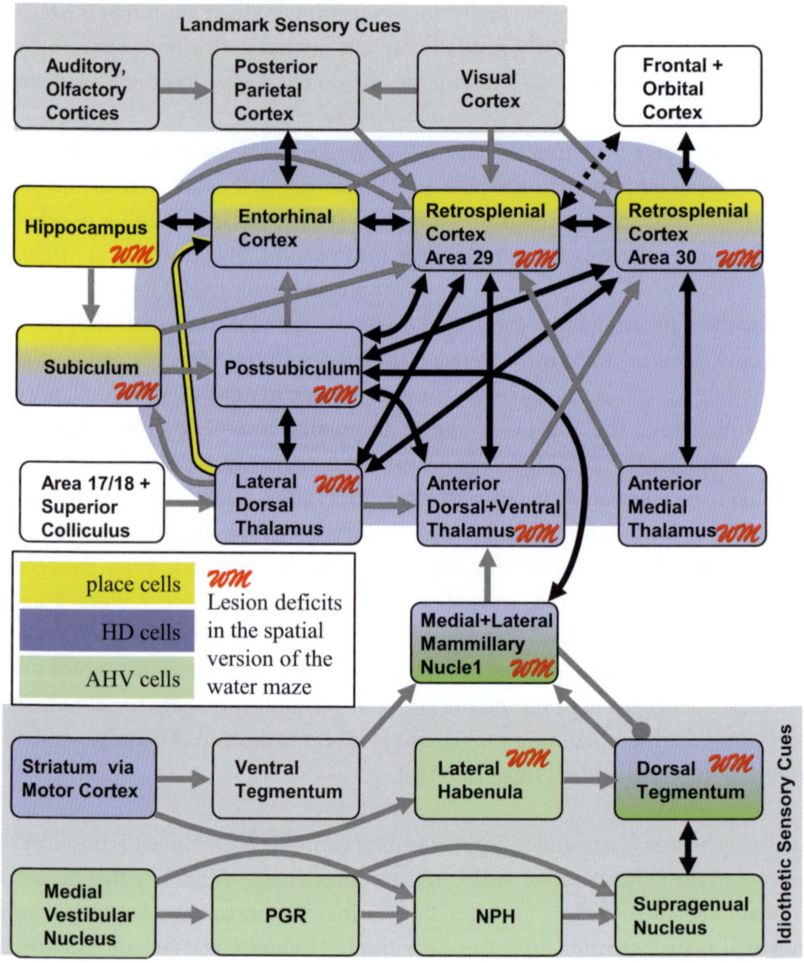

Fig. 7.3 Locations in the brain from which place, head direction (HD), and angular head velocity (AHV) cells have been recorded (shaded boxes) and locations at which lesions have been shown to impair spatial learning (WM). The figure also shows the connections between these areas and the hippocampal formation and areas that are likely to provide the sensory information driving the head direction cells (adapted from Taube et al., 1996; Taube, 2007; with data from Tsanov et al., 2011; van Groen et al., 2002; Clark et al., 2013; Frost et al., 2021; Mao et al., 2017; Sugar et al., 2011; Aggleton et al., 2021; and citations in the text). *Abbreviations:* NPH = Nucleus Prepositus Hyoglossi; PGR = Nucleus ParaGigantocellularis Reticularis

> areas 29 and 30, along with their convergent influences on cortical and thalamic targets. Consequently, despite their differences, both areas 29 and 30 are necessary for an array of spatial and learning problems.
>
> (Aggleton et al., 2021, abstract, our emphasis; see also Lomi et al., 2021)

Taube et al. (1996) concluded that a 'motor efference copy' is important in generating HD cell discharge, but that sustained discharge when the animal is stationary requires more complexity. Knierim and McNaughton (commentary following Taube et al., 1996, p. 484; see also

Knierim et al., 1995) note that 'both place cells and HD cells do maintain their tuning properties when the animal is passively rotated, as long as the animal is not tightly restrained. It thus appears that some type of 'motor set'—the preparedness for motion—has an influence over the responses of these cells, rather than any copy of actual motor commands'; and, as we quoted earlier, that 'hippocampal neuronal activity may reflect the [learned] association of movements with their spatial consequences' (Foster et al., 1989, p. 1580; see also O'Mara et al., 1994 on the effects of passive movement of a monkey on hippocampal cells).

> Motor set, intention, and goals embedded within HD fields are consistent with the fact that the responses of vestibular neurons within the vestibular nuclei are markedly attenuated when an animal makes a volitional head turn compared to passive rotation. This finding presents a conundrum in that if vestibular responses are suppressed during an active head turn how is a vestibular signal propagated forward to drive and update the HD signal? [There are] four possible mechanisms that could resolve this problem. These mechanisms are:
> (1) the ascending vestibular signal is generated by more than just vestibular-only neurons,
> (2) not all vestibular-only neurons that contribute to the HD pathway have firing rates that are attenuated by active head turns,
> (3) the ascending pathway may be spared from the affects *[sic]* of the attenuation in that the HD system receives information from other vestibular brainstem sites that do not include vestibular-only cells, and
> (4) the ascending signal is affected by the inhibited vestibular signal during an active head turn, but the HD circuit compensates and uses the altered signal to accurately update the current HD. Future studies will be needed to decipher which of these possibilities is correct.
>
> Shinder and Taube (2014, p. 123)

We would rephrase option 4 in more goal directed terms. The superficially complex (and often reciprocal) circuits of Fig. 7.3 are consistent with a system where idiothetic, land mark, and motor information send convergent sources of upcoming goal information clamped onto a system that is informed as to what goals are upcoming (with eye blink fields, and place fields being similar in this respect) and the function of which is higher order control via the inhibition of goals not their activation.

7.6 Path integration

The sandwiching of the core place/HD structures (yellow highlight in Fig. 7.3) between landmark and idothetic systems fits with the idea that the hippocampus

> can encode relative spatial location, without reference to external cues, by the integration of linear and angular self-motion (path integration). . . .
>
> Each place cell receives two different inputs, one conveying information about a large number of environmental stimuli or events, and the other from a navigational system which calculates where an animal is in an environment independently of the stimuli impinging on it at that moment. The input from the navigational system gates the environmental input, allowing only those stimuli occurring when the animal is in a particular place to excite a

> particular cell. One possible basis for the navigational system relies on the fact that information about changes in position and direction in space could be calculated from the animal's movements. When the animal had located itself in an environment (using environmental stimuli) the hippocampus could calculate subsequent positions in that environment on the basis of how far, and in what direction the animal had moved in the interim ... In addition to information about distance traversed, a navigational system would need to know about changes in direction of movement either relative to some environmental landmark or within the animal's own egocentric space ...
>
> (O'Keefe, 1976)

> Today, more than thirty years after the discovery of spatially selective place cells in the hippocampus and the proposal that the hippocampus is the neural substrate of a 'cognitive map', it would be difficult to write a more concise and accurate summary of our current understanding of hippocampal spatial encoding dynamics. .... Nevertheless, the history of the last 30 years of research aimed at characterizing the determinants of hippocampal neuronal activity in freely behaving animals has been rich with controversy, the central debate being whether location *per se* or sensory and cognitive factors provide the best predictor.
>
> (McNaughton et al., 2006a, p. 663).

One sensory/cognitive alternative is that path integration, in the sense of maintenance in memory of a fixed location through the process of dead-reckoning, is a special case of the sequencing of successive goals to achieve some final objective (Wiener and Korshunov, 1996), since:

> hippocampal neurones discharge selectively as the subject ... responds during successive phases of a behavioral task [to] stimulus and reward presentations as well as task-related behaviors ... [so that] *all of the behavioral components of the experimental task can be comprehensively represented.* [For example, in] a water search task ... [specific] neurones discharged when the rat performed [specific] task-related behaviors at several locations in the arena, each of which were virtually identical both in appearance and in significance with respect to the task requirements.... Thus the motor components of these behaviours were not the principal correlate of the unit activity. The fact that some of these neurones were selective for either trajectories towards the corners or the center also argues against a simple relation to sensory cues or rewards.... It appears then that this discharge selectivity depended on the behavioral context, that is, the rat being engaged in only one of the phases of a cycle of actions that it had adopted to satisfy the exigencies of the task.
>
> (Wiener, 1996, pp. 346, 348, our emphasis)

This seems true even with nictitating membrane response conditioning, since trace conditioning (a hippocampal lesion-dependent task) can have specific hippocampal cells firing in relation to specific components of the task, with essentially all components of the task covered (Weiss et al., 1996); and, as we note in Appendix 6, the same appears true even in the simple conditioning of this response (Berger et al., 1983).

Let us look closely at the idea of a hippocampal cell being activated by a specific goal within a sequence of task-related goals (Wang et al., 2020). For both the non-spatial and spatial cases, we found that two units with apparently the same type of correlate under one set of conditions could have different correlates from each other when the conditions changed. Also, spatial and HD fields appear to be seen, not when the animal *is* about to move, but whenever it *could* do so.

The firing of an individual cell must, therefore, be related to the available goals, with many such being signalled in the hippocampus simultaneously. For example, cells which signal the presence of a left-hand goal and cells which signal the presence of a right-hand one will fire simultaneously when the subject reaches a T junction. This fits with the fact that changing the location of reward changes the position of the place fields of only some cells. The goal fields have remained constant and the change in location of reinforcer has shifted the position of goals related to that reinforcer, but not goals related to other reinforcers. The notion that hippocampal cells are activated by available goals is consistent also with the one case where place fields seem predictable from apparatus to apparatus: a set of varying sized rectangular boxes. Here, the available goals (or paths to be integrated) should be strongly related from apparatus to apparatus. The idea of 'available goal' fields can also account for the lack of topographic mapping of 'place fields' (§7.8) and the fact that, when the location of 'place fields' is altered, closely related fields tend to stay together and to show similar changes in size (Hampson et al., 1996).

There are many possible models of path integration (McNaughton et al., 2006a), and many possible hypotheses as to where in the brain the actual integration is carried out. Such models may or may not involve a true cognitive map in O'Keefe and Nadel's (1978) sense. But, whatever the precise means used by the hippocampus to obtain information about the alternatives that can be chosen at any particular point in space or time (but note that odour is more stable Taxidis et al., 2020), such information should allow it to 'select and test hypotheses, or strategies, concerning the solution [to a problem]' (O'Keefe and Nadel, 1978, p. 2). Such selection and testing by the hippocampal system would be particularly important when a novel short-cut between two points can be substituted for a prior longer route by comparison of alternative immediately available goals or when remembered sequences must be correctly ordered in time (Umbach et al., 2020). It has been argued by Bennett (1996) that the capacity to select short cuts in this way can be computationally simple and can account for all the current evidence for cognitive maps of the type proposed by Tolman and by O'Keefe and Nadel (see also McNaughton et al., 1991). If so, this brings our account of hippocampal fields very close indeed to that required by O'Keefe and Nadel's (1978) cognitive mapping account.

7.7 Topographic mapping of single cell fields

As we have seen, positions of 'place fields' are not topographically mapped into the hippocampal formation; and in large environments not really mapped at all (Harland et al., 2021). Yet when their location alters, closely related fields tend to stay together and to show similar changes in size (Hampson et al., 1996; see also Pavlides et al., 2019). Given its small size, relative to neocortex, it seems unlikely that spatial coding is compounded, as has been suggested, with social dimensions (Dorfman et al., 2021). This all suggests the hippocampus has a topography but that it is not spatial in the geographic sense.

We should expect topography; brain organization is fundamentally topographic (Swanson, 2018). The afferents, efferents and internal structure of the hippocampus are themselves strongly topographically ordered (see e.g. Fig. 9.7, Fig. 10.4, and Appendix 4). We also have a ready candidate for the type of entity that might provide the basis for topographic mapping.

We proposed earlier that hippocampal cells code for 'available goals' and so must be organized in a map of 'goal space'. But, on what psychological dimensions could available goals be simply mapped? We will look at cells' mapping in neural terms; and the suggest one way this *can* be interpreted by psychology in a simple fashion.

We think that the hippocampal cells fire because they receive efference copies from one or more distinct goal processing areas in the brain; and their inputs to, and outputs from, the hippocampal formation are topographically mapped. With the subcortex this can relate to response organization (amygdala, accumbens, basal ganglia, hypothalamus) or internal adjustments related to the anticipation of action (amygdala, hypothalamus). For example, 'different hippocampal regions map in an orderly way onto hypothalamic systems mediating the expression of different classes of goal-oriented behaviour' (Risold and Swanson, 1996, p. 1484). That is, the septal-temporal aspect of the hippocampal formation maps topographically to dorsomedial-ventrolateral in the septum and caudal-rostral in the hypothalamus, while also retaining the distinction among hippocampal fields (Fig. 9.7; Risold and Swanson, 1996).

Likewise, the amygdala is more strongly connected to the temporal hippocampus and to the subicular-CA1 border (Appendix 4).

The main cortical areas that interlink with the hippocampal formation are concerned with planning (prefrontal cortex, cingulate cortex). The topography of these connections gives the hippocampal formation a simple functional organization. The septal end of the hippocampus receives more dorsal trend ('where') information and the temporal end more ventral trend, 'what', information (Fig. 10.4; Appendix 4; see also McNaughton et al., 1989). Consistent with this, relative to the septal end, the temporal hippocampus has fewer place cells (from about 50% to 20%) with larger fields (Jung et al., 1994; but see also Poucet et al., 1994). We have already noted that some goals are more easily distinguished in response terms (approach/avoidance) and others in stimulus terms (left lever/right lever), although any goal representation must combine situational and motivational properties. We argue that the hippocampus is organized in relation to these properties, from particularly situation-oriented (with tight place fields) to particularly motivation-oriented (with broad place fields) with essentially a steady gradient, at least in terms of connections (Moser and Moser, 1998; Strange et al., 2014; but see also Chockanathan and Padmanabhan, 2021). This accommodates 'lamellar' organization with similar computations (but see also Houser et al., 2021) being carried out on inputs that have varying emphasis on situation versus motivation. But note that the essence of the dorsal/ventral trend distinction is that the representation of goals is distributed, resulting in phenomena such as the man who mistook his wife for a hat (Sacks, 1985). There is also, for example, a superficial (novelty replay, entorhinal output) versus deep (ensemble activation/consolidation, prefrontal output) distinction for CA1 pyramidal layer cells (Harvey et al., 2023). It follows that one should not see hippocampal cells as operating in isolation but rather as parts of a distributed, extended, network (Strange et al., 2014); such a network may be as much concerned with prediction in partially novel situations as about 'recall' of unchanged ones (Miller et al., 2023).

> By simultaneously recording up to 620 principal neurons in the hippocampal area CA1 of freely moving rats, we could evaluate single-cell and population-level perspectives on how local objects influence representations of space. Some cells fired at the object (object cells),

> others at fixed distances and directions from it (object-vector cells, reminiscent of landmark-vector cells). In addition, the majority of the CA1 cells changed their spatial firing patterns when the object was introduced, moved, or taken out from the environment. At the level of neural populations, the heterogeneous responses were coherently organized across cells so that the amount of reorganization of the hippocampal map depended on distance from the object in a graded manner. The reorganization of the hippocampal map in the presence of objects was widely distributed and did not require specific subsets of cells or the presence of object cells and object-vector cells. Although past studies have already raised the possibility that the hippocampal representation of objects may be non-factorized, we here demonstrate how by describing (1) a strikingly smooth change in population activity according to object distance, and (2) an emergent property of the code, where the distance-based representation becomes more evident as sample sizes are increased. Our findings hint that some aspects of *hippocampal cognitive maps may not be understood through properties of dedicated functional cell types—such as object cells, object-vector cells, or place cells—but through emergent properties of cell populations* whose activities appear random and disorganized when viewed individually.
>
> (Nagelhus et al., 2023, pp. 2100–2101, emphasis added)

Note that the septal/temporal dimension appears to be truly dimensional and not, as would be implied by the dorsal/ventral distinction, categorical. The 'where'/'what' separation within the hippocampus reflects variations only in the *proportions* with which dorsal and ventral trend information arriving in the entorhinal cortex is mixed as the two streams are transferred to the hippocampus (hence the motivation-dependence of hippocampal place fields of all types and the, albeit coarse, location-dependence of even the largest fields). It is in the nature of the concept of a goal that it must combine 'what' and 'where' to some extent; hence, perhaps, the otherwise peculiar anatomical fact that the hippocampus (which can be thought of as a remnant of the primordial evolutionary and developmental origin of the dorsal trend) receives a confluence of both dorsal and ventral trend information.

What of the orthogonal dimension (CA3–CA1-subiculum) in the hippocampal formation? In discussing the habituation and simple conditioning results of single-unit recording experiments earlier (and see Chapter 10 for greater detail), we suggested that there is a fairly complex set of logical gates which takes a relatively non-specific septal signal and combines it with a specific entorhinal/dentate signal and with aminergic input to determine the extent to which each stage of the trisynaptic pathway will be activated, and the extent to which such activation has functional consequences. Place fields, on this scenario, are recorded with both the dentate-CA3 and CA3–CA1 gates open. The effects of lesions on place fields suggest that septal input relates to the local presence of important stimuli (and hence rather gross response tendencies, consistent with the multimodality found in septal firing repertoires in the simpler single-unit recording paradigms); while entorhinal input, once processed in the dentate (see also Lian and Burkitt, 2021), provides more specific positional information (e.g. distinguishing routes within an environment, Wilmerding et al., 2023). So entorhinal input relates to the more detailed organization of response programs—consistent with the modality-specific firing repertoires of entorhinal cells found in the simpler paradigms; and with the attraction of entorhinal grid cells to goals (Boccara et al., 2019). We presume that CA3 activity is the result of the integration of dentate with septal input. Consistent with this assumption, as we go from dentate to CA3 (Jung and McNaughton, 1993) to CA1 and then subiculum (Barnes et al., 1990; Sharp and Green, 1994), spatial specificity decreases. This second dimension of hippocampal mapping may then reflect 'level of processing' in some sense or other.

7.8 Conclusion

We will now draw some general conclusions about 'spatial' and 'non-spatial' fields since they must be based on the same neural computations.

First, pure stimulus-oriented descriptions (line/edge/head direction/place) are easy but *incorrect*.[2] The response elicited by the stimulus must be taken into account. For example: 1) with the nictitating membrane *field*, the firing pattern can model the *response* so closely that the hippocampus was earlier suggested to be the 'neuronal substrate of classical conditioning' (Berger and Alger, 1976)—a similar result is obtained with conditioned freezing, where 50% of freeze-related cells may have no spatial correlate (Schuette et al., 2020); 2) firing can predict an upcoming choice and flag whether a specific choice has just been rewarded (Takamiya et al., 2021); and, 3) when 'novel' stimuli fire hippocampal cells, they are not *just* novel but must be motivationally significant enough to elicit a response in the form of an orienting reflex (Appendix 6, §A6.2.1.8, §A6.2.2; McNaughton & Bannerman, 2024).

Second, responding *per se* is not critical: 1) there may be no firing in relation to an unconditioned response; 2) cells fire during a delay even when the upcoming response is indeterminate; 3) place and HD fields disappear when the rat knows a physical response is impossible, but fields remain with passive movement if the rat thinks a response is possible.

Third, fields depend on importance not position: 1) in areas CA3 and CA1 firing to neutral stimuli swiftly habituates, but firing to important stimuli that predict events like reward increases (§10.3); 2) place fields are unevenly distributed, they cluster on a goal (Hollup et al., 2001); 3) the position of a 'place field' can shift, *independent of other cell fields*, to a new geographic location that reward has moved to; and, 4) field existence, directionality, and spatiality depend on task demands and responding (Schuette et al., 2020), not just with place fields (Hollup et al., 2001) but also with HD and eyeblink fields—adaptive organisms must care about functional results. This cannot be due to *spatial* mapping by the cell.

Fourth, even a clear response correlate is not related to response control. With CA1 or CA3 firing (e.g. the modelling of the nictitating membrane response to the CS; Berger and Thompson, 1978a; Berger and Thompson, 1978b), the unconditioned response and the conditioning are controlled outside the hippocampal formation, and are unaffected by hippocampal lesions. Likewise, 'place fields' are particularly clear in runways but learning in a runway (where directional *interference* is low) is not affected by hippocampal lesions. Conversely, posterior cortex cells provide a precise representation of space, the formation of which requires an intact hippocampus (Esteves et al., 2021).

Fifth, fields signal exactly the same general class of feature under all circumstances. We agree with Wiener (1996, p. 355) that

> the discharge correlates for location and for task-related behaviours appear to be extremes of a continuum of responses in a single population of neurones. In intermediate cases,

[2] This is a general truth for visual cortex, hippocampus, or anywhere.

the discharge correlate is for conjunctions or recombinations across certain information domains, while generalizing over others. These responses seem to originate in a single population of neurones since cells with location-selective discharges can, in different circumstances, also have task-related behavioural correlates.

Sixth, the small hippocampus cannot possibly encode the complex information normally attributed to it. It may provide an index to information elsewhere (e.g. Goode et al., 2020) or integrate such information into predictions (Miller et al., 2023); but this idea ignores its non-memory functions. Importantly, in these cases, complex hippocampal-cortical machinery must be invoked in contrast to more simple Hebbian solutions (McNaughton and Wickens, 2003).

In conclusion, it is undoubtedly possible to demonstrate correlates of hippocampal cellular firing repertoires that are suitably and succinctly described as 'place fields'. However, the correlates of hippocampal firing are not uniquely spatial. A hypothesis that is able to encompass the bulk of the data from both spatial and non-spatial tasks is that the firing repertoires of hippocampal neurones represent available goals. The goals of a rat are often located in a particular place, giving rise to the place field as a correlate. But cells also signal upcoming choices, and so the bringing to mind of distinct future goals—which are then correlated with the location of *the choice point*. In such cases the spatial correlate of the cell firing is radically different from the reward location that is generating the firing.

The hypothesis we will adopt in the remainder of the argument pursued in this book is that hippocampal cell firing reflects an efference copy from a future goal that is coded in other brain areas, with feedback from the hippocampus during consolidation affecting future goal-oriented behaviour (Berners-Lee et al., 2021). Thus, the hippocampus and orbital frontal cortex contain related, interactive, cognitive maps that vary with both situation and motivation (Wikenheiser and Schoenbaum, 2016; Wikenheiser et al., 2021). Rather than storing information. the primary function of the hippocampus is to maintain in a meaningful form information that is stored elsewhere (Theves et al., 2021). This information can include sequences of events (Reddy et al., 2021), selection of specific versus general coding (Brunec, 2016; Brunec et al., 2020), evaluation of future possibilities (Kovács, 2020), egocentric space (Kunz et al., 2021), and hierarchical integration of concepts (Theves et al., 2020; Theves et al., 2021).

8
Memory and the septo-hippocampal system

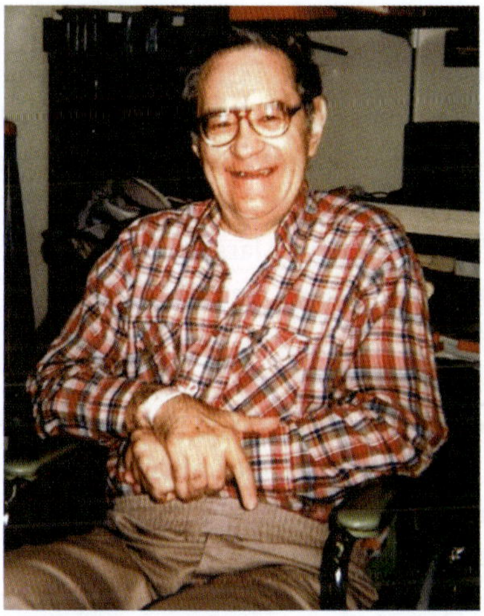

Henry Gustav Molaison, aged 60, at MIT in 1986.
Photograph (adapted with permission) and copyright: Jenni Ogden, author of *Trouble In Mind: Stories from a Neuropsychologist's Casebook*, Oxford University Press, New York, 2012

H.M., Whose Loss of Memory Made Him Unforgettable, Dies

He knew his name, that much he could remember.

He knew that his father's family came from Thibodaux, La., and his mother was from Ireland, and he knew about the 1929 stock market crash and World War II and life in the 1940's.

But he could remember almost nothing after that.

In 1953, he underwent an experimental brain operation in Hartford to correct a seizure disorder, only to emerge from it fundamentally and irreparably changed. He developed a syndrome neurologists call profound amnesia. He had lost the ability to form new memories.

For the next 55 years, each time he met a friend, each time he ate a meal, each time he walked in the woods, it was as if for the first time.

And for those five decades, he was recognized as the most important patient in the history of brain science. As a participant in hundreds of studies, he helped scientists understand the biology of learning, memory and physical dexterity, as well as the fragile nature of human identity.

On Tuesday evening at 5:05, Henry Gustav Molaison—known world-wide only as H. M., to protect his privacy, died of respiratory failure at a nursing home in Windsor Locks, Conn.

Benedict Carey, *The New York Times*, Friday 5 December 2008, Page A35

The Neuropsychology of Anxiety, Third Edition. Neil McNaughton and Jeffrey A. Gray, Oxford University Press.
 DOI: 10.1093/oso/9780198843313.003.0008

You have likely experienced the tip-of-the-tongue phenomenon. You know you know something but your mind is a total blank. Often you don't even have the feeling of knowing. Critically, later, you recall the thing—and often the reduced pressure to remember is why you now do so. We think you just shared H.M.'s day-to-day experience except he had no later recall.

So, what is amnesia? Our first edition (Gray, 1982) extracted three major principles that have stood the test of time:

1. amnesic patients remember a lot (see §8.1.1) even with massive temporal lobe lesions (see §8.1.2); and what they remember fits the non-human data (see §8.1.3);
2. consolidation, per se, does not appear to be disrupted—a contentious issue that we will also analyse in detail;
3. memory problems in 'amnesics' derive largely from interference—a detailed analysis of this is crucial to the core of our theory (see §8.4).

But these define amnesia by exclusion. What is included? Do amnesics lack a certain type of memory? If the tip-of-the-tongue failure involved memory *loss*, how could you later retrieve it? The number and variety of supposed 'hippocampal' types of is bewildering (Table 8.1)—this requires explanation. In many cases there is no doubt about the existence of the type. But we will argue that none have evidence for specific hippocampal dependence.

One key reason so many types have been postulated is that many effects of hippocampal lesions imply changes in more fundamental processes than memory. Analyses of 'types of memory' should first exclude these as causes of the observations; but they seldom make the attempt.

A second reason is that memory theories ignore many behavioural effects of SHS damage that are unrelated to these specialized forms of memory, or to memory at all (Gray and McNaughton, 1983). The idea that the hippocampus is primarily a memory control structure, then, ignores a large literature; and neither the older age of this literature, nor 'memorial' preconceptions justify implicit or explicit (Eichenbaum et al., 1996) exclusion. Nonetheless, here we will address memory theories on their own ground, ignoring the non-memorial data.

A third, key, reason is that no type has captured hippocampal function even within the memory domain—so the search for the one true grail continues. All the postulated types suffer from both positive and negative failures (§8.2). We suggest this is most easy to understand if *apparently minor* procedural features of training and testing regimes are what render retrieval, formation, or consolidation of memories hippocampal-sensitive or hippocampal-insensitive (see e.g. §8.2.8, 8.4.4 and Rawlins, 1985 for an analysis of time as a simple but general confound).

To start with all the available data, and try to integrate them, would need many volumes. Instead, we critique earlier distinct views. Some of these have been elaborated at book length (e.g. Baddeley, 1986; Cohen and Eichenbaum, 1993; Fuster, 1995) and extend to including hemispheric differentiation between spatial and semantic 'maps' (O'Keefe and Nadel, 1978, p. 3, p. 410). We highlight the data that distinguish our approach from others—producing the equivalent of a comprehensive review of the memory literature and its mapping to our theory, but in minimal space.

First, we critique some myths about 'amnesia' that confuse the literature (§8.1). Second, we use critical experimental data to critique some of the more influential past theories—using

Table 8.1 Types of memory that have been postulated to be differentially sensitive to hippocampal damage. From McNaughton and Wickens (2003).

Hippocampal sensitive	Hippocampal insensitive
fact	skill
conscious recollection	skills
conscious	automatic
memory	habit
knowing that	knowing how
representational	dispositional
declarative	procedural
declarative	nondeclarative
explicit	implicit
locale	taxon
cognitive mediation	semantic
episodic	semantic
elaboration	integration
memory with record	memory without record
autobiographical	perceptual
conceptual	perceptual
working	reference
instance	rule
data based	expectancy based
contextual	associative
relational	associative
configural	associative
intermediate	long term

the latter as summaries of the vast body of literature (§8.2). Third, we provide a preliminary theory of hippocampal 'catastrophic hypermnesia' (§8.3). Finally, we discuss in more detail interference and its relation to different past views of the hippocampus and amnesia (§8.4).

We focus heavily on basic ideas that appeared over 20 years ago in their purest form because modern theories that have been built on them have similar problems and for similar reasons. The modern literature has added virtually no new fundamental ideas (but see §8.2.10), with new theories essentially combining sets of older ones. Interestingly, there still seem to be two separate camps: a non-human spatial perspective (§8.2.1) based on single cell recording albeit with complexities provided by 'remapping' (Chapter 7, Kubie et al., 2020) and restriction to the dorsal hippocampus; and a human relational perspective (§8.2.7) albeit with complexities provided by the addition of context (§8.2.6) and binding (Sadeh and Pertzov, 2020). Muddying the waters, there has been a trend for the first camp to refer to spatial arrays or environments inappropriately (§8.1.5) as 'contexts': giving the word a quite different meaning to that of both the second camp and the dictionary.

We will argue: 1) that the effects of hippocampal lesions in tests of memory are the result of changes in more fundamental processes that are *not* specific to memory; 2) that 'amnesia' is better viewed as 'catastrophic hypermnesia' (a failure to suppress the remembering of inappropriate information); 3) that the hippocampus is not a site of long-term memory storage; and 4) that, even if it were, the properties of long-term potentiation (the current best accepted basis of 'Hebbian', i.e. purely associative, learning and memory) are not appropriate for such storage. Indeed, we unashamedly ascribe to a Hebbian view of reference and working memory (Hebb, 1949) and to his focus on the Conceptual Nervous System (Hebb, 1955). In particular we, (like others, Moscovitch et al., 2016) agree with his view that information is encoded by cell assemblies that involve much the same cells in both perception and memory (see §8.1.2, §8.2.2; see also Nadel and Maurer, 2020 for an overview of Hebb and his debt to Lashley, Lorente de Nó, and other earlier workers).

8.1 Hippocampal amnesia myths

8.1.1 Myth 1: Amnesia is *loss* of memory

This myth saturates the available literatures. We cannot easily ignore the 'practically irresistible' clinical impression that these patients 'cannot form a durable record of their new experiences' (Weiskrantz, 1978). So, in this section, we will address the myth of amnesia as being a loss of memory or of a failure to form memory traces.

The emphasis on *amnesia* in this literature arises because of the relatively normal IQ and other intellectual functions of many such patients. For example, Jenni Ogden

> decided to assess H.M.'s ability to measure time and told him that he would be left alone for a period, and then asked to estimate the time that had elapsed. [She] left the room at 2.05 pm and returned at 2.17 pm. When H.M. was asked how many minutes had passed, he replied, without hesitation, '12 minutes; got you there!'. There was a large clock on the wall and H.M. had noted the time when [she] left, and continued to rehearse it while looking at the clock. When asked how many minutes had passed, he simply subtracted the time he was rehearsing from the time shown on the clock. This anecdote illustrates more about H.M.'s sense of humour, his willingness to cooperate with anything experimenters may come up with, and his intact intellect, than about his ability to estimate time without memories!
>
> (Ogden and Corkin, 1991, p. 199)

Superficially, then, H.M. appears to have a quite specific problem with memory, while general lexical and grammatical processing are intact (Kensinger et al., 2001). Yet this very anecdote shows that, at least by rehearsing (and rehearsing why he is rehearsing), he can under some conditions produce apparently intact memory performance.

Such intact learning and memory in 'amnesics' is seen across diverse conditions. Consistent with §7.1, they can show eyeblink conditioning with a 24-hour retention interval

(Weiskrantz and Warrington, 1979). As with hippocampal rats (§4.6.2, Table 4.2) H. M. had good learning of simple motor tasks such as pursuit rotor and sequential tapping (Corkin, 1968), operant discrimination of circles from ellipses and matching-to-sample with trigrams and ellipses (Sidman et al., 1968). More generally, as reviewed by Ogden and Corkin (1991), H.M.'s intact memorial functions include immediate memory (e.g. digit span); remote memory (factual information learned before he was 17 years old); and implicit memory (e.g. the simple motor tasks described earlier). In contrast, his long-term, explicit memories from 17 years old onwards were largely absent (the exceptions seem to be items that have been for one reason or another extensively rehearsed). H.M.'s explicit memory was faulty for both semantic (general knowledge) and episodic (specific experience-related) items. His memory for verbal and nonverbal items was equally bad, which can be attributed to the bilaterality of his lesions.[1] It is consistent with our theory that H.M. also appeared unusually lacking in anxiety (J. Ogden, pers. comm.)—but this observation can hardly be construed as proof!

It is this contrast between the dramatic 'amnesia' and the normal learning and memory in specific tasks that has generated a large literature devoted to the analysis of 'types' of memory that are 'hippocampal-dependent' or not. This has clinically pragmatic utility (Butters et al., 1995); but it implies that the hippocampus stores one categorical type of memory, and another brain area stores another type. But why has this single area of literature spawned so many types (Table 8.1)?

Our simple explanation is that dichotomies of memory type are being applied to a non-memorial continuum; but that the fundamental intractability of 'types' is not the only reason for doubting their validity. We believe there is a fundamental flaw: the hippocampus does not store even intermediate, far less long-term, memories of any type (although it may store 'program-like' information that alters its own processing). Instead, as implied by Hebb (1949), memory proper is distributed throughout the brain. Here, we also agree with Fuster (1995, pp. 1–5) that:

> Memory is a functional property, among others, of each and all of the areas of the cerebral cortex, and thus of all cortical systems. This cardinal cognitive function is inherent in the fabric of the entire cortex and cannot be ascribed exclusively to any of its parts.... Because of the multiplicity of actual and potential connections in the cortex, each neuronal ensemble may be part of multiple networks and, thus, part of multiple representations. What most critically defines a network (i.e. a memory representation) is the ensemble of connections that has formed it. Relationship is of the essence and, in this sense, *all memory is associative*.... Association is an attribute of all memories, at the root of their genesis as well as their evocation.... [As a result] perceptual [declarative, episodic, and semantic] memory is mainly represented in posterior cortex.... Motor memory consists of representations of motor action in all its forms, from skeletal movement to the spoken language. It too is acquired and evoked through the senses but, once acquired, it is largely represented in the neocortex of the frontal lobe, which comprises roughly one third of the human neocortex. The most automatic and firmly established aspects of motor memory are represented outside the neocortex, notably in the basal ganglia and the cerebellum.

[1] Verbal memory is usually affected more by lesions of the hippocampus/amygdala of the language-dominant hemisphere, non-verbal more by similar lesions of the opposite hemisphere, with bilateral damage producing more severe effects than the sum of the unilateral effects. It also appears that 'interpretation of language involves widespread distributed systems bilaterally' (Bottini et al., 1994, p. 1241)

To this we can add affective memory in the amygdala (Chapter 6) and, by implication, the potential for memory (but not necessarily conscious retrieval) in all subcortical areas.

8.1.2 Myth 2: Amnesia is purely hippocampal

This myth, most common in the human neuropsychological literature, is that that the hippocampus proper is the primary locus at which damage gives rise to amnesia. This is clearly not true in the exclusive sense given the occurrence of diencephalic amnesia (e.g. Dalrymple-Alford et al., 2015) and the evidence for the control of memory by the anterior thalamus (Barnett et al., 2021). But with diencephalic amnesia it seems hippocampus can be involved (Nelson et al., 2020) with the subiculum likely to be a key mediator (Frost et al., 2020; Frost et al., 2021) and, even with 'hippocampal' amnesia, other structures tend to be involved and one source of apparent species difference is the supposed site (or rather variable sites) of damage in amnesic patients; making it unclear what is the appropriate lesion for a non-human model.

Here, the nature of the clinical data presents major problems, not least to know what they are. There are three major collections to choose from, each with its attendant sources of confusion.

8.1.2.1 Deliberate bilateral surgical removal of the hippocampus

There are a few individuals (such as H.M.) with bilateral extensive (but not entirely complete; Annese et al., 2014) removal of the hippocampus and adjacent areas. Most reports are from the late 1950s and 1960s (Milner, 1970) because the resulting huge amnesic deficit essentially rules out such surgery for relief of temporal lobe epilepsy. Less complete resection is still used for drug-resistant cases but remains infrequent (Jobst and Cascino, 2015).

The hippocampus may make an important contribution to temporal lobe amnesia (Milner, 1970; Milner, 1971; Butters and Cermak, 1975); but all such patients had extensive damage to overlying temporal cortex and amygdala. More distal damage from the long duration of their seizures is likely; but animal studies suggest that prior convulsions do not add to hippocampal deficits (Vanderwolf, 1995); and O'Keefe and Nadel (1978, p. 416), p. 416) note that profound amnesia can occur with hippocampal damage absent prior seizures.

Some patients with lesions mainly restricted to area CA1 have extensive memory deficits and the severity of the amnesia increases with additional hippocampal formation damage (Zola-Morgan et al., 1986; Rempel-Clower et al., 1996)—suggesting truly hippocampal involvement in amnesia. However, such involvement may be through interaction with other brain areas that code the key information (Bonnici et al., 2012) and these can be the sole source of some deficits (see §8.2.2).

8.1.2.2 Korsakoff's syndrome

Korsakoff's syndrome is often the result of prolonged drinking, and remains unsurprisingly prevalent (~2% in the USA); so, it has provided the test bed for views of amnesia. Although superficially similar to the surgical patient group (see Weiskrantz, 1978), Korsakoff patients usually lack hippocampal pathology (compare Mair et al., 1979; Victor et al., 1971) and are more likely to be an example of diencephalic amnesia (see, e.g. Dalrymple-Alford et al., 2015). Their deficits, then, could result from mammillary body lesions (Squire et al., 1990; Aggleton et al., 1990), restricted thalamic lesions (Markowitsch et al., 1993; Daum and Ackermann, 1994; Parkin et al., 1994), or damage in multiple related systems (see Markowitsch, 1982).

Korsakoff patients cannot represent human *hippocampal* amnesia, whatever links one might want to make between hippocampal and mammillary body, or hippocampal and thalamic, damage on anatomical or theoretical grounds.

8.1.2.3 Senile dementia of the Alzheimer type (SDAT)

The bulk of the population will contract SDAT with age (interacting with a range of primary triggers, Herrup, 2010); so SDAT availability is large, increasing, and a major target of health research. For hippocampal neuroscience, SDAT is slightly less problematic than Korsakoff's syndrome: the hippocampus and other temporal lobe structures are a prime site of degeneration.

Unfortunately, SDAT involves diffuse, sometimes extensive, damage all over the brain. So, specific conclusions about hippocampal involvement are impossible. Also, a primary source of the memory deficit in SDAT, as opposed to temporal lobe patients, is loss of cholinergic function. SDAT certainly cannot, therefore, be viewed as an example of pure hippocampal damage.

8.1.2.4 Human 'hippocampal' amnesia, an overview

All of our human amnesia data sources have problems and so we do not provide a detailed review of them (for early reviews, see Weiskrantz and Warrington, 1975; Weiskrantz, 1978; Butters and Cermak, 1975; Baddeley, 1981; Squire and Zola-Morgan, 1991). We will lump the data into a general 'amnesic syndrome'; but concentrate mostly on surgical cases, which allow fairly direct comparison with the animal data at the anatomical level. We will then use the animal data for an attempted functional dissection of amnesia.

The clinical material, with the possible exception of cases such as R.B., who appears to have bilateral damage limited to area CA1 (Zola-Morgan et al., 1986), does not tell us which structures are crucial for the amnesia, nor what specific contribution is made by the hippocampal formation. For example, the damage sustained by H.M. involves the large *but incomplete* loss of hippocampus plus amygdala plus adjacent cortex including the bulk of the entorhinal cortex. There was also minor frontal damage to left lateral orbital gyrus, likely caused during surgery (Annese et al., 2014).

A large animal literature has investigated the different aspects of H.M. type lesions, usually labelled H+ A+ (for hippocampus + surrounding cortex plus amygdala + surrounding cortex). It has become clear that the contribution of the amygdala itself to the observed memory effects was greatly overestimated in the early literature, because of incidental damage to fibres of passage (see Murray, 1996). Conversely, damage to perirhinal and parahippocampal cortex alone can produce major memory deficits (e.g. Suzuki et al., 1993; Zola-Morgan et al., 1989; Murray, 1996); in some tests, damage limited to the hippocampus proper may have little effect (see Murray, 1996); and a single test can show clear effects of rhinal cortex lesions under conditions where there is no effect of hippocampus + amygdala lesion (Mumby and Pinel, 1994; Mumby et al., 1992; for direct comparison of the two see Fig. 11.15 in Pinel, 2011). Such dissociations do not exclude a role for the hippocampus proper since, within the temporal lobe, the effects of damage appear to summate to a large extent across structures (e.g. Zola-Morgan et al., 1994; Meunier et al., 1993; but see Meunier et al., 1996); however, they emphasize that the full-blown temporal lobe amnesic syndrome depends to a large extent on damage to extra-hippocampal structures and less to hippocampus proper.

The latter point will also be important when we come to consider the effects on memory of the anxiolytic drugs (§13.2.4). Blocking theta can block hippocampal-sensitive learning; and reinstatement of theta with a 'brain bypass' reinstates learning (McNaughton et al., 2006b). A key fact for our theory is that the anxiolytics impair the control of theta rhythm (McNaughton et al., 2007; Appendix 5) and their injection into the supramammillary area changes theta and behaviour to the same extent as systemic injections (Woodnorth and McNaughton, 2002b). From this we infer that the drugs should produce an impairment equivalent to that seen after modest damage to the hippocampal formation (including entorhinal cortex and posterior cingulate). But, at present, we have no evidence that theta is crucial for perirhinal or parahippocampal function. A lack of action on these structures, and/or only modest reduction in hippocampal formation function generally, would account for the relatively mild amnesic effects of the anxiolytics when these are given at the lower doses that are effective in treating clinical anxiety. That said, doses well above those used for clinical anxiety produce an amnesia similar to that of patients such as H.M., with intact short-term memory, anterograde amnesia limited to the affected period, and no retrograde amnesia (Brown et al., 1982).

8.1.3 Myth 3: Amnesia is unlike 'animal' memory failure

This myth, most common in the human cognitive literature, is that the gulf between ourselves and other animals is so great as to make comparison irrelevant. This false belief allows many theorists to retain concepts that fit their preferred data domain but that are false with other data or species. This is a vital myth to eliminate, since the bulk of detailed data on brain processes underlying memory (and the key data in the previous section) come from non-human subjects.

In the past, a key problem has been methodology. As noted by Tulving (1985, p. 67), non-human and human memory research

> seem to represent separate cultures: they begin with different pre-theoretical assumptions, they are concerned with apparently different problems, they employ different methods, and they speak different languages. In the animal literature, there are few references to work in human memory; in human memory literature there are even fewer mentions of work in animal learning.

Tulving argued, therefore, for a need to concentrate on the classification of tasks so as to be able to translate between the literatures (see also Steckler and Muir, 1996; Roberts, 1996). However, a CNS (Hebb, 1955) approach is easier since animal physiological psychology and human neuropsychology differ much less than do human cognitive psychology and animal learning. That said, Macphail (1996) made a non-physiological argument for homology of human and non-human learning; and McNaughton and Corr (2008) detailed nine fallacies underlying a separation of the species for cognition, emotion, and personality: 1) primary anthropocentrism; 2) cognitive anthropocentrism; 3) language = cognition; 4) cognitions are emotionally neutral; 5) cognitions are unconstrained; 6) cognitions are hardware-free; 7) radical behaviourism (i.e. thou shalt not talk about anything internal); 8) cognitions are behaviourally silent (i.e. animal cognition can never be demonstrated behaviourally); and,

9) the cortex is the seat of cognition (so, e.g. fish cannot feel pain, Rose, 2002). In relation to (9) in particular, note that the highest order cognitive processing in humans is undertaken in the phylogenetically most primitive areas at the boundaries of the neocortex (Pandya and Barnes, 1987; Nauta and Feirtag, 1986) with progressively more recently evolved zones adding progressively novel cytoarchitectures for ever-more-peripheral filtering of the input.

It is now clear that, provided the methods used to test a non-human subject share key *conceptual* features with those used to test a human being, the results are essentially the same. Indeed, the same translation problem exists between say rats and pigeons as between either and humans. For example, in tests of spatial working memory, rats and humans use similar coding strategies (Kesner and DeSpain, 1988) and suffer similar hippocampal lesion deficits (Morris et al., 1996b). Similarly, rats can show primacy and recency effects (Gray and McNaughton, 1983; Kesner et al., 1994a; but see Deacon and Rawlins, 1995 and references cited by them). Monkeys and human beings use similar attributes and dimensions in visual discrimination learning and its reversals (Roberts et al., 1988); and, provided that they have similar prior experience, lesioned monkeys show 'impairments of object memory . . . analogous to the impairments of episodic memory seen in human amnesic patients' (Gaffan, 1994, p. 305; see also Vnek and Rothblat, 1996). Non-verbal testing of humans shows that 'animal memory is similar to, at least, the nonverbal part of human memory' (Wright, 1994; see also Gilboa and Moscovitch, 2021).

It is also clear that the neural bases of various memory impairments are similar across species (see Kesner, 1996). For example, hippocampal lesioned rats and monkeys can learn simple motor tasks like running down a runway or pressing a lever; and H.M. (Henry. G. Mollaison, see opening chaper quotations, whose brain has now been reconstructed post mortem by Annese et al., 2014), the famous case of bilateral (but not entirely complete) removal of hippocampus, amygdala, and other parts of the temporal lobe, could learn and retain motor tasks such as mirror drawing as easily as intact people. Korsakoff patients tested with a standard associative 'animal' task, concurrent object discrimination, show the same severe impairment as do animals (Kessler et al., 1986). Prefrontal lesions produce similar dissociations of item and order memory in rats and human beings (Kesner and Holbrook, 1987). Interestingly, when a rat test of *non-spatial* declarative memory was constructed, it was as sensitive to hippocampal damage as the human tests (Bunsey and Eichenbaum, 1996); conversely, a rat test of complex remote spatial memory showed that this was intact after hippocampal lesions, matching H.M.'s intact remote memory (Winocur et al., 2005); and, when human lesions have been found that approximate the discrete lesions made in animals, similar results and similar dissociations have been obtained (Bechara et al., 1995).

Importantly, successful performance does not necessarily match verbal report. Amnesics such as H.M. can learn and retain certain tasks; but appear unaware, in terms of verbal report, that they have undertaken them before or that they are progressively improving. This is a key source of confusion in the literature: the testing of human beings via the verbal channel (which is of course not available in animals), coupled with inappropriate inference from verbal results to memory in general.

Conversely, great care must be taken to use stimuli that cannot be verbally encoded. For example, verbal rehearsal can provide a human subject with a non-memory strategy to solve a particular problem and hence give rise to quite different results from those seen in the rat or pigeon, even though the truly memorial performance of all three species is the same (White, 1985; Kirk et al., 1988a; Money et al., 1992). Note that related care is required to prevent rats using position habits to bridge the memory gap and so appear un-pigeon-like (Kirk et al., 1988a; Mumby, 1995). Whatever the two species being compared, one must always be on the look-out for species-specific reactions or bias that can distort the data. When verbal mediation is excluded, human beings solve radial-arm maze problems in a similar fashion, and with the same implied memory capacity, as do rats (Glassman et al., 1994). Human infants also lack the verbal channel but can show excellent memory given appropriate means of response (Diamond, 1995; Hayne et al., 1997; Hayne, 1998). In all tests, therefore, one must be careful to exclude species-specific factors before comparing memory systems as such and be careful not to be caught out by one of the fallacies detailed by McNaughton and Corr (2008). Appropriate comparison and theory application can then unify the non-human and human memory literatures (Winocur et al., 2010).

8.1.4 Myth 4: Amnesia is faster forgetting

The fourth myth we must dispel is the idea that amnesia necessarily involves faster forgetting.

In matching-to-sample tasks, H.M.'s performance deteriorated badly when a delay was introduced. In delayed matching of ellipses, his deficit was severe at delays greater than 24 seconds; with trigrams, his retention was normal for as long as 40 seconds. In the latter task, it was noted that he achieved good performance at this longer delay only with the aid of constant verbal rehearsal (Sidman et al., 1968). Matching based on ellipses and similar visual stimuli, by contrast, usually eliminates the possibility of verbal rehearsal.

Verbal rehearsal is particularly significant in the context of White's (1985) theory of direct remembering. In his view, stimuli in memory have similar properties to stimuli in a visual field, 'memory decay' is a direct result of the *temporal distance* at which the item is 'viewed'. Verbal rehearsal, so long as it can be continued, provides a means of retaining at least some aspects of the original information (those which can be verbally encoded), while by-passing the 'viewing' of the richer memory stimulus itself. White's model predicts that memory decay will follow a single exponential function, provided: (a) strategies such as rehearsal are eliminated; and (b) response bias is eliminated by signal detection analysis. In particular, the rate of decay will be the same independent of the point in time at which it is estimated. His model accounts for over 95% of the variance in memory decay in experiments with, for example, pigeons performing delayed matching to sample and rats performing delayed conditional discrimination (Kirk et al., 1988b, who took care to prevent position strategies).

We have found that, when undergraduate subjects perform delayed matching to sample with swastika-like stimuli and random checker boxes, as with rats allowed to adopt positional strategies, there can be virtually no memory decay. In the checker board case, this is true even when the difficulty of the discrimination is increased to the point where overall performance becomes very poor. However, when verbal rehearsal is prevented by adding a competing verbal task in the delay interval (R. Kirk and N. McNaughton, unpublished data) or by using a circle size discrimination which is not amenable to verbal encoding (Money et al., 1992), then the expected exponential decay is observed. What is particularly important about this result is that the exponential function allows estimation of the discriminability of the positive versus the negative stimulus at a nominal zero delay (note that this is *not* the same as the discriminability obtained in a simultaneous matching-to-sample task). When amnesics, diagnosed as SDAT, are tested on this task they show perfectly normal memory decay rates, but their capacity to discriminate the alternatives at nominal time zero is greatly reduced (Fig. 8.1). This result is consistent with the fact that, if the level of initial learning is equated, rates of forgetting in amnesics can be similar to controls (e.g. Freed et al., 1987).

We have the interesting situation, then, that amnesics can carry out concurrent matching to sample provided stimuli are maintained in iconic or similar storage, or provided any delay is bridged by rehearsal or a similar strategy, but not if the delay must be bridged by 'direct remembering' (White, 1985). Most obviously in Fig. 8.1, faulty direct remembering in amnesics need not involve an increased rate of memory decay. Rather, it is the result of a confusion of stimulus alternatives, a confusion that is present even at the very smallest delays (e.g. 0.1 s). This is also the pattern of results seen in rats treated with either the anticholinergic scopolamine (Kirk et al., 1988b) or the anxiolytic chlordiazepoxide (Tan et al., 1990). This suggests a fault in encoding, retrieval, or related processes.

Whether, hippocampal lesions in non-humans produce an increased rate of decay of memory has been debated (see also Mayes et al., 2019, for a discussion of accelerated long-term forgetting versus classic organic amnesia). Many early reports of faster decay have one or more confounds: 1) use of per cent correct (which has a Christmas pudding rather than normal distribution)—a bias free measure like log d, or d', is preferable; 2) there may be delay-related response biases (Herremans et al., 1995); 3) control values across shorter delays are at ceiling and so forced down to similarity with hippocampal values, which are often close to 90% (see Squire and Zola-Morgan, 1984); 4) more contentiously, few studies fit an exponential decay model to assess rate (as noted earlier, we found that departures from the model resulted from species-specific, non-memorial strategies).

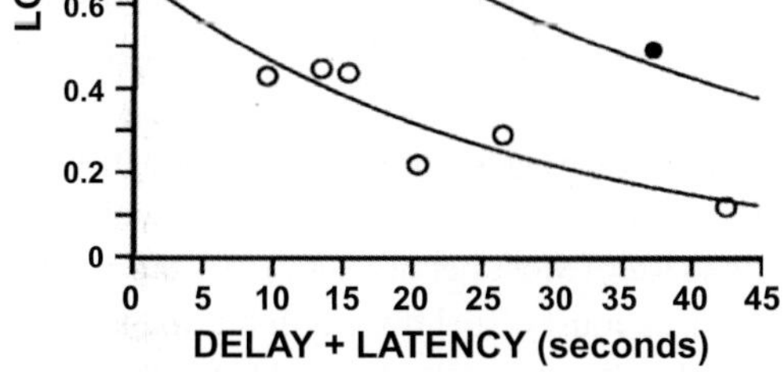

Fig. 8.1 Performance of patients diagnosed with Senile Dementia of the Alzheimer Type (SDAT) and age-matched controls (CON) on a delayed matching to sample task. Performance was assessed using a bias-free measure (log d) derived from signal detection theory and plotted as a function of the actual delay between stimulus presentation and response (i.e., experimenter-imposed delay plus subject-imposed latency to respond after presentation of the choice stimuli). The curves show simple exponential decay functions fitted to these data (see text). SDAT showed a clear decrease in the parameter log d at nominal zero delay but no decrease in the parameter b, i.e., the rate of memory decay (From Money et al., 1992).

However, beyond simple decay, time can have a range of effects on 'forgetting of hippocampus-dependent memories'; and when Sadeh and Pertzov (2020, p. 386) took into account, the relational nature of memory (§8.2.7), encoding duration, top-down processes such as reward, and gradual versus all-or-none loss, they concluded that

> time-dependent forgetting across short and long timescales is reflected in progressive degradation of hippocampal-dependent relational information. This evidence provides an important extension to a growing body of research accumulated in recent years, showing that— in contrast to the once prevailing view that the hippocampus is exclusively involved in memory and forgetting over long timescales—the role of the hippocampus also extends to memory and forgetting over short timescales. Thus, we maintain that similar rules govern not only remembering but also forgetting of hippocampus-dependent information over short and long timescales.

8.1.5 Myth 5: Amnesia is contextual

Definition of *context*

> 1: the parts of a discourse that surround a word or passage and can throw light on its meaning
> 2: the interrelated conditions in which something exists or occurs: ENVIRONMENT, SETTING
> //the historical *context* of the war
>
> https://www.merriam-webster.com/dictionary/context

The fifth myth we must dispel is that what is lost in hippocampal amnesia is *de facto* a 'context'.

As normally defined, a context is a background in which a discrete stimulus occurs (even this requires careful spelling out as in Miller, 1991, pp. 1–6). Thus, *the box in which* a CS-UCS pairing *occurs* is the 'context' for that pairing. But many, starting with that fact, then describe the box itself as a 'context' even when there is no explicit CS (e.g. Gidyk et al., 2021). They may even emphasize that the presentation of the shocks is *un-signalled* and unpredictable as a means of ensuring that the box is a 'context' (Luyten et al., 2011). But it should be obvious that pairing a box with a shock is not contextual conditioning but merely simple CS-UCS associative conditioning where the CS is complex and extended in space and time. Indeed, if a simpler box is compared with a more complex one, hippocampal lesions impair conditioning less to the former than the latter (Moses et al., 2007). To call the box a 'context' is a plain misuse of language. We said we must dispel this myth but the usage is so common now that the meaning of the word in this literature has changed for many to mean simply an extended space (e.g. Kubie et al., 2020). This incorrect usage, and the mixing of the meanings, has only increased the theoretical confusion as to the nature of the learning and memory involved. More recent theories combine true context-dependence of memory with the requirement, in effect, for this to be complex—but even they can mix the meanings (§8.2.10).

Phillips and LeDoux (1994) present a more truly contextual view of hippocampal function in an experiment involving three conditions:

> forward pairing of a phasic tone conditioned stimulus (CS) with a footshock unconditioned stimulus (US), unpaired presentations of the CS and US, or presentations of the US alone. All three procedures resulted in the acquisition of conditioned freezing to the box in which these manipulations took place. Lesions of the dorsal hippocampus prevented the acquisition of contextual conditioning in the paired procedure, as also reported previously, but not in the unpaired or US alone procedures.

Despite the authors' description of the box as a 'context' in all three cases, their results show that it is only when the box provides a true context for the CS-UCS conditioning that hippocampal lesions have an effect.

Note, however, that Phillips and LeDoux did not show that hippocampal lesions impair the use of a context to enable the CS-UCS conditioning. Instead, they showed that when both a discrete and a non-discrete CS-UCS association can be formed, then hippocampal lesions selectively impair conditioning to the non-discrete but not discrete CS. By contrast, when a context is explicitly used to enhance the effects of conditioning, hippocampal lesions have no effect (Gisquet-Verrier and Schenk, 1994; Hall et al., 1996). Conversely, hippocampal lesions do impair fear conditioning to a simple but diffuse stimulus—food deprivation—even when this cannot be viewed as a 'background' to some other conditioning and when conditioning to a continuous auditory tone was intact (Davidson and Jarrard, 1993). All of these data argue against a role for the hippocampus in conditioning to context, in the strict 'background-to-a-foreground' sense, and suggest that some interaction of the stimulus parameters (diffuse nature, temporal continuity, etc.) with the response system is important in making the tasks sensitive to hippocampal lesions via, perhaps, a requirement for 'binding' (§8.2.3).

One particularly detailed development of this general contextual orientation was Gaffan's analysis (e.g. 1994) of 'scene specific memory for objects'. He used computer generated 'objects' and 'backgrounds' to create 'scenes'. This allowed careful variation of the precise relationships of objects to backgrounds and, crucially, permitted testing of monkeys after learning of many hundreds of discriminations against a multitude of backgrounds—experience approximating the normal human situation. As with Myth 3, the monkeys in these experiments showed the same deficits as human beings when this experiential background was matched. But, in relation to the role of context, his manipulation of backgrounds produced key results.

> The animals learned four types of discrimination problem: (1) object-in-place discrimination learning, in which the correct (rewarded) response was to a particular object that always occupied the same place in a particular unique background, (2) place discrimination learning, in which the correct response was to a particular place in a unique background, with no distinctive object in that place, (3) object discrimination learning in unique backgrounds, in which the correct response was to a particular object that could occupy one or the other of two possible places in a unique background, and (4) object discrimination learning in varying backgrounds, in which the correct response was to a particular object that could appear at any place in any background. The severest impairment produced by fornix transection was in object-in-place learning. Fornix transection did not impair object discrimination learning in varying backgrounds. The results from the other two types of learning task showed intermediate severity of impairment in the fornix-transected animals' (*op. cit.*, p. 305).

Gaffan argues that the varying background case makes background irrelevant and so eliminates interference from previous background-related learning. In the object-in-background case, the control subjects learned particularly well. Gaffan argues that this is because they can use the specific background and spatial contextual information to eliminate the interference from previous background-related learning; and that this active removal of interference is prevented by the fornix lesions. This is a specific form of a more general hypothesis that we discuss in §8.4. Gaffan also suggests that 'if different features of a complex scene are represented in the various cortical areas that are linked together via the hippocampus-fornix-mammillary system, then this system might connect those features together into a widespread cortical distributed representation of the scene' (*op. cit.*, p. 314). Later, as with our treatment of other theorists (see especially §8.2.7 and §8.4.2), we suggest the opposite: that the hippocampus *prevents* connection of unwanted features that would otherwise confuse the distributed representation of the scene.

8.2 Theories of hippocampal amnesia

These myths cut across theories of hippocampal-dependent amnesia. With §8.1 as background, let us now look at some of the more distinctive theories that have attempted to account for hippocampal amnesia in terms of types of memory. As in §8.1, we focus on gross temporal lobe lesions (in essence H + A+ lesions) but allow, e.g. fornix-fimbria lesions, which produce a major disconnection of the SHS. We discuss selective lesions to specific parts of the SHS in Appendix 9 (see also Moscovitch et al., 2016, for a memory-oriented discussion of hippocampal subfields).

Some detail is necessary; but past views of 'hippocampal function' often derive from just a few experiments and can be encapsulated in a single adjective or a sentence or two. The bulk lack detailed learning theory, cognitive psychology, neuroanatomy, neurophysiology, etc. but there are some key exceptions and these share some important details that we will flag. To a large extent we can see the content of the smaller scale theories as supplementing the spatial theory (§8.2.1; Chapter 7) to generate the relational theory, which we will treat as a paradigm example (§8.2.7); with all of these, in a sense, being combined in the more recent Trace Translation Theory (§8.2.10).

Even the detailed theories share a failure to deal with a range of what, for us, are key issues. First, is long-term potentiation (LTP). As argued in Appendix 7, LTP *in the hippocampus* is likely to be a general attention-like, or programming-like, mechanism. There are significant difficulties in seeing it as the basis of detailed hippocampal storage of large volumes of complex sensory information (although indexing is a partial solution to this, Teyler and Rudy, 2007; Goode et al., 2020), this is likely achieved by LTP in the cortex (Sumner et al., 2020). Second, is innate responding. It is difficult to reconcile a role for the hippocampus as an active creator of memory with its involvement in innate responses (e.g. innate conflict, Blanchard and Blanchard, 1972) or its strong engagement with hormonal systems (Lathe, 2001). Third is unlearning (§8.3). Memory theories seldom account for the contrast between runway acquisition (intact after hippocampal lesions) and extinction (impaired) or simultaneous discrimination (intact) and its reversal (impaired). Fourth, is *suppression* of interference (§8.4). For many situations, if the hippocampus were to inhibit the formation or the recall of incorrect memories, this would produce similar (but not identical) results to its actively forming correct ones. The differences occur in subtle details: we have already noted that errors made by amnesics are frequently intrusions of items that would have been correct on previous trials (a fact not dealt with by, e.g. the relational theory).

8.2.1 Theory 1: Spatial memory

The earliest theory of hippocampal function that attempted to integrate the bulk of the anatomy, physiology and psychology of the hippocampus was O'Keefe and Nadel's (1978) spatial theory of hippocampal function.

This was, and remains, an impressive piece of work. Its evidential base is much greater than that of most of the other theories covered in the present chapter: single unit recordings showing place fields of hippocampal cells (critiqued in Chapter 7); the extreme sensitivity of spatial tasks to hippocampal lesions; a coherent account of the role of theta in hippocampal function; consideration of the detailed anatomy of the hippocampal formation; and derivation of the underlying concepts from the philosophical works of Newton, Leibniz, Berkeley, and Kant. It has also achieved greater longevity than any of the other theories discussed here. The full version of the theory (which had been developing for some time previously) was published in 1978 and is still being strongly defended now, over 40 years later—recently garnering a Nobel prize (Burgess, 2014).

As summarized at the time of our second edition, O'Keefe and Nadel's theory is based on

> the view that the hippocampal system is quite specifically a spatial mapping system. [But] the cognitive map theory of hippocampal function is, first and foremost, a theory about *memory* for spatial layouts and the ways in which animals use such a memory system for adaptive behaviour in the world. . . . Adherence to such a multiple memory system view has now become the accepted norm [but at that time our view] was sufficiently different from the standard view that cognitive map theory was considered merely a theory about space, not memory.
>
> We assumed that there were two classes of learning systems, corresponding roughly to the notions of 'knowing that' and 'knowing how'. We created names for these two classes of learning systems: *locale* and *taxon*. These names were chosen to represent certain critical features of each of the learning systems. In the case of the locale system this was the fact that the memories it contained incorporated information about place and time; in the case of the taxon system, it was the fact that they were governed by the rule of category inclusion. Memories in taxon systems were organized in terms of features and their similarity/ dissimilarity, while those in the locale system were not. There was also an important distinction between these learning systems in terms of the role of time/place context—it played a central role in locale-based memories, but was absent from taxon-based memories.
>
> The foundation for . . . the locale system lies in its inclusion of spatial information. In the years since our formulation of this theory, there has been much support for the view that the hippocampus is crucially important in the processing of spatial information. What has been rejected is our insistence that this spatial signature is the best way of describing hippocampal function.
>
> Finally, and very briefly, I will toss in the towel and admit, as we did in 1978, that at least in the case of the human hippocampal system, there is more than merely spatial mapping going on. . . . Why not admit [also] a more abstract representational system into the monkey, rat, or

even bird hippocampus? The answer, then as now, is simply that we did not, and still do not, see the need for such hypothesis drift.

(Nadel, 1991, pp. 221–222)

The range of the home database for the spatial theory is impressive. At the time of its proposal this range was so much greater than that of any other theory that a few problematic items around the edges (e.g. accounting for the effects of hippocampal lesions on DRL, i.e. differential reinforcement of low rates, performance) did not detract from its appeal.

Since then, competing theories (e.g. Eichenbaum, 1996) have responded to perceived deficiencies of spatial theory but, necessarily, attempted to incorporate the spatial results. The purely spatial theory can be viewed as a special case of the relational theory (§8.2.7) and the 'toss in the towel' cognitive map version as one of the systems of Multiple Trace Theory (§8.2.10). However, there is one important point of difference. For O'Keefe and Nadel, the hippocampus is itself the place where the permanent *cognitive* map is stored. It is difficult to reconcile this with the limited retrograde amnesia observed in subjects such as H.M. and intact remote spatial memory in rats (Winocur et al., 2005). This would surely require, in addition to the hippocampal map, considerable extra machinery for transferring maps from hippocampus to neocortex while also assuming that the cortex has a similar mapping capacity, in which case the hippocampus, as hypothesized, should not be strictly necessary (see also §8.2.9).

More importantly, non-humans with hippocampal system damage can acquire some forms of spatial task and fail to acquire some forms of non-spatial task (see particularly §8.2.3). Within the memory domain the clearest non-spatial tasks affected by hippocampal system damage in humans and non-humans alike are various forms of delayed matching and delayed non-matching in which, except in the special case of matching or non-matching to position, spatial strategies are deliberately excluded as a means of solution.

Intact spatial learning is shown in hippocampal lesioned rats under interesting circumstances. Eichenbaum et al. (1990) trained fornix-lesioned rats in the standard water maze apparatus, but starting them always from the same position rather than from randomized positions. The lesioned rats learned the task as well and as quickly as controls. When switched to the conventional randomized start procedure, the controls immediately swam directly to the platform, but the lesioned rats demonstrated a deficit (although this was not so large as the deficit observed with similar lesions when acquisition is with randomized multiple start positions). A crucial point is that 'performance of fornix rats was indistinguishable from that of sham rats on the standard transfer test; both groups spent most of their time in the [correct] half of the pool . . . [with] no significant difference between groups in the distribution of swim times among quadrants' (Eichenbaum et al., 1990, p. 3535).

From this we can conclude that the fornix-lesioned rats had learned the position of the platform in a truly spatial fashion, as opposed to simply learning to swim towards some specific cue (taxon learning in O'Keefe and Nadel's terms). But when they were required to approach the platform from novel directions, they suffered significant problems. It could be argued that it is the representational flexibility (see Fig. 8.5) required by multiple starts that causes the problem. However, Whishaw (personal communication) has shown that fornix-lesioned rats can learn even the multiple start version of the water maze as well as controls provided that their initial training prevents them from making errors (and hence presumably adopting incorrect initial response strategies, see Fig. 8.3). In this experiment, the rats were initially placed on the platform, then placed in the water close to and facing the platform, and so on, with farther starting positions on each trial, until they had become the conventional starting points at the edge of the pool. Whishaw (1998, p. 209) 'describes a series of studies using swimming pool spatial tasks that show that hippocampal rats have considerable place learning ability, which includes the abilities of finding, remembering, and searching for places'.

We may appear to have dismissed O'Keefe and Nadel's theory in a somewhat cursory fashion. However, the reasons we have found to reject a *purely* spatial view of the hippocampal formation (see also Appendix 8) are ones that also compelled Nadel's own, essentially similar, view quoted earlier, except that we have included further data that extend the view to non-human animals. Should we also reject a fuller cognitive map theory? We return to this in §8.2.10.

Whatever the merits of a uniquely spatial view of the hippocampus, any alternative theory of hippocampal function must provide an account of the overwhelming impression from many studies that the hippocampus is concerned with space; and, also, for the data indicating that hippocampal neurones are capable of forming 'place' fields (which we critiqued in Chapter 7). Importantly, even now, O'Keefe and Nadel's is one of the few theories designed as a modern theory should be: it attempted to account for all the available data at the time, not artificially restricting the explicanda to those few that can be accommodated by the theory; it provides detailed anatomical and physiological machinery (see Hunsaker and Kesner, 2018, for a recent multicomponent system model), and a prescription for the functions of each part of the machine; it allots roles to LTP and RSA/'theta' rhythm. All provide opportunities to falsify the details as well as the main thrust of the theory. It is surprising that, despite this glowing example, few of the theories of Table 8.1 have followed suit; most state a theory in a few words or sentences, apply it to only a carefully selected set of data, with no specification of the detailed underlying machinery at all. We review a selection of alternatives to the spatial view next.

8.2.2 Theory 2: Working memory

At the same time that O'Keefe and Nadel were producing what is in essence a spatial reference memory theory, David Olton (Olton, 1978a; Olton et al., 1979a; Olton et al., 1979b) suggested that hippocampal lesions specifically disrupt working memory (spatial and non-spatial). The key distinction is that, where information is constant from trial to trial or moment to moment, it is held in 'reference' memory; but when it varies it is held in 'working' memory.[2] The nature and function of working memory has received quite extensive analysis by cognitive psychologists over many years (see Baddeley, 1986; Baddeley, 2011, for reviews). Currently, 'fluid' working memory can be seen as including visuo-spatial, episodic, and phonological modules, each of which can not only control current action but also can interact reciprocally with equivalent 'crystallized' reference memory modules (Baddeley, 2011).

The paradigm example of a test of working memory is the delayed matching-to-sample task. Here, the animal is presented with a sample stimulus and then, after a delay, must

[2] This might be better termed 'active memory' see (Fuster, 1995, p 5)

choose it from a pair of stimuli. From trial to trial (each trial consisting of the sample presentation followed by the choice test) the sample stimulus is changed (the stimuli can be trial-unique, or the sample can be randomly chosen from a fixed pair of stimuli, or some variant between these two extremes), so that the animal can only make the correct choice by remembering the specific sample presented at the start of the current trial. This job is done by working memory, and is attributed by Olton et al. (1979a) to the hippocampus. Conversely, according to their proposal, the hippocampus is not concerned with memory of those features of the matching-to-sample task that are constant from trial to trial (e.g. the nature of the reward, the required motor response, the matching-to-sample rule itself).

The initial experiments were conducted in the radial-arm maze, where the rat's task is to obtain a piece of food from the end of each of the arms. The working memory component of this task comes from the necessity to remember which arms have already been visited within any one trial. The normal rat shows an impressive capacity to remember which arms it has already visited, even in a 17-arm maze (Olton, 1978a). To achieve this high level of performance it appears not to rely on marking strategies (i.e. odour trails), response chaining, or consistent response strategies (e.g. go to the next arm on the left). When intra-maze cues are pitted against the general spatial environment provided by the experimental room, the latter usually dominate performance. There is a recency effect, in that errors increase the closer the first choice of an arm is to the start of the trial. But this recency effect is eliminated if the rat is confined to the centre platform of the maze for 20 seconds after each arm entry. There is no primacy effect in the standard version of the maze, that is, no tendency for the first trial to be relatively immune to later error (but see Kesner and Novak, 1982 for primacy and recency effects in a modified form of the test, with hippocampal lesions disrupting primacy, but not recency). If the animal is exposed to several trials within the same day (at a one-minute intertrial interval), there is an increase in errors across trials; but the first visits at the start of each new trial are made with perfect accuracy. Thus, although there is proactive interference between trials, the rat distinguishes between the end of one trial and the beginning of the next. The distribution of errors in space is random.

Based upon these observations, Olton (1978a, p. 365, our emphasis) describes working memory as having 'limited capacity, *interference among contents*, lack of decay for periods up to several minutes, little if any serial ordering, and no generalization or confusion among items'. If the hippocampus is the site of this memory system, performance on the radial-arm maze should obviously be impaired after hippocampal lesions. But note that the same prediction is made by Gaffan's (§8.2.4) recognition memory view (since the rat must recognize the locations it has just visited), by O'Keefe and Nadel's (§8.2.1) spatial memory view, and several others.

Given this convergence of predictions, it is not surprising that lesions of the hippocampus, the fornix-fimbria, the entorhinal cortex, or the septal area all profoundly impair performance in the radial-arm maze (Jarrard, 1978; Olton et al., 1978b; Olton and Werz, 1978; Walker and Olton, 1979). When unilateral destruction of the fornix is combined with unilateral destruction of the entorhinal cortex, performance is essentially normal if the lesions are made on the same side of the brain, but as impaired as with a bilateral lesion if they are made on opposite sides of the brain (Olton, 1978b). Thus, for successful performance in the radial-arm maze, the hippocampus has to have access to both its cortical and subcortical connections on at least one side of the brain.

We can eliminate at least one explanation of these results—the spatial one (§8.2.1)—with a version of the task that depended for its solution on the use of intra-maze, not spatial, cues (Olton et al., 1979a).

> Intramaze cues were made salient by having the sides of the arms 10 cm high and placing a unique set of visual and somatosensory stimuli in each arm. For example, one arm had black and white stripes in the floor and sides, and a groove 2 cm deep cut into the arm at each black stripe. Another arm had a diamond pattern painted on the sides and a smooth floor and sides. Extramaze cues were minimised by lighting the inside of the maze, covering the top of the maze with cheese cloth and reducing room illumination to a low level . . . An opaque guillotine door was placed between the centre compartment and the entrance to each of the arms. By lowering the doors, the experiment could confine the rat to the centre.
>
> All rats were first shaped to run out the arms with the maze in stationary position in the room. They were then placed in an 'interchange' procedure as illustrated in Fig. [8.2]. After the rat had chosen an arm and returned to the centre, the guillotine door in front of each arm was lowered confining him to the centre compartment. While the rat was confined, the arms were moved and their topological relationship changed . . . After the arms were moved, the guillotine doors were raised and the rat allowed to make a choice. When he returned to the centre, the guillotine doors were lowered and the arms were interchanged again.
>
> (Olton et al., 1979a, p. 317) (our figure reference)

These procedures ought effectively to have prevented the construction of any kind of spatial map and it certainly made the task much harder for the rats. However, the impairment produced by destruction of the fornix-fimbria was as profound as it is in the usual radial-arm maze (Olton et al., 1979a).

Of course, the deficits described so far could be the result not of a failure of working memory, but of a failure to remember the rule on which the working memory task is based (i.e. the reference component of the task). To show a specific working memory deficit, Olton and Papas (1979) made use of a 17-arm radial maze in which eight of the arms (the same on every trial) were never baited. Thus, the rat had two things to remember: (1) the eight arms that were never, and the nine arms that were always, baited at the start of the trial (reference memory); and (2) the arms in the baited set that it had already visited on a particular trial (working memory). On Olton's theory, damage to the hippocampus should disrupt the latter

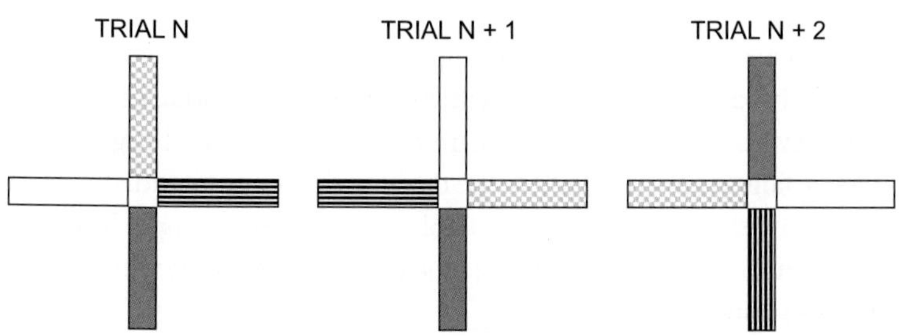

Fig. 8.2 A diagram of the experimental 'interchange' procedure modified from Olton et al. (1979a). Each arm of the maze is indicated by a different pattern. After each choice the rat was confined to the centre compartment and the arms were moved while it was so confined.

but not the former. Lesions of the fornix-fimbria severely disrupted the working memory component of this task, as predicted. The reference memory component was also disrupted, but only transiently. Thus an animal with fornix lesions can learn not to enter arms that are never rewarded (Olton and Papas, 1979) and it can also remember which objects have been followed by reward or non-reward (Gaffan, 1974).

Despite its elegance, there are at least two problems with a pure 'working memory' view of hippocampal function. The first is the severe deficit obtained when rats are required to swim to a submerged platform in a fixed location in the water maze, a reference memory task. An *ad hoc* solution to this problem would be to argue that determination of one's current position in space requires working memory and, without this, the reference memory task can never be solved. This would appear to be stretching the original idea of working memory rather a long way. The second problem is the fact that not all working memory tasks are sensitive to hippocampal lesions (and the bulk of H.M.'s working memory appears intact too §8.1.1). Delayed matching to sample of objects is sensitive to hippocampal lesions *only* if a limited set of repeated objects is used, *and not* if trial-unique objects are used. Even trial-uniqueness *per se* does not appear to be the critical factor behind this difference. Rawlins et al. (1993) found no deficit with delayed matching to sample using stimuli that were not trial-unique but which repeated only seldom; a modest deficit with a single trial-repeating pair of complex stimuli; and a much greater deficit with a single trial-repeating pair of simple stimuli. Likewise, Yee and Rawlins (1994) found no deficit in delayed non-matching with four choice alternatives when (a) four complex stimuli were used; and (b) four complex stimuli were used with the three to-be-rewarded choices constituting novel stimuli on every trial. But they demonstrated a deficit when (c) four simple stimuli were used. (Comparison of (a) versus (b) demonstrated the presence of interference effects that did not appear to be exacerbated by the lesions; we discuss this point further in §8.4.).

Overall, the hippocampus has 'been shown to be implicated in short-term memory and working memory, especially if precision and relational binding are required. [However,] patients with hippocampal lesions rarely complain of perceptual or WM deficits but always complain of episodic memory deficits.... The complexity of the items and the precision of the discrimination determine hippocampal involvement on tests of perception and short-term/working memory... [With increased] *susceptibility to interference*... the impact on memory is more keenly felt' (Moscovitch et al., 2016, p. 121, our emphasis).

8.2.3 Theory 3: Configural memory

We now turn to a theory based largely on a single experimental result: hippocampectomized animals failed to solve a discrimination in which a light (L) and tone (T) were reinforced if presented separately (L+, T+) but were non-reinforced if presented together (LT–). As we will see, the theory fails even with some of the data to which it is intended to apply; and only applies to a very limited selection of the available data on hippocampal lesions. However, it is important as a kind of simplified building block for later theories; which tend not to fully explain its founding result.

On the basis of this result, Rudy and Sutherland proposed that the hippocampus is necessary for configural associations, i.e. for 'the acquisition of a representation of a compound stimulus that is distinct from its elements' (Rudy and Sutherland, 1989, p. 97; Sutherland and

Rudy, 1989). An equivalent hippocampal sensitivity was found (Alvarado and Rudy, 1995b) with 'transverse patterning' (i.e. A + B–, B + C–, C + A–), which was dissociated from a lack of failure on a set of equivalent elemental problems (i.e. A + B–, C + D–, E + F–).

Critically, as they note, their experimental result is inconsistent with any spatial view (§8.2.1), working memory view (§8.2.2), or temporal buffer view (§8.2.8) of hippocampal function. It is also difficult to fit to the procedural/declarative distinction, since it is not clear whether the tasks studied are declarative, given that the simple associative version of the task with the same stimuli is taken not to be. They note, however, that their results are largely consistent with Hirsh's contextual view (§8.2.6), and to this we can add also the relational view (§8.2.7) and Trace Transformation view (§8.2.10). But they provide a simple paradigm example that makes us ask how far the engram complexity fundamental to these other views is necessary.

Hippocampal lesions do not always produce an impairment in configural discrimination. In particular, Whishaw and Tomie (1991) showed that, while some of their rats (all of which had massive hippocampal lesions) were impaired in learning a configural discrimination, others were not, the fastest learner of all being one with lesions. They also showed that, with a lesion made after acquisition of the task, there was excellent postoperative retention. They point to a number of features of their procedure that might account for this: they used a string-pulling task which maximizes the contiguity of cues; they used a tactile-olfactory compound rather than a tone-light one; and the rats had a choice between a correct and an incorrect response (rather than the go/no-go of Rudy and Sutherland's experiment). Cue contiguity does not appear to be the crucial factor, as a visual-tactile version of the task is also not impaired (Whishaw and Tomie, 1995). None of the variations, of course, change the configural nature of the task from a theoretical standpoint. Other differences from the original study by Rudy and his collaborators, which Whishaw and Tomie do not mention, were that all of the stimuli used were compounds formed from one of two alternative tactile stimuli and one of two alternative olfactory stimuli, and that hence both positively and negatively reinforced compound stimuli were presented (rather than the L+, T+, LT- of the original experiment).

Cohen and Eichenbaum (1993, pp. 165–171, 260–263) provided a detailed critique of the configural view. Their main points are that 'although Sutherland and Rudy have attempted to extend the proposal beyond the initial paradigms of interest to them, it remains a limited-domain account . . . [and] it is in the *absence* of the hippocampal system that animals fuse perceptually distinct stimuli into configurals, at least in some circumstances' (Cohen and Eichenbaum, 1993, pp. 261–262). Davidson and Jarrard (1992, p. 90) also point out that in fact 'rats solve serial-compound discriminations because stimulus B comes to modulate the capacity of stimulus A to elicit a response [rather than by compound formation]. Hence, although it appears to be the basis for solving a task purportedly explained by Sutherland and Rudy's (1989) theory, [the actual mechanism of] conditioned modulation does not seem to be encompassed by either their configural or their simple association view' (but see also Rudy and Sutherland, 1992).

Even the original finding may not hold. Davidson et al. (1993) found that neither the kainate/colchicine hippocampal lesion originally used (Rudy and Sutherland, 1989) nor ibotenic acid lesions affected the negative patterning task. Although they do not remark on this, the likely reason for the discrepancy is that Rudy and Sutherland used continuous reinforcement of the positive stimuli while Davidson et al. (1993) used what appears to have been a variable ratio (VR3) schedule. This increases the problem for configural theory, but suggests that the deficit, when it occurs, may result from the degree of response competition since, with continuous reinforcement, the secondary positive reinforcement accruing to the elements that make up the negative compound will be higher than with VR3 (see also Whishaw and Tomie, 1991).

Interference from response competition is a particularly obvious explanation for the transverse patterning result (Alvarado and Rudy, 1995b); and comparison over a number of configural tasks that did, or did not, show lesion effects led Alvarado and Rudy (1995a, p. 183) to conclude 'that hippocampal formation involvement depends on the degree to which the elements of a compound (e.g. A and B) provide sources of generalized excitation that oppose the inhibitory control conditioned to a configural unit (AB)' rather than on configural association as such. In what follows it will be useful to remember not only the key distinction between conditioning to elements and conditioning to a compound but also generalized excitation and the consequent need for inhibitory control.

8.2.4 Theory 4: Recognition memory

David Gaffan (Gaffan, 1972; Gaffan, 1974; Gaffan, 1977a; Gaffan, 1977c) proposed that hippocampal damage disrupts 'recognition' memory. This has much in common with David Olton's (Olton, 1978a; Olton et al., 1979a; Olton et al., 1979b) 'working' memory theory (§8.2.2) and Olga Vinogradova's (1975) view that the hippocampus subserves both orienting responses to novelty and, importantly for memory, their habituation as the stimulus becomes familiar.

Gaffan proposed that hippocampal lesions disrupt only recognition memory (familiarity) and (as Rudy & Sutherland) not the simple associative memory that is responsible for turning stimuli into secondary reinforcers. He proposed that hippocampal lesions disrupt only the former and tested this with lesions of the fornix/fimbria, a key input/output tract. In a T-maze with one black and one white arm, when one arm is changed, normal rats choose it; except when there is also a frightening stimulus (loud noise) when they choose the familiar arm. Rats with fornix lesions chose at random under both conditions (Gaffan, 1972).[3] Gaffan attributes these findings to a failure on the part of rats with fornix lesions to discriminate the familiar from the changed arm.

Gaffan (1974) used monkeys to more clearly separate recognition from associative memory. One task presented a set of 10 objects, one at a time, five of which were followed by food and five not. To test retention the monkey was faced with pairs of objects, with one constant and the other selected from the initial set. The monkey had to choose the latter if it had initially been paired with food, and choose the constant object otherwise. Essentially, it was asked, 'Do you remember which objects were paired with food and which were not?' As predicted by Gaffan, fornix-lesioned animals were not different from controls on this task. A second task was similar, except that the animal was initially presented with only five objects, all followed by reward. These five, and five new ones, were each then paired with the constant object. If the non-constant object had previously been presented (and paired with reward, as in the first experiment) the animal was required to choose it. If the non-constant

[3] Note the similarity to the effect of anxiolytic drugs (Ison et al., 1966); see also Appendix 1.

object had not previously been presented (unlike the first experiment) the animals was required to choose the constant object. Essentially, it was asked, 'Do you remember seeing this object before?' This time, but still as predicted, fornix-lesioned monkeys were inferior to controls. Furthermore, controls were better in the recognition task than in the test of associative memory, whereas the lesioned animals were better at association than recognition.

This kind of task is very similar to many used to study human memory, e.g. presentation of lists of words or pictures, and a request to identify if an item in a second list did or did not figure in the first. To match the model even closer, Gaffan (1977b) showed the monkey 25 pictures (on slides) per daily session, each picture occurring twice. Order of presentation was randomized but the same slides were used each day. The task was to press a panel only on the second appearance of any slide. This is analogous to asking a human subject to answer 'yes' or 'no' to the question 'Have you seen this picture earlier today?'. Two rhesus monkeys achieved over 90% accuracy even when an average of nine slides were presented between the first and second occurrence of any one slide. After fornix section, they were able to achieve accurate performance only up to an average of three intervening slides. Note that it is precisely on this kind of yes-no recognition task that the human amnesic impairment is particularly pronounced.

Gaffan (1977d) compared a spatial and a non-spatial version of list learning. In the non-spatial version, the monkey was successively shown three colours (transilluminated discs) followed three seconds later by one of six possible colours. Its task was to press one response panel if the test colour had been presented in the sample set of three, or another if it had not. The spatial version consisted of the successive illumination of three out of six discs, followed three seconds later by the illumination of one of them. The task was to press one panel if the test disc was in one of the positions first illuminated and another panel if it was not. Fornix-lesioned monkeys were impaired on the two tasks to the same extent and in the same manner: they made a great number of omission errors ('forgetting'), but only when the test stimulus was the first to have been presented in the initial list of three colours or positions. Both normal and lesioned monkeys showed a pronounced 'recency' effect, that is their recognition was better the more recently the test stimulus had appeared (i.e. the later in the list). These results show the operation of retroactive interference (see §8.4.3).

Gaffan's recognition view is to some extent a special case of the relational view (although it is not discussed by Cohen and Eichenbaum, 1993), in that what distinguishes items is their relation in time (i.e. more or less recent). It probably did not find favour because of the relative difficulty it has in accounting for spatial (location of a submerged platform, impaired) versus non-spatial (location of a visible platform, unimpaired) performance in the water maze, and for the fact that deficits in delayed matching to sample (see §8.2.2) are obtained with trial-repetitive but not with trial-unique stimuli—where recognition as such is held constant, so the greater difficulty of trial-repetitive stimuli must lie in some other factor. Conversely, hippocampal lesioned rats can make recency discriminations (inherently more taxing in recognition terms than pure familiarity), provided the items as a whole are fairly recent and there are not too many intervening items (Fig. 3 in Chiba et al., 1994). Also, like the configural and working memory theories, the recognition hypothesis has trouble with simple tasks like extinction and DRL; is intended to apply only to the memory data; and makes no attempt to provide a theory in terms of the known anatomy and physiology of the hippocampal system.

8.2.5 Theory 5: Semantic encoding

This next theory is somewhat of an outlier and derives from verbal learning experiments and can be applied to non-linguistic tests only with difficulty. Butters and Cermak (1975) suggested that amnesic subjects suffer from a disturbance in the process of 'semantic encoding'. (But note that this may be in interaction with episodic memory, Moscovitch et al., 2016.) Put like this, the encoding hypothesis is almost necessarily limited to testing with language, since the notion of *semantic* encoding is closely tied to the details of experiments on verbal learning. It is supposed that, when a subject is presented with a word, this word can be committed to memory after being subjected to one or more of (at least) three different kinds of analysis: acoustic (what the word sounds like), associative (what it is associated with), or semantic (what it means). If semantic encoding were the chief deficit in the amnesic syndrome, the problem of relating linguistic to non-linguistic data would be acute indeed.

The bulk of the evidence for the semantic encoding hypothesis is from Korsakoff patients required to learn serial lists of words (Cermak and Butters, 1972; Cermak et al., 1973; Butters and Cermak, 1975). Initially, the list consisted of eight words, with two from each of four different semantic categories (animals, professions, etc.). Cueing by category name improved recall among controls, but not among Korsakoff patients. This is consistent with a failure of adequate semantic encoding at the time of learning in the patient group. Cermak et al. (1973) compared the improvement in recall with associative (e.g. 'table' as a cue for 'chair'), rhyming, or semantic cues. Association and rhyme helped controls and amnesics equally; category names helped amnesics less than controls—suggesting that semantic encoding was specifically deficient. This also seemed true when participants were asked to detect repetitions in a long list of words. Besides genuine repetitions, the list contained some homonyms, synonyms, and associates. Korsakoff patients made *as many correct identifications* as controls, and no more false recognitions of either synonyms or neutral words; but they made *more false recognitions of both homonyms and associates*.

Butters and Cermak (1975, p. 393) concluded that 'the Korsakoff patients were encoding the words on acoustic and associative dimensions, but were not encoding the semantic dimensions of the words to the extent that would allow the rejections of acoustically identical or highly associated words'. They took this further with a test of 'release from proactive interference'. Wickens (1970) found that normal subjects had reduced proactive interference if the semantic category to which successive items belong is changed for a particular item in the list. Cermak et al. (1974) found this true also for Korsakoff patients, provided that the change in category was relatively gross (from letter sets to number sets); but, unlike controls, the amnesics derived no benefit when the category shift was more subtle (from sets of animal names to a set of names of vegetables). So, there is a strong case, for a role for semantic encoding as an important parametric feature in making a task sensitive to the amnesic syndrome.

Does this imply that a deficit in semantic encoding is the key feature of amnesia in human beings? This would re-open a substantial gulf between human and non-human data and separate linguistic from non-linguistic human data. Before accepting this, we need to show that a deficit in semantic encoding can explain all the features of the amnesic syndrome; and, also, that there is not some more general principle, consistent with the non-human data that could account for the apparent deficits in semantic encoding.

We have already detailed (§8.1.4) experiments that prevented verbal rehearsal (so eliminating semantic encoding). They found an amnesic deficit with the form predicted by previous non-human experiments. Amnesics can, also, benefit from semantic cueing (Winocur and Weiskrantz, 1976; Winocur, 1981) potentially as much as controls (Mayes et al., 1980). The semantic encoding hypothesis thus fails to account for all the data on the *human* amnesic deficit.

What of consistency with *non-human* data? Butters and Cermak (1975, p. 393, our emphasis) suggest that 'the Korsakoff patient's encoding deficit may be related to *a general impairment* in their ability to attend to the relevant dimensions of stimuli'. Faced with stimuli differing simultaneously in form, colour, size, and position, Korsakoff patients were shown, in transfer tests, to use fewer of the available stimulus dimensions (none of which was distinctively 'semantic') than other brain-damaged patients, or controls (Oscar-Berman and Samuels, 1973; Oscar-Berman and Samuels, 1977). The Korsakoff patients concentrated especially on colour, ignoring the other possibilities. This is like hippocampal lesioned rats who are poorer than controls at transferring from a simultaneous discrimination in which brightness and position are perfectly correlated to brightness alone (Samuels and Valian, 1968). Similarly, amnesic patients have an excessive dependence on environmental context (Winocur and Kinsbourne, 1978) as do rats with hippocampal lesions (Winocur and Olds, 1978). So, change in a dominant environmental cue can produce a retention deficit; while provision of such a cue can eliminate it. In human and non-human alike, hippocampal damage produces a general problem in multidimensional stimulus analysis that prevents the control of behaviour by more subtle, or additional, cues in the environment.

Given the Oscar-Berman and Samuels results, the amnesic impairment has to be of multidimensional stimulus analysis that underlies a deficit in semantic encoding rather than the other way round. So, even those cases where semantic coding appears important depend on more general processing deficits similar to hippocampal deficits in non-human subjects.

8.2.6 Theory 6: Contextual memory

In §8.1.5 (Myth 5), we rejected 'context' as a synonym for an extended space; we also argued that contextual conditioning *per se* is not hippocampal; and the hippocampal sensitivity of conditioning depends on the complexity of the box used as 'context' (Moses et al., 2007). But earlier work used the word context according to the dictionary definition—and in a sophisticated manner that cannot be ruled out of hand as misguided. Indeed, this perspective is having a renaissance (Yonelinas et al., 2019); with additions such as the idea that space often provides the key context so hippocampal damage leads to abnormal generalization across context (Nadel, 2008; Winocur et al., 2007); and that context is the basis for relational binding (Sadeh and Pertzov, 2020) in a form similar to earlier relational theory (§8.2.7). There are also new tests designed to assess different effects of distinct forms of context-specific recall (Prodan et al., 2022). We discuss these hybrid developments further in §8.2.10 and deal with more restricted ideas about context here.

First, and simplest, is the idea of context-dependence of memory. Winocur (1981) proposed that, *under conditions of high interference*, animals with hippocampal lesions are unable (for whatever reason) to extract enough information from cues that are typically sufficient for controls. In consequence, they become abnormally dependent on 'contextual cues' (i.e. background stimuli that can be used to determine which of several possible responses to a common stimulus is correct in a particular context).

In support of this view, Winocur and Olds (1978) trained rats on a simultaneous discrimination between horizontal and vertical stripes and then tested them after a seven-day retention interval either in the same or a different apparatus, and either under the same (food) or a different (water) drive. There was a retention deficit only when conditions were changed between acquisition and retention testing. When reversal learning was substituted for retention testing, the opposite occurred: there was a large deficit in the unchanged conditions, and only a nonsignificant one in the changed conditions. Thus, in accord with Winocur's hypothesis, the lesioned animals were excessively dependent on contextual cues for the maintenance of the behaviour that they had first learned. (Note that this result is opposite to that predicted if hippocampal lesions *impair* conditioning to context.)

A rather different suggestion, also concerning context, has been made by Hirsh (1974). According to this proposal, hippocampal lesions disrupt the 'contextual' retrieval of information from memory. Since this proposal has been somewhat neglected, and is rather technically defined, we cover it in detail, largely in Hirsh's own words.

> Contextual retrieval is defined as the retrieval of an item of stored information initiated by a cue which refers to but is not necessarily described within the information that is retrieved. An example is the indexing of library books according to their authors. This concept has strong implications for theories of how the brain controls behaviour. Understanding these implications requires defining and exploring the metaphysiological concept of the performance line. A performance line is defined as a system mediating the series of events or processes initiated by the overtly observable stimulus and resulting in the occurrence of the overtly observable response. It is considered to exist in real time and real space and ultimately to be physiologically observable.
>
> S-R theories, as usually interpreted by physiological psychologists, hold that memory is stored upon the performance line. The stimulus is defined as activation by an environmental event of a neural system sensitive to it. Memory, or more exactly learning, is held to result from the formation of a functional connection between the neural elements sensitive to the stimulus and those responsible for producing the response. This connection becomes the key part of the performance line for that particular combination of stimulus and response elements and is unique to it . . .
>
> When contextual retrieval is present it is no longer necessary to store acquired information upon the performance line. Information can be stored in a sequestered place or state free from interference by information processing being carried out on the performance line. Schematic representations of systems with and without contextual retrieval are presented in Fig. [8.3]. In a system with contextual retrieval, information can be moved from storage to the performance line independently, and thus before the occurrence, of the stimulus described within the retrieved information . . .
>
> It is assumed that when an item of information is contextually retrieved it is placed upon the performance line. Perceptual systems are adjusted to be particularly receptive to the stimulus described within the information. The object of attention is specified. In such a system behaviour is no longer completely controlled by environmental events because the perceptual systems are adjusted prior to the occurrence of the overtly observable stimulus. The potential of the retrieved stimulus description for controlling behaviour is considerably greater than that of non-retrieved descriptions . . . By contrast, when memory is stored upon

the performance line, no stimulus "description' has more potential for controlling behaviour than any other until the event described actually occurs and initiates retrieval . . .

It is also assumed that motor systems are adjusted to more readily produce the response described within the retrieved information as a result of contextual retrieval . . .

When behaviour which conflicts with previous learning is acquired, the previous acquisition must be made inoperative when learning involves altering the performance line. The new and previous acquisitions cannot both be retained, as both would be activated by the stimulus. To avoid conflict at least part of the previously acquired learning must be removed from the performance line, usually by inhibiting one of its stages.

Systems utilizing contextual retrieval do not require deletion of previous learning. The conflicting items of information can be differentiated by the addition of a contextual label indicating that the previously acquired information was formerly true . . .

The effects of hippocampal lesions are held to result from the disruption of contextual retrieval. In the normal brain, storage is considered to be separate from the performance line. When the hippocampus is absent storage is held to occur within the performance line.

(Hirsh, 1974, pp. 422–426) [our figure reference]

Hirsh applies this theory to the whole gamut of behavioural changes seen after hippocampal lesions. But, since we are concerned here with purely memorial approaches to hippocampal function, we note only that the general theory of septo-hippocampal function that we present has much in common with Hirsh's ideas, except that we would see the *ordering* of contextually retrieved goals as being the job of the prefrontal cortex rather than the hippocampus; with the hippocampus becoming involved only when there is significant conflict between goals at a specific point in time. As applied to the particular problem of memory, Hirsh's theory treats the hippocampal deficit (when it occurs) as arising from an inability to use contextual labelling to decide between competing response tendencies under conditions of high interference (see also Yonelinas et al., 2019). This emphasis on interference is very different from the simple contextual views discussed earlier and is a key to our own account in §8.3.

As far as the concept of context goes, Hirsh's (1974) view of its role in the behaviour of animals with hippocampal lesions seems very different from Winocur's (1981). Indeed, Winocur himself (personal communication, 1981) originally saw the two approaches as diametrically

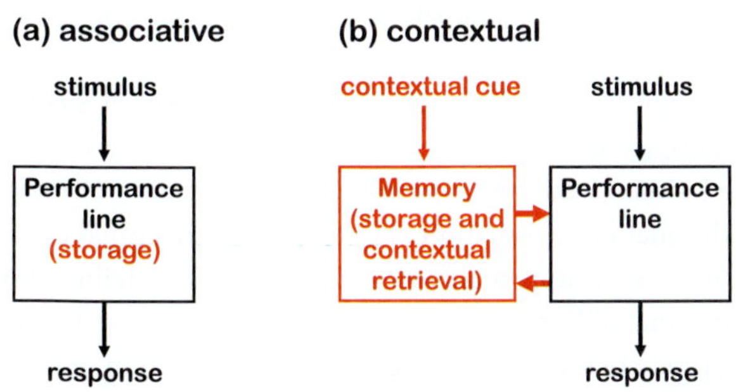

Fig. 8.3 Schematic diagrams of systems using either associative (a) or contextual (b) retrieval. In the associative case, memory storage is on the performance line. In the contextual case, both stimulus and contextual information are stored off the performance line and placed on it as required. (Redrawn following Hirsh, 1974).

opposed. But now, 'as it happens, Hirsh & I are no longer as apart as we thought we were in 1981. Hirsh was right to argue that the HPC is necessary for processing contextual information to form episodic memories; I was right to argue that without the HPC, the animal (person) relates distinctive contextual cues to an event to form schematic or non-context-dependent, memories that can be remembered' (Winocur, G. personal communication by email, 27 October 2021). Thus, they used the term 'context' in different ways. For Hirsh, this was something the animal puts into the description of the stimuli to which it responds; for Winocur, it was out in the environment. The process that Hirsh ascribes to the hippocampus would play a particularly critical role in the control of behaviour when there are no large changes in the environmental context (Winocur) to assume this control. Thus, *both* Hirsh and Winocur should predict that a large difference in the environmental context between initial acquisition and reversal training would help the animal to overcome its usual deficit in reversal learning, as was in fact found by Winocur and Olds (1978). Conversely, when controls benefit from a large difference in context, lesioned animals show a deficit (Winocur et al., 2007). So, from this point of view, rather than being opposed to each other, the two hypotheses are mutually complementary. Hirsh's mechanism can be seen as specifying the reasons why, as postulated by Winocur, animals with hippocampal lesions are unable to extract enough information from cues that are typically sufficient for controls: they lack the process of contextual labelling and retrieval. In line with this suggestion, Brown (1982) found single units in the hippocampus that, in rhesus monkeys trained on a conditional discrimination, responded, or failed to respond, to particular stimuli depending on the context in which these were presented (see Smith et al., 2022, for review).

As we have noted, Hirsh's views are very close to our own and quite close to the relational view of Cohen and Eichenbaum (1993; see §8.2.7); but, as with a number of other theories of hippocampal function with which we contrast our position, we believe that his argument should be turned exactly upside down. In our view, hippocampal lesions do not so much cause the animal to fail to label a particular stimulus with its context, but rather permit too many stimuli to be so labelled. Contextual errors occur, then, not because the key item is not retrieved by the context, but because many other items are concurrently retrieved and the correct item is then lost in the Hebbian pandemonium (§8.3; see also Smith et al., 2022). On this view, contextual errors should be 'intrusion' errors: the retrieval of information associated with the context but which is currently incorrect. In contrast, from a pure contextual labelling point of view, errors should be random. We take the same position with Miller's (1991) theory, which sees the hippocampal theta rhythm as indexing contextual information in the brain.

Probably the most explicit case of contextual control of retrieval is conditional discrimination. This is usually impaired in animals by hippocampal lesions, as it is also in human beings with temporal lobe lesions (Daum et al., 1991). The dissociation of intact non-conditional and disrupted conditional discrimination is clear even with simple classically conditioned responses (Ross et al., 1984; Daum et al., 1991). One interesting failure, however, to produce a deficit of this kind is that of Whishaw and Tomie (1991), who used a string-pulling task in which size of string predicted the position of reward. Observation of the rats suggested that they were not turning the task into a simple go/no-go discrimination by adopting a position bias, and that some feature of the stimuli (such as their contiguity to the rat) may have removed the normal deficit through the loss of some source of interference. Similarly, with delayed conditional discrimination, the size of the deficit appears to depend on the extent to which there is interference (Wan et al., 1994). All of this is consistent with Hirsh's general position and so with our inversion of it.

A very similar view of context has recently been taken as important for some aspects of relational memory (see next section) and, in particular, forgetting. In an appendix to a detailed review arguing that hippocampal-sensitive forgetting occurs at both short and long time scales Sadeh and Pertzov (2020, p. 396) say:

> Time-dependent forgetting of hippocampal-based, relational representations is readily accounted for by the notion of contextual drift. The hippocampus binds item information (e.g. a face, word, picture) with the context in which the item was encountered. Context refers to any information peripheral to the study item, including external information (e.g. the spatial location) and internal information, such as an individual's mood and her thoughts and associations. The bound item-context entity constitutes the memory trace. Successful retrieval of an item depends on the degree to which the study context is reinstated during retrieval. Therefore, according to the contextual drift notion, forgetting is the result of a change or drift in context between study and test. Indeed, models of episodic memory, such as the temporal context model, highlight the short-lived nature of context, such that contextual information continuously fluctuates over time. Relatedly, forgetting may be further advanced by contextual interference, such as intervening activities or physical changes.

This kind of process may also be important for consolidation and for therapeutic attempts to alter context-based fear memories (Ressler et al., 2021).

8.2.7 Theory 7: Relational memory

Despite covering context and item-in-context in detail, Sadeh and Pertzov (2020) emphasize more general 'relational binding' as a key to hippocampal sensitivity of a test—using examples such as intact object and location memory but impaired memory for object-location associations. In this section, we look in detail at an earlier book-length synthesis of the animal and human literature on the hippocampus and memory (Cohen and Eichenbaum, 1993; Eichenbaum et al., 1994) that sees relational memory as critical.

Key features of their proposal, with which we agree, are that:

- the hippocampus is not concerned with very short- or very long-term memory storage (see Sadeh and Pertzov, 2020 for a discussion of potential confounds, particularly with tests of short retention), these being functions of cortical areas;
- the hippocampus is not concerned with simple associative learning (of the type we ascribed in Chapter 6 to, for example, LTP of sensory input to the amygdala);
- the entorhinal cortex carries multimodal information to the hippocampus;
- an intact hippocampus is necessary if an animal is to learn many tasks (Eichenbaum et al. would say all tasks) that require relational processing.

However, as we noted in a commentary on the Eichenbaum et al. paper (McNaughton, 1994), we believe that their theory (along with others) is flawed because of the specifically memorial perspective they take to the data. They deliberately and quite explicitly excluded from consideration much of the data on behavioural inhibition that have been central to our own approach. They also excluded all consideration of septal and monoaminergic input to the hippocampus and of subcortical output (a surprising omission since this is a major output in neuronal terms). Further, in common with other memory theories, they view the hippocampus as a form of intermediate store and do not make it entirely clear (Cohen and Eichenbaum, 1993, pp. 68–72) how information stored in the hippocampus can be transferred to distributed networks (and distributed they must be, given the complex polymodal associations usually involved) in the neocortex. (See Inostroza and Born, 2013 for a recent account of transfer including a role in sleep-based consolidation.)

At root, Cohen and Eichenbaum (1993) base their theory on the declarative-procedural distinction ('knowing what' as opposed to 'knowing how'), which is essentially the same as the locale/taxon separation §8.2.1. They propose 'that the hippocampal system plays a critical role in mediating declarative memory, one of the memory systems of the brain' (*op. cit.*, p. 60). What is distinctive is their elaboration of the critical features of declarative memory: 'input to the hippocampal system consists of highly processed data from many higher-order cortical processing areas, each representing *functional descriptors* of the perceptually distinct objects and events encountered during learning, plus information about the affective and behavioural responses elicited' (*op. cit.*, p. 61). A crucial point is that 'representation of scenes, events, and complex ideas in our proposed declarative memory system is *not* as blends . . . and does *not* involve conjoining of the multiple individual stimuli or constituent pieces of knowledge into unified knowledge structures . . . [It] preserves the status of the constituents of the larger structure while still permitting the larger structure to be appreciated' (*op. cit.*, p. 64). Thus, declarative memory, within their theory, consists of a wide variety of informational entities (not just objects or qualities but also, e.g. behavioural responses) all interconnected by the relations that each holds to the other: e.g. bird—[is an]—animal; canary—[is]—yellow. Storage of items belonging to the declarative system is presumed to be located within the neocortex.

A declarative memory system with these properties must suffer from a 'binding' problem. Within perception, the equivalent problem is: given the multiple unimodal systems, each dealing with a separate aspect of the visual world (e.g. colour), how do we obtain a unified picture of the world—how are the separate parts bound back together again? The declarative memory system (and a variety of other types of complex parallel associative memory systems, c.f. §8.5) suffers from the memorial counterpart to this problem. With each node representing an entity and connections between nodes representing relations, how, at any one time, do we ensure that the right combination of nodes and connections is active?

In Cohen and Eichenbaum's version, 'the hippocampal system . . . apparently stores—for a time after learning—a representation from which declarative memory of the event or scene can be *reconstructed* from the permanent representations of the various attributes or features of the event or scene stored within the various neocortical processors' (Cohen and Eichenbaum, 1993, p. 288). This resolution appears rather neat until we notice that it does not solve the binding problem as such. If the neocortical networks can, through strengthening of connections, ultimately represent the declarative memory then, intrinsically, they have no need of a separate processor to produce the binding itself—all of the necessary bonds are potentially there already. Alternatively, if the hippocampus is necessary for binding as such, its removal should degrade all memories, whatever their age.

An alternative solution to this problem is that there is an independent (hippocampal) indexing system (Teyler and Discenna, 1986)—though indexing could also occur in the prefrontal cortex (Fiebig et al., 2020). On this view the hippocampus stores (via LTP) the 'index of neocortical areas activated by experiential events' (Teyler and Discenna, 1986, p. 147). A pure indexing view fails because loss of the index should eliminate *all* declarative memory; yet, for example, H.M.'s longer-term memories are intact. However, it is likely that with replay during sleep, for example, 'continual reactivation of a particular hippocampal index would have a slowly incrementing effect on the cortical circuitry it indexes [and] the hippocampal index, with time, would become redundant' (Teyler and Discenna, 1986, p. 150; updated by Teyler and Rudy, 2007; see also Goode et al., 2020). We will return to these ideas in §8.2.10.

These criticisms of the relational memory theory treat it as a paradigm case and apply to the other alternative memory theories, which often reduce to special cases of the relational theory (see Cohen and Eichenbaum, 1993, their Chapters 11 and 12); and translate to our theory in the same way. We now move on to cases that relate more to mechanical type of memory process than cognitive type of engram.

8.2.8 Theory 8: Temporal buffer

A theory superficially similar to the working memory theory (§8.2.2) is that the hippocampus constitutes a high-capacity, intermediate-term memory store (Rawlins, 1985). Rawlins's approach has a major similarity with our own, in that he argues strongly against 'the idea that the hippocampus is required to process items only of some qualitatively specifiable kind, and is not required to process items of some complementary set. In contrast, it is now proposed that the hippocampus is needed to process stimuli of all kinds, but only when there is a need to associate those stimuli with other events that are temporally discontiguous' (Rawlins, 1985, p. 479).

The basis of Rawlins' theory is a careful analysis of the tasks that purport to distinguish different types of memory; with the conclusion that 'the sensitivity of these tasks as indicators of hippocampal dysfunction is not well predicted by existing task classifications based on current views of hippocampal function.... Existing theories need to be significantly modified. They need to explain why increasing or decreasing the degree of temporal discontiguity within their paradigmatic designs concomitantly increases or decreases the tasks' sensitivity to hippocampal dysfunction' (Rawlins, 1985, pp. 496–497). We agree.

Rawlins goes on from this to the stronger claim 'that the hippocampus functions as an intermediate memory system. Information is normally admitted to this store in parallel with admission to a much more limited short-term store. When the intermediate-term system is incapacitated, any task in which information must be given temporary storage will become insoluble once the storage duration or the number of items to be stored exceeds the residual short-term storage capacity. This view holds for information of all kinds and suggests that the critical determinants of task sensitivity to hippocampal dysfunction are temporal discontiguity and number of items requiring temporary storage' (Rawlins, 1985, pp. 496–497).

We remarked in a commentary on Rawlins's paper that his 'reanalysis of previous experiments and the results of his own experiments make an impressive case for the importance of temporal discontiguity in the effects of hippocampal lesions. However, his success in substituting temporal discontiguity for previous constructs prompts the question: Does temporal discontinguity itself mask some other factor? Rawlins himself identifies one possibility. He states that 'the time over which storage is required *and the number of items needing storage* can be seen as trading off against each other' (our emphasis). However, increasing temporal discontiguity increases the probability of interference from extraneous stimuli' (McNaughton, 1985c, p. 508). We (McNaughton, 1985c) then reviewed data on passive avoidance, extinction, and taste aversion conditioning, all of which were incompatible with Rawlins's theory. Since then, Rawlins's own laboratory has produced data that effectively demolish a time-capacity view of the hippocampus: hippocampal lesions impair delayed matching to sample most with a pair of simple stimuli, less with a pair of complex stimuli, and not at all with pairs of pseudo-trial-unique stimuli, distinctions that do not involve the temporal domain (Rawlins et al., 1993).

Unlike many of the other theories we have looked at, Rawlins's theory is not intended to be limited in its domain, though it was not supplied with any detailed physiological or anatomical machinery. However, from the data briefly reviewed earlier, we must conclude that, while the strong parametric influence of time on the effects of hippocampectomy must be accounted for by any successful theory, time itself is not of the essence. We return to this point next.

8.2.9 Theory 9: Intermediate memory

Rawlins's view of a temporally-limited intermediate store is very similar to the standard consolidation theory (for additional critique, see Moscovitch et al., 2016, pp. 115–117; Moscovitch and Gilboa, 2021), which allows many of the 'memory type' (hippocampal vs. non-hippocampal) theories to account for the limited retrograde effects seen in amnesics. For these variations of the standard consolidation theory, the 'hippocampal store' is not strictly limited in the time that it can hold information. Rather, the hippocampus is specialized to hold certain types of complex information, and does so for as long as is necessary for cortical circuits to consolidate that information (see Fig. 2 in Inostroza and Born, 2013 for a detailed mechanism for this). The great variety of proposed memory typologies of this kind, noted earlier, suggests that they may all suffer from some kind of fundamental intractability. But there are additional reasons to doubt the validity of any intermediate store approach: serious problems are raised by the nature of the processes that must be attributed by this class of theories to the 'intermediate hippocampal memory store'.

H.M. had an intact long-term memory for information acquired preoperatively. It follows that the putative hippocampal-dependent memories are distinct from non-hippocampal memories not only in terms of their 'type' but also in that, if they require storage in the hippocampus, they do so only for a relatively brief period of time. So, if memories are temporarily stored in the hippocampus they must ultimately be copied into cortex (or wherever is their final repository). Wilson and B. McNaughton (1994), for example, explicitly suggest that the hippocampus contains a fast flexible store that can then replay information into cortical circuits during consolidation (particularly during sleep, see Inostroza and Born, 2013 and Appendix 7). This idea of a specialized store, ultimately transferring its information to other parts of the brain, can certainly account for an initial sensitivity of only certain classes of memory to hippocampal damage, and for the later lack of such sensitivity. It is also a superficially attractive notion when one thinks of the ease with which areas of memory can be copied in computers.

However, let us ask *why* computers need to copy memory information, and whether what we know of neural plasticity is compatible with such copying. Computers copy 'memories' from place to place with great facility; and hippocampal and cortical synapses both show LTP, which might store information in a computer-like fashion. But the analogy breaks down when we note that copying of memory areas, one to the other, is easy in a computer because, in memorial terms, it is unnecessary. Memory is copied when one area is to be modified and another is required to retain the original information. But the process is only possible because *both* areas are equally good repositories of the original information (which is coded by bit pattern rather than location); and what is copied to where is completely arbitrary and involves exact replication of the original source by the copy. The analogy with the brain breaks down in two separate ways. First, a supposed significant difference in the fundamental nature of hippocampal and non-hippocampal storage is the only reason for postulating a particular 'type' of hippocampal memory in the first place. *Ex hypothesi*, therefore, the uniformity between memory areas in the computer is not true of the brain. Second, the brain codes information positionally (the point in the brain, e.g. visual cortex, defines the nature of the information), not in terms of bit patterns.

Let us consider, for a moment, the formation of simple, hippocampal-independent, memories. There is good evidence (Chapter 6; Appendix 2) that active avoidance depends on LTP (or some similar process) of input from sensory systems to the amygdala. Likewise (§7.1; Appendix 6), conditioning of the nictitating membrane response involves plasticity of sensory inputs to cerebellar circuits. Much of what we term memory must, therefore, involve CS-response program associations, produced by LTP or something like it, in a bewildering variety of different places in the brain. Given the fact that hippocampal-dependent memories are not sensitive to hippocampal lesions once they are fully consolidated, it follows that even these types of memory must ultimately be instantiated in strengthened connections between and within appropriate extra-hippocampal areas creating an appropriate cell assembly (Hebb, 1949 used visual cortex as his example of a memory store). Why, if the cortex (or other final long-term repository of intermediate 'hippocampal' traces) can store the relevant information after consolidation does it need the hippocampus as a temporary store?

There is a further fundamental logical flaw in the idea of the hippocampal formation as an intermediate memory store, which follows from the general nature of hippocampal-dependent memories. Whatever the specific type postulated to be hippocampal-dependent, they all have in common that they are seen as being more complex than simple associative memories, and usually (most clearly in the case of relational, declarative, contextual, spatial and configural theories) that they involve combinations of elements that can separately enter into hippocampal-independent associations.

Consider relational memory. Neocortex is held to support simple associations of the 'B will follow A' type, which we can represent as A–B. It is only when some specific more complex relation (e.g. A–B–C, as distinct from A–C–B, B–A–C, B–C–A, C–A–B, and C–B–A) must be encoded that the hippocampus is required. Note that, if the hippocampus is to be the location where such relational information is encoded, this implies that the hippocampus can duplicate all the possible associative connections of those other parts of the brain that deal with the same information but at a non-relational level (since A–B and B–C are elements of A–B–C). This type of theory implies also that the hippocampal input and output connections can, in principle, carry the factorial combination of all the embedded simple associative connections taken N at a time, where N is the largest number of simple elements normally combining to form a distinct relational memory. This is inherently unlikely. With minor changes of detail this same conclusion can be drawn for all the current 'memory-type' theories.

Thus, the hippocampus should be bigger than the totality of those parts of the brain with which it interacts in the formation of memories. Not only is this clearly not the case, but the relative increase in size of the hippocampus with encephalization (four times the size of an average insectivore's) has been nothing like as great as the increase in the size of the neocortex (150 times). The aye-aye lemur has a larger hippocampus than you. Unlike prosimians, in simians 'the wide scattering of the hippocampal indices for similar neocorticalization indicates further that there is no close size relationship between hippocampus and neocortex. Very high indices, up to 3.8, have already been reached in . . . progressive insectivores with a still poorly developed neocortex' (Stephan and Andy, 1969, p. 379; see also Weisberg and Ekstrom, 2021). The problem gets worse when we note that the temporal/ventral/anterior hippocampus has expanded much more than the septal/dorsal/posterior hippocampus; but the dominant view in the field is 'that dorsal parts of the hippocampus mediate cognitive functions—particularly spatial memory—whereas ventral portions of the hippocampus are involved in emotional responses' (Strange et al., 2014, p. 655).

8.2.10 Theory 10: Transformation of multiple traces and contextual binding

The size problem we have just outlined automatically occurs with standard consolidation theory:

> the traditional view . . . that the hippocampus is necessary for retaining memories until they are consolidated in their original form in the neocortex. An alternative view is that the original memory, which is hippocampus- and context-dependent, becomes transformed with time to one that is more schematic and independent of the hippocampus.... Initially memories are inextricably linked to details of the environment in which they were formed (for example, a specific room with unique cues, spatial configuration, lighting, etc.). With the passage of time, contextual sensitivity is diminished, and the learned response can be elicited by new environments that share general, but not specific, features of the original learning situation.
>
> (Winocur et al., 2007, p. 555, 556).

This suggestion offers, instead of a simple background view of context (§8.2.6), a complex, configured, view where 'relational binding is required to represent the link between a certain item and its location, the association between two items (e.g. two words), and the relation between an item (e.g. a sentence) and the context in which it was experienced (e.g. where we heard that sentence)' (Sadeh and Pertzov, 2020, p. 388). On this view, consolidation of the key memory in a hippocampal-independent form is directly linked to its transformation to a schematic.

Trace transformation theory (TTT), then, includes elements of space, configuration, context, relation, and the variation of memories with time that we discussed separately earlier. We discuss some complex aspects of TTT in detail here since it can be seen as a starting point for both contextual binding theory (Yonelinas et al., 2019) and for our approach; with all of these rejecting standard consolidation theory (§8.2.9; see also Winocur and Moscovitch, 2011).

The whole gamut of types of representation are likely to be formed at the time of an event (Gilboa and Moscovitch, 2021), with distinct types of episodic, semantic, and spatial memory involving different brain areas and subject to dynamic change (Sekeres et al., 2018). Further, there can be varying capacities to reduce a context-based memory to a schematic. So, it can be argued

> that retention and retrieval of detailed, vivid autobiographical memories depend on the hippocampal system no matter how long ago they were acquired. Semantic memories, on the other hand, benefit from hippocampal contribution for some time before they can be retrieved independently of the hippocampus. Even semantic memories, however, can have episodic elements associated with them that continue to depend on the hippocampus. Likewise, we distinguish between experientially detailed spatial memories (akin to episodic memory) and more schematic memories (akin to semantic memory) that are sufficient for navigation but not for re-experiencing the environment in which they were acquired. Like their episodic and semantic counterparts, the former type of spatial memory is dependent on the hippocampus no matter how long ago it was acquired, whereas the latter can survive independently of the hippocampus and is represented in extra-hippocampal structures. In short, the evidence reviewed suggests strongly that the function of the hippocampus (and possibly that of related limbic structures) is *to help encode, retain, and retrieve experiences*, no matter how long ago the events comprising the experience occurred, and no matter whether the memories are episodic or spatial. We conclude that the evidence favours a multiple trace theory (MTT[4]) of memory over two other models: (1) traditional consolidation models which posit that the hippocampus is a time-limited memory structure for all forms of memory; and (2) versions of cognitive map theory which posit that the hippocampus is needed for representing all forms of allocentric space in memory.
>
> (Moscovitch et al., 2005, p. 35; our emphasis)

The idea that the hippocampus helps encode, retain, and retrieve experiences is also a key feature of the more general theory we will present. However, we will depart from the TTT/MTT solution to the problems of intermediate memory:

> the episodic memory trace or engram consists of a bound ensemble of hippocampal-neocortical neurons with a sparsely coded hippocampal component. This is envisioned as a spatial scaffold or matrix (Nadel, 2008; O'Keefe and Nadel, 1978) that acts as a pointer or index (Teyler and Rudy, 2007) to neocortical components that together represent the totality of the experience, including not only the perceptual, emotional, and conceptual details that form the content of the experience, but also the processes that imbue it with a sense of autonoetic consciousness. Because hippocampal binding is obligatory, storage is random, and only close temporal contiguity, or close contiguity with a reinstated context, determines the elements that are bound to each other.
>
> (Moscovitch et al., 2016, p. 107)

[4] See also (Moscovitch et al., 2005). For a recent critique of MTT see (Sutherland et al., 2020).

We will also disagree with TTT/MTT and agree with Lynn Nadel (email 28 October 2021) when he says:

> The problem I have with Trace Transformation Theory . . . is that it leads readers to think that a given trace has actually been transformed. This is, quite simply, wrong in my view. Instead, the traces that are used to inform memory recall/retrieval change over time—so what comes out as memory seems different. Any given trace (say the one in hippocampus, or the one in PFC, etc.) is what it is, and stays that way throughout, at least in terms of its underlying semantic/episodic content. There can be more or less of it (through forgetting or strengthening) but there cannot be transformation of it, at least not in my view. The point of MTT is that there are multiple traces and what is 'transformed' over time is which one gets to dominate retrieval.
>
> I remain a firm believer in Johannes Muller's 'theory of specific nerve energies'—it was good enough two centuries ago and it still seems good enough now. Of course, development can determine what a given circuit comes to represent, but a neuron's inputs remain a neuron's inputs once the system has matured, and that means it's 'content' so to speak cannot be transformed. It can just be attended to or ignored in what eventually becomes a memory 'report'.

In sum, we see TTT/MTT as a useful amalgam of several of the key early theoretical ideas that has the added advantage of at least partially solving the intermediate memory problem (§8.2.9). However, we see the idea of a change in the content of the memory trace as suffering from similar computational problems to the idea of a hippocampal intermediate memory—it breaks the positional coding that appears fundamental to normal brain function; and it is incompatible with a Hebbian perspective on perception/working memory/reference memory as supported by activation of fundamentally the same cell assembly and of consolidation involving recurrent re-activations (Dudai et al., 2015). Such reductive consolidation could well result in older autobiographical memories being processed more like semantic memories (Norman et al., 2021).

These problems are reduced by the modifications to TTT/MTT made by contextual binding theory, where 'forgetting is largely due to contextual interference, episodic memory remains dependent on the hippocampus across time, contextual drift produces post-encoding activity and sleep benefits memory by reducing contextual interference' (Yonelinas et al., 2019, p. 364; see also Lerner et al., 2021). But we must ask how far this binding of complex elements involves true context and how far it fits a more general hippocampal 'role in integrating multiple stimulus elements in a memory trace' (Moses et al., 2007, p. 333). The complexity of the proposed engrams and the proposal that the hippocampus acts to *positively bind* elements seem to us to be incompatible with the data on configural association and transverse patterning (§8.2.3)—where interference from excessive simple 'binding' appears to be the problem, not a lack of complex binding.

As with all the other theories, therefore, we will invert the 'binding' views of hippocampal function. Rather than *activating* a cortical engram (via, e.g. an index Teyler and Rudy, 2007; Goode et al., 2020), we see the hippocampus as *suppressing* unwanted, wider, cell assembly activity that would otherwise corrupt the engram. On this view reduction of an engram to a schematic would be the sculptural result of progressive removal of original parts of the cell assembly by consolidation.

8.2.11 Theory 1–10: Our points of agreement

We agree that there are metaplastic, iconic, short, medium, intermediate, and long-term stages on the way to production of the long-term trace. These stages are clearly present at the biochemical level (Abraham and Bear, 1996; Rosenzweig et al., 1993; Raymond, 2007; Çalışkan and Stork, 2018)—but reflect stages of electrical or biochemical cascades at a single location (node) not trace transfer from one location to another.

We also agree that existing stored information can form new durable traces. This must occur when memories are integrated to form novel concepts—but here the new information is of a form quite different to the old and is a conjunction of prior networks not a new network with additional copies of the original information. True information transfer between areas must occur with interhemispheric transfer—but here the transfer is between areas that are essentially isomorphic, and the transfer is required because of lateralization of inputs or outputs, not because either area is in principle incapable of forming the associations initially encoded in the other.

We also see a clear distinction between working and long-term memory. Working memory can be conceptualized as depending on continuous *active* interaction between the frontal cortex and other areas of the brain, holding information actively in mind (Chapter 6; Appendix 3; Fuster, 1995; see Baddeley, 2011, for a complex modular view of working memory systems; and Gilboa and Moscovitch, 2021 for a matching picture of reference memory). Working memory reflects iterative processing (rather than a process like LTP) that can be viewed as involving a 'working' component supported by activity in the frontal cortex and a 'memory' component, resident within the area of cortex currently interacting with frontal cortex. Thus, in agreement with Hebb (1949), the specific details of the information being processed depend on essentially the same neural circuitry as was activated by the original perceptual information now actively being recalled. Here too, then, we can view memory itself as unitary, with working memory reflecting the reactivation by frontal cortex of the circuitry (in, e.g. posterior cortex) that contains the long-term trace (in a distributed form). Critically for hippocampal analysis, working memory is clearly associated with frontal cortical function (see, e.g. Selemon et al., 1995; Funahashi and Kubota, 1994) and is not associated with hippocampal function (except incidentally, as we discuss next).

In summary, we agree with many of the basics shared by memory theories of the hippocampus—including acceptance of many of the types listed in Table 8.1. Where we part company is that we do not see the hippocampus as linked to any specific type of memory, nor as a temporary store of information that is then transferred to cortical areas during consolidation. Rather, we see it as a device that interacts with storage, which is always elsewhere (cortical, subcortical or cerebellar), to allow consolidation of the extra-hippocampal traces to proceed without degradation. This is very close to the recent contextual binding theory (Yonelinas et al., 2019) except that context is neither necessary (§8.2.3) nor sufficient (§8.1.5) and we see binding as an automatic Hebbian process that the hippocampus functions to suppress when in excess.

8.3 A preliminary theory of hippocampal 'hypermnesia'

Substantial parts of the text of this section are quoted from McNaughton and Wickens (2003), which presents in much greater detail the idea that Hebbian association in the cortex can result in catastrophic hypermnesia that is prevented when the hippocampus suppresses inappropriate associations.

Here, we will present an initial overview of the memory-related aspects of our counterintuitive countertheory. This has extensive detail (see Chapter 9) and specific machinery (see Chapter 10); but, briefly summarized in the context of amnesia, is as follows.

The hippocampus is at the core of the Goal Inhibition System (GIS), which detects and eliminates conflict between nearly equally primed incompatible goal representations (see Fig. 1.7). These representations (perceived from reality or retrieved from memory) can conflict in terms of distinct motivations (attraction/repulsion) or of distinct situations (such as a left/right lever) to which a response can be made. Memory experiments will usually involve the latter. The detection of conflict often results in external information-seeking behaviour (e.g. risk assessment), but can also result in internal re-assessment of older information via an increase in the valence of affectively negative features or associations of stimuli. In memory experiments, risk assessment behaviour is likely to be minimal, as measured by standard tests; and with consolidation during sleep there will be no external evidence for conflict control at all. Under these circumstances, the most obvious result of output from the GIS is that of goal inhibition itself, in the form of suppression of any prepotent tendencies to make the same motivated response to incorrect alternatives (including verbal alternatives). In experiments involving threatening stimuli, increased attention to such stimuli and increased negative valence of the associations to them on future trials each give rise to anxiety.

This hypothesis is intended to apply equally to all species. That does not mean that all species will show the same sensitivities to hippocampal lesions in the face of any specific experimental paradigm. For example, reliance on the verbal channel in human beings or on olfactory stimuli or position habits in rats will greatly modify how any particular problem is solved (allowing performance that appears consistent with infinite memory).

The hypothesis implies that removal of the hippocampus does not cause a loss of memory as such (as opposed to failed retrieval Miller, 2021). It implies also that the amnesia following hippocampal damage does not necessarily involve an increased rate of forgetting (unless increasing delay increases some source of conflict—for some examples, see Sadeh and Pertzov, 2020).

To get a further flavour of the implications of this hypothesis, let us look at the challenge to a truly memorial view of amnesia raised by the ancient method of cued recall (Weiskrantz, 1978). Participants are given partial information about an item they are to recall and then asked to name the complete item. The partial information can be fragments of a picture, the first few letters of a word, a semantic clue, or the first of a pair of words that rhyme. With repeated exposure of the incomplete cue followed by the complete item, participants need less and less partial information to identify the item (or identify it more rapidly) thus providing a learning curve. Alternatively, the cue can be presented at the time of retention testing. Milner et al. (1968) showed that H.M. had normal learning and retention using incomplete pictures (see also Ogden and Corkin, 1991, p. 200; see Krueger et al., 2020 for equivalent effects with progressive hippocampal dysfunction in mice). The normal or nearly normal performance of amnesic participants in general is not simply due to the task's being easier, since they are disproportionately aided by the provision of cues (Warrington and Weiskrantz, 1970; Warrington and Weiskrantz, 1974).

As with the delay data (§8.1.4), cued recall suggests that in amnesics the stored memory as such remains largely intact, but that there is some problem with the capacity to place it into storage or to retrieve it correctly. This further suggests that what characterizes amnesic-sensitive, and potentially also hippocampal-sensitive, tasks is not a particular type of memory at all. Rather, it is some specific task demand, unrelated to type of memory *per se*, that makes these tasks sensitive to temporal lobe damage. The most obvious effect of partial cueing is to reduce the number of potentially correct answers and, as a mirror image of this argument, our theory is that the hippocampal formation normally functions, in the absence of partial cueing, to eliminate the clamour of incorrect alternatives (as in the tip-of-the tongue phenomenon).

The key problem may not be the number of choices but the strength of an alternative choice.

> The animal literature is replete with cases where a hippocampal lesioned animal can learn to discriminate between two stimuli, but cannot unlearn when the positive and negative valence of the stimuli is reversed (Gray and McNaughton, 1983). For an equivalent demonstration in human beings, one requires both relatively intact amnesic patients (i.e. those that do not have widespread damage in areas outside temporal cortex) and also a task the difficulty of which has been adjusted for the amnesic group in question so as to allow normal acquisition. The evidence is that, under these conditions, the form of the amnesic deficit is similar to that shown with reversal learning in animals.
>
> Fig. [8.4] shows data from Warrington and Weiskrantz (1978) on a task that involves verbal 'reversal learning'. They presented a list of words to be learned, with each word cued by its first three letters. It is important for the conclusions to be drawn from the experiment that task difficulty and level of brain damage were such that learning of this list by the amnesics was no different than controls (A in Fig. [8.4]). The words were carefully chosen so that the first three letters were shared by only one other word in English. Reversal was accomplished by presenting a new list made up of these exclusive alternate words. The key point being that, of necessity, the same set of three-letter recall cues had to be used as for the first list. As can be seen from the figure, both amnesics and controls showed a large impairment learning this list of second alternatives relative to their learning of the first list. Learning of the first list had clearly created interference. However, the amnesics not only learned the original list as well as controls but also were no more sensitive to interference *per se*. Critically, and consistent with the failure of hippocampal rats in extinction (or reversal) to give up their initial response, with further training controls' recall improved quickly to the level of the first list. The amnesics, by contrast, showed only very slow recovery from the effects of interference. As with the very large body of much better controlled animal data, we have evidence that when the appropriate type of information (in this case words cued by trigrams) can be learned as easily by amnesics as by controls then there is a selective impairment of unlearning or switching response alternatives.
>
> (McNaughton and Wickens, 2003, pp. 1143–1144, our figure reference)

But where do the conflicting choices normally come from in situations that give rise to amnesia? We argue that the core of the issue is the catastrophic forgetting that can occur with neural nets that use Hebbian (purely associative) learning to store information. 'The distributed nature of memory storage in these networks means that regardless of specific network architecture, network activity generated by a new input pattern can be adversely influenced by connections modified by previously stored patterns' (Hasselmo and Bower, 1993). Critically,

> Hebb's view was, essentially, that percepts and active memories (as well as imagination and visualisation) reflect specific patterns of activity in specific cell assemblies (Hebb, 1949). The main distinction between a percept and a memory, at the neural level is, on this view, the means of activation. According to Hebb, presentation of a dot in one part of the visual field would activate a particular cell (A) because of input from the retina. Activation of cell A would result in perception of the dot. Presentation of a dot in an adjacent part of the visual field would activate a different cell (B) and result in perception of this other dot. The key part of Hebb's theory of associative memory was that presentation of both dots together would also activate a cell or cells (C) connecting cell A to cell B. This co-activation would strengthen any connections between C and B so that, later, presentation of a dot that activated A alone would tend to fire B. Our use of the term 'purely Hebbian' is intended to emphasise, in particular, Hebb's view that simple coincidence of activation of the neural representations of two stimuli (or strictly stimulus elements) will be sufficient for association. Unlike Pavlov, he did not see strengthening of connections as requiring a 'reinforcer'.

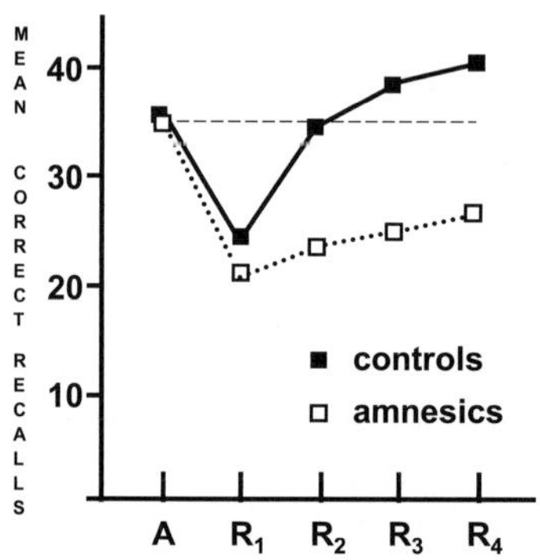

Fig. 8.4 Recall of words from a list by amnesics and controls. Recall was cued by the presentation of the first three letters of the word and words (and cues) were chosen so that there were only two possible alternative answers. Controls and amnesics showed similar memory for an initial list of words (A). Controls and amnesics were equally impaired in the initial learning (R1) of a second list of words consisting of the second of the two possible alternatives and cued by the same 3-letter cues as for the list tested in A. Over successive trials on the second "reversal" list (R2, R3, R4), controls, but not amnesics, overcame the effects of interference (intrusion errors from the first list). (Legend from McNaughton and Wickens, 2003; Figure redrawn from Warrington and Weiskrantz, 1978).

There are three important points to note about Hebb's original proposal.

1) 'Cell B' would normally be a vast conglomerate of neurons forming a cell assembly and not all parts of the conglomerate encoding a particular percept would necessarily be activated by input from the cell assembly equivalent to 'cell A' via the multiple connections equivalent to 'cell C'.
2) The level of activation of cell B (or cell assembly B) would usually be less for associative input than for perceptual input and would always be less than when perceptual and associative input was concurrent. (When the two dots are presented together cell B will receive associative input from cell A, but recall of the memory as such will be masked by the direct perceptual activation of the assembly.)
3) Association is a property of neuronal circuits. C (at the level above A and B) mediates the association of A and B.

(McNaughton and Wickens, 2003, pp. 1145–1146)

McNaughton and Wickens (2003) explain in detail how this view can account for the *intact learning* but *impaired extinction* of running in a straight alley seen in hippocampal rats—a dissociation that, by itself, is hard for most standard memory theories to explain. (In what way is failed extinction a case of episodic amnesia?) Importantly, they then provide results from a simulation of behaviour in the water maze (a classic test of hippocampal learning and memory) that shows that, if only pure associations of the standard Hebb type are allowed, a rat will essentially be incapable of learning the maze even with a massive number of trials. Instead, as is actually observed in hippocampal rats (and untrained intact rats), the pure Hebb rat will swim semi-randomly with a bias to circling around the edges (Fig. 8.5).

The problem, as the values read out of the model show, is that the rat is faced on the current trial with promiscuously remembering too many currently incorrect alternatives. It does not fail to store the trial-by-trial information. (This can be rephrased as a version of the relational problem discussed next.)

The same will be true of relational memory generally. Let us run the conventional argument (§8.2.7) backwards. Suppose that all of the necessary connections and potential bindings for a relational memory are present in neocortex *from the start* (see, e.g. Lindsay et al., 2017). What will happen during the initial phases of learning (or of consolidation, which we can view as a form of internal rehearsal of a specific learning experience)? With items A, B, and C, all with potential relations just subthreshold, and with the particular desired relation (perhaps temporally ordered) A–B–C, how do we prevent the coactivation of A, B, and C from generating B–A–C or C–A–B or, even more likely, the higher-order structure where all possible binary and ternary links between A, B, and C are equally strengthened? The binding problem in memory, then, is not about how we take inherently separate units of information (as in perception) and ensure that they are bound together; for these units will be bound by simple associative coincidence (Lindsay et al., 2017) based on a Hebbian process such as LTP (Linden, 1999). Rather, the problem is about how we take the multitude of potential relations (which must exist as sub-threshold connections before the start of learning, if the relation is *ever* to be formed in the neocortex) and *prevent* excessive binding. In other words, how do we inhibit the formation of incorrect linkages, how do we prevent a superfluity of incorrect memories? We believe the theory of this book supplies the answer to this question as part of a more general answer to the question of conflict between goal representations.

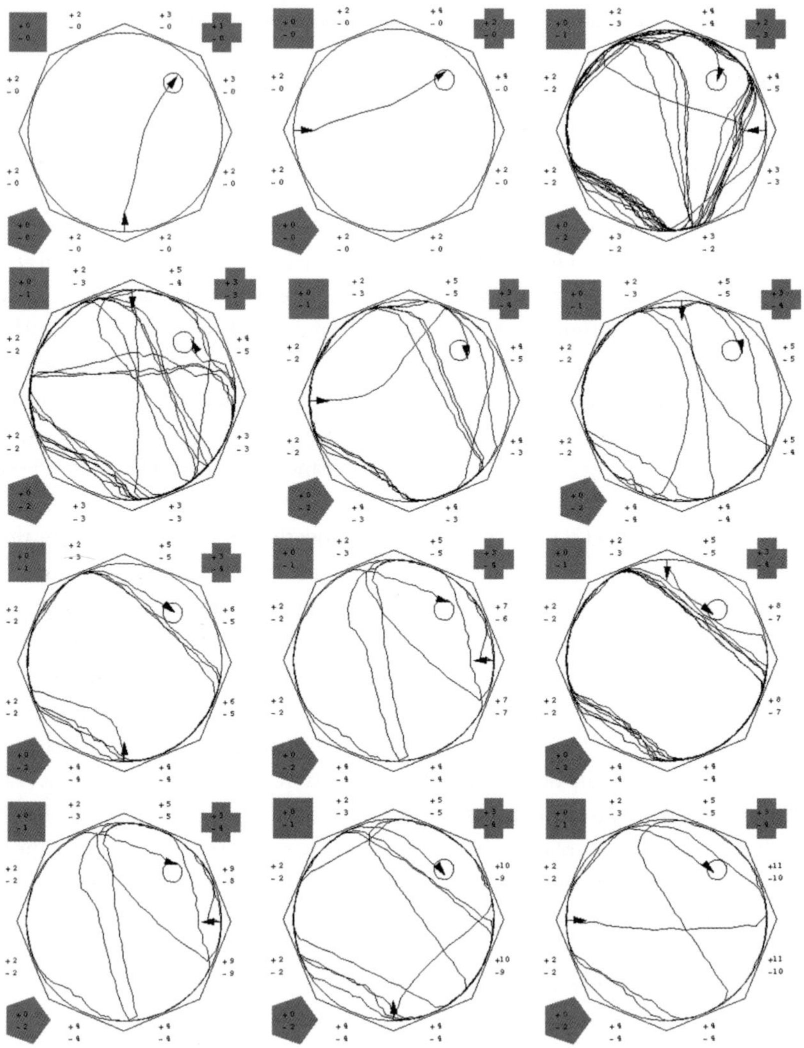

Fig. 8.5 Computer simulation of a "pure Hebbian rat" in the water maze. The solid trail represents the path of the rat. The arrows indicate the rat's position and heading at the start and finish of each run. The maze wall is treated as a set of 8 identifiable segments arranged to approximate a circle. Three additional objects are located outside the maze. Each of the segments and objects is a potential goal, with positive and negative values. The wall segments are initially positive (+ 2, – 0) and the external objects are initially neutral (+ 0, – 0). The rat has a field of view of +/– 25 degrees. Objects are totally invisible unless in the field of view. The motion of the rat is determined by several factors: the sum of the vectors representing the direction of the objects in view and their net values, an intrinsic source of nondirectional movement, the rat's inertia, and a wobble representing the rat's locomotor movements. Each miss (that is, running into the wall when heading to a positive target) increases negative strength of the objects in view by 1. Each hit (that is, contacting the platform) increases the positive strength of the objects in view by 1. The results of 12 successive runs from different starting points are shown. Figure and legend from McNaughton and Wickens (2003).

A second experiment (Winocur and Kinsbourne, 1978) derived more explicitly from the concept of context. Amnesics were tested on paired associate learning: a) in a standard experimental room with normal sound and illumination levels; or, b) in a room illuminated only by a bright red lamp and with background music. When both learning and retention were tested in the more unusual environment, the amnesic deficit was greatly reduced. Conversely, if amnesics learned two successive lists in the two different rooms, this reduced the degree to which learning of the first list impaired subsequent learning of the second list. In neither experiment was the performance of normal subjects affected by the context of learning. These results parallel those reported in hippocampal lesioned rats by Winocur and Olds (1978); (but see Winocur et al., 2007; Gidyk et al., 2021): the amnesic, like the hippocampal, deficit is reduced by a strong context common to the conditions of learning and recall; the reversal deficit is reduced by a change in context between learning and reversal.

In sum, the provision of a strong cue for the correct response aids the amnesic to select it from among the possible competitors. But there is no good reason, either empirical or theoretical, to distinguish between the cases in which the cue is intrinsic to the item to be retrieved (cued recall by partial information) or extrinsic to it (contextual cueing). There is also no good reason to see the cueing process as being memorial. For example, cues provided only at the time of learning, do not affect recall; but provided only at the time of retention testing, greatly reduce the amnesic deficit (Warrington and Weiskrantz, 1970; Warrington and Weiskrantz, 1974)—implying that the material has been stored, though not necessarily stored normally.

On this basis, contextual cues (in Winocur's as opposed to Hirsh's sense, §8.2.6) reduce the effects of interference (Smith et al., 2022); but other cues can do the same. So, interference appears the more general concept.

8.4.3 Interference, recognition memory, and working memory

Careful analysis of working and recognition memory tasks suggests that hippocampal deficits do not result from failure of memory but from interference. Thus, with delayed matching to sample of colours and spatial positions fornix-lesioned monkeys show a deficit only with the first item in the list, the one most likely to suffer from retroactive interference (Gaffan, 1977d; see also Kesner and Novak, 1982). Likewise, after reversal learning was complete (Fig. 8.4), subjects were asked to produce two words in response to each cue; and amnesics produced significantly fewer list 2 responses, although they actually produced more list 1 responses than controls. But if the amnesic deficit lies only in recognition (§8.2.4), or only in working memory (§8.2.2), there should be no difference between amnesics and controls in *generating* items from either list. The use of trial-unique as opposed to trial-repetitive objects in a working memory task such as delayed matching to sample should reduce interference; and, as predicted, this procedure eliminates the lesion deficit in the conventional form of this task. Presumably for the same reason, hippocampal lesioned rats may show an impairment in delayed non-matching to sample if the information (lever-press) response is rewarded, rendering it more similar to the choice trial, but not if it is not rewarded (Rawlins and Tsaltas, 1983).

8.4.4 Interference and spatial memory

As delineated by Nadel (1991), the spatial memory theory of hippocampal function is intended to be purely spatial only in the case of non-human animals, or possibly non-primates. That is, in the case of human beings, the functions of the hippocampus are presumed to be lateralized, with one hemisphere producing 'cognitive' rather than 'spatial' maps. However, even 'in rodents, lesions of hippocampus or related structures impair odor discrimination learning, the ability to time a short interval, and performance in configural discrimination tasks that require remembering unique combinations of stimuli' (Squire and Cave, 1991, p. 269). So, we will consider the role of interference in the more general case of cognitive mapping next, when we consider relational memory tasks.

In the specifically spatial case, it is clear that, where a spatial task is normally sensitive to hippocampal lesions (excluding therefore, e.g. simple position discrimination in a T-maze), there will be ample opportunity for interference from the many different alternatives available in the task (e.g. Fig. 8.5). More importantly, there are a number of cases (see §8.2.1) where hippocampal lesioned animals show apparently normal spatial location learning when training procedures remove the effects of competing response tendencies. It could be argued that these procedures have encouraged taxon (persistent, inflexible) as opposed to locale (flexible) learning and so rendered the tasks non-spatial (but probe tests suggested otherwise). For our present purposes the critical point, however, is that removal of presumed sources of interference rendered the tasks insensitive to the lesions.

8.4.5 Interference and temporal memory

As we have already discussed, in many tasks increasing delay coupled with increasing information load will result in increasing interference. In most cases, the separate contributions of time and interference will be impossible to disentangle. However, there is at least one clear case where delay does not usually result in a hippocampal deficit: taste aversion conditioning. Here the 24-hour delay over which conditioning can be obtained is itself unusual, and there is good evidence that this is because most other paradigms have much greater levels of inherent interference (Revusky, 1971; Wixted, 2004; Sadeh and Pertzov, 2020). For this reason, we predicted that 'taste aversion would become sensitive to hippocampal lesions if the animal were presented with a variety of non-novel tastes during the conditioning interval' (McNaughton, 1985c, p. 509). To our knowledge this (fixed interval, more tastes) prediction has still not been tested; but both dorsal and ventral hippocampal lesions impair taste aversion conditioning if a long but not short interval is used between taste and illness generation (Koh et al., 2009).

8.4.6 Interference and relational memory

We discussed relational memory, *per se*, in §8.2.1. Here we subsume this with cognitive mapping and similar theories (e.g. §8.2.10). The key point for all of these is the argument that the relation A–B–C can only be formed if A, B and C are concurrently activated; and, hence, there is a high probability that relations such as B–A–C and C–A–B will be formed incidentally. As a result, relational memory tasks are likely to be inherently high-interference tasks, with recent theories (including ours) differing in how they explain the role of the hippocampus in coping with that inherent interference (Moscovitch et al., 2016; Koolschijn et al., 2019; Sadeh and Pertzov, 2020).

8.4.7 Interference and behavioural inhibition

The idea that the hippocampus mediates behavioural inhibition is not strictly a memory theory; nor, as we saw in Chapter 6, can it account for all of the effects of hippocampal lesions. But even a fairly loose idea of behavioural inhibition encapsulates a feature of the data often ignored by memory theorists and which certainly presents unusual difficulties for such theories. As we saw in Chapter 6 (see also Appendix 8), the animal literature has many examples of cases where learning of a simple task is intact in hippocampal lesioned animals but where unlearning, which should be as simple or even simpler if considered purely in terms of the learning requirements themselves, is impaired.

Human amnesics have not usually been tested in the tasks that show apparent losses of behavioural inhibition in animals. However, the animal data themselves show that behavioural inhibition *per se* is not lost after hippocampal lesions. Thus, hippocampal lesioned animals can, for example, learn a DRL task, provided that no prior training has been given on a competing response. Similarly, fornix-lesioned rats can learn locomotor passive avoidance as quickly as controls, provided the initial baseline tendency to respond is low, whereas they show a deficit when transferring from active to passive avoidance dependent on the same response (i.e. if they have to shift from producing the response to inhibiting it; e.g. see Okaichi and Okaichi, 1994).

Thus, the requirement for behavioural inhibition *per se* is not critical; it seems that an intact hippocampus is required only when substantial interference from a competing alternative must be eliminated.

8.4.8 Interference as separate from memory

Conversely, if interference is a critical element of tasks sensitive to hippocampal lesions, its effects are not limited to memory tasks. On the contrary, we have seen several examples of a heightened susceptibility to interference in lesioned animals under conditions in which memory plays a minimal role (Chapter 6; Appendix 8). Indeed, in some experiments the difficulty experienced by the lesioned animal seems to arise because it is *more* strongly dependent than intact controls on what it has already learned. Thus, if anything, these experiments suggest that the lesioned animal forgets too little rather than remembers too little.

This is obvious in the case of extinction and reversal deficits. However, a more subtle interference was demonstrated by Winocur and Mills (1970): hippocampal lesioned rats were impaired in learning a simultaneous pattern discrimination only if they had first learned a brightness discrimination. Likewise, Donovick et al. (1979) first trained rats on a simultaneous discrimination with either brightness or position as the relevant dimension; then used the other dimension to add a second, redundant cue. Transfer of behavioural control to the added cue was impaired by septal lesions. Such interference can also be self- rather than experimenter-generated (Kimble, 1975). Rats trained under various conditions of reinforcement in a Y-maze with one arm lit and the other unlit can show position or brightness hypotheses in their successive choices of arm. Hippocampal lesioned rats clung longer to whichever response strategy they first happened upon, and their subsequent behaviour in a changed environment was dominated by this strategy to an abnormal degree.

8.4.9 Interference and 'rat knows best'

The necessity to determine how the control animal is in fact solving a problem is brought into sharp relief by Eichenbaum's experiments in which fornix lesions affected *simultaneous* discriminations with olfactory stimuli, whereas such discriminations are usually unaffected by hippocampal damage when other stimulus modalities are employed. With simultaneous olfactory discrimination there was

> a qualitative distinction between normal and [fornix-lesioned] animals in their response latencies. Normal animals had bimodal distributions of latencies, with one peak corresponding to left-port responding and the other peak to right-port responding, suggesting that the animals sample both ports and make some comparative judgement at the time of their response decision. By contrast the responses of animals with hippocampal system damage had shorter latencies and a single-peaked distribution, suggesting that these animals made their choices without comparative judgements at the time of their response decision.
>
> (Cohen and Eichenbaum, 1993, p. 140)

Thus, in 'simultaneous' olfactory discrimination there is in actual practice a strong successive or conditional element in control rats' responding,[5] and the evidence shows that the lesioned rats fail to inhibit responding, fail to correctly sample and assess the alternatives, and hence make errors. Brown (1992) made a similar analysis of the detailed behaviour of rats in the radial-arm maze. He found that control animals oriented towards arms and made a number of 'go/no-go microchoices' before choosing to fully enter a target arm. This switching to and fro is very similar to that observed by Cohen and Eichenbaum in the simultaneous olfactory discrimination case. In all of this we must take Skinner's advice to Lindsay as paramount (§0.3).

8.5 The role of the hippocampal formation in memory and sleep

We have compressed rather a large body of data into a single chapter, mostly by the device of using a number of theoretical positions to act as summaries of substantial parts of these data. These summaries leave us with a number of pragmatic requirements for any theory of the role of the hippocampal formation in memory.

Any theory must account for the roles of time, task complexity, space, working memory, interference, etc. in determining the sensitivity of tasks to hippocampal formation damage.

[5] It is also possible, however, that olfactory stimuli are processed differently than other modalities and, in particular, more easily elicit affective associations (Herz and Cupchik, 1995)

In all of the cases that we have considered the critical aspect of interference in relation to amnesic performance appears not to be a degradation of initial information or increased decay of the memory trace. Rather it consists in a failure on the part of the lesioned animals or human patients to engage in the same active suppression of competing incorrect responses as intact subjects. Where the correct response is not in competition with a prepotent incorrect response, then normal (or even superior) performance can be obtained.

Further, it seems well established that the hippocampal formation is not the final repository for any long-term memories. While it remains possible that it is an intermediate repository for some restricted types of memories, an indexing or sculpting function is much more likely. On this view, hippocampal ripples would both aid retrieval from cortex of complex (semantic, autobiographical) information (Norman et al., 2021) and strengthen cortical representations during slow wave sleep, with REM sleep and the related RSA/'theta' activity acting to suppress unwanted information (Brodt and Born, 2021)—so 'that sleep rescues memories after interference has occurred' (Zhang et al., 2022, p. 1). There is certainly no type of memory for which it could be even the intermediate repository. For all of the 'types of memory' that we have considered, there are clear examples (see Rawlins, 1985) of insensitivity to hippocampal formation damage. It is in any case extremely difficult to envisage a means of holding and transferring intermediate memories in a manner consistent with the known facts of brain architecture and operation.

We believe that the plethora and continued development of memory theories arises from their exclusively memorial perspective. We have good evidence that hippocampal lesions affect tasks (or innate situations) that are intrinsically non-memorial (Appendix 8). Rather than excluding these from consideration, in the hope of simplifying the memory problem, let us include them in the hope of solving this as a special case of a more general problem. Our proposed solution (§8.3) views the hippocampal deficit as unitary, the same in simple conflict situations as in memorial tasks. Specifically, hippocampal damage removes the capacity to eliminate strongly competing, conflicting alternatives as the result of a loss of the capacity to amplify the negative associations of the diverse stimuli that lead to those alternatives, or the negative associations of alternatives concurrently primed by some single stimulus (see Clewett et al., 2022, on hippocampus and retrograde memory effects of fear conditioning). In the case of an approach-avoidance conflict, such damage weakens the avoidance component of the conflict. In the case of a memory task, it weakens the capacity to eliminate competition from incorrect alternatives for encoding, recognition, or recall. Given a pandemonium model of memory retrieval (see also Miller, 2021), the hippocampal damaged subject chooses too quickly among the available goals (Meck, 1988; Fig. 6.2 in Cohen and Eichenbaum, 1993) and hence chooses incorrectly.

The strength of this goal-conflict hypothesis resides in the fact that it essentially conflates many of the previous hypotheses and is able to account for the data upon which they variously rested. Its weakness is that it often requires us to know special species-unique, and indeed situation-unique, details of the experimental design or of the animal's specific solution to a problem, details not necessarily mentioned in the methods or results sections of the papers concerned. However, this weakness in applying the theory to the data currently available is a fault in experimenter-centric designs and does not entail that the theory is not testable with future experiments and we have made above a range of quite specific predictions; particularly general ones about the effects of removal or introduction of interference.

9

Fundamentals of the septo-hippocampal system

We started our *Neuropsychology of Anxiety* with a sketch of the ethology (Chapter 2), behaviour analysis (Chapter 3), and pharmacology (Chapter 4) that define the Goal Inhibition System (GIS; Chapter 5). We also provided a map (Chapter 6) of the 'survival circuits' involved in the GIS and its key inputs: the Goal Attraction System (GAS) and Goal Repulsion System (GRS). However, before we detail our theory (Chapter 10), we need to cover the fundamentals that will place the septo-hippocampal system (SHS) at its centre.

Our ultimate goal is an integrated neuropsychology of anxiety that intentionally blurs the separate languages of brain process and mind. We aim for a true Conceptual Nervous System (a further step in the direction taken by Hebb, 1955). Our concept of anxiety derives as much from pharmacology and neurophysiology as from psychology; conversely, our neurology of the GIS derives as much from ethology and learning theory as from neuroanatomy. We can, and will, use different terms for different levels of explanation within the theory—but the different levels are intended to be consistent with, and able to challenge, each other (except where some property is truly emergent, McNaughton, 2020, pp. 9–10).

Such conceptual amalgamation already occurs in computer models that attempt to have both neurally realistic architecture and outputs that can be tested neurologically, psychologically, or even robotically (Whelan, 2020). The marriage of psychology and neurology via such cybernetic models forces out many of the hidden false assumptions buried within each discipline (e.g. Hinton et al., 1993). In the previous edition, we thought that analysis of the SHS might have reached the stage where computational models would be profitable (e.g. *Hippocampus* 1996, volume 6, issue 6). However, we still see the lack of certain critical data (such as the detailed nature of the subcortical systems that control rhythmicity; and the detailed interactions of the SHS with areas like the prefrontal cortex) as making a 'whole SHS' model premature. Current models will be driven by preconceptions rather than being predictive; so, they are unlikely to go against the preconceptions. Instead, we present a skeleton (Chapter 10) that we hope can later be fleshed out in such a model.

This neuropsychological overview leads on to our subtitle: *An Enquiry into the Functions of the Septo-Hippocampal System*. A key idea, so far, has been that anxiolytic drugs define the GIS; and that these drugs then indicate a key role for the SHS (see Chapter 4). Until recently (and even now with the dorsal hippocampus), this was not at first sight compatible with other views of SHS function; nor is it central to other views of anxiety systems (Calhoon and Tye, 2015). So, our enquiry started with general critiques of the data on hippocampal single cells and a spatial map (Chapter 7); and on the hippocampus as a specific type of memory store

The Neuropsychology of Anxiety, Third Edition. Neil McNaughton and Jeffrey A. Gray, Oxford University Press.
 DOI: 10.1093/oso/9780198843313.003.0009

that is lost in amnesia (Chapter 8). In this chapter, we summarize other key data-driven conclusions about the SHS[1] framed as a set of principles. These principles are often phrased so as to be easy to apply to the theory in Chapter 10, but are tightly constrained by the available data. We think that any current theory of the SHS or of anxiolytic action should be consistent with them. To provide a coherent background for Chapter 10, we briefly reiterate some points from previous chapters.

9.1 Anxiolytics and the SHS—an overview

At the core of our theory has always been one major premiss: that selective anxiolytic drugs as a class (including both novel and classical) can identify both neural and psychological processes underlying anxiety—and provide a tracer that allows mapping between these levels. As a result, we emphasize in our theoretical scheme many data that others would simply ignore. This is because the most important single fact for this book is that *all known clinically effective centrally acting anxiolytics* produce *the same characteristic changes in the SHS*, and these changes are not duplicated by any drugs that have not been shown to be anxiolytic in the clinic. Moreover, anxiolytic drugs produce these common changes through a wide number of pharmacologically and anatomically different routes and have confirmed our predictions about new anxiolytics for over 40 years (see McNaughton et al., 2007 for review) including, most recently, ketamine (Engin et al., 2009). Translation of these results has now delivered the first theoretically based biomarker for an anxiety disorder (Shadli et al., 2021a; Chapter 13). These are objective data. Whether or not you share our particular perspective, the consistent effects of these drugs on the SHS (and the similar behavioural effects of the drugs to SHS lesions, Table 4.2) must be accounted for by any theory of hippocampal function, or anxiety systems (e.g. Calhoon and Tye, 2015), that attempts to be complete.

9.1.1 Anxiolytic action on the SHS

The anxiolytic drugs share two quite distinct actions on rhythmical slow activity (RSA/'theta'[2]) in the SHS. These are demonstrated in freely moving animals by septal and reticular stimulation, respectively. We discuss the control of RSA/'theta' in detail in §9.2.

Septal driving: The first action of anxiolytics on RSA/'theta' to be reported, and the one on which the theory of the first edition was primarily based, was an action on septal driving of hippocampal RSA/'theta'. With this driving, stimulation is at RSA/'theta' frequency and the threshold for elicitation is assessed. As shown in Fig. 9.1C, anxiolytics increase this threshold (Appendix 5) predominantly in the middle of the frequency range. This anxiolytic effect can

[1] These conclusions are more fully justified in our appendices and recent reviews, see lists on pages xxix–xxxi. A number of parts of Chapter 10 of the previous edition that were speculative are now substantiated and have been moved to the current Chapter 9 with the related assumptions converted to principles.

[2] RSA in the rat hippocampus runs from ~4 to 14 Hz and so covers the human EEG theta (4–7Hz) and alpha (8–12 Hz) bands. The word 'theta' can then cause confusion between these literatures and with human EEG need have no relation to hippocampal activity at all. Human hippocampal RSA appears from 2 to 14Hz; predominantly in two bands, 1–4 Hz and ~8 Hz, that may vary with task demands and appear to occur in anterior (temporal) and posterior (septal) hippocampus, respectively (Watrous et al., 2011; Goyal et al., 2020; see also Jacobs, 2014; Joensen et al., 2023).

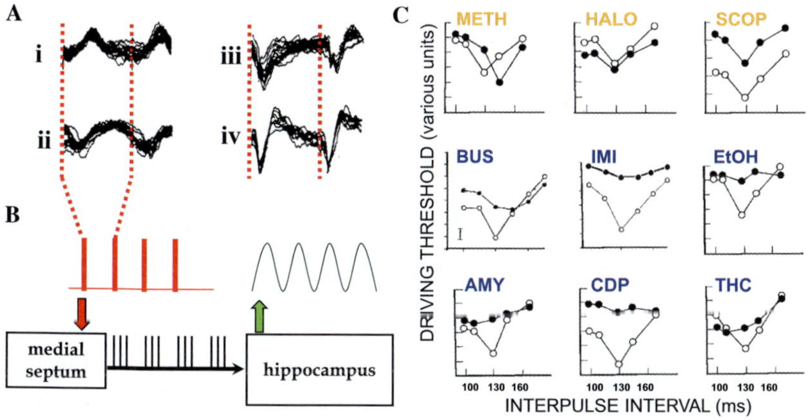

Fig. 9.1 Septal driving of RSA/'theta' rhythm—common effects of **anxiolytic** compared to **non-anxiolytic** drugs. **(A)** Trains of low frequency (5-12 Hz) stimulation delivered to the medial septum can induce synchronous activation of the SHS. Each panel is the superimposition of about 10 successive sweeps with two stimuli from the train within each sweep (waveforms from James et al., 1977). The responses shown in **i** and **ii** are examples of RSA/'theta' driving in two different rats: the synchronous responses are sinusoidal and have the same conformation as spontaneous RSA/'theta' waves of the same frequency (7.7Hz) in that rat. **ii** and **iv** are driven RSA/'theta' and non-RSA/'theta' evoked potentials obtained in two animals which only showed driving or evoked potentials respectively. **i** and **iii** show a shift, with an increase in stimulation intensity, from driving to evoked potentials within a single rat. To detect the effects of anxiolytic drugs it is important that the stimulation should only produce RSA/'theta' driving. **(B)** Diagrammatic representation of RSA/'theta' driving. The imposed electrical pulses (red) activate the septum and cause it to produce the *bursts* of impulses (shown between the septum and hippocampus) of the same type as are produced in the generation of spontaneous RSA/'theta' activity. These entrain similar activity in the hippocampus which, because it is synchronous in many cells, can give rise to a high voltage (up to about 1mV) sinusoidal wave form—RSA/'theta' rhythm (green). Note that each pulse, burst of septal firing, and RSA/'theta' wave is synchronous. **(C)** The effects of anxiolytic drugs on the threshold for driving RSA/'theta' rhythm. Septal driving stimulation (see panels A, B) produces RSA/'theta' rhythm at a threshold that varies in a U-shaped fashion with frequency in male rats (open circles; see James et al., 1977; see Drewett et al., 1977 on female rats). Treatment with anxiolytic drugs (**BUS, IMI, EtOH, AMY, CDP, THC**) increases the threshold for driving (filled circles), particularly in the middle of the frequency range (McNaughton et al., 1977; Zhu and aMcNaughton, 1994). Treatment with drugs that are not anxiolytic (**METH, HALO, SCOP**) does not produce this effect but can alter the location of the minimum of the curve (METH, see also McNaughton et al., 1980a; McNaughton et al., 1980b; Valero et al., 1977) or reduce thresholds generally (HALO, see McNaughton et al., 1977). Treatments that impair noradrenergic function have similar effects to anxiolytics (Gray et al., 1975). Scopolamine (**SCOP**) does not affect thresholds as such. Rather, as it does with spontaneous and reticular-elicited RSA/'theta', it totally blocks RSA/'theta' that is not accompanied by movement. Possibly as a result of this block, it can reduce anxiety symptoms in patients with uni- or bi-polar depression (see Furey et al., 2010) but has not be tested in generalized anxiety. As a result, it increases the average threshold for driving. *Abbreviations:* METH, methysergide; HALO, haloperidol; SCOP, scopolamine; BUS, buspirone; IMI, imipramine; EtOH, ethanol; AMY, amylobarbitone; CDP, chlordiazepoxide; THC, Δ-9 tetrahydrocannabinol. *Note:* THC is not conventionally used as an anxiolytic (particularly given previous legislative problems) but see (Murkar et al., 2021) for a recent review of cannabinoids and fear/anxiety.

be reproduced by specific lesions of the noradrenergic input to the hippocampus from the locus coeruleus (Gray et al., 1975; see §9.1.2 for comment on the behavioural effects of these lesions; and Table 4.2 for details).

Reticular elicitation: The second action of anxiolytics on RSA/'theta' to be reported was an action on the frequency of reticular-elicited RSA/'theta'. With this elicitation, stimulation is at high frequency (often 100 Hz) and the frequency of theta is related (Fig. 9.2A, B) to the intensity of the stimulation (whether amplitude, train frequency, or pulse width). As tabulated in Fig. 9.2C, anxiolytics reduce this reticular-elicited frequency (and they also reduce spontaneous frequency while the rat engages in a range of behavioural tests as well). This frequency change is not specific to any part of the frequency range, and cannot be reproduced by depletion of noradrenaline. It can, however, be reproduced by injections of anxiolytic benzodiazepines into the supramammillary nucleus (McNaughton et al., 1995a; Woodnorth and McNaughton, 2002b) and the dorsomedial nucleus of the hypothalamus (Woodnorth and McNaughton, 2002a).

Thus, anxiolytic drugs are unique in impairing these two independent aspects of the control of hippocampal RSA/'theta' rhythm. Conversely, these two tests are essentially unique in demonstrating similar dose-related physiological effects of the different classes of anxiolytic drugs. These data strongly suggest, therefore, that anxiolytic drugs achieve their clinical effects by impairing the control of RSA/'theta' rhythm in the hippocampus and related structures such as the entorhinal cortex and posterior cingulate cortex (Appendix 5). It should be noted that both of these electrophysiological tests are carried out in essentially motionless animals. Theta can also be elicited by running and, in this case, there is a dissociation (Wells et al., 2013; for review see Korotkova et al., 2018) between the slope of the

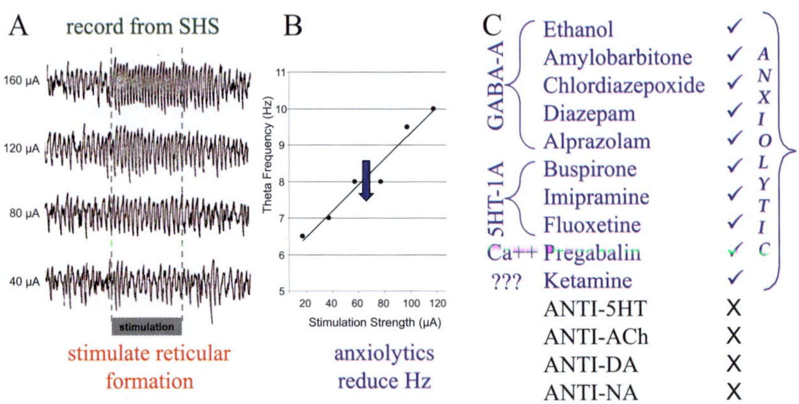

Fig. 9.2 Reticular-elicited RSA/'theta' rhythm—all classes, no false positives, no false negatives predictive validity for over 30 years common effects of anxiolytic drugs. **(A)** Increasing levels of reticular stimulation produce a linear increase in the frequency of RSA/'theta' rhythm. **(B)** anxiolytic drugs decrease the frequency of RSA/'theta' (blue arrow) while sedative but non-anxiolytic drugs do not (McNaughton et al., 1986). **(C)** this reduction is produced by all known classes of clinically effective anxiolytic drugs and is not the result of reduced activity in cholinergic, serotonergic, dopaminergic or noradrenergic systems (McNaughton and Sedgwick, 1978; Coop et al., 1990; McNaughton and Coop, 1991; Coop et al., 1991; Coop and McNaughton, 1991; Coop et al., 1992; Zhu and bMcNaughton, 1994; Zhu and McNaughton, 1995a; Munn and McNaughton, 2008; Siok et al., 2009; Engin et al., 2009; see McNaughton et al., 2007 for review).

frequency relationship[3] (reduced by novelty, and linked to changed hippocampal spatial representations) and its intercept (reduced by anxiolytics, and linked to changed anxiety-like behaviour). Across anxiolytics as a whole, reticular stimulation also has a reduced intercept (measured at the centre point of the control curve) but not necessarily slope.

9.1.2 Anxiolytics share the behavioural effects of septo-hippocampal lesions

If RSA/'theta' activity is important for hippocampal function, the impairment of RSA/'theta' control produced by anxiolytic drugs should make them act like weak and/or selective hippocampal lesions. This prediction holds true over a surprisingly wide range of behaviour (Chapter 4, Table 4.2), given that the drugs do not eliminate RSA/'theta', far less eliminate the whole hippocampus.

Of particular note, is the fact that anxiolytic drugs impair behaviour in tasks such as delayed matching to sample and spatial navigation that are often thought of as being particularly 'mnemonic' or 'hippocampal' tasks. Of equal note is the fact that the effects of hippocampal lesions include retarded extinction without change in acquisition of simple running in an alley way; and include impaired passive but intact one-way active avoidance (and so *improved* 2-way avoidance). These results show that hippocampal lesions do not affect memory in any simple way; indeed, we argued in Chapter 8 that they do not directly affect memory at all.

9.1.3 Changes in RSA/'theta' control mimic anxiolytic action and hippocampal damage

The fact that anxiolytics impair hippocampal function and that they produce behavioural effects like hippocampal lesions provides only correlational evidence for the view that the drugs produce their behavioural effects because of their action on RSA/'theta'. Direct tests have also been conducted.

A direct test of the role of the anxiolytic change in the threshold of septal driving of RSA/'theta' is provided by investigation of the behavioural effects of noradrenergic depletion. As noted earlier, neurotoxic lesions of the dorsal ascending noradrenergic bundle reproduce the anxiolytic effect on septal driving (Gray et al., 1975). As can be seen from Table 4.2 (and less extensively in Table 9.1), such lesions reproduce a large part, but not all, of the common behavioural profile of anxiolytic drugs and SHS lesions (see also Appendix 10).

Similarly, a direct test of the role of the anxiolytic reduction in reticular-induced RSA/'theta' frequency is provided by investigation of the behavioural effects of injections of benzodiazepines into (and neurotoxic lesions of) the supramammillary nucleus and the dorsomedial hypothalamic nucleus. Only a few such studies have been carried out, but the evidence from the supramammillary area (Table 9.1) is that, together with dorsal bundle lesions, they could account for the bulk of the common behavioural profile of anxiolytic drugs and septo-hippocampal lesions. Particularly in tests insensitive to dorsal bundle

[3] This slope is usually reported as a speed-frequency value but this may in fact be artefactual with acceleration (coupled with a slow decay of frequency during deceleration) being the key factor (Kropff et al., 2021).

Table 9.1 Complementary effects of dysfunction of SuM compared to DANB on behaviour. Measure increased (🡅), decreased (🡇), or unchanged (⇔). More arrows mean larger effects

Task	measure	SuM	DANB	ANX	HPC
Open field Activity	activity	🡅**	⇔	🡅	🡅🡅
Fear conditioning (CS)	activity	⇔		⇔	⇔
Fear conditioning (context)	activity	🡅	🡅/⇔	🡅	🡅🡅
Passive avoidance	activity	🡅	🡅/⇔/🡇	🡅	🡅🡅
FI (rate of response)	activity	🡅	⇔/🡇	🡅	🡅🡅
DRL (rate of response)	activity	🡅	⇔	🡅	🡅🡅
Spatial-conditional Learning	learning	⇔	🡇*		🡇🡇
Water maze Learning	learning	⇔/🡇🡇	⇔	🡇	🡇🡇🡇

Data from Table 4.1, Table 2 of Pan & McNaughton 2004, and Langlais et al. (1993)*. ** no change in theta rhythmicity observed.

Abbreviations: ANX = anxiolytics; DANB = neurotoxic lesion of the dorsal ascending noradrenergic bundle; HPC = hippocampal lesion; SuM = medial supramammillary neurotoxic lesion or cellular blockade.

lesions but involving classic behavioural inhibition, injections of benzodiazepines into the supramammillary nucleus can have effects on RSA/'theta' frequency and on behaviour that are as large as those of systemic injections of the same drug (Woodnorth and McNaughton, 2002b).

A further way to test the causal role played by hippocampal RSA/'theta' in mediating the effects of the anxiolytic drugs is with changes in behaviour produced by septal driving of RSA/'theta' rhythm. Experiments of this kind, focusing on resistance to extinction of both running and lever-pressing responses, have shown that such 'RSA/'theta' driving' at frequencies close to 7.7 Hz (the frequency at which systemic anxiolytic administration maximally elevates the driving threshold) produces, as predicted, behavioural effects opposite in sign to those of systemic administration of the drugs themselves (Williams et al., 1989; Appendix 7).

So, when the characteristic changes in hippocampal electrophysiology produced by anxiolytic drugs are reproduced by highly selective intracranial manipulations, these appear to reproduce the bulk of the behavioural profile of systemic anxiolytics; and, conversely, when electrophysiological changes of opposite sign to those caused by the drugs are experimentally induced, so the behavioural profile, too, is opposite in sign. This leads us to:

> *PRINCIPLE 1: the SHS mediates anxiolytic drug action and hence at least some aspects of anxiety.*

9.2 The control of SHS RSA/'theta' activity

So far, we have focussed on the 4–12 Hz gross extracellular local field potentials recorded from the hippocampus. This RSA/'theta' *rhythm* results from the summation of currents linked indirectly to approximately synchronous RSA/'theta' *activity*—that is, burst firing of cells (see Petersen and Buzsáki, 2020 on variation in phase with position in hippocampus). This synchronous bursting is thought to be an important functional state of the hippocampus and related brain structures (see Grossberg, 2021 for a review and model; see Mitchell et al., 2008 for the view that frontal midline theta is distinct; see Buzsáki and Vöröslakos, 2023, for the general view that 'brain rhythms have come of age'). A key question is how RSA/'theta' frequency is determined. So far, we have taken this to be by the supramammillary nucleus, dorsomedial hypothalamic nucleus, and other nuclei linked to them. Here we look at the complex ramifications of additional aspects of RSA/'theta' control—and at gaps remaining in our understanding of the fundamental mechanisms involved. For a more wholistic view of brain rhythms, their interactions (including multiplexing), and their functions, see Buzsáki (2006)

9.2.1 An 'ascending' view of the subcortical control network

We will start with the ascending reticular→hypothalamic→septal→hippocampal system that underlies the manipulations discussed in §9.1. The key circuit details are shown in Fig. 9.3 (see also Appendix 5). Activation of distinct but interconnected reticular areas such as nucleus reticularis pontis oralis and nucleus incertus sends tonic input to multiple, distinct but interconnected sites in the hypothalamus, of which the best understood (and the only one obviously present under urethane anaesthesia) is the medial supramammillary area (Fig. 9.3C). These sites co-operate to generate a common-phase rhythmic output where the frequency is proportional to the strength of reticular input. In freely moving animals, lesions of the supramammillary area reduce frequency but do not eliminate rhythmicity (McNaughton et al., 1995b).

This interconnected set of hypothalamic nuclei, then, embodies a *distributed frequency integrator* that provides phasic input to areas such as the medial septum. Anxiolytic drugs act on hypothalamic sites to reduce theta frequency (McNaughton et al., 1995a; Woodnorth and McNaughton, 2002b; Woodnorth and McNaughton, 2002a; §9.2.4). This signal is passed via the medial forebrain bundle to a *distributed synchronizer*[4] in the medial septum (Appendix 5; Nerad and McNaughton, 2006; Varga et al., 2008) and also direct to the hippocampus (Li et al., 2023).

The septal synchronizer includes distinct cell sub-populations that vary in their rhythmicity and hippocampal targets. The most rhythmic, '*Teevra* cells' (Fig. 9.4, Joshi et al., 2017), are GABAergic, fire coincidentally with hippocampal excitation and, as shown by labelling with Neurobiotin, preferentially innervate CA3 GABAergic interneurons (axo-axonic and CCK), controlling hippocampal theta activity via disinhibition. (Note that the direct glutamatergic projection from SuM also preferentially targets these interneurones, Li et al., 2023.) These are distinct from '*Komal*' cells that show less variation in firing rate between rest and running and have longer burst durations.

[4] We refer to a hypothalamic *frequency integrator* and medial septal *synchronizer* to avoid the ambiguity (and other associations) of the word 'pacemaker'. As discussed in §9.2.3, we would emphasize that the system is chaotic (as with the control of heart rate) and not harmonic, which allows its large dynamic range.

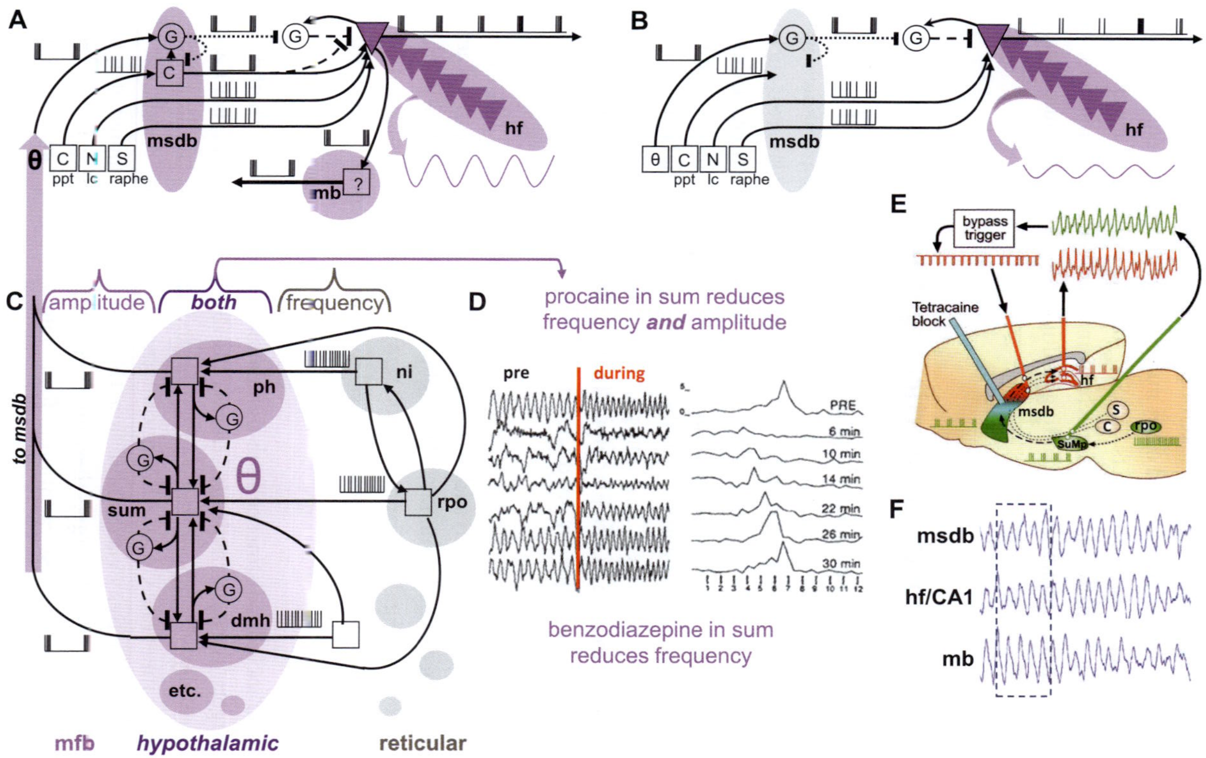

Fig. 9.3 Ascending circuitry controlling theta rhythmicity (Based on Vertes and Kocsis, 1997; Lee et al., 1994; Ryan et al., 2011; see also Kowalczyk et al., 2021). Circuits involved in feedback and descending control are omitted, see §9.2.2.

(A) The medial septum/diagonal band complex (**msdb**) contains gabaergic (G) and cholinergic (C) cells that project to the hippocampal formation. The G cells are thought to synapse on G interneurones via inhibitory (- - - -|) connections. The C cells are thought to excite principal cells (filled triangles) of the hippocampal formation (**hf**) and to inhibit the G interneurones which, in turn, inhibit principal cells. Phasic drive of the **msdb** arrives via the medial forebrain bundle (**mfb**) from a network that determines theta frequency (θ, see also panel C) and a cholinergic input which can gate theta activity arrives from an ascending cholinergic network of which the pedunculopontine tegmental nucleus (**ppt**) is part. (The transmitter for the sum-msdb pathway is not well-established, see §9.2.2). When the animal is stationary the phasic and cholinergic inputs are sufficient for phasic G and C input to be transferred to **hf** and so produce cellular theta activity (regular bursting action potential patterns shown schematically above the principal cell axons) and, in many areas, a gross extracellular hippocampal theta rhythm (wavy line shown to below the principal cell layer) including output targets such as the mammillary bodies (**mb**, see also panel F). Serotonergic (S) input from the raphe can also act to gate theta activity when the animal is moving so that, in this case, loss of the C input from ppt does not result in a loss of theta activity. Noradrenergic (N) input from the locus coeruleus (**lc**) can alter the threshold for **msdb** activation of **hf** but does not appear to produce the more extensive gating effects of the S and C inputs. The interactions of N and S inputs with **hf** may be as complex as those proposed for C inputs but there are insufficient data to be sure.

(B) Cholinergic-specific lesions of the C cells of the **msdb** produce a reduction in the amplitude of theta rhythm. This effect is not produced by blockade of the ascending C system from **ppt** and is likely to be the result of a reduction of phasic activity in the G cells of **msdb** and the principal cells of **hf**. Amplitude can also be reduced by blockade of the output from the theta frequency control network (θ, see also panel C).

(C) The theta frequency control network (pale oval labelled θ). The **msdb** receives phasic input from hypothalamic areas such as the medial supramammillary nucleus (**sum**), which are in turn activated by reticular inputs. For example, high-frequency stimulation of nucleus reticularis pontis oralis (**rpo**) in urethane anaesthetized rats sends tonic input to **sum** where it is recoded to phasic theta activity. Frequency is increased by any increase in afferent drive (by changing amplitude, pulse width, or frequency of stimulation). Injections of procaine at different points in the ascending pathways affect frequency when caudal to **sum**, amplitude when rostral, and both frequency and amplitude when in **sum** (see panel D). Frequency is decreased by injections of benzodiazepines into **sum** (Woodnorth and bMcNaughton, 2002); but amplitude and not frequency is decreased by injections of GABA (Jiang and Khanna, 2004). This suggests that frequency is encoded by recurrent gabaergic interneurones synapsing on $GABA_A$ receptors. There is evidence that, in freely moving animals, areas other than **rpo** (e.g., nucleus incertus, **ni**) can provide tonic drive and that theta frequency transduction can occur in areas other than **sum.** Injections of benzodiazepines and benzodiazepine antagonists (Woodnorth and aMcNaughton, 2002; Woodnorth et al., 2003) suggest that the dorsomedial and posterior hypothalamus (**dmh/ph**) may contain such areas but there are also likely to be others (**etc.**). These areas appear to act in concert (see also see §9.2.2). Circuits between the nuclei similar to those required within any one of them would allow both joint summation of inputs and phase-locking across the network (which would account for theta not showing the 'beats' that would be expected with multiple harmonic sources, see also see §9.2.3).

(D) Effects of procaine injected into **sum** (data from Kirk and McNaughton, 1993). Spontaneous (pre) and stimulus elicited (during) hippocampal local field potentials are shown before and at 6-30 minutes after procaine injection. The power spectra show that frequency and amplitude change in parallel.

(E) Brain bypass. **msdb** tetracaine blocks normal theta. SuM recording is fed through a trigger to stimulate the fornix superior and generate **hf** theta. (Modified journal issue cover image from McNaughton et al., 2006b).

(F) Concurrent local field potentials recorded from **msdb**, **hf**, and mammillary bodies (**mb**) in a rat running in an open field. These show clear theta rhythm (as do **sum** and prefrontal targets of **hf**). Note that hf and mb are synchronous (vertical dashed lines) with msdb phase-locked to them and about 270° ahead. It is clear that amplitude can vary at each site to some extent independently of the others. Given the data of panel B and D, therefore, the amplitude of theta rhythm (and hence the number of principal cells firing and/or their rhythmicity) can be adjusted at each of θ, **msdb**, **hf**, and **mb** (see also Fig. 9.5). Data provided by Luděk Nerad.

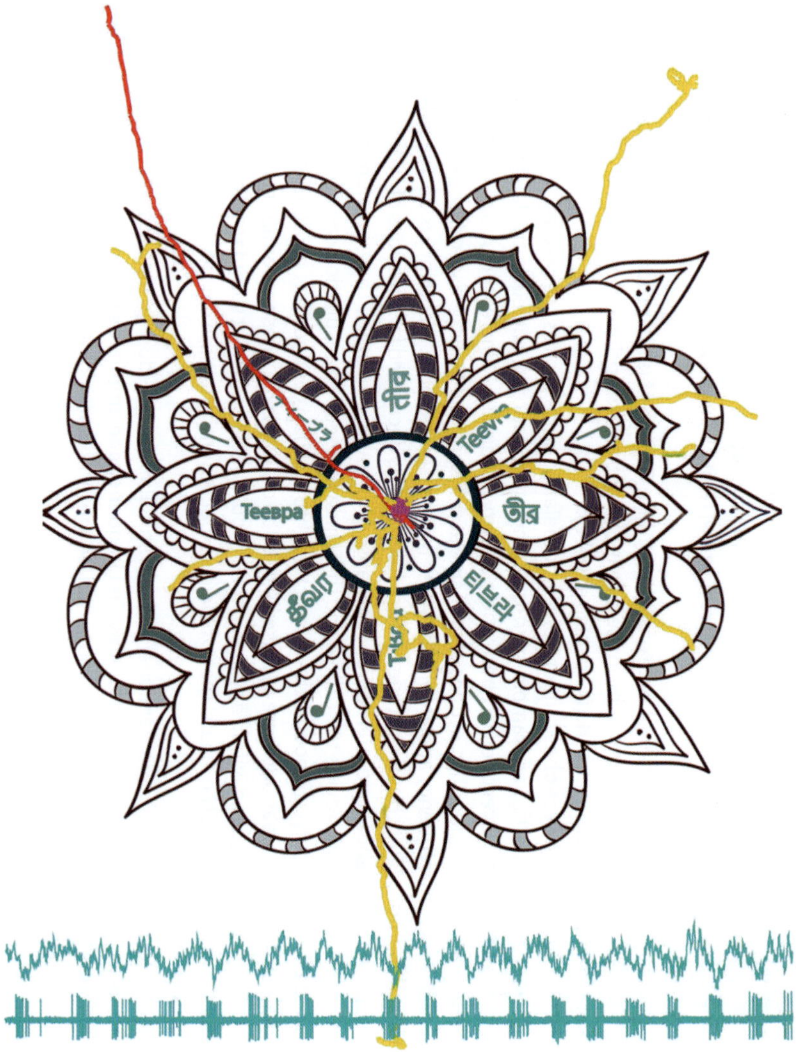

Fig. 9.4 'A Teevra neuron (yellow), named in Sanskrit and inspired by classical music after the 'sharp' sound of signalling by the neuron as recorded electrically and displayed as sound. Visualised in the medial septum, the cell integrates information from many areas of the brain, just as scientific insight progresses through knowledge created and accumulated over millennia by curiosity driven scientists from many cultures. The Mandala, a South-Asian symbolism, depicts the complexity of signatures of the distinct features that define neuronal types in the brain. Hidden amidst the lines and curves of the Mandala are musical notes reminding us of the songs of neurons as they communicate through electrical signals, and "Teevra"; written in major scripts of the world expressing the sharing of scientific knowledge and co-operation of scientists.
Abhilasha Joshi discovered at Oxford . . . that the information integrated by the cell is transmitted through the axon (red) to a small area of the hippocampus of the brain to a select few key neurons, which in turn influence large neuronal assemblies encoding memories. Below the Mandala is the electrical recording of brain waves (theta oscillation, blue) as the mouse explores the world and the rhythmic electrical signals sent by the Teevra cell (yellow) as it participates in information representation.' Somogyi & Joshi (Personal Communication 10 March 2021) Transliteration by Rimjhim Dobhal and artwork by Anuja Gopidas.

Stimulation of the medial septum (including optogenetic pacing of GABAergic cells Zutshi et al., 2018) or fornix superior at RSA/'theta' frequencies can produce a rhythm, indistinguishable from spontaneous activity but phase-locked to the stimulus (Appendix 5; see Fig. 9.1A). Notably, unlike the hypothalamus, high-frequency tonic stimulation of the medial septum blocks rhythmicity (phasic gaps can drive theta). Hypothalamic RSA/'theta' recording can be used to trigger a phase-locked 'brain bypass' stimulation that reinstates lost RSA/'theta' in the hippocampus (Fig. 9.3E) and repairs hippocampal-dependent memory (McNaughton et al., 2006b; see also §9.2.4). Fixed frequency stimulation also produces some recovery of function. This shows that theta rhythmicity, in and of itself, is functional—and acts to enable synchronous processing of information that is provided by other inputs to the hippocampus (see also §9.2.3).

The subsequent generation of hippocampal rhythmicity is complicated by the fact that there appear to be two pharmacological gates—an ascending serotonergic one related to movement and an ascending cholinergic one related to non-movement—which enable (separately or together) the entrainment of the hippocampus by the phasic septal impulses, the frequency of which is determined independently of the gates (Appendices 5 and 6; Fig. 9.3A, C). There are also separate cholinergic septal cells that contribute to theta amplitude (Fig. 9.3B).

The integration of RSA/'theta' frequency appears to be through small numbers of intrahypothalamic inhibitory interneurons that regularly clamp the output of much larger numbers of hypothalamic projection neurones (Pan and McNaughton, 2004; Appendix 5); with stronger excitatory reticular input overcoming inhibition earlier and so giving rise to shorter inter-burst intervals and so higher burst frequencies. Given this mode of organization, changes in the control of RSA/'theta' frequency, *per* se, should modify the temporal packaging of information in targets of the RSA/'theta' system, but will not necessarily change any topographic encoding of that information (see also Li et al., 2023, on targeting of hippocampal interneurones rather than pyramidal cells). Similarly, alteration of the frequency or presence of RSA/'theta' in the hippocampus and entorhinal cortex would be presumed to leave intact the (much richer) topographic encoding of information in these areas. Of course, where the loss of RSA/'theta' has resulted from medial septal lesions, and especially electrolytic medial septal lesions, there would be an additional loss of the specific information transferred to the hippocampus via the septum, on top of the loss of temporal packaging of all hippocampal-entorhinal information by RSA/'theta'. However, even under these conditions, many of the important cortical connections of the SHS would remain intact.

Thus, neither medial septal lesions nor injections of anxiolytic drugs would be expected to have effects identical to those of hippocampal lesions. In particular, RSA/'theta' would not be expected to be essential to all hippocampal function (but see McNaughton et al., 2006b for evidence that theta pattern activity, *per se*, is crucial for water maze learning).

PRINCIPLE 2: RSA/'theta' activity in the hippocampal formation is the result of phasic inhibitory input from subcortical systems coupled with excitatory (potentially tonic) inputs from the cortex and other areas. These provide the foundation for hippocampal rhythmicity that is then enabled by tonic cholinergic and/or serotonergic inputs acting as gates.

9.2.2 Adding subcortical and cortical iteration

Fig. 9.5A–C shows the anatomy of the supramammillary (SuM) and septal areas in more detail. The areas involved in the control of RSA/'theta' are shown in purple. Reticular input is to the most medial (parvicellular) portion of SuM (SuMp) but output to the medial septum is from the grandicellular portion (SuMg). Injection of GABA reduced the amplitude but not the frequency of RSA/'theta' when injected into either SuMp or SuMg (Jiang and Khanna, 2004). So, both the ascending reticular input to the supramammillary area and the supramammillary input to the septum are polysynaptic.

The septal synchronizer (Fig. 9.5D) has additional complexity (see Fig. 9.5E for a schematic diagram).

> Individual neurons in the medial septum and diagonal band fire in phase with … the hippocampal theta rhythm … [and] most septal sites showed theta rhythm concurrent with hippocampal theta during locomotion. However, periods with theta at hippocampal but not septal sites were more frequent than the reverse. Theta waves in different parts of the septum were synchronized with each other but medial septal sites showed less frequent theta than other sites. The phase delays between medial and lateral septal sites were < 10 ms, suggesting that the hippocampus does not act as a simple relay between the two.… Our data suggest that the pacemaker of hippocampal theta may best be thought of as a set of functionally differentiated components rather than as a single homogenous unit.
>
> (Nerad and McNaughton, 2006, p. 155).

This picture, as with the hypothalamic control of frequency, and the input from the ascending reticular activating system, involves an apparent paradox. In each case, multiple areas operate in parallel, with primary control switching between them but with both phase-locking and amplitude integration coordinated among them. We will discuss how this can occur in §9.2.3.

There is a (close to ubiquitous) mass of potentially iterative return pathways within the supramammillary-septal-hippocampal system. Similarly, the main subcortical output from the hippocampus to the mammillary bodies is the start of the Papez circuit (Papez, 1937; Fig. 9.5C, Fig. 9.9) and we will argue (§9.9.2) that iterative processing by this circuit is a key mechanism for goal conflict resolution by the hippocampus (see Vann, 2013 for evidence that the mammillary bodies are also important for processing that does not involve hippocampus).

The more immediate return pathways challenge the idea of a simple unidirectional circuit (§9.2.3; Fig. 9.3) that would have a supramammillary input and a mammillary output as unidirectional relays. Both single-unit data from anaesthetized rats (Kocsis and Kaminski, 2006; Kirk et al., 1996) and field potential data from free-moving ones (Ruan et al., 2017) show that 'SUM neurons effectively drive theta oscillations in the hippocampus during epochs of sensory-elicited theta rhythm and short episodes of theta acceleration, whereas spontaneous slow theta in the SUM is controlled by descending input from the [SHS]. Thus, in certain states, rhythmically firing SUM neurons function to accelerate the septal theta oscillator, and in others, they are entrained by a superordinate oscillatory network (Kocsis and Kaminski, 2006, p. 531). It is likely that a similar organization applies to all the hypothalamic areas where

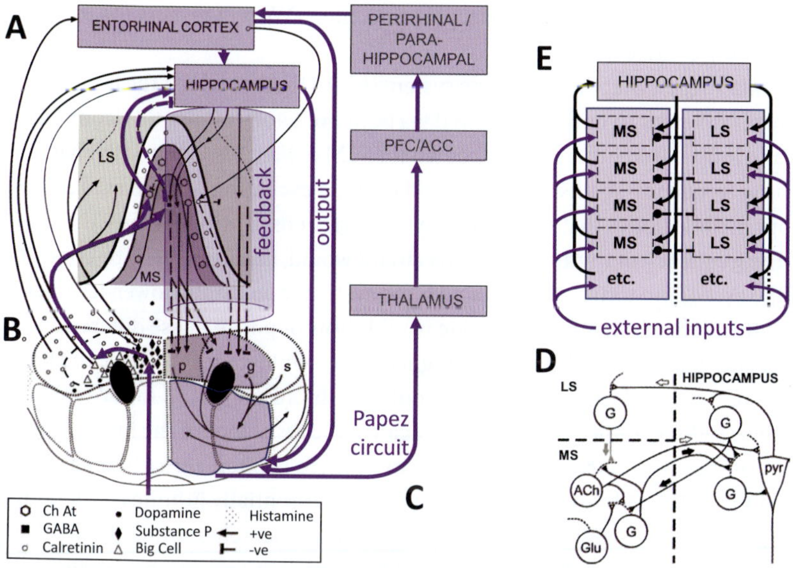

Fig. 9.5 **(A)** Interconnections of parts of SuM with the septum and hippocampus (simplified). Excitatory connections are indicated with solid lines and arrows and inhibitory ones with dashed lines and rectangles. The medial septum is divided into three distinct zones with an intermediate zone characterised by presumed cholinergic cells and an outer zone characterised by calretinin containing cells that receive projections from the entorhinal cortex.
(B) The parts of SuM in relation to its cell types and their connections to the entorhinal cortex, septum and hippocampus. Cells are indicated by symbols indicating specific characteristic histochemical markers but with no indication of co-localisation of multiple markers. SuM as a whole contains calretinin-containing cells. The most medial portion of SuM contains small cells (and is therefore termed by us the parvicellular portion) and is distinguished by having substance P containing cells and a high density of dopamine-containing cells. Around the pm fibre tract (solid black) is an area most clearly distinguished by containing large cells (and is therefore termed by us the grandicellular portion) that has projections to the medial septum as well as to the hippocampus. More laterally is an area with much more loosely packed cells (and so termed by us the shell portion) that is most clearly delineated by containing cells that project to the entorhinal cortex. The parts of SuM as described by us occupy approximately the same medio-lateral positions as the parts of the mammillary bodies.
(C) Output to the cortex from the mamillary bodies via the Papez circuit (see Fig. 9.9 for more detail).
(D) Neuronal interactions in the SHS. The MS and hippocampus are mutually interconnected and the activity in one structure can affect EEG in the other structure both by excitatory (Δ) and inhibitory (▲) synapses. G, GABAergic neuron; ACh, cholinergic neuron; Glu, glutamatergic neuron; pyr, pyramidal cell.
(E) A schematic illustration of connections within the SHS that determine the kind of EEG activity that occurs in the target structure. Various parts of both the LS and MS are drawn separately and mutually interconnected. They are not identified with any specific subregion of the septum or a class of septal neurons here but the parcellation reflects the fact that such diversity exists. Purple arrows represent the afferents from sources extrinsic to the SHS (e.g., panel B). In this model, different rhythms can co-occur in the septum and have their sources in the septum, hippocampus or hypothalamus. Figure and legend modified from: A-C, Pan and McNaughton (2004); D-E, Nerad and McNaughton (2006).

the frequency is sensitive to benzodiazepine injections. We will discuss the precise nature of this descending control in §9.2.3.

These data suggest that the ascending system (§9.2.1) acts to adjust the frequency of rhythmicity that is inherent to nodes connected via both excitatory loops and a combination of recurrent and loop-based inhibition (as shown for SuM in Fig. 9.3C); but with phasic inhibition accelerating frequency against a background of tonic excitation (Zutshi et al., 2018). Where such loops include nodes that tend to retain the current oscillation pattern, there will be hysteresis. The frequency of rhythmicity of the circuit would, then, normally be controlled by the level of the ascending tonic reticular activating system input to the lower-level (clock) node but it and the higher (synchronizer) node would show opposite phase differences during acceleration and deceleration. That is, the higher node would *appear* to drive the lower during deceleration; but the deceleration itself would be the result of the lower (frequency integrator) node 'pulling' rather than 'pushing' against the resistance of the higher node.

In the absence of acceleration or deceleration there is often zero phase lag (compare **hf** and **mb** in Fig. 9.3F). While this might seem to imply essentially infinite conduction velocity, '[zero-lag] synchrony is an inevitable property of delay elements similar to dendrites joined by long-range couplings with relatively rapid transmission and can be explained by simple linear models operating on uncorrelated inputs' (Clare et al., 2002, p. 73). Zero-lag synchrony would time-lock processing across what could be large networks (which is important for our theory. see §1.12.7, Fig. 1.6). It should also be noted that field potential coherence can result from post-synaptic potentials being generated in parallel in the local region of firing neurons and in their distal targets (Schneider et al., 2021).

9.2.3 Inhibitory circuits

§9.2.2 raises the issue of where the hysteresis in the RSA/'theta' circuit comes from. One obvious source is the recurrent inhibition that is present in all the structures in the circuit and which could give rise to auto-rhythmicity given appropriate tonic afferent drive. It should also be noted that the hippocampus also has quite complex intrinsic inter-neuronal circuitry (Fig. 9.6) that may be necessary to maintain stability in what, otherwise, could be essentially unlimited positive feedback loops.

Consistent with this, isolated slices of either septum (Vinogradova et al., 1980) or hippocampus (Bland et al., 1988; Fellous and Sejnowski, 2000) can show clear RSA/'theta'-like activity. However, it should be noted that simple tonic high-frequency stimulation of septal or hippocampal afferents does not result in RSA/'theta' but, instead, blocks it; that synchrony across structures at a common frequency is the general rule (e.g. with septal parcels, Fig. 9.5E), with only occasional exceptions; and that the observed rhythmicity does not show the 'beats' that would result if there were separate oscillators running in parallel at somewhat different frequencies.

9.2.4 The role of intracellular oscillations

Recent reports suggest a role for Hyperpolarization-activated, Cation Nonselective (HCN) channels. These appear to contribute to the stability of, e.g. cardiac automaticity and

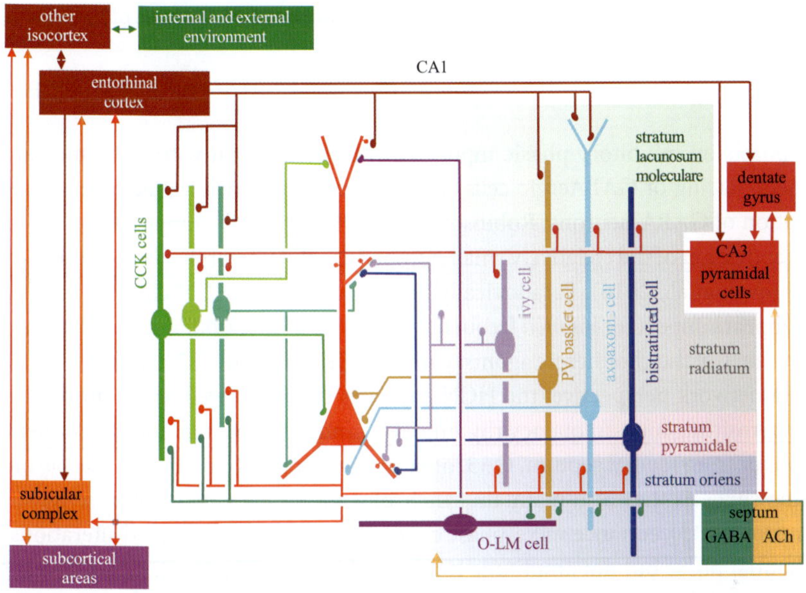

Fig. 9.6 Schematic of the spatial relationships between pyramidal cells and eight types of GABAergic interneuron in the CA1 area. The main synaptic connections of pyramidal cells (red, middle), three types of CCK-expressing cells (basket cell, perforant path-associated cell, Schaffer collateral-associated cell), ivy cells and PV-expressing basket, axo-axonic, bistratified and O-LM interneurons. The other 13 defined types of interneuron are not shown; ACh, acetycholine. Connections among interneurons are not shown for clarity. Figure and legend from Somogyl et al. (2014) with permission.

> in the CNS [play] three distinct roles in the generation of spontaneous activity: [a] as a primary pacemaking current, [e.g. in thalamo-cortical neurons, where] an organic antagonist either completely blocks pacemaker activity or substantially slows the rate of spontaneous firing.... ; [b] to modulate the inherent spontaneous activity generated [e.g. increasing stability of cerebellar Purkinje cells, where antagonism] fails to alter the rate of spontaneous firing or enhances the rate of firing, or leads to bistable membrane potentials;[c] support [of] subthreshold oscillations. Entorhinal cortex neurons . . . that fail to fire action potentials spontaneously do show subthreshold oscillations, especially in response to depolarizing current injections. Subthreshold oscillations at a frequency of around 2–4 Hz are a prominent component of activity at potentials between −60 and −50 mV.... These neurons also play an important role in the generation of hippocampal theta rhythm.... [HCN] lags behind the voltage change by slightly more than half a cycle, because of its opposite voltage dependence and slower kinetics. Although the function of these oscillations is not clear, they may be needed to integrate the many convergent inputs from association cortex to a synchronous output from an entorhinal stellate cell to the hippocampus.
>
> (Robinson and Siegelbaum, 2003, pp. 468–469)

Importantly, analysis of inhibitory synaptic input on EC layer II neurons shows that inhibitory postsynaptic potentials, which EC stellates are likely to receive during [RSA/'theta'] can very efficiently reset the intrinsic oscillations. In addition, theoretical, experimental and

> modeling studies also indicate that the intrinsic subthreshold oscillations of individual cells can engender synchronized population activity.
>
> (Dickson et al., 2000, p. 2577)

This emphasis on inhibitory phasic input fits with the fact that within the medial septum optogenetic pacing of GABAergic cells (Zutshi et al., 2018) or of glutamatergic cells (and so activation of GABA neurons; Robinson et al., 2016) can drive hippocampal rhythmicity; whereas activation of the (relatively small number of) glutamatergic fibres in the fornix does not (Robinson et al., 2016). Paradoxically, *inhibitory* reset of HCN channels in the medial septum appears important for *high* frequency (8 Hz) RSA/'theta' but not low (6 Hz) especially in the presence of the cholinergic agonist carbachol (Kocsis and Li, 2004).

From a network perspective, the HCN channels can be viewed as a high pass filter, selectively permitting high-frequency rhythmicity—and are important for entrainment of area CA1 to input from medial septum, CA3, or entorhinal cortex (Combe and Gasparini, 2021). Modelling suggests they also maintain synchrony within extended dendritic trees (Vaidya and Johnston, 2013), enhance spike-phase coherence, and produce graded alterations in local field potential phase but not amplitude (Sinha and Narayanan, 2015). The simplest explanation of residual rhythmicity in the total absence of HCN is that the low-frequency theta (like that induced by carbachol in hippocampal slices) is due solely to tonic cholinergic input with no phasic component (an imbalance that may not occur normally in intact rats). Critically,

> HCN-expressing neurons represented a subpopulation of GABAergic cells in the [medial septum (MS)] partly overlapping with parvalbumin (PV)-containing neurons. Rhythmic firing in the [RSA/'theta'] frequency range was characteristic of all HCN-expressing neurons. In contrast, only a minority of HCN-negative cells displayed theta related activity. Microiontophoretic blockade of HCN channels resulted in the reduction of discharge frequency, but [RSA/'theta'] rhythmic firing was perturbed only in a few cases. Our data imply that HCN-expressing GABAergic neurons provide rhythmic drive in all phases of the hippocampal theta activity. In most MS theta cells rhythm genesis is apparently determined by *interactions at the level of the network* rather than by the pacemaking property of HCN channels alone.
>
> (Varga et al., 2008, p. 3893; our emphasis)

HCN channels may also provide an explanation of the effects of septal cooling. Petersen and Buzsáki (2020, p. 731) found that 'cooling of the MS reduced both theta frequency and power and was associated with an enhanced incidence of errors in a spatial navigation task, but it did not affect spatial correlates of neurons. MS cooling decreased theta frequency oscillations of place cells and reduced distance-time compression but preserved distance-phase compression of place field sequences within the theta cycle. Thus, the septum is critical for sustaining precise theta phase coordination of cell assemblies in the hippocampal system, a mechanism needed for spatial memory'. Their cooling was locally about a 20° drop. HCN are very temperature-sensitive with a Q_{10} for activation and deactivation of about 4.5 (Magee, 1998). Their time constants would, therefore, have changed from ~20 ms before cooling to ~200 ms at maximum cooling and so permitting the 1 Hz drop (and flattening of the running speed-frequency relationship). So, the current carried by the HCN channels, 'I_h is a potential mechanism of the cooling effect' (Buzsáki, Personal Communication, 23 November 2021).

Do medial septal HCN channels act as primary pacemakers, modulators, or subthreshold oscillators? The entorhinal example (Dickson et al., 2000), and the differentiation of multiple parcels in the septum (Fig. 9.5E) suggest that the main role of the HCN is to maintain subthreshold oscillations that, via GABA inputs, maintain membrane synchrony across the medial septum even in the absence of the firing of individual neurons. Similar effects in the hippocampus would account for the tendency of cells to fire in relation to global theta rhythmicity, even when they do so only occasionally in, e.g. place fields. As with the entorhinal case, ascending (RPO-SuM-medial septal) inhibitory GABAergic inputs would reset the phase of subthreshold oscillation to achieve higher overall RSA/'theta' frequencies. Local phase variation relative to global synchrony could then be important for, e.g. symbolic processing (Do and Hasselmo, 2021). Ascending cholinergic systems (originating in the pontine tegmentum) would enable low frequency (4–6 Hz) rhythmicity but with increased input altering amplitude more than frequency (Vertes et al., 1993). Such low-frequency RSA/'theta' may not be functional (Pan and McNaughton, 1997; Petersen and Buzsáki, 2020) with a critical threshold value in the region of 6.5 Hz independent of the type of treatment (Pan and McNaughton, 2004, p. 154). It may be significant that the midline cortex shows strong synchrony with the hippocampus only at higher frequencies (Young and McNaughton, 2009).

PRINCIPLE 3: ***The phasic aspect of RSA/'theta' represents synchrony coded by inhibition and stabilized by HCN channels across structures at a large scale (including zero phase lag between structures) that influences when packets of cells are likely to fire more than whether they fire. This synchrony is likely to be most important for hippocampal function when intense iterative processing is involved.***[5]

9.2.5 Multiple sites of anxiolytic action

In interpreting PRINCIPLE 1, we should remind ourselves (§9.1.3) that

- the behavioural effects of the anxiolytics are sometimes mediated by changes in the threshold control of RSA/'theta' (as evidenced by the effects of dorsal bundle lesions)
- and they are sometimes mediated by changes in RSA/'theta' frequency (as evidenced by experiments on the hypothalamus)
- but also, *behaviourally significant* changes in frequency may be mediated by different parallel strands (Fig. 9.5E) of the ascending system under different behavioural conditions (Fig. 9.7).

PRINCIPLE 4: ***Multiple topographically organized functionally-distinct parallel threads pass through the SHS with RSA/'theta' ensuring whole-system synchronous processing by them with sub-system phase variation.***

[5] For a review of interplay between HCN, RSA/'theta', memory formation, and dementias see Kazmierska-Grebowska et al. (2023).

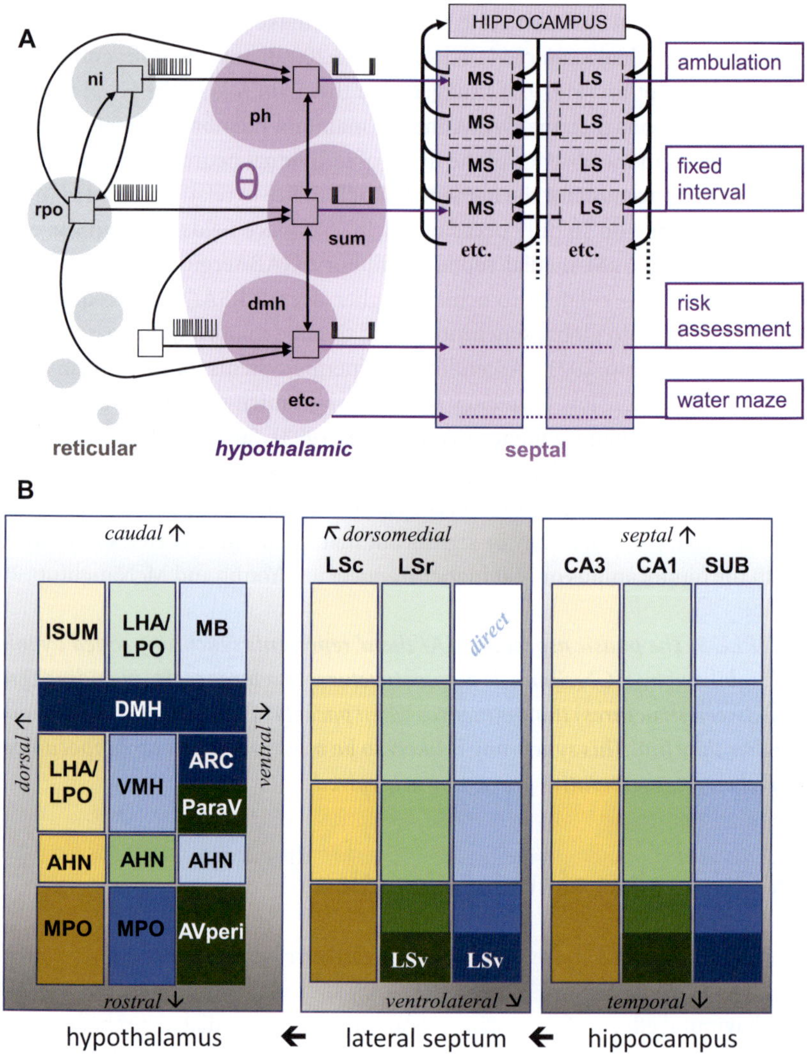

Fig. 9.7 Topographic mapping and functional differentiation of the control of RSA/'theta' and behaviour. **(A)** Ascending topographic control of rhythmicity and behaviour (simplified to 1 dimension). Different hypothalamic areas project via different medial septal (MS) modules to a different part of the hippocampus and, in turn, different parts of the lateral septum (LS) and the hypothalamus (see B)—ultimately controlling different aspects of behaviour. For example, injections of benzodiazepines into **sum** reduce the frequency in a fixed interval schedule and change behaviour as much as does systemic injection. However, they reduce frequency and affect behaviour much less than systemic injections in the water maze test of spatial navigation and do not reproduce either the frequency reduction or the behavioural effects of systemic injections in the open field. Thus, different activating and frequency controlling nuclei appear to be involved to different extents in different behavioural tasks (Woodnorth and McNaughton, 2005). **dmh**, dorso-medial hypothalamus; MS, medial septum/diagonal band complex; **rpo**, nucleus reticularis pontis oralis; **sum**, medial supramammillary nucleus.
(B) Return (descending) topographic mapping of hippocampal formation into the lateral septal area and hypothalamus. The hippocampal formation (right) can be viewed as a two-dimensional sheet (right hand panel) with unfolding of the cell layers and removal of the curvature of the hippocampus resulting in the top of the sheet being the septal pole of the

9.3 Sensory processing and the SHS

As one follows a sensory system from the periphery, deeper into the brain, the information encoded is initially unimodal, but then, for example in parietal cortex, this gives way to multimodal encoding. If we follow, say, visual information, from V1 to V2, V4, inferotemporal cortex, perirhinal and parahippocampal cortex, entorhinal cortex and, finally, hippocampus, we could, by extrapolation, conclude that the hippocampus is concerned with producing the very highest order abstractions from multimodal sensory information. However, the bulk of the evidence is as much against a purely perceptual as against a memorial or motor function for the hippocampus. Further, the bulk of the single cell data suggest that many hippocampal cells are non-specifically multimodal. Rather than firing to only one stimulus which has a specific combination of, say, visual, auditory, and olfactory properties, the cell fires to any of several stimuli whether visual, auditory, or olfactory (Appendix 6). Furthermore, anatomically and developmentally, the hippocampus appears distinct from the higher levels of association cortex.

An important route by which this modulation of sensory processing can take place is via the nucleus accumbens (to which the SHS projects from the subiculum and entorhinal cortex), and thence on successively (via a series of GABAergic pathways) to the ventral pallidum, nucleus reticularis thalami, and the whole array of thalamocortical sensory processing loops. Analysis of the likely mode of operation of this circuit suggests that activation of the subiculo-accumbens projection can boost thalamocortical sensory processing in all modalities; while analysis of the likely behavioural effects of such activation suggests that it is particularly novel stimuli and stimuli with strong associative significance that are picked out for enhanced sensory processing in this way (Gray et al., 1997). It is possible that this route is

---

Fig. 9.7 (*continued*)

hippocampus and the bottom being the temporal pole, the left-hand side of the sheet being CA3 and the right-hand side being subiculum (SUB). The central portion is labelled CA1, but evidence for distinct functionality of CA2 (see Lehr et al., 2021; He et al., 2021) and that the amygdala connects to an area which is essentially the CA1/SUB border suggests that there should be more strips than the three shown. The hippocampus is topographically mapped into the lateral septal area which can also be viewed as a two-dimensional sheet which with the proper bending and orientation (middle panel) provides a direct correspondence with the hippocampal sheet (e.g., the dark temporal portion of CA1 and SUB projects to LSv). The floor of the brain in the region of the hypothalamus can largely be viewed similarly, with the sheet essentially standing on edge (lSUM is largely dorsal to MB) with septal portions of the hippocampus projecting via the septum to caudal hypothalamic areas and temporal portions to rostral (giving approximately similar path lengths in the two cases). The most septal quarter of SUB appears to project directly to MB without relaying in the septum. The labelling of nuclei and the colours indicating the source of septal connections are only approximate. Abbreviations as for Fig. 9.7. c, l, r, v, caudal, lateral, rostral, ventral; AHN anterior hypothalamic nucleus; MPN medial preoptic nucleus; PV periventricular nucleus. (Based on Risold and Swanson, 1996; Rizzi-Wise and Wang, 2021).

responsible for conscious processing of anxiety-related stimuli (Gray, 1995); but we will not pursue that possibility here.

> *PRINCIPLE 5: the hippocampus is best viewed as a device that modulates activity in sensory systems, but is not itself a higher level of the classical sensory systems.*

9.4 Working/active memory—frontal/posterior iteration

We have already noted that the SHS is a key node in the Papez circuit that passes through anterior cingulate and prefrontal cortex (Fig. 9.5); and will discuss its role in this next. However, the prefrontal cortex is involved in quite separate loops that allow it to interact with posterior cortex and limbic cortex (Chapter 11).

The prefrontal cortex as a whole can be seen both as providing high level (essentially inhibitory) control of the ordering of ongoing motor programs, and as having mapped into it a variety of types of working memory.[6] What distinguishes this region from areas such as the amygdala or cingulate is the high degree of flexibility of the resultant motor output. Given the parcellation of prefrontal cortex (Fig. 11.2A), it is likely that different types of working memory are uniformly topographically mapped into different parcels of prefrontal cortex. Thus visuo-spatial information is transferred from posterior parietal cortex in direct projections to the principal sulcus, where it provides the basis for visuo-spatial working memory; and object attributes are transferred from visual association areas to below the principal sulcus, where they provide the basis for visual working memory.

At first sight, working memory and motor programming might seem quite distinct entities. But, in line with McKay's (1987) equation of perception with action, the information held in working memory effectively defines the way motor programs will run. This is particularly the case if the working memory holds temporary versions of motor programs recalled from long-term storage, as well as temporary versions of stimulus items. In one of the standard tasks used to test working memory in monkeys, where the monkey must move its eyes to a new position after a delay, it should be noted that the 'memory of the stimulus' is *identical* to the 'goal of the upcoming motor act' (Fig. 11.5). This intertwining of stimulus and response aspects is something which, in relation to the hippocampus, has caused many attempts at pure stimulus or pure response theories to come to grief, and constitutes one of the reasons we have preferred the term 'goal' to describe the nature of the encoded information.

If we view motor cortex as an area where specific movements are organized, then the supplementary motor area (to which it is reciprocally connected) is where anticipated movements (plans) are organized. This is in turn reciprocally connected to the prefrontal cortex, which is hierarchically organized with reciprocal connections between levels (Fig. 11.2A). Each level of this hierarchy (working back from motor cortex) appears (Appendix 3) to organize an aspect of motor performance one step more anticipatory than the previous one. Thus, the frontal eye fields represent a system that controls the direction of gaze so that the direction of the next motor act can then be computed. Similarly, the area in the region of

[6] This might be better termed 'active memory' see (Fuster, 1995, p. 5).

the principal sulcus can be thought of as controlling the direction of 'gaze' into the memory stores of the posterior cortex, so that, for example, future eye movements can be computed.

This same hierarchical organization is seen, in very close parallel, in the separate dorsal ('where') and ventral ('what') trends in frontal cortex. These are reciprocally connected with each other, thus binding the what and where information together into a distributed representation of a goal (situation + motivation). Further integration appears to occur with the connection of postrhinal/parahippocampal cortex to *both* lateral and medial entorhinal cortex.

> ***PRINCIPLE 6: At the level of operation of the prefrontal cortex and the SHS no distinction should be made between 'stimulus'/situation and 'response'/motivation. Both should be conflated into a term such as 'goal' (hippocampus) or 'plan', i.e. the ordering of successive goals and subgoals (prefrontal cortex).***

Theoretically, all that is required for the use of working memory is iterative 'refreshing' of activity (see Fig. 11.5 for more detail) by reciprocal connections between some area of prefrontal cortex ('working') and the equivalent area of more posterior cortex ('memory' in the form of a reactivated cell assembly that echoes the original percept). In many cases, sensory input will take the form that only one such circuit will control behaviour. However, there exist multiple possibilities for the co-activation of different prefrontal-posterior cortical networks so as to produce different working memories.

As with the hierarchical ordering of the motivational systems (Chapter 6), the hierarchical organization of frontal cortex (in terms of progressively higher levels of anticipation) can normally provide a means of resolving goal subgoal conflicts or, which is computationally the same thing, organizing sequences of goals in time. However, at any individual step in a complex motor sequence there may be uncertainty as to which of two concurrently activated goals is correct. (This would be particularly true in, for example, a working memory task with a high level of interference from earlier trials.) Uncertainty of this kind would involve a conflict between areas coding for different goals *within* a specific level of prefrontal cortex (i.e. at the same nominal step in the upcoming action sequence) rather than *between* levels of the system (i.e. at different steps in the upcoming action sequence). We propose that, when two or more such goal representations are highly and equally active at the same sequence step, the hippocampal formation can become engaged in order to resolve the conflict between the incompatible upcoming goals.

The prefrontal system has major links to the perirhinal and parahippocampal cortices (Fig. 9.5), links that provide the main basis for its interactions with the hippocampal formation. There may be cases when only the entorhinal, perirhinal and parahippocampal cortices interact with prefrontal cortex (as, perhaps, with concurrent discriminations; see Appendix 9, §A9.3). These purely cortical interactions are likely to involve conflicts between goals, the distinction between which is related more to the stimulus to be acted on than to the specific actions to be taken with respect to the stimulus (see G3 and G4 in Fig. 1.7): conflict, in essence, between memory items. But there are also cases where the hippocampus proper is involved. These appear to consist in conflicts between goals that differ more in the action to be taken than in the stimulus to be acted on (see G2 and G3 in Fig. 1.7), though the relevant stimuli may also be quite different, e.g. food in one location versus safety in another.

On this view, the iterative connections of the hippocampus and the frontal cortex would allow the hippocampus to do two things. First, the hippocampus could alter processing in the working memory system (for example, producing an increase in negative bias of the type ascribed by Eysenck, 1992a, to generalized anxiety disorder), and hence affect motor programming indirectly. Second, it could actively interrupt ongoing motor programs and replace them with specific information gathering (e.g. risk analysis) programs. The same logic can be applied equally well to higher-order, more anticipatory, computations (planning) and lower-order, less anticipatory, computations (attention/gaze direction).

Here it will be seen that our view of frontal cortex follows closely those of Goldman-Rakic, Fuster, Pandya, and Barbas, as well as many others (Appendix 3). However, as with our view of the threat system, what generally distinguishes our theory are the ideas: (1) that all memory is located outside the hippocampus (see also §9.3); and (2) that the hippocampus is a quite specialized structure that acts solely to resolve conflicts between incompatible goals (Chapter 10). Conflicts of this kind are fundamentally linked to response programming. However, there are cases in which working memory holds a goal for which the critical information is predominantly stimulus-related (determining, e.g. towards what object to direct the eyes next). Here, the distinction between response competition and memory competition may be hard to make; and there is nothing about the machinery we attribute to the wider hippocampal formation, including the entorhinal cortex, which would prevent it resolving a pure stimulus competition, in the sense of a conflict between two goals both of which can be acted upon by what is fundamentally the same response. Certainly, the hippocampal formation does receive some purely stimulus information, which, however, it appears to use predominantly for response control purposes.

In addition to the resolution of conflicts between concurrently activated goals (dealt with by the hippocampus), a task may require resolution of conflicts between different subgoals contributing to an overall goal (essentially the problem of ordering the different subgoals into an appropriate sequence). We see this latter resolution as the business (perhaps, in essence, the only business) of the prefrontal cortex. Thus, the hippocampus and prefrontal cortex deal with different kinds of goal conflict. In some cases (e.g. delay tasks), however, it is difficult to distinguish between opposing response requirements (to respond on the one hand and withhold responding on the other) and sequencing (withholding responding now while aiming to respond later). In such tasks performance could depend on both the hippocampal formation and the prefrontal cortex.

Note also, that frontal cortical systems are in parallel to the defence and eyeblink systems that we are about to discuss (§9.5), in the same sense that each of these is in parallel to the other. Each of these systems can be concurrently and separately active, with each determining some course of action on the basis of the information available to it. The eyeblink system is the most fundamentally reflexive, the defence system is to a large extent based on fixed action patterns (in the most flexible sense of this term), while the frontal cortex (with primary and secondary motor areas viewed as the lowest levels of the system) appears to deal with the least reflexive of motor outputs.

PRINCIPLE 7: Motor control, attention, working memory, and planning reflect successively deeper levels of processing in otherwise fundamentally similar processing units located in the frontal cortex. The hippocampus has no necessary involvement in any

of these functions. Rather, it operates to modulate the activity in frontal circuits only under conditions where concurrent goals conflict.

9.5 Conditioning and the SHS—from eyeblink to fear

We discussed eyeblinks and eyeblink conditioning in §7.1. Critically we noted that trace conditioning is sensitive to hippocampal lesions (Ivkovich and Stanton, 2001) but simple and delayed conditioning are not (Berger et al., 1986a; Logan and Grafton, 1995; Blaxton et al., 1996; Steinmetz, 2000). Eyeblink control appears to be a paradigmatic case of a hierarchically organized system. The lowest level (nucleus interpositus) is all that is required for the simplest conditioning, but is also the final common path for more complex conditioning. In this system the cerebellar cortex stands in about the same relation to interpositus as do hypothalamus and amygdala to the dorsal periaqueductal grey (PAG, Chapter 6), providing a capacity for more anticipatory responses. Finally, occupying the same logical position in both systems, is the hippocampus. This provides the higher level eyeblink circuits with the additional capacity for inhibition of the previously correct lower order response during reversal; and for inhibition of the multiple incorrect alternatives that will arise through simple conditioning to multiple parallel cortical delay lines during trace conditioning (Appendix 6).

This provides a general model where, superimposed on the most basic conditioning circuits, are higher-order circuits (that can provide simple output from detectors of progressively more complex stimulus configurations), including those that can deal with delays and relations between stimuli. Despite the complexity of the networks involved, all of the resultant conditioning is, from the point of view of the target structure, identical to that of the simplest possible stimulus input; all that differs is the source of the afferent impulses, and the receiving cell has no way of telling what that is. Depending on the precise conditions of the experiment, these multiple parallel circuits will on occasion tend to produce concurrent activation of two incompatible goals. It is the business of the hippocampal system to detect this conflict between proposed goals and send out signals that are designed to devalue all but the correct one.

Let us now apply this basic model to the example of simple avoidance and its conditioning that we have already considered (§6.5; Fig.6.3B. Unlike the uni-dimensional eyeblink, this involves a hierarchical set of structures that control complex motor patterns. The hierarchical circuits of interest (Fig. 6.5B) start with the PAG. The dorsal PAG is activated by an immediate predator, by an immediate dominant conspecific, by pain, and by high levels of carbon dioxide. Graeff (1994) suggested that activation of this region is the basis of panic attacks. It is important to note that the flight (escape) elicited by activation of the PAG is undirected. Above this is *directed* escape controlled by the medial hypothalamus, and, above this, is simple active avoidance controlled by the amygdala. Given adequate stimuli, all of these nuclei will be concurrently pre-programming a range of quite independent potential responses. This multiplicity of potential responses may seem complicated, but it can easily be controlled by a system which depends on release (inhibition of inhibition), rather than activation, to select responses (see, e.g. Chapter 2 in McNaughton, 1989b). In all these cases, activation of a higher level by an appropriate *innate* stimulus will cause output from the lower levels to be restricted, and controlled by the higher level. Note that this should not normally result in what we would term goal conflict. The goal is the same for each system (i.e. achievement of a place of safety); it is only the selection of responses to achieve that goal that must be controlled, and this can be achieved within the hierarchical system without the need for outside influence.

We argued (Chapter 6, Appendix 3) that the anterior cingulate represents several additional levels of the active defence system and hence is directly above the amygdala in an 'active defence' hierarchy. By contrast, the hippocampus and, above it, the posterior cingulate appear to be parts of a parallel inhibitory system principally concerned with the approach into dangerous situations (Fig. 6.5B). It should be emphasized that all these areas are reciprocally interconnected, but that the connection from the amygdala to the hippocampus appears to be feedforward, while that from the hippocampus to the amygdala appears to be weaker and feedback (Appendix 2).

With simple fear conditioning (LeDoux, 1994) an initially neutral input from the thalamus comes to elicit freezing or avoidance due to long-term potentiation of its input to the amygdala. As with simple eyeblink conditioning, this simple avoidance conditioning is not sensitive to hippocampal lesions.

However, the organization of the sensory inputs to the defence system raised an interesting question. Is the hippocampus, rather than the anterior cingulate, the top of the 'motor' threat system (receiving sensory input as do the amygdala and PAG, and controlling responses when these structures do not), or is it the top of the 'sensory' threat system (sending a particularly highly organized type of sensory information, such as context, to the amygdala, which instead controls the response to threat)? Both points of view appear to be correct to some extent (LeDoux, 1994). The hippocampus needs to be engaged in the organization of avoidance responses when these conflict with other classes of goal (e.g. approach) and hence require inhibition of a prepotent response. However, the hippocampus is also required when there is competition between incompatible specific goals (stimulus sources) to which to direct the same appropriate avoidance response (as with contextual or reversal learning).

At this point we depart from the views of LeDoux and Graeff (see Chapter 6 and Appendix 2). We differ from them in thinking that the hippocampus should not be viewed as a source of contextual stimuli that can come to control the amygdala (for then there should be strong hippocampo-amygdalar connections rather than, as is the case, the other way round). Rather, we think of the hippocampus as a device that can resolve conflicts, not only between programs concurrently activated within the amygdala, but also between programs in the amygdala and those elsewhere. Thus, the hippocampus does appear to be important in dealing with some cases where contextual stimuli determine defensive behaviour but only when the contextual stimuli elicit conflict (e.g. Gemzik et al., 2021). Equally, the hippocampus is also important for the way in which the amygdala deals with non-contextual stimuli. It will be involved in all cases, for example, where the stimuli generate approach-avoidance conflict. While contextual stimuli, being diffuse, will often have this effect, this is a correlational rather than necessary relation. That is why, on our view, contextual or configural views of the hippocampus can appear to provide satisfactory accounts of many of the hippocampal effects in memory-oriented experiments, but do not account for all such effects and lacks of effect (Chapter 8), and do not account for the non-memorial effects of hippocampal lesions.

The commonalities of these two 'simple conditioning' systems (fear and eyeblink) lead to our next important principle.

PRINCIPLE 8: Conditioning, as such, reflects simple changes in associative strength at single synaptic junctions in relevant systems distributed throughout the brain

(amygdala for fear conditioning, interpositus for eyeblink). These changes can take the form of increases as a result of long-term potentiation (or equivalent plastic changes) or decreases as a result of long-term depression. Long-term potentiation and depression in the hippocampus, on the other hand, do not represent conditioning (or storage of sensory information), but the reprogramming of a system that modulates conditioning (or storage of sensory information) in other structures.

9.6 The 'emotion' system—cingulate cortex

Following Papez, and by direct analogy with classical sensory systems, it is tempting to view the anterior cingulate gyrus as being emotional sensory cortex (receiving its input fairly directly from e.g. the pain system). By analogy with other sensory systems, its reciprocal links with the prefrontal cortex would then be viewed as supporting emotional working memory. However, the input to the anterior cingulate gyrus from the amygdala and hypothalamus, and its immediate links with motor cortex and dorsal and ventral striatum, speak of a motor-programming role, making it akin to a second ventral prefrontal cortex (see also §6.7; Chapter 11).

In the case of the classical perceptual systems, we found that we could equate perception with action only at the very highest levels of these systems, at the point where they are involved in working memory. However, this equation is much easier to make in the case of emotional perception, since the detection of an emotional state of affairs can reasonably be presumed to imply immediate action of a quite specific type. There is also evidence that cingulate cortex is not primary pain-receiving cortex, but rather is concerned with the organization of responses to pain. Cingulate lesions in human beings do not eliminate the capacity to detect pain and report changes in its level, but they do rob it of its emotional, imperative quality.

Let us consider further the fact that the cingulate cortex receives information not only from the hypothalamus (which can be presumed to relate to innate motor programs activated by current internal states), but also from the caudate nucleus and amygdala. According to Rapoport (1989), these pathways allow information about innate motor programs (grooming, checking territory, etc.) to gain access to the frontal cortex. She proposes that, in at least some cases of obsessive-compulsive disorder, an abnormality in the basal ganglia (of a type which gives rise to choreas and tics in a variety of other disorders) releases such innate programs. The resultant activity in cingulate and frontal cortices then gives rise to the compulsions and obsessions, these being perceived, at least initially, as 'intrusive and senseless' (*op. cit.*, p. 63). This line of thought leads to two, mutually compatible, ways of regarding obsessive-compulsive disorder. First, one can treat the symptoms of this disorder as reflecting activity in the highest goal-setting levels of the motor-programming system; on this view these symptoms consist of affective action programs repetitively released despite stimulus conditions that would normally inhibit them. Second, one can treat obsessive-compulsive symptoms as reflecting activity in the highest levels of the affective perceptual systems; on this view, they consist of affective percepts occurring in the absence of a normally adequate stimulus and hence giving rise to inappropriate behaviour that, because it cannot correct a condition that does not objectively exist, is remorselessly repeated. Since, at this level of the nervous system, the distinction between action and stimulus is, as we have emphasized, arbitrary, these are two different ways of saying exactly the same thing.

In this light, anterior cingulate cortex is concerned with the control of relatively innate motor programs that each fulfil phylogenetically distinct functions. Hence it has strong links with the amygdala, dorsal and ventral striatum, and motor cortex. It functions, therefore, very much like ventral frontal cortex, except that the latter is concerned with the production of novel flexible motor programs rather than innate ones.

What of posterior cingulate cortex? This appears (Appendix 3) to be a somewhat ambiguous structure. It is tightly and reciprocally linked to anterior cingulate, and yet stimulation does not elicit affective responses as it does in anterior cingulate. It is placed in the cortex close to the subiculum, receives largely unidirectional links from subiculum, as does subiculum from other hippocampal areas, and shows the RSA/'theta' activity and local field potentials that are characteristic of the hippocampal formation. Yet it is not usually treated as simply another module of the SHS. We argue in Appendix 3 that posterior cingulate is in fact tightly related to both anterior cingulate and the SHS. Its reciprocal links with the anterior cingulate mirror the reciprocal links between the dorsal and ventral trends respectively of frontal cortex, with anterior cingulate mirroring the ventral 'what' trend and posterior cingulate, the dorsal 'where' trend. The distinction between posterior cingulate and dorsal prefrontal cortex would then be the same as the distinction already proposed between anterior cingulate and ventral prefrontal cortex: posterior cingulate cortex deals with more stereotyped, and dorsal prefrontal cortex with more flexible, motor programs. Both are primarily concerned with prediction and anticipation (hence the lack of motor output when posterior cingulate is stimulated), and with the inhibition of ongoing programs.

It is in this anticipatory and inhibitory role that we can see a link with the hippocampal formation. The posterior cingulate receives many inputs that match those of prefrontal cortex (from the anterior thalamus, the anterior cingulate, the mammillary bodies, the subiculum). However, as we argue in Appendix 3, it seems to have a particularly close relationship with rhinal cortex. Matching the architectonic mapping of posterior sensory cortical areas into prefrontal cortex, we can see an apparently similar architectonic mapping of rhinal isocortex into the most differentiated layers of posterior cingulate and of subiculum into the least differentiated (Fig. 11.2A). The direction of flow of cingulate information, predominantly from least to most differentiated, matches that in frontal cortex, while the flow of hippocampal information from most differentiated to least matches sensory cortex. Thus, the projection from parahippocampal cortex to the final output stage of posterior cingulate could be a direct 'quick and dirty' route for information that can also be processed through the 'slow and sophisticated' circuitry running through all the levels of the hippocampal formation and then all the levels of the posterior cingulate to arrive at the same final destination (comparable to the direct and cortical sensory inputs to the amygdala; LeDoux, 1994; Fig. 6.1).

Posterior cingulate, then, as anticipatory, inhibitory, affective, innate premotor cortex, is in receipt of information from a variety of levels of the hippocampal formation and is in direct receipt of at least part of the isocortical input to the hippocampal formation. Yet we cannot view posterior cingulate as the sole or even primary cortical recipient of hippocampal output. The subiculum projects to anterior cingulate (matching its projection to the amygdala) and both directly and via the anterior thalamus to the prefrontal cortex (Fig. 11.2A).

PRINCIPLE 9: The dorsal trend of prefrontal cortex, the posterior cingulate, the hippocampal formation and the basal ganglia all deal with different aspects of response inhibition. The dorsal prefrontal cortex is primarily involved in the sequencing of sub-goals, the cingulate cortex in the achievement of a range of innate goals, the hippocampus with concurrently conflicting goals, and the basal ganglia with the selection (or prevention) of an action to achieve a specific goal.

9.7 How to approach the SHS

We believe a modern theory of hippocampal function must present a picture that is consistent with the position of the hippocampal formation within each of the very many distinct neural systems of which it is a component. The temptation, of course, is to ascribe to the hippocampus a different function with respect to each of them. However, the internal anatomy of the hippocampus (Fig. 1.4D) suggests a high degree of uniformity in its processing; while its external connectivity (Appendix 4) suggests a high degree of topographic mapping (see also §9.2, Fig. 9.7).

In constructing our own theory, therefore, we have searched for fundamental cybernetic principles of operation of the hippocampus that are the same for its relations with all its afferent and efferent connections. We have also attempted to derive, for each of the several levels of the hippocampal formation, a single principle of operation that is consistent with the principles ascribed to the other levels. The apparently different psychological functions of the SHS in different situations should then derive mostly from the particular structures with which it interacts at different times rather than the operations it performs on their activity.

PRINCIPLE 10: any theory of hippocampal function should account for all the different effects of SHS disruption and all of the observed correlations of cellular activity in terms of a single consistent set of principles. It should also relate these to the known functions of the structures immediately afferent and efferent to the SHS.

9.8 The general anatomy of the SHS

If we are to relate hippocampal function to its afferents and efferents, we must first highlight some key aspects of the anatomy of the SHS and of the structures most closely related to it. In this section we will present an overview—in Chapter 10 we will discuss in more detail differences between the septal/dorsal/posterior hippocampus and temporal/ventral/anterior hippocampus.

We can trace our way (antero- or retro-gradely) ever deeper into the brain from several different starting points via a large number of independent routes all leading to the hippocampus:

- dorsal PAG–hypothalamus–amygdala–hippocampus (Chapter 6, Appendix 2)
- primary sensory systems—association cortex—parahippocampal cortex—entorhinal cortex—hippocampus (Appendix 4)
- nucleus reticularis pontis oralis—supramammillary nucleus—medial septum—hippocampus (Appendix 5)
- hypothalamus—cingulate cortex—hippocampus (Chapter 6, Appendix 3)

- primary motor cortex—supplementary motor cortex—prefrontal cortex—hippocampus (Chapter 6, Appendix 3)
- cerebellum—retrosplenial cortex—hippocampus (Appendices 3 and 5).

There are several general points to notice about this anatomy.

First (Fig. 9.8) **the SHS has important connectivity with many motor-programming areas** (highlighted in green), characterized by low-level input and high-level output, including extensive subcortical loops. The mapping of these motivation-focussed areas into the different levels and parts of the hippocampus (Fig. 9.7; e.g. Risold and Swanson, 1996) provides the only clear source of topographic organization within the hippocampal formation.

Second, the SHS sends output (often from the subiculum) to more sensory levels of many of these systems (or to polymodal association cortex) and receives input (often to the entorhinal cortex), not only from those sensory levels, but also from the more motor levels of many of those same systems. Relatively speaking, then, hippocampal links with pure sensory processing, and potentially with such memory as can be dissociated from action, are modest, although not negligible, until we look at the Papez circuit (or rather the set of parallel Papez-like circuits, Fig. 9.9).

Third, in parallel with the more direct cortical connections, the hippocampus sends long loop output through a range of onion-like layers of Papez-like circuits (§9.2.2) that allow its output to be modified by subcortical motivation information as it is recirculated to the cortex. These circuits (long and short loop) provide a substrate for complex iterative processing.

Fourth, the hippocampal formation has many levels. This led to the greatest uncertainty in the previous version of our theory and is still a matter of some speculation. A complete theory should explain the functions carried out by each of the entorhinal cortex, dentate gyrus (including CA4), CA3, CA2, CA1, subiculum, and posterior cingulate cortex—and reconcile these functions with their anatomy. The different levels are unlikely to exist simply so as to pass unaltered information on to one another; each must allow some particular transformation or integration of its inputs (compare CA3 and CA1 in Dong et al., 2021). We propose that the hippocampus is a system of logical gates that allows different types of information to progress to different points of the circuit and hence to produce (or in many cases not produce) outputs from different levels of the system subject to different conditions. We are fairly certain that the hippocampus constitutes a set of such logical gates. On the other hand, we are far from certain that our specific assignments of input values to, transformations produced by, and outputs from the different levels will prove accurate when there are sufficient new data to test our ideas directly. Our detailed specification of functions for particular components (Chapter 10) is made quite consciously, therefore, to encourage experiments able to disprove the specific details, and to make clear the nature of the theory itself.

While the mechanisms we postulate later are speculative, it should be noted that other current theories (with the sterling exception of the original O'Keefe and Nadel spatial mapping model) do not assign an integrated set of specific information processing functions to the different parts of the hippocampal formation at all. Linked to the details of the onion-like organization of, at least, the Papez-like circuits (§9.8.2, Fig. 9.9), we currently see the levels of the hippocampus as reflecting hierarchical levels of processing (and reflecting hierarchical additions during phylogeny)

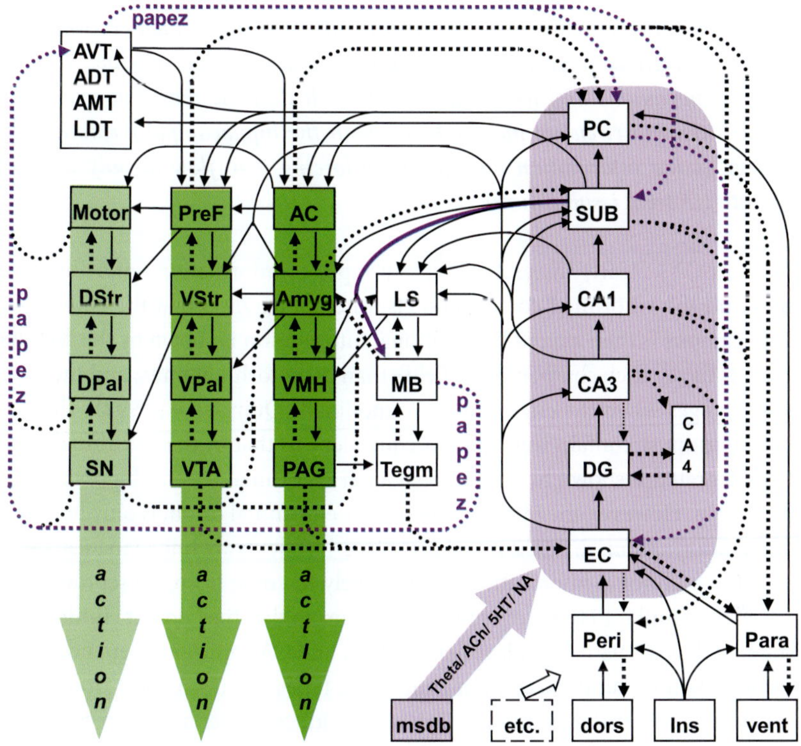

Fig. 9.8 The general organization of the hippocampal formation and its connections (see also Fig. 10.2). The hippocampal formation can be viewed as an essentially linear, unidirectional set of modules (EC, DG, CA3, CA1, SUB, PC) embedded in systems which have largely bi-directional connections. It receives (purple large arrow), as a whole (purple area), phasic RSA/'theta'-controlling GABAergic input together with cholinergic, serotonergic and noradrenergic inputs that gate or modulate the occurrence of RSA/'theta'. (DG, CA3, CA1, SUB and PC can also be viewed as receiving parallel input from the subcortical RSA/'theta' controlling systems and from EC.) CA3, CA1, SUB and PC all provide feedback to EC. The hippocampal formation is also embedded in a range of external loops of the which the Papez circuit (papez, purple lines) is the most famous example and can be viewed here as potentially involving EC, DG, CA3, CA1, SUB, LS, MB, AVT, PC thence back to EC. We view the hippocampal formation as interacting with a range of modules (oriented vertically in the diagram) each with nodes at a number of cortical and subcortical levels (shown by the rows in the diagram, where lower rows are more caudal in the brain than the higher rows). We see these modules as principally concerned with the organization of goal-directed action. (Systems such as the cerebellar circuits involved in the control of eye-blink conditioning are omitted here for simplicity, but can be viewed as having an essentially similar organization.) EC receives input from the lower stages of most of these systems and it and PC also receive input from the higher stages. EC also receives input, usually relayed by Peri and Para from the higher levels of the dorsal and ventral streams of sensory cortex and has a connectivity that allows combinations of their 'where' and 'what' information (Nilssen et al., 2019; §10.5). *Abbreviations:* AVT, anteroventral thalamus; ADT, anterodorsal thalamus; AMT, anteromedial thalamus; LDT, latero-dorsal thalamus; Motor, motor and premotor cortex; DStr, dorsal striatum; DPal, dorsal pallidum; SN, substantia nigra; PreF, prefrontal cortex; VStr, ventral striatum; VPal, ventral pallidum; VTA, ventral tegmental area; AC, anterior cingulate cortex; Amyg, amygdala; VMH, ventromedial hypothalamus; PAG,

(Contd.)

PRINCIPLE 11: Major connections of the hippocampus (like the hippocampus itself) are phylogenetically old and often provide links to systems, many of which are subcortical, directly concerned with complex motivated action. Further, the anatomy of the hippocampus and its connections is such that the most important information will tend to circulate in long loops, with the hippocampal formation as a key element gating information and generally forcing it to flow in only one direction (dentate-CA3-CA1-subiculum).

Fifth, CA1 and CA3 clearly integrate divergent types of information—arriving from both the septum and the entorhinal cortex (and elsewhere, Fig. 7.3). That the entorhinal input to the hippocampus is then altered by additional information is shown by the fact that CA1 and CA3 units have much sharper 'place field's than do entorhinal units, and they show different field changes when the environment is modified (Quirk et al., 1992). That the non-entorhinal input must contain information equivalent to that of the entorhinal input with which it is integrated is shown by the fact that, after entorhinal lesions, hippocampal place-like fields remain. However, the information of non-entorhinal origin is only loosely similar to entorhinal information, since these residual place-like fields are linked to local rather than distal cues. The additional information is most likely to come from the septum. Fornix lesions have effects similar to those of entorhinal lesions in that they do not eliminate all place fields (Miller and Best, 1980). The place fields of CA1 and CA3 appear to depend, then, on the combination of somewhat different, but congruent, types of information from the septum and the entorhinal cortex that, when they interact, produce tighter field than can either input alone. That this interaction occurs within the hippocampus proper is suggested by the fact (Kita et al., 1995) that, in monkeys, lateral septal neurones (which receive output from area CA3) are more likely to have spatially-related fields than are medial septal neurones (which provide input to area CA3). The effects on hippocampal firing repertoires of the septal or entorhinal lesions may, then, be the simple result of a reduction in the amount of information available to areas CA1 and CA3 for their computations. The lesion-induced effects are similar to the changes produced by blinding and deafening the rat (Hill and Best, 1981), and also appear to match the effects on place fields of testing rats in the dark (see Markus et al., 1994). So, CA1 and CA3 place fields depend on septo-entorhinal interactions in much the same way as we have described for non-place fields (§7.2), and that loss of either input coarsens a property akin to sensory acuity.

PRINCIPLE 12: Each separate level of the hippocampal formation represents a separate logical gate. A distinct function must be assigned to each of these gates and must account for the outflow of the resultant information from areas CA3 and subiculum, in particular.

Fig. 9.8 (*continued*)

periaqueductal grey; LS, lateral septum; MB, mammillary bodies; Tegm, dorsal and ventral tegmental nuclei; PC, posterior cingulate; SUB, subiculum; CA1, CA3, CA4, subfields of Ammon's Horn (Cornu Ammonis)—CA2 and CA4 have been omitted for simplicity but, particularly with CA2 (see Lehr et al., 2021; He et al., 2021), are functionally important and distinct; DG, dentate gyrus; EC, entorhinal cortex; Peri, perirhinal cortex; Para, parahippocampal cortex; dors, vent, dorsal and ventral streams of sensory cortex; Ins, Insula.

9.9 Long-term memory and the SHS

9.9.1 Connection building or connection pruning?

It is now generally agreed that, for very long-term memories (we think for all durations of memory), the relevant associations are located outside the hippocampal formation. The role of the hippocampal system in memory is then usually seen as involving interaction with sensory, particularly polymodal, cortex (for direct evidence, see Esteves et al., 2021). We agree that this will often be the case. But, if one equates the formation of memory with learning, subcortical areas such as the amygdala and nucleus interpositus should also be included together with neocortical areas as sites of memory formation. Whatever distinctions might be made at the psychological level, the plasticity seen in the amygdala during avoidance conditioning or in the nucleus interpositus during eyeblink conditioning does not seem to differ in any fundamental way from cortical plasticity. In many respects, then, we can see memory as being distributed throughout much of the brain.

Given this view of simple associative memory, what could be the function of the hippocampus? We rule out working memory, both because of the data reviewed in Chapter 8 and because (following Goldman-Rakic, 1992) we have attributed this function to the prefrontal cortex (§9.3; Chapter 6; for more detail, see Chapter 11, Fig. 11.5, and Appendix 3). We rule out long-term memory of all types, as this is intact in H.M. and related amnesic cases. We rule out intermediate memory, because (Chapter 8) of the presence of intrusion errors in amnesics' responses and the effects of interference. We can also rule out consolidation of at least some contextual conditioning (Gidyk et al., 2021).

We propose the following scenario. The associative rule instantiated in long-term potentiation requires that a stimulus representation of a goal be activated if any strengthening is to occur. Where only one such stimulus representation is available for conditioning, then only the connections of that stimulus can be strengthened. If, therefore, the task (e.g. in an eyeblink conditioning paradigm) is set up so that there can be no possible strengthening also of inappropriate connections (or so little possibility that no inappropriate response is generated able to compete with the one required), then memory formation can occur, without hippocampal involvement, in the region where the relevant sensory-motor connections are located as in Hebb's original (1949) model of memory. However, where the task demands become sufficiently complicated, the distributed activity in the extra-hippocampal networks will represent a number of incompatible concurrent goals. Hence, a range of different and functionally conflicting pathways could have their connections strengthened. It is the business of the hippocampal system to resolve this conflict between goals and to prevent widespread strengthening of associative links that could produce catastrophic forgetting (§8.3; McNaughton and Wickens, 2003). This will also be true with the special form of goal conflict that arises with extinction (Szadzinska et al., 2021).

> ***PRINCIPLE 13:** The hippocampal formation is at no time a memory store, intermediate or otherwise. Nor does it aid in the formation of specific strengthened connections. The primary function of the hippocampus is inhibition. In the context of memory experiments this inhibition represents the suppression of incorrect alternatives and pruning of unwanted connections and is necessary in some variants of some paradigms*

if consolidation is to result in the correct recall of only a single alternative. In effect, output from the hippocampus enhances the negative associations of inappropriate stimuli.

9.9.2 Incompatible cell assemblies and their resolution

On this view, where a set of neural links A-B-C is required in contrast to A-C-B, the hippocampus would act, during the initial formation of the A-B and B-C links, to prevent the (extremely likely) formation of the highly undesirable A-C and C-B links. The A-C and C-B links are likely because simple associative rules, like those embodied in long-term potentiation, will operate whenever items A, B and C are all concurrently present (in the environment or in active memory), as they must be if a relation between them is to be perceived. Thus, the hippocampus acts asymmetrically. It interacts with the formation of all current possible relations to suppress those that have more adverse results. That is, it *enhances the value of the negative reinforcement* that will accompany activation of the A-C or C-B links. Even in memory, then, the hippocampal formation acts to increase negative bias and, consequentially, produce inhibition.

A process of this kind has some of the flavour of lateral inhibition, but its iterative mechanism is inherently much more powerful and distinctive in producing non-linear results. Hippocampal iteration need not result in a simple 'winner-take-all' output, in which the initially most active link would be enhanced and others suppressed. The hippocampal formation will act to increase only affectively negative associations of a particular goal, and hence to inhibit that goal in a fashion unrelated to its prior level of activation. Further, the effects of the hippocampus on any particular cycle (locked to ongoing theta rhythmicity) of an iterative sequence will depend on the results of the immediately preceding cycle, which will change the weights of the inputs fed back to the hippocampal input units. Thus, the end result depends on the pattern of weights of negative associations enhanced by the hippocampus across a range of different efferent targets and would not depend on the initial level of activity in any target.

Active iteration is likely to have an additional advantage over simple lateral inhibition. The extent of the resultant inhibition can be adjusted from occasion to occasion in relation to the requirements of the task. This means both that its effects will be independent of the intensity of the individual inputs to the hippocampal formation, and that they can be gated out if this is required (hence, we believe, the requirement for long-term potentiation in the hippocampus). Hippocampal cell assemblies expand with better neural and behavioural learning (Leake et al., 2021). This suggests to us an increased suppression of competing incorrect engrams (stored elsewhere); not an expansion of the cell assembly coding the correct engram or of one indexing (e.g. Goode et al., 2020) the correct engram elsewhere (since both of these would be likely to increase the chances of catastrophic forgetting).

We have just suggested that the hippocampal formation is a device that can resolve conflicting memory representations in other structures (e.g. Esteves et al., 2021). But our earlier equation of perception with action implies that a precisely similar hippocampal operation in relation to neural networks that code for movement would have the net effect of behavioural inhibition. Although we did not detail the machinery earlier, the mechanism suggested for memory processing by the hippocampus is sufficient to support the functions already proposed for its interactions with both the defence and eyeblink conditioning systems.

The connections of the hippocampal formation with each of amygdala, cingulate cortex (and hence nucleus interpositus), prefrontal cortex and rhinal cortex can then be viewed as operating in the same basic way in which it interacts with polymodal association cortex. The hippocampus would circulate information between itself and those areas so as to sharpen peaks of activation in a way roughly equivalent to lateral inhibition in sensory systems, but with a power and sophistication equivalent to that of the global stereopsis network (Fig. 1.6) or the linguistic network Hinton et al. (Hinton et al., 1993) discussed in Chapter 1 (with, in both cases, 'clean up' units able to extract figure from ground), and a non-linearity dependent on the fact that it acts mainly to increase existing negative biases and does not interact directly with current positive biases.

PRINCIPLE 14: ***The longer-term effects of hippocampal function are achieved through the iterative circulation of information between it and its efferent targets. This processing is essentially identical whether the target is an area that processes predominantly sensory/situation or predominantly motor/motivation information. The iterative operation of the hippocampal formation is akin to the extraction of a figure from a ground and depends on amplification of affectively negative associations.***

9.9.3 The role of iteration in memory formation and consolidation

Together with the fundamentally linear flow of information within the SHS itself (§9.7), this leads us to a picture of the hippocampus as a device that circulates information iteratively through its target structures. This is reminiscent of the prefrontal circuitry involved in the 'rehearsal' that constitutes working/active memory (see §9.4, Appendix 3, and McNaughton and Vann, 2022). But we believe the 'Papez circuit' has essentially opposite functions: prefrontal-posterior iteration *maintaining* neural activity in the short term and hippocampal-neocortical iteration *suppressing* neural activity (albeit selectively), particularly in the long term. Critically, even simple iteration in parallel networks has immense computational power, that can be expressed at multiple levels. Iteration, *per se,* was discussed extensively in §1.9, with Marr and Poggio's global stereopsis algorithm as an exemplar (Fig. 1.6).

So, a possible model for the operation of the hippocampus is suggested by *analogy* with the models of global stereopsis and language processing discussed in Chapter 1. In iterative processing models, input is clamped onto a network. Iteration of the information around a circuit allows a figure to be extracted from a ground, or a correct item to be selected from a pandemonium, in a process that progressively restricts the output from the network. The iterative links of the hippocampus with all its closest neighbours would, with suitable connections, allow it to 'sharpen up' the encoding of stimulus information or its recoding during consolidation, and hence to resolve the conflict between the alternative possibilities. Note that this processing would be required in the encoding case only when there is interference; and in the consolidation case only transiently while the engram is being stabilized (for an example with goal processing, see Bradfield et al., 2020).

Further, this overall class of processing will occur *concurrently* in hierarchical, onion-like, 'Papez' circuits (Fig. 9.9) that can apply quick and dirty or slow and sophisticated processing as required (McNaughton and Vann, 2022) as well as in the more direct hippocampal-cortical circuits and via their bidirectional connections with, e.g. nucleus reuniens (Ferraris et al., 2018; Angulo-Garcia et al., 2020; Ferraris et al., 2021; Griffin, 2021; Rahman et al., 2021).

This leads to:

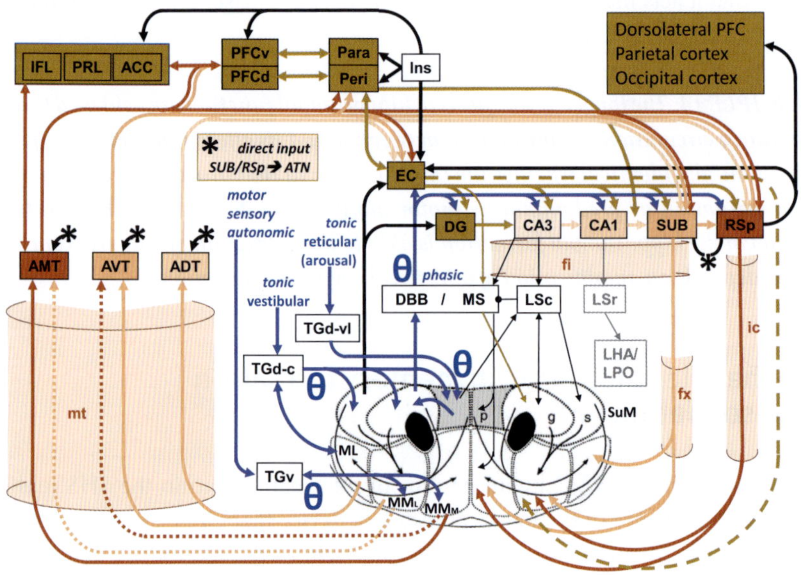

Fig. 9.9 Overview of long and short loop connections from the hippocampus via mammillary area to the frontal cortex and back present in mammals ranging from rodents to primates. The mammillary bodies (MB) and supramammillary area (SuM) have aligned medial, mediolateral, and lateral parts. MB targets prefrontal and anterior cingulate cortex, which target the hippocampal formation, completing the Papez circuit. Tonic arousing reticular input to medial (p = parvicellular [28]) SuM is converted to phasic theta rhythmicity (θ), passed to mediolateral (g = grandicellular) SuM, then diagonal band of Broca (DBB)/medial septum (MS) complex then hippocampal formation. Lateral (s = shell) SuM project to entorhinal cortex (EC). The fimbria (fi), fornix (fx), and internal capsule (ic) return hippocampal formation output to SuM/MB in onion-like, nested loops. EC, dentate gyrus (DG), CA3, CA1, subiculum (SUB), and retrosplenial cortex (RSp) connect unidirectionally. Successive loops are similar, but outside loops have greater delays and more highly processed information. There is a similar 'onion' with mammillothalomic tract (mt) output from MB and output from AMT/AVT/ADT to infralimbic (IFL), prelimbic (PRL) and anterior cingulate (ACC) cortex. Dorsal and ventral prefrontal (PRFd, PRFv) then perirhinal (Peri) and parahippocampal (Para) cortex complete the Papez circuit in entorhinal cortex (EC). We have not included, e.g., the AMT-CA1 connection [129], to keep the fundamental architecture of the loop circuits clear. Abbreviations: ADT, AMT, AVT = anterior thalamus, dorsal, medial, ventral, respectively. ML, MML, MMM = mamillary nucleus, lateral, medial pars lateralis, medial pars medialis, respectively. Figure and legend from McNaughton and Vann (2022).

PRINCIPLE 15: Iteration round external and internal loops (Fig. 9.9), carried out in parallel across multiple, hierarchical, levels in the hippocampus allows for functionally sophisticated output as a result of very simple, albeit repetitive, computations.

9.10 Mismatch detection and the SHS

Conflict between goals, in the simplest sense, will occur when two incompatible goals are concurrently present. We will present a model in which the hippocampus (or strictly its interaction with its target structures) can detect, as well as resolve, such conflict. There is reason also to believe that the hippocampus detects the more subtle conflict that occurs when there is a mismatch between observed and expected events. In all these cases, the conflict is anticipatory of action—and is predictive (Stachenfeld et al., 2017). It is not the 'outcome conflict' generated by feedback from an incorrect response (Botvinick, 2007; Yeung et al., 2004; Botvinick et al., 1999).

The idea of mismatch detection is inherent in Vinogradova's (1975) view that the SHS mediates the orienting response and its habituation (Appendix 6). This view is close to the more general one proposed by Douglas (1967) that the hippocampus gates out redundant stimuli from the control of behaviour. Both these views are in many respects complementary to the view that the hippocampus is involved in motor components of behavioural inhibition (Kimble, 1969).

Vinogradova's view gains support from the association of low-frequency RSA/'theta' with responses to novelty and her (Vinogradova, 1975) observations of hippocampal and lateral septal unit responses to novel and familiar stimuli. These show that the SHS receives the information it would require if it were indeed to organize *orienting behaviour* or eliminate responses to unimportant stimuli. On the other hand, only a few of the findings in lesioned animals support this specific position, e.g. the loss of Kamin's blocking effect (Solomon, 1977; Rickert et al., 1978) or of latent inhibition (Ackil et al., 1969; Weiss et al., 1974; Solomon and Moore, 1975; see Buhusi et al., 1998 for review). Indeed, a critical point against the most substantive version of Vinogradova's hypothesis is that there is very little evidence of change in simple orienting responses or their habituation after damage to the SHS (Appendix 8); and it seems more that the lesions release from inhibition motor responses to novel stimuli (as they do to stimuli of other kinds).

It seems likely, then, that the apparently simple neuronal habituation described by Vinogradova (1975) underlies something more complex than simple habituation at the behavioural level. This inference is strengthened by a consideration of the experiments on Kamin's blocking effect. The normal animal fails to develop an association to a second CS if this is added to a first one that already predicts the same UCS (Mackintosh, 1974); but animals with lesions of the hippocampal formation respond to the added CS (Solomon, 1977; Rickert et al., 1978; Buhusi et al., 1998). This is probably not due to a simple delay in the habituation of the response to the first CS, since Rickert et al. (1978) failed to alter the effect of hippocampal lesions by doubling the number of trials of training on the first CS. It is possible that, in the normal animal, blocking depends on a process that one might call 'instructed habituation'; that is, as a result of the discovery, on the first compound-stimulus trial, that reinforcement conditions have not changed, the redundant stimulus is identified as one to which attention need not be paid (Mackintosh, 1978). Thus, hippocampal lesions may disrupt this more complex type of habituation. This hypothesis is consistent with Douglas's (1967) description of the hippocampal formation as a device for gating out stimuli that are not predictive of reinforcement.

Let us consider precisely how, according to Vinogradova, the hippocampus could perform this function. We summarize her position in Appendix 6 (see also McNaughton & Bannerman, 2024): it is that the hippocampal formation receives sensory information by two independent routes. Stimuli encoded by the reticular formation are relayed by the medial septum to the hippocampus (where they represent a highly general alerting signal that has lost much of the specific qualities of the initiating stimulus). The *same* stimuli are processed by the cortex and, *if a model of the stimuli is already present in the cortex*, the actual occurrence of the predicted stimulus is also sent via the entorhinal cortex to the hippocampus, where, according to Vinogradova, long-term potentiation of the perforant path input to the dentate gyrus prevents further processing by the latter structure. On this view, the hippocampus acts in this case as a comparator of observed with expected input. If there is input via the medial septum but not entorhinal cortex, the stimulus can be classified as novel. Equally, if there is input from entorhinal cortex but not from the septum, an expected stimulus can be classified as absent. Given either type of mismatch, output is required from the hippocampus. Note that, while the input from the medial septum here permits the hippocampus to detect novelty (and hence to detect potential conflict with ongoing motor programs), we need not regard it as a signal of novelty *per se*. Rather, in keeping with the reticular origin of the information, it should be viewed merely as a signal that some important stimulus has occurred and, as we emphasize in Appendix 6, that some response may be required. The entorhinal signal can then be viewed as indicating that an appropriate response will be forthcoming, and the devaluing of a redundant stimulus would be equivalent to the suppression of the competing responses to which it might otherwise give rise.

Although this is not emphasized by Vinogradova, the septal signal must be of a fairly crude type, as the medial septal area has very few neurones with which to encode fine distinctions and, moreover, sends its output fairly diffusely to all fields of the hippocampal formation, including the entorhinal and posterior cingulate cortices. Indeed, given the known properties of the reticular system and the reaction of the RSA/'theta' system to stimulation of the midbrain, it is possible that the septal signal carries no specific information at all. Certainly, replacement of lost theta rhythmicity without replacing specific neuronal coding is sufficient to restore lost function (McNaughton et al., 2006b). Rather, at all times, the input from the reticular formation via the septum can be seen as providing an indication of the general level of activation summed across a number of subcortical systems. However, given the topographic organization of the septal input to the hippocampus, the topographic mapping of the hippocampus into hypothalamic 'goal space' (Fig. 9.7), and the detailed variations in the firing patterns of individual septal neurones, it seems likely that some aspect of goal type or at least valence is encoded as well. In a novel situation, therefore, the hippocampus receives information that something is going on (and in essence how important that something is), but has no information as to what. This discrepancy, if unchecked, results in the activation of behaviour designed to make good the information deficiency. Operation of the output from the subiculum via nucleus accumbens, and more directly, to thalamocortical sensory processing systems, as indicated in the previous section, may in part underlie this reaction pattern. However, the elicitation of information-seeking behaviour more generally appears to depend on the ascending supramammillary-medial septum pathway (Kesner et al., 2022).

The Douglas-Vinogradova 'attentional' view of the generation of behavioural inhibition by the hippocampus is closely related to two other hypotheses.

The first is the hypothesis that the SHS mediates responses to omission of expected gain (Gray, 1970b), depending on omission of an expected stimulus, this hypothesis is probably not fully dissociable logically from Vinogradova's. Empirically, Amsel (1972) has provided a strong case for the view that novelty and gain omission elicit essentially similar responses. Since these responses include inhibition of ongoing behaviour and increased attention to the environment, the gain omission hypothesis is equally close to the motor and attentional versions of a general behavioural inhibition theory.

The second close relative of the Douglas-Vinogradova position is Gaffan's (1972) recognition memory hypothesis of hippocampal function (§8.2.4). Since this proposes that the hippocampus is a mechanism for detecting novelty/familiarity, it is at first sight indistinguishable from Vinogradova's orienting reflex hypothesis. It can be distinguished, however, from Douglas's (1967) position because, according to Gaffan, the hippocampus is involved in the recognition of familiarity, whether this results in the production or the inhibition of responses, whereas Douglas supposes it to be concerned only with the latter. The data (Chapter 8; Appendix 8) give greater support to Douglas: hippocampal memory deficits consist largely of false positives rather than false negatives, and these are heavily influenced by sources of interference in the experimental task. In particular, trial-unique delayed object discriminations are intact after hippocampal lesions despite their requirement for a relative familiarity discrimination.

Gaffan's concept of recognition memory is very close to Olton's working memory hypothesis (§8.2.2). While we reject both, there is an important feature that they share, which sets them apart from Vinogradova's simpler treatment of novelty, and with which we agree: that is, their concern with renewable lists. These consist of a sequence of items that recur, require a response when they first occur, then for a period of time or during certain experimental circumstances do not require a response, and then again require a response on some later occasion. (An example is the radial arm maze, in which during one trial the animal needs to visit each arm in turn, without re-entry into any given arm, and is then required to repeat this process on a later trial.) In Gaffan's case, renewable lists are a feature of experimental practice, rather than, as in Olton's, central to the theory; but it is the experimental results that we must accommodate. Renewable lists require the subject to answer, not just the question 'is this stimulus novel or familiar?', but also 'is this stimulus more or less familiar than that one?' or 'is it *relatively* novel (within the last day, hour, or few minutes)?'. Thus, if the hippocampus is the organ responsible for successful performance in tasks of this kind, it must be given additional properties besides those required for its higher-order control of habituation. We must ask, therefore, what is it about lists, and especially renewable lists that require recognition memory as defined by Gaffan (1977a); (Gaffan, 1977c), which provokes a particularly profound and enduring deficit in the performance of hippocampal animals (Olton et al., 1979b; Olton and Pappas, 1979)?

A natural link exists between Gaffan's recognition memory hypothesis and earlier research on the orienting reflex (Sokolov, 1960). This research showed that, although the response to a repeated neutral stimulus habituates, habituation can be prevented for an indefinite period by turning the stimulus into a Pavlovian CS. Note also that this treatment guarantees that the stimulus continues to evoke unit responses in the hippocampal formation (Appendix 6). Observations such as these imply that the habituation of the orienting reflex (both behavioural and 'hippocampal') is under higher controls that are sensitive to the associative significance of stimuli. These controls might be of cortical origin (Sokolov, 1960) or they might form part of the hippocampal circuitry itself; and there are of course other possibilities.

Performance on a renewable list, of the kind used by Gaffan or Olton, might depend, then, on a type of higher nervous control over a hippocampal circuit whose basic function is that of mediating the production or habituation of orienting responses under simpler conditions. For this kind of control to work, it would be necessary that habituation of the orienting reflex could be both cancelled (at each new presentation of a previously encountered list) and expedited (when an item within a given list presentation has been sufficiently processed for the current trial). It is possible that the second of these processes is also responsible for 'instructed habituation' in the Kamin blocking effect, as discussed earlier. By analogy, therefore, we can call the first process (cancellation of habituation) 'instructed dishabituation'.

In all of the above, matching of septal input with a 'model' coming from entorhinal cortex can be seen as preventing the behavioural inhibition, orienting, and information gathering that would otherwise occur. This implies

> ***PRINCIPLE 13: Matching input from the medial septal area and entorhinal cortex will normally result in output (or lack thereof) which, in effect, constitutes a 'familiar-ignore' signal. Mismatch (either septal input in the absence of entorhinal, or entorhinal in the absence of septal) will result in information gathering behaviour to resolve the discrepancy.***

Note that familiarity, *qua* familiarity, is encoded elsewhere. Also note that this familiar-ignore signal, while it is fundamental for at least some aspects of hippocampal processing, represents a combined septal-entorhinal *input* to the hippocampus proper. Hence it cannot reflect the major purpose of the circuitry of this structure. The entorhinal cortex, then, allows for instructed habituation, latent inhibition and for at least some aspects of the partial reinforcement extinction effect (which can be viewed as a special case of latent inhibition to the stimuli of gain omission; see Appendix 9 for a discussion of the relevant data). However, a system capable of forcing response programming mechanisms to ignore all familiar stimuli could itself be a liability; it will require suppression when the stimuli are, in fact, important. We turn to this problem in the following section.

9.11 Neuromodulatory systems that gate the SHS

Even when viewed as a means of reducing interference between conflicting goals rather than as a full-blown memory system, our description of the hippocampal formation has provided a highly cognitive, memory-oriented view of the hippocampal formation. However, 'goals' and 'plans' are not affectively neutral. It is time, therefore, to reaffirm the links of the hippocampus with emotion, and to consider the contribution of the diffuse ascending subcortical systems to its operations.

As reviewed in Chapter 6 (§6.9–6.15; for more detail on the monoamines see Appendix 10), ascending neuromodulatory inputs to the hippocampus (serotonin, noradrenaline, dopamine, histamine, acetylcholine, relaxin-3) originate in small nuclei that send massively divergent collaterals to much of the forebrain. Chapter 6 attempted to identify the *common*, fairly simple, signal that each neuromodulator sends to all of its target structures, and to account for the different uses to which this is put by the different targets. In particular, we noted that the serotonergic input appears to shift control from fast reflexive systems to slower 'planful' systems (Carver et al., 2008) and so, for example, has opposite effects on the dorsal PAG and the amygdala—helping coordinate the hierarchical elements of the defence system (Chapter 6). We will argue that all the neuromodulatory systems are concerned, but in somewhat different ways, with the focusing of 'attention' or, better, with reduction in signal-to-noise ratios within the SHS. We will also argue for a similar modulatory function for the descending habenular control of all these systems (which we argued represented important feedback control) and, but in the temporal domain, for the ascending RSA/'theta' system, particularly its GABAergic component (§6.16–6.17).

Where the simple associative significance of stimuli is the crucial feature, the noradrenergic input to the hippocampus appears to be important (Appendix 10). Thus, this sends to the hippocampus a signal that indicates that an attractor, repulsor, or novel stimulus is present. In all these cases, the stimulus must be treated as important and its occurrence must be able to interrupt ongoing motor programs. Simple *occurrence* of an important stimulus need not generate output from the hippocampus. With an attractor, we note in Appendix 10 that input from the locus coeruleus could prevent input from the entorhinal cortex from affecting subsequent elements of the hippocampal trisynaptic circuit. Thus, it is only an *unexpected* attractor, or unexpected omission of an expected attractor that will affect later stages of hippocampal processing—linked, in particular, to increased or decreased, respectively, moderate-latency dopamine input[7] from the 'Reward Prediction Error'[8] system (Schultz, 1998; Schultz, 2016). The same requirement for unexpectedness will be true, of course, of the capacity of a novel neutral stimulus to produce hippocampal output, linked to short-latency dopamine release (Redgrave and Gurney, 2006), which does not distinguish between different affective valences (Schultz, 2016).

Repulsors, require rather different treatment. The noradrenergic input to the hippocampus appears (Appendix 10) functionally more concerned with gain and novelty, while the serotonergic input appears more concerned with loss, despite the fact that their final effects on hippocampal electrophysiology seem fairly similar and neither is tied to a particular affective valence (see next). Here, we should notice an asymmetry. It is possible to present a CS for loss (CS-LOSS+; see Chapter 3 for terminology) in the absence of prior conditioning; however, a CS for gain omission (CS-GAIN−) can be presented only against a prior conditioning history of gain. The hippocampus, therefore, needs to be able to distinguish between presentation of gain and loss. While it could do so via cortical inputs, it might do so also by comparison of noradrenergic and serotonergic inputs. Thus, both loss and gain activate the former but, since loss but not gain activates the latter, the ambiguity can be resolved.

This brings us to the issue of the distinction between CS-LOSS + and CS-LOSS− (Chapter 3). The serotonergic input to the hippocampus is from collaterals of neurones that innervate, among other structures, the PAG and amygdala. The information it carries, therefore, must be fairly nonspecific. In the case of the PAG, release of serotonin blocks functional output, whereas in the amygdala and hippocampus such release increases it. This

[7] From distinct cell populations (Liu et al., 2022).

[8] As discussed in Chapter 3, we prefer to avoid the word reward because of the ambiguities it creates. But, in this case, it is too embedded in the relevant literature to avoid.

differentiated pattern of change is consistent with the requirement to inhibit undirected escape when directed escape or avoidance is possible (Chapter 6).

What, however, of conjoint serotonergic input to the hippocampus and the amygdala? Whether this input is essentially inhibitory, excitatory, or increases the signal-to-noise ratio, it is only of concern to the hippocampus if it is associated with a CS-LOSS + and not a CS-LOSS–. Here we can postulate a function for the link between the amygdala and the hippocampus. Serotonergic input, as suggested by Graeff (1994), signals the anticipation of an aversive event (CS-LOSS + *or* CS-LOSS–) to both hippocampus and amygdala (or, better, it signals the readiness to respond to whatever event is currently predicted, while the amygdala codes the aversive nature of the event; see Appendix 10). In the presence of a CS-LOSS–, the amygdala will be activated to produce an avoidance response and can signal this to the hippocampus. From the point of view of the hippocampus, then, CS-LOSS + could, in principle, be signalled by input from the raphe, which lacks concurrent input from the amygdala. However, a more likely scenario is that CS-LOSS + will be signalled by concurrent activation of the amygdala and some other area that is activated to produce an incompatible approach response. The hippocampus can then act to inhibit this approach response.

The rather glib terms attractor, repulsor, and novel stimuli that we have applied to the noradrenergic and serotonergic systems, respectively, need closer inspection. First, we should note the non-specificity implied. In the noradrenergic case, we presumed that the hippocampus (or any other target structure) could not differentiate between the three different relevant types of important event on the basis of this input alone. Even in the serotonergic case, the small number of neurones in the raphe suggests that there will be little differentiation between different classes of negative reinforcer; and we argued that it is planfulness in general, not aversion, which is being coded. We are clearly, therefore, dealing with modulatory systems rather than ones that carry specific information. The supramammillary system may be a partial exception, with a capacity to signal contextual and social novelty via distinct output systems (Chen et al., 2020).

We have also been talking as if the ascending inputs to the SHS (and the amygdala, which also receives both noradrenergic and serotonergic input) were simple unidirectional inputs. However, the key architectural feature of the SHS and the structures closely related to it is their capacity for iterative processing (§9.2.2). We have already discussed the general properties of such iterative architectures; and will discuss in Chapter 10 the specific properties of this architecture in the context of the SHS. For the present we should note that, while the monoaminergic inputs may carry signals *resulting from* attraction, repulsion, and novelty, they should not be perceived as signalling attraction, repulsion, or novelty as such. Rather, their capacity to *increase signal-to-noise ratios* should be seen as setting parameter values at various points in the hierarchical iterative loops that have the SHS as a key set of nodes. So, they determine what information these loops preferentially process and in what way. Thus, for example, the monoaminergic afferents might allow other inputs more specifically related to the particular eliciting stimulus to have a greater control over behaviour than they would otherwise be able to exert.

In Chapter 6, we pointed out that lesions of the amygdala impair active as well as passive avoidance, while hippocampal lesions impair only the latter. This is best accounted for by the notion that the amygdala is not only the source of action in the form of avoidance, but also the source of perception of threat. It can be viewed, then, as passing to the hippocampus highly specific information, which the hippocampus then uses for inhibitory purposes.

Equally, the hippocampus could be seen as passing back to the amygdala cleaned up versions of the same information, which would have the net effect of increasing avoidance responses in cases where conflict is present. Thus, the specific signals of negative reinforcers (and probably, in some cases, of positive reinforcers) can come to the hippocampus from the amygdala, while activity in the noradrenergic and serotonergic systems reflects increases in more general aspects of 'sensory attention' and 'planfulness', respectively, without which hippocampal processing cannot operate efficiently.

> *PRINCIPLE 14: The neuromodulatory inputs to the SHS provide largely undifferentiated signals (perhaps translatable in psychological terms as 'arousal' or 'attention' of different types). Each signal flags a different type of event or requirement.* ***They alter various aspects of the signal-to-noise ratio within the SHS, within the defence system as a whole, and among the hierarchical iterative processing circuits that pass through the SHS.***

9.12 Hormones and the SHS

The aminergic systems can, in one sense, be viewed as neurohormonal systems. That is, they release hormone-like compounds (noradrenaline is released by the adrenals also; and the noradrenergic system releases noradrenaline into the cortex via varicosities more than conventional synapses, Descarries et al., 1977); and, as we have just argued, they have information-poor, modulatory functions.

The role of hormones is similar—but with an involvement of the hippocampus in their control, surprising were it to be a purely memory-related structure. Indeed, the hippocampal

> role in memory may be ancillary to physiological regulation. Molecular studies demonstrate that the hippocampus is a primary target for ligands that reflect body physiology, including ion balance and blood pressure, immunity, pain, reproductive status, satiety and stress. Hippocampal receptors are functional, probably accessible to their ligands, and mediate physiological and cognitive changes. This argues that an early role of the hippocampus may have been in sensing soluble molecules (termed here 'enteroception') in blood and cerebrospinal fluid, perhaps reflecting a common evolutionary origin with the olfactory system ('exteroception'). Functionally, hippocampal enteroception may reflect feedback control; evidence is reviewed that the hippocampus modulates body physiology, including the activity of the hypothalamus–pituitary–adrenal axis, blood pressure, immunity, and reproductive function. It is suggested that the hippocampus operates, in parallel with the amygdala, to modulate body physiology in response to cognitive stimuli. Hippocampal outputs are predominantly inhibitory on downstream neuroendocrine activity; increased synaptic efficacy in the hippocampus (e.g. long-term potentiation) could facilitate throughput inhibition. This may have implications for the role of the hippocampus and long-term potentiation in memory.
>
> (Lathe, 2001, p. 205)

The role of the hippocampus in hormonal control has been extensively studied in relation to corticosterone/cortisol (CORT). As reviewed by McEwen and Akil (2020), the

Table 9.2 Partial list of metabolites, hormones, ligands, and other factors interacting with the hippocampal formation. Receptors, ions, and likely neurotransmitters are not included (adapted from Lathe, 2001)

Acidic fibroblast growth factor	Glucocorticoid (cortisol, corticosterone)	PACAP
Activin	Glucose	Plasmin
Adrenaline (epinephrine)	Gonadotrophin-releasing hormone	Platelet activating factor
Aldosterone	Growth hormone	Pregnenolone
Angiotensin	Heparin-binding neurotrophic factor	Progesterone
Atrial natriuretic peptide	Hepatocyte growth/scatter factor	Prolactin
Basic fibroblast growth factor	Inhibin	Prostacylin
BCA/BLC	Insulin	Prostaglandin
Bombesin	Insulin-like growth factor (IGF-I, IGF-II)	RANTES family
Bradykinin	Interferon (rat)	Relaxin
Cannabinoids	Interleukin (IL-1, IL-2, IL-3, IL-6, IL-8)	Renin
Carbon dioxide	IL-1 receptor antagonist (IL-1Ra)	SDF1
Cholecystokinin	Leptin (Ob)	Secretin
Complement C3a, C5a	Luteinizing hormone	Somatostatin
Corticotrophin-like peptide	Melatonin	Testosterone
Corticotrophin-releasing factor	Midkine	Thrombin
Dehydroepiandrosterone	MIP (-1β, -3β)	Thyroid hormone
Fractalin	Neurokinin	Thyrotrophin-releasing hormone
Galanin	Neurotensin	Transferrin
Gastrin	Neurotrophins (BDNF)	TRH potentiating peptide (PS4)
Gastrin-releasing peptide	Nociceptin	Tumour necrosis factor
Gastric inhibitory polypeptide	Oestrogen (oestradiol)	Vasoactive intestinal polypeptide
Glucagon	Oxytocin	Vitamin D
Glucagon-like peptide		

hippocampus is rich in glucocorticoid receptors; and activation of these receptors causes output, via the bed nucleus of the stria terminalis, to suppress expression of corticotropin releasing factor mRNA in the paraventricular nucleus, a key centre for stress control. Thus 'environmental and psychosocial factors that disrupt the hippocampus can also lead to excessive levels of glucocorticoids, which can in turn further damage the hippocampus' (p. 14, see also their Figure 2)—making the hippocampus a key locus for stress related disorders (see, e.g. Sapolsky, 2004). This limbic control of the hypothalamic-pituitary-adrenal axis is phylogenetically old—present in a homologous form in fish (Nagpal et al., 2019).

The hippocampus is clearly not just a stress controller, but also involved in a much wider range of motivation-related systems. Glucocorticoids are just one of a wide range of factors with hippocampal involvement (Table 9.2).

> *PRINCIPLE 15:* ***The SHS is a key detector and controller of hormonal systems and particularly stress. Its current functions will be expansions of this primordial role in physiological regulation driven by the subsequent development of the neocortex.***

9.13 Postscript

We have now enunciated a series of principles that we believe are solidly based on the available data and against which, therefore, all theories should be judged. While these place severe limits on the assumptions and machinery (§9.2.2) of a theory, they are not sufficient to provide a theory in and of themselves. There are also clearly relevant areas, like symbolic processing, where we have not attempted to produce such principles in relation to the SHS and would plead 'insufficient data.' 'The ability to use symbols is a defining feature of human intelligence. However, neuroscience has yet to explain the fundamental neural circuit mechanisms for flexibly representing and manipulating abstract concepts' (Do and Hasselmo, 2021, p. 1). In the next chapter, therefore, we develop our own theory through the addition of some further assumptions to the principles outlined earlier.

10
A theory of the septo-hippocampal system (SHS)

In Chapter 1, we promised a theory of anxiety that would flow out of a theory of the SHS. Given the complexity of the SHS, this might seem to have put the cart before the horse. But, much of this neural complexity involves parallel mechanisms (particularly multi-nodal loops, e.g. §9.9.3), all of which serve the same class of purposes. Moreover, a neural systems approach resolves the problems of varying definitions of anxiety (§1.2; McNaughton, 2018). So, our theory is simply that the SHS resolves *conflicts between concurrent goals*; with this resolution most obviously representing anxiety when an attractor goal overlaps with a repulsor, and least obviously when memory of a correct goal suffers interference from memory of an incorrect one. Here we will flesh out this summary with detailed mechanisms.

The SHS receives input from neocortical (planning circuits—Chapter 11) and subcortical (survival circuits—Chapter 6) areas concerned with goals, not simple acts or actions (Chapter 11). If more than one goal is concurrently highly activated and none predominant, the SHS detects conflict; returns to the active areas a signal that blocks current behavioural output; and increases repulsion. Where a strong attractor is counterbalanced by a strong repulsor (e.g. previous association of the attractor situation with delivery of shock), repulsion will increase. This is most obvious with approach-avoidance conflict.

With competing positive goals, anticipatory frustration (from attractor omission) will create repulsion, which will increase—although uncertainty will also have a role. In sum, prepotent behaviours (including escape and avoidance) will be inhibited but repulsion favoured via an increase in negative bias (Fig. 1.7).

This process of conflict detection and increased goal inhibition continues, with iterative/progressive memory scanning, until the conflict is resolved and the animal approaches an attractor or retreats from a repulsor. Where information in memory is insufficient to quickly resolve the conflict (i.e. all iteratively updated goals remain with their output blocked), the SHS elicits slower external-information-gathering behaviours (e.g. exploration, risk assessment).

On this view, an amnesic subject with SHS damage is failing to assign sufficient negative valence to unwanted alternatives and hence failing to eliminate incorrect (retrieval) goals (Chapter 8). A cue will face the subject (either explicitly/recognition or implicitly/recall) with alternative goals. In the recall case, both specific retrieval cues and their context can act on links created by Hebbian association to activate a number of goal representations including those that would have been correct on previous trials. 'Goal inhibition' here is a filter that allows only one of the pandemonium of alternatives, each demanding attention, to control behaviour. In our theory, a balance between the strongest competing tendencies of any origin (including species-specific competing responses) will render any task sensitive to malfunction of the SHS, while a predominance of one goal over others will render a task insensitive,

The Neuropsychology of Anxiety, Third Edition. Neil McNaughton and Jeffrey A. Gray, Oxford University Press.
 DOI: 10.1093/oso/9780198843313.003.0010

whatever the nominal psychological class of paradigm to which the experimenter supposes the task belongs.

The disturbance experienced in generalized anxiety disorder is the reverse of the consequences of hippocampal damage (see Chapter 11). The associations of stimuli *that elicit a goal conflict* are assigned *excessive* negative valence. In particular, cases of approach-avoidance conflict have the balance shifted in the avoidance direction. More colloquially (and in agreement with the data; see Chapter 13), the subject's perception of threat is increased. From this perspective, the principal clinical effect of anxiolytic drugs is to decrease the assignment of negative valence and hence decrease perceived threat. It is an important feature of our theory that this decrease will normally take some time to become fully effective, since previously acquired negative associations have, first, to be extinguished. The apparent immediate clinical effect of benzodiazepines probably represents a special case where temporary euphoriant and muscle relaxant actions mask the lack of a truly anxiolytic effect (Chapter 4, §4.4; Appendix 1). Note also that the effects of hyperfunction in the SHS will be evident only in cases in which there is in fact conflict, i.e. a source of threat that has to be approached, not when active avoidance (motivated by pure fear) is engaged, as in simple phobias.

Despite over 20 years of research since the second edition, the theory still reflects work in progress and is still necessarily incomplete. Detailed mechanisms proposed in the second edition have here been adjusted to new data; more adjustment will be necessary in another 20 years. Important details are still all largely unknown, such as: 1) the extent to which novel and classical anxiolytics differ because of muscle relaxant and euphoriant side effects of the classical anxiolytics, or because of the corticosteroid-releasing side effects of the novel anxiolytics; 2) the precise number and type of gates within (and outputs from) the SHS; 3) the behavioural functions of specific components of the system, such as the output from CA1; and, indeed, 4) the detailed anatomy of crucial parts of the system, such as much of the ascending theta control network. So, our proposed detailed mechanisms are often inference or guesswork, and other schemes could be built of the same general type.

Nonetheless, in all key respects the theory is still fundamentally that of the first edition—which itself retained roots in much older ideas (see McNaughton, 2011, for historical review). We still see the SHS as, in Simonov's lapidary phrase, 'an organ of hesitation and doubt'. The primary business of the SHS is still to act as a comparator; although we now see this comparator function occurring at more levels than before and in a simpler form. The most significant functional output from the SHS is still 'behavioural inhibition'; although we now prefer to term this 'goal inhibition' and have made the links with memory more explicit and increased the emphasis on information gathering and goal processing. The SHS still represents the core of the (renamed) Goal Inhibition System (GIS); although in the second edition we altered the precise weightings of some of the inputs (e.g. downgrading the medial septum and upgrading the dorsal noradrenergic bundle in relation to frustration). The SHS is, also, still the final common path through which anxiolytic drugs, as a chemically disparate class, produce the majority of their effects; with the second edition adding, e.g. the amygdala as where anxiolytics can alter the 'increment arousal' and 'negative bias' outputs of the GIS; and the current edition adding areas like the PAG (§6.2; Silva and McNaughton, 2019) and insula (§11.7).

Overall, our theory has stood for over four decades. It accounts for the role of the SHS in memorial tasks as well as do the most recently formulated memory theories; and (uniquely) uses the same fundamental mechanisms to account for the role of the SHS in non-memorial tasks. It accounts also for the fact that all currently known clinically effective anxiolytic drugs (including many recently discovered ones) impair SHS function. No other theory of the SHS or of anxiety has this breadth and depth.

10.1 The theory: some basic assumptions

The theory did not start with all the ideas just outlined. We gathered many small pieces of information, considered many alternatives and built up extensive dossiers (Gray, 1977; Gray and McNaughton, 1983; McNaughton and Mason, 1980; Gray, 1971; Gray, 1975) that provided evidence for and against particular points of view. This continued for the publication of the second edition (Gray, 1987b; Gray and McNaughton, 2000, see Appendixes 1–10, reprinted with the 3rd edition) and since (McNaughton and Corr, 2004; Pan and McNaughton, 2004; McNaughton et al., 2007; Mitchell et al., 2008; Corr and McNaughton, 2012; Stevenson and McNaughton, 2013; McNaughton et al., 2016; Frost and McNaughton, 2017; Silva and McNaughton, 2019; McNaughton and Vann, 2022). It has been like living in a detective novel, trying to decide whodunit, or rather what it—the SHS—does. As in all the best detective stories, the real culprit will fully emerge only when we have constructed a theory to account for 'all' of the evidence—which remains a moving target. Since our theory remains unconventional, let us begin where the detective always begins, by eliminating some of 'the usual suspects'. This will provide context for our specific proposals.

10.1.1 Consolidation?

The first suspect to come to the detective's notice is usually innocent. Here, it is Milner's hypothesis that the hippocampus is a store where memories are actively consolidated (Milner, 1970; Milner, 1971). As discussed in detail in Chapter 8, this is not consistent with the nature of the animal and human deficits in recall or recognition after hippocampal damage. These appear to result from catastrophic hypermnesia rather than amnesia (McNaughton and Wickens, 2003). From this we derive the first assumption for our theory.

> *ASSUMPTION 1*[1]*: **there is no long-term storage of information in the SHS. The SHS may seem an intermediate store (Rawlins, 1985; Cohen and Eichenbaum, 1993; Inostroza and Born, 2013) but this is a side effect of its interactions with other areas of the brain where it normally ensures that incorrect items are not retrieved or stored concurrently with correct items during the intermediate phases of consolidation.***

Thus, the SHS is not required once the requisite connections in these other areas have been consolidated, nor is it necessary for consolidation that is uncomplicated by interference. This view sits comfortably both with what is currently known about synaptic plasticity and with theories of memory that share Hebb's (1949; and Lashley's, see Nadel and Maurer, 2020) general approach to the neural basis of associative learning. Importantly, both a percept and its

[1] A number of 'assumptions' in Chapter 10 of the previous edition that were speculative are now substantiated and have been moved to the current Chapter 9 and converted to principles.

recall at all durations activate part or whole of a single cell assembly (for a related recent view, see Gilboa and Moscovitch, 2021). Its active memory ('working' memory) is supported by recurrent loops (Fig. 11.5) and the capacity to retrieve from long-term memory results from prior plastic changes in inputs to the assembly, which is located outside the SHS.

10.1.2 Voluntary movement?

Another suspect that can be rapidly eliminated is Vanderwolf's (1969) voluntary movement hypothesis. Experiments on the behavioural correlates of theta activity in the rat SHS (Fig. 10.1; Appendix 6) suggest a strong relation between theta and movement through space. 'Bypass' stimulation experiments (Fig. 9.3E; McNaughton et al., 2006b) show that theta is functional, in and of itself, so the SHS must be doing something when the rat moves. However, neither theta, nor its frequency, are *necessarily* related to movement, since not only low but also high-frequency theta can be observed in unmoving animals (Sainsbury and Montoya, 1984). Critically, lesion of the entire hippocampal formation has no obvious effects on the control of movement as such.

10.1.3 Habituation?

A similar discordance between activity correlations and lesion results occurs in single-unit experiments (Chapter 7 and Appendix 6). For example, if a stimulus achieves special significance for the animal (as when it is turned into a Pavlovian CS or the cue for an instrumental response), habituation of the hippocampal unit response is prevented; indeed, such stimuli appear to receive a privileged passage around the hippocampal circuit. But experiments reviewed in Appendix 8 demonstrate that precisely those tasks (simple classical or instrumental conditioning) which protect stimuli from habituation in the hippocampal circuit are immune to disruption by hippocampal lesions. This leads to our second assumption.

> *ASSUMPTION 2: the SHS receives and integrates much information about behaviour that it does not at that time control. More specifically, our theory postulates that the matching of subcortical with cortical goal information within the SHS indicates that an appropriate response is already programmed to occur (and hence there is no conflict) and so produces no output from the SHS comparator. Much of the time, therefore, the hippocampal formation is busy 'just checking', but producing no functional output.*

10.1.4 Spatial mapping?

The elimination of our next suspect is more controversial. This is the theory (O'Keefe and Nadel, 1978; Nadel, 1991) that the SHS constructs and stores spatial (or cognitive) maps.

The spatial mapping theory accounts for the voluntary movement data; with the SHS doing something important (laying down and/or utilizing spatial maps) *while* the animal is moving, but not controlling movement. It accounts for a vast amount of SHS lesion data showing disruption of spatially complex tasks; and is consistent with our ASSUMPTION 2,

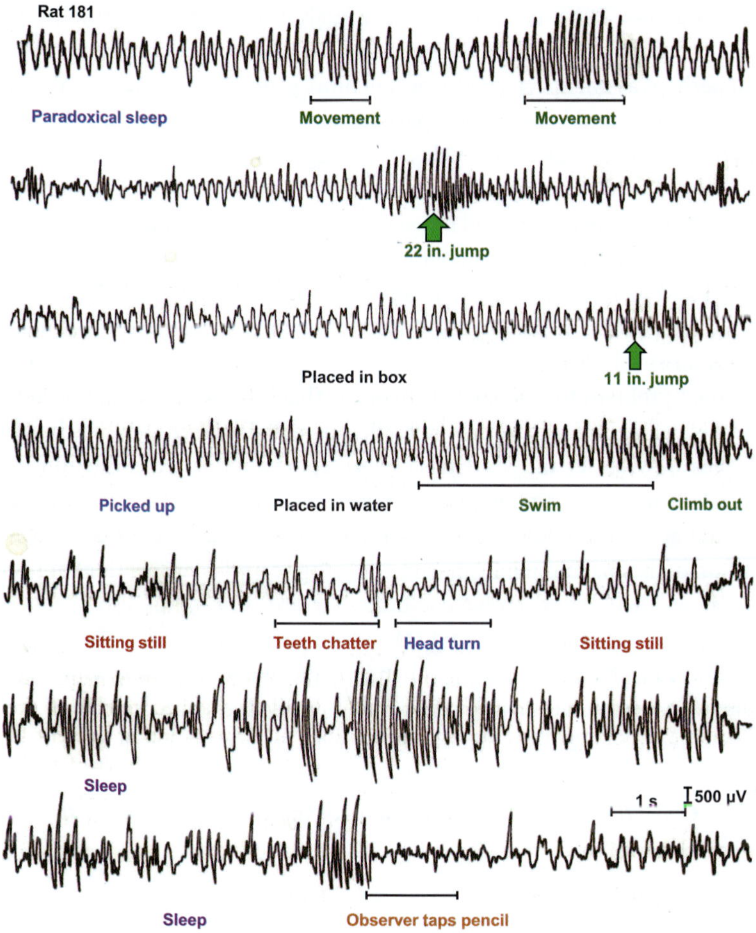

Fig. 10.1 Electrical activity in area CA1 of the hippocampus during sleep and various types of behaviour in the rat. Note the following: a)[blue text] *theta* during paradoxical sleep, struggling when held in the hand, swimming and head movement; b)[red text] *large-amplitude irregular activity* during sitting while alert, and while chattering the teeth; c) [purple text] *irregular slow activity and 'spindling'* during slow wave sleep; and d)[orange text] *small-amplitude irregular activity* when the rat was awakened but did not move about. Theta frequency increases with increasing movement (see the changes with twitching movements during paradoxical sleep, when making an 11 in. and, more so, a 22 in. jump); and theta amplitude increases with increasing vigour of movement (see the 11 in. and 22 in. jumps and swimming). Calibration: 1 s, 500μV; half amplitude filters, 0.3 and 75 Hz. Enhanced version of supplied original, with permission of I. Q. Whishaw, see Whishaw and Vanderwolf (1973) for a published version.

allowing encoding of spatial information even when the SHS need not produce behaviourally effective output. However, the affirmation that spatial memories are *stored* in the SHS (Nadel, 1991) contradicts ASSUMPTION 1, unless this is temporary (e.g. Inostroza and Born, 2013; see also §8.2.7, §8.2.8, §8.2.9).

The spatial mapping theory was inspired by the discovery of 'place fields'; with recent recognition by a Nobel Prize for 'discoveries of cells that constitute a positioning system in the brain' (Burgess, 2014, p. 1120). But our analysis of single-unit studies (Chapter 7, McNaughton & Bannerman 2024, and Appendix 6) finds little evidence for true spatial mapping, except perhaps as one specialized aspect of more general SHS function. Many cells have non-spatial correlates; and 'remapping' (particularly 'flicker', Jezek et al., 2011) and prediction of upcoming choices (Takamiya et al., 2021) suggest the SHS receives efference copies of spatially-correlated goals from other areas, rather than indicating in any unambiguous way the animal's location in space—indeed much remapping is incompatible with any contiguous 3D representation, with the equivalent of the single city of Edinburgh suddenly disappearing from Scotland and then reappearing half-way between Lyon and Marseille in France. Even the entorhinal grid system distorts in response to new reward locations reflecting goal representation (Boccara et al., 2019).

An additional problem for the spatial theory is that lesions to the hippocampal formation disrupt behaviour in tasks from which all apparent spatial content has been removed. Good examples are Webster and Voneida's (1964) report of impaired extinction and reversal (but not initial learning) of a simultaneous tactile discrimination; the many reports of an extinction but not acquisition deficit in the Skinner box; and Gaffan's (1977d) experiment on the recognition of lists of colours. Damage to the hippocampus proper does appear to affect spatial tasks more than exteroceptive cue tasks (Jarrard, 1991), but also affects interoceptive cue tasks with no spatial component (Davidson and Jarrard, 1993). So, in concordance with Squire and Zola-Morgan (1991), Cohen and Eichenbaum (1993), Gaffan (1994) and many others, we assume that most spatial paradigms involve some critical feature that renders them sensitive to SHS lesions that they share with some non-spatial tasks.

ASSUMPTION 3: the SHS plays no necessary role in learning, including spatial learning, as such.

However (see Chapter 8), spatial discriminations, relational discriminations, and the like are particularly likely to generate conflict between explicit or implicit alternative goals. Implicit alternative goals will often constitute what we call 'interference', but also often involve species-specific reactions or other unplanned effects of particular experimental configurations. It is the business of the SHS to eliminate this conflict, where possible. Effects of hippocampal lesions will not be seen either where there is insufficient conflict *or where the unlesioned control animals have been unable to overcome the conflict.*

10.1.5 Multiple possibilities?

Our analysis rejects, then, each of memory consolidation, voluntary movement, and spatial mapping as *complete* accounts of SHS functions. Alas, no other major suspect can be so readily eliminated. One problem is even to know how many suspects there are. Several shade into one another: interference/context; non-reward/novelty; familiarity/recognition; all of these/relational memory. We have attempted to deal with each of these one by one already (Chapters 8 and 9); but perhaps we are dealing with a master of disguises; or a conspiracy. Non-reward or novelty might be responsible for the break-in, but goal inhibition for the break-out; and they might both have inside help (from attention, multidimensional stimulus analysis, or one of the other servants). Careful scrutiny of the suspects we have just listed suggests, indeed, that we could be dealing with a whole gang, of somewhat flexible membership, who usually work together rather than against each other.

A pattern recurs. This congeries of hypotheses, all previously promoted in the literature, each explains some things well (hence its adherents), but none explains more than a small part of the data. Even when they merge it is not with all the other required explanations. Accepting a 'gang' solution is a counsel of despair, defying the principle of parsimony, and providing no good basis for predictions. The SHS is a mass of similar 'slices' (Fig. 1.4C), with (when placed in a dish) the same fundamental circuits as we go from end to end and from mouse to human (Franck et al., 1995; Schwartzkroin, 1994). It has expanded 40 times less between basal insectivores and humans than the neocortex (Stephan and Andy, 1969) with the dorsal hippocampus expanding less than the ventral. Such a simple, highly conserved, structure must have a simple fundamental function—current views of the SHS are like those of the blind people holding different parts of an elephant.

Our fourth and central assumption, then, is a metatheory rather than a theory.

ASSUMPTION 4: the SHS has an essentially single function that combines with its multifarious inputs to generate superficially complex outputs via simple algorithms.

10.2 The theory: goal-conflict detection basics

We propose (as we have argued in the previous chapters) that the SHS acts as a detector and resolver of conflict between concurrent incompatible goals. This conflict-related role explains both transience and context-dependence of goal processing by the SHS (e.g. Bradfield et al., 2020). What precisely is meant by the term 'goal' is crucial to the theory and so, before proceeding, we should make clear what we mean.

First, we separate learning about goals from learning to make responses. This is discussed in more detail in Chapters 1 (§1.12.4) and 3. But note, while well-learned responses may appear stereotypical, blocking of these usually results in immediate appearance of completely new responses that achieve the same goal (McNaughton et al., 2016). It does not result in a period of new learning 'of the response'. Second, a goal is the end-point of a *response sequence* and has no direct connection with any specific element within the sequence. Thus, the *response* conflict that can occur in tasks such as mirror drawing (where there is only a single goal, but there is conflict between the expected and actual outcome of particular motor patterns) should not engage the SHS. Third, the concept of a goal is a compound of situation + motivation (with the absence of either, what is coded ceases to be 'a goal'; see §1.12.4). For example, a mouse may continue to run past identical cues on a track but lose its 'place cell' firing as it loses its motivation (Pettit et al., 2022). Hence, goal conflict can result both from an apparent conflict between situations (as in a delayed matching to sample task, where essentially the same motor response must be addressed to one of two distinct physical stimuli) and from an apparent conflict between quite distinct motivations that are elicited by the same situation (as in the classic approach-avoidance conflict where the end of the straight alley affords both a positive and a negative goal; McNaughton et al., 2016). In both cases the animal must choose between two conflicting, mutually incompatible goals, and it makes little sense to suggest that we can ignore either the stimuli to which responses must be directed or the responses that must be directed to the stimuli.

10.2.1 Types of conflict

There are a number of different types of conflict with which we suppose the SHS deals, each engaging its circuits somewhat differently (§10.4). We will now describe these, but first we must emphasize that they do not equate with 'conflict' in general.[2] We see the SHS as responsible only for the detection of conflict between *concurrent goals*, where one goal is correct and a second incorrect. Conflict in execution of *successive goals* (where both goals are in a sense correct but must occur in a particular order) is dealt with in the prefrontal cortex (Chapter 11; Appendix 3); conflict between different *motor patterns* that can achieve a single goal is dealt with by the motor system (see also discussion of the defence system in Chapter 6), particularly the basal ganglia; and action conflict that requires simple stopping is dealt with by supplementary motor cortex and right inferior frontal gyrus (Aron et al., 2014a, see also Chapter 11). These anticipatory forms of conflict are also distinct from the conflict between actual and expected outcomes (Schoenbaum et al., 2003; Nieuwenhuis et al., 2005; Ostlund and Balleine, 2007). This is not to say that these different conflict resolution systems are totally independent. Cortical systems, including in particular the prefrontal cortex and anterior cingulate cortex, furnish predictions about upcoming events/actions, many of which are funnelled through the entorhinal cortex. They are, therefore, essential to at least a subset of hippocampal operations (as it is, in turn, essential to a subset of their operations).

10.2.2 Detecting goal conflict

According to the theory, the function of the SHS is to detect conflict between goals, quite generally. It does so by indirectly monitoring information, not only about currently activated motor programs (necessarily directed towards specific goals and so directly represented in the SHS as such), but also about the stimulus representations that are at any time seeking to gain access to motor mechanisms. Such stimulus representations are also directly represented in the SHS as goals, but remain potential rather than actual at the motor level. In this monitoring capacity, the SHS functions continuously; but it controls other brain systems directly only under certain special conditions. Thus, it has two principal modes of operation: 'just checking' (not controlling other brain systems) and 'control' (directly controlling other brain systems). These labels represent extremes of a continuum rather than distinct categories.

The principal function of the hippocampus proper in control mode is to narrow the focus of processing in extrahippocampal networks and to increase negative affective bias. An additional control function is provided by an instructed habituation/latent inhibition function of the entorhinal cortex (see Appendix 9). At some times, a small amount of control mode operation will be sufficient for adaptive behaviour; at other times, extreme amounts will be required. As with many emotional systems, we presume that continuous high levels of control mode activity are maladaptive, consistent with the fact that there are tasks where hippocampal lesioned animals produce superior performance to controls. If this were not the case there would not be any need for the complex gating of information within the hippocampal formation that we describe in §10.4. Further, we shall argue in Chapter 13 that

[2] We are grateful to Dr Lynette Tippett for pointing out to us the necessity to make the distinctions clear.

the primary *pathology* in generalized anxiety disorder is *excessive* control mode activity of the SHS and so maladaptive negative bias.

There are two basic conditions where goal conflict can occur. These involve two, or one, primary goal, respectively.

The first, paradigm, case is when two incompatible goal representations are concurrently highly activated. Here, in essence, detection of conflict requires a comparator that is also an integrator—detecting when opposing activities are similar in size, summing them, and producing output when the sum exceeds some threshold. The coding of response tendencies appears to be topographically mapped into the SHS (Appendices 4 and 6; Fig. 9.7B), and so, at present, we view this comparator/integrator function as likely to depend, in part, on the fibres that carry information along the septo-temporal axis of the hippocampus. This form of goal conflict comes in two flavours one where situations differ and the motivation is the same (go left/right for food) and the other where motivations differ and the situation is the same (classic food/shock approach/avoidance).

The second case is when responding to a prepotent goal is subjected to unexpected salient circumstances: the occurrence of an unexpected event or the omission of an expected event. Here detection requires a comparator that produces an output when there is a discrepancy between observed and expected inputs. This can still be viewed as reflecting goal conflict, but not limited to a choice between two alternatives that remain the same from trial to trial. The unexpected event is likely to generate a number of potential response tendencies directed to a number of environmental stimuli. Both the response tendencies and the stimuli to which they are directed are likely to vary from trial to trial or from moment to moment. Further, the precise treatment of each must be adjusted by the comparator in relation to the relative importance of the expected outcome of the specific action directed to specific environmental stimuli. As a result, in these cases a more situation-oriented description of the operation of the comparator will often be appropriate. We will deal with this familiarity comparator first.

10.2.3 Area CA3—the familiarity comparator

The hypothesis that the SHS contains a familiarity comparator was originally developed in detail by Vinogradova (1975; see Appendix 6; §7.2). According to her, the CA3 region of the hippocampus acts as a detector of novelty or of omission of expected events by comparing actual sensory input (via the septum) and predicted sensory input (via the entorhinal cortex). But, as we discuss in Appendix 10, the SHS does both less and more than detect novelty. Less, because lesions do not disturb the orienting reflex; more, because lesions disrupt other comparisons besides simple judgements of familiarity.

However, if the SHS makes other comparisons, it is unlikely that they only involve the CA3 comparator described by Vinogradova (1975). First, she showed that information processing in area CA3 is only sufficiently detailed to distinguish 'novel' from 'familiar'. Second, all of the subfields of the hippocampus appear to receive equivalent information from both the medial septum and the entorhinal cortex. Thus, although the theory we shall develop here incorporates a version of Vinogradova's CA3 novelty comparator, it treats this as only part of a more extensive system that can produce output from additional comparators in CA1 and subiculum as well as CA3 (and which can also produce output from integrators in the entorhinal cortex and other areas such as the subiculum).

10.2.4 Area CA1, subiculum, etc.—troubleshooting

The elements of what we propose can be viewed as a second class of comparators, additional to Vinogradova's. These are described next; but note, at the outset, that the anatomy suggests that each output from the SHS may be from a separate (CA3, CA2, CA1, subiculum, retrosplenial cortex) comparator (or logical gate). The outputs from these comparators each addresses different subcortical, particularly hypothalamic, structures. They also address different cortical structures, each part of its own parallel Papez microcircuit (McNaughton and Vann, 2022). However, we can speculate on, but cannot yet unambiguously identify, the function of any of these potential comparators. (For example, CA2 may be specially tuned to environmental novelty, Bhasin and Nair, 2022; social memory; or more general gating for consolidation, Lehr et al., 2021; while also acting as a filter for replay of information between CA3 and CA1 during ripple events, He et al., 2021.)

For the CA1 and subicular comparators, the CA3 familiarity comparator (and CA2) is auxiliary—sending on to them only signals that have special importance that allow, e.g. rapid changes in CA1 coding (Priestley et al., 2022). The function of the subicular comparator is, essentially, troubleshooting when the animal's proposed goal is faced with other, conflicting, goals. These latter can be elicited, notably, by novelty, the threat of non-reward, the threat of aversive stimulation, and relational processing. The task of the subicular comparator is to iterate increases in negative affective bias in all of the active and conflicting goal processing areas until only one alternative is clearly dominant. In this way existing plans can be applied again or new ones substituted as appropriate. Where there is insufficient information for resolution of the conflict to occur, all of the alternative goals will be suppressed. Under these conditions, output from the first, CA3, comparator will initiate general information gathering behaviour (and particularly risk assessment); or output from the subiculum to the posterior cingulate cortex will initiate more complex forms of risk assessment, checking and safety-seeking behaviour, including, for example, innate routines that do not depend for their termination on the achievement of a specific reinforcer. The conflict should then be resolved once the existing internal positive and negative affective associations have been updated with external information. These ideas directly reflect the psychological concept of the GIS developed in detail in Chapters 2 and 3. They also resemble closely everyday notions of anxiety and much of clinical ideas of anxiety. But the purpose of the theory at this point is to account for the data on the SHS, not for anxiety.

10.2.5 Goals as efference copies, 'just checking', 'control', and the release of risk assessment

The idea of conflicting goals is easiest to understand with respect to motor programs. The SHS is connected, directly or indirectly, to all major areas in which general goal-oriented motor programs can originate. In many situations the current stimuli (from both the internal and the external environment) will strongly activate only one such area and only one goal within that area. The SHS receives, as an efference copy, the information that a specific goal is being processed; and this will activate a subpopulation of hippocampal cells. Since, in the case of a single such input, there is no conflict, the subject's motor behaviour can be released by the goal processing area and will be directed towards the current goal. This is the 'just checking' mode of operation of the SHS.

Let us suppose now, however, that more than one goal is strongly activated, requiring 'control' mode. The SHS as a whole will receive much greater input than it would in the single goal case. (This could involve either a greater strength of total input to the SHS, or a wider topographic spread of activation within the SHS.) Integrating these inputs, probably via intrinsic excitatory connections such as the longitudinal connections that run along its septo-temporal axis, the hippocampus will 'detect conflict' when the integrated sum effectively passes some threshold (in practice there may simply be an output that is proportional in strength to the degree of conflict detected).

The output of the detector must then take active control of the ongoing motor output, either inhibiting output from one of the conflicting goals or inhibiting both goals and commanding appropriate exploratory or risk analytical action. These last might range from simple adjustments of autonomic or sensory organs (e.g. dilation of the pupils) to complex patterns of locomotion. In certain cases, a compromise might be possible (e.g. the animal might continue to run towards the goal-box of an alley to obtain food, but do so more slowly while sniffing at the side-walls to gather information).

Given the anatomical simplicity of the SHS and the complexity of the outputs we have just described, it is important to note, however, that 'inhibition' and/or 'exploration' are not postulated to be controlled in detail by the SHS as such. Instead, they are a consequence of the impact on other brain areas of the increases in negative bias which *are* produced directly by SHS output. In particular exploration and risk assessment, controlled by their own dedicated circuits (McNaughton and Corr, 2018), will be released by the SHS not actively directed by it.

10.2.6 Adding the 'faulty' tag

An important feature of the theory is that, when conflict is detected, output from the SHS will influence, not only current behaviour, but also future behaviour (see also Robinson and Brandon, 2021) by adding what is, in effect, a 'faulty' tag to one or more programs. Hippocampal output should achieve this tagging automatically, as an incidental though important consequence of the increase in negative bias through which it alters the balance between current goals—a distinct hippocampal output is not required for this. The inhibition of future behaviour is likely to depend upon outputs from the subiculum to the higher levels of goal processing systems. In this way, the subiculum would be able to alter the affective bias of information arriving in specific goal processing systems from, e.g. polymodal association cortex. Again, the complexity of the processing just described is presumed to reside, not in the SHS itself, but in the responses of its many output targets (some active, some not) to a modulatory signal from the SHS, a signal that need have no target specificity at all except in that the target is active (and so will support association via long-term potentiation).

Note also that the final effect of inhibition of a specific prepotent appetitive goal is likely to be the result of hippocampal excitation of a competing aversive goal. The greater the competition and the greater the hippocampal output, the greater will be the arousal and attentional concomitants of hippocampal activity. Critical for the anxiety-related aspects of the theory is the idea that hippocampal excitation of specific nodes will result in long-term potentiation in extra-hippocampal targets that would not otherwise have occurred; and that this in turn results in subsequent retrieval of affectively negative (in the approach-avoidance case, 'threatening') associations at greater strength than would have occurred in the absence of functional hippocampal output.

The 'faulty' tagging in memory must involve an asymmetry between reward, on the one hand, and punishment on the other. If the current motor program is interrupted by an unexpected reward, it may need to be modified; but the plan elements up until the reward was obtained can be retained. However, if it is interrupted by an unexpected punishment, it is likely that the whole program must be treated as faulty. Thus, the conflict detector needs, not only information about the presence of conflict, in a purely cognitive sense, but also information about the general affective value of unexpected stimuli.

10.2.7 Complex results from simple mechanisms

The capacity to resolve conflict between two incompatible goals that we ascribe to the SHS is, then, inherently very simple. The SHS is functionally activated simply by increases in the topographic spread of the inputs to it from cortical and subcortical goal processing areas, and so requires little in the way of specific complex information. It needs to know only that there is more than one incompatible goal, but does not need to identify each specifically. This is consistent with the fact that the hippocampal formation is phylogenetically very ancient. In animals such as fish it represents a major part of the cortex (Gastaut and Lammers, 1961). It is unlikely that sharks, for example, have as great a need for relational (or whatever) memory as do human beings, but easy to believe that they have as great a need to resolve conflicts between concurrent incompatible goals (since these can as well be innate as learned).

We have talked about detection and resolution of conflict between goals in a way that is easiest to understand if the goals differ in the nature of the response to be made (e.g. approach, avoidance). But the model can be applied equally well to the resolution of conflict between goals that differ in the stimulus to which to direct a particular type of response (e.g. a choice between levers to press). There will be conditions where two stimuli, assigned as positive and negative by the experimenter, may appear to be equally attractive goals to the subject (depending on the nature and history of the stimuli and of the contexts in which they have been presented). On detecting conflicting items, each priming a response system, the SHS will selectively dampen activity (via increased negative bias *in both structures*) so as to leave only one item available for transfer to working memory. It will also tag incorrect retrievals, so that their probability of occurrence in a similar context is reduced in future.

We should also note the special case of novel 'neutral' stimuli. Here the stimulus itself need not be an innate elicitor of some incompatible response. Nor does the stimulus necessarily conflict with a second stimulus for access to the upcoming response. Rather, the presence of the stimulus (independent of the response it elicits), since it is unexpected, has the capacity to inhibit any ongoing response. To the cases of nominal response-response and nominal stimulus-stimulus conflict considered in the previous paragraph we must, therefore, add nominal stimulus-response conflict. All of these, however, can be recombined as different flavours of goal–goal conflict. In particular, according to the theory, a novel stimulus will only produce functional output from the SHS if it is *not merely novel but also is the goal of an orienting response.*

10.3 The theory: goal-conflict resolution basics

We ascribed a fairly large number of quite complex functional outputs to an anatomically simple structure. However, the actions we assign to the SHS have been simple; it is the response of the target structures when they receive functional SHS output that generates psychological complexity. In this section we describe specific SHS operations that enable this complexity.

10.3.1 Iteration

Most fundamental is iteration[3]: the 'cycling' of information around loops as new input. This cycling does not hold information unchanged, unlike active memory (see §9.4 and Fig. 11.3). At each cycle the information is modified not only by the consequences of SHS input for the relative weighting of affectively different classes of information in the source of the original information, but also by the current state of the SHS circuitry and the interaction of its output with hypothalamic (emotional) and thalamic (cognitive) nodes of Papez-like circuits (McNaughton and Vann, 2022, Fig. 9.9).

The function of this looping can be understood by analogy with the global stereopsis and language models that we described in §1.12.7. The SHS as a whole appears to do a great deal of 'talking to itself', that is, it sends out and gets back messages via the systems with which it is reciprocally connected (systems whose higher levels receive e.g. subicular output, and whose higher and lower levels return information to e.g. the entorhinal cortex); and, since it sends out its message by various different routes, it also gets 'the message' back again (modified) in multiple copies.

As we discussed in §7.4.9, this can involve flickering between representations on the way to full 'remapping' (which we argued there and in §10.1.3 contradicts any idea of a true map). Consistent with this, 'the ability to recall discrete memories is thought to depend on the formation of attractor states in recurrent neural networks. In such networks, representations can be reactivated reliably from subsets of the cues that were present when the memory was encoded, at the same time as interference from competing representations is minimized' (Jezek et al., 2011, p. 246). That is, if the SHS-to-goal area circuits recycle information to resolve conflicts using processes analogous to the global stereopsis model (Fig. 1.6), one would expect initial conflicting retrieval (biased to the earlier representation) to be reprocessed to progressively suppress the older/incorrect information and allow the new to become the primary representation of goal space.[4] This reprocessing likely involves 'a key role for hippocampal ripples in orchestrating hippocampal-cortical communication across large-scale networks involved in conscious recollection' in humans (Norman et al., 2021, p. 2767). 'From this perspective, sharp waves may be the means of internally organized hippocampo-neocortical

[3] 'Recursion' used in the 2nd edition is technically incorrect in this case, as pointed out to me by Brendan McCane.

[4] Likely equivalent to 'rich' coding with orthogonalized coding axes. 'In humans, we found that dorsal portions of the PFC and posterior parietal cortex share a neural geometry and dimensionality with [artificial] networks that are trained in the rich regime. This solution involves representing distinct tasks as low-dimensional and task-specific neural manifolds in a way that minimizes interference and maximizes robustness among potentially competing responses' (Flesch et al., 2022) p. 1259.

transfer of neuronal information. Beneath all the turbulence, sharp waves retain *and replay* the information embedded in the synaptic network that gives rise to the event' (Buzsáki, 2006, p. 347, emphasis added).

We must also account for the fact that within the hippocampus proper, by contrast to its extrinsic connections, there is an essentially linear, unidirectional flow of information; and must bear in mind that, as far as the septal and entorhinal inputs are concerned, all levels of the hippocampal linear array appear to receive essentially the same information in parallel—while with respect to other connections there is a hierarchical onion-like topography (McNaughton and Vann, 2022, Fig. 9.9), necessary for the proper functioning of a series of logical gates (§10.4). Each module receives much the same septal and entorhinal input as the others, but each performs a different calculation on this input, integrating in particular the septal and entorhinal inputs with other signals, especially those from the ascending aminergic systems and medial frontal cortices.

10.3.2 The internal cascade

The major terminal point of this cascade of processes within the SHS is, essentially, the subiculum. This is not only the final point where unidirectionality is largely maintained (output from the retrosplenial cortex is generally reciprocated by the areas to which it projects), but is also a major source of efferents from the SHS.

Information reaches the subiculum from CA1/CA2 after passing from the entorhinal area to the dentate gyrus via the perforant path, thence to CA3 via the mossy fibres, and on to CA2/CA1 via the Schaffer collaterals. It recirculates through the fornix to the mammillary bodies then anteroventral thalamus and cingulate cortex, back to the subicular area. (There is also a smaller loop providing direct two-way connections between the subiculum and anteroventral thalamus.)

Given this architecture, the subiculum is a prime candidate for the role of goal-conflict detector (in contrast to the mismatch comparator in CA3). It receives general information ('arousal') via the septum and aminergic inputs; information that predicted stimuli (goals) have occurred via the entorhinal cortex; details of motor programs/working memory (goals) from the prefrontal cortex; and details of innate programs (goals) from the cingulate cortex, amygdala, cerebellum, etc. But note that CA3, CA1, and retrosplenial cortex support similar Papez-like loops (Fig. 9.9; McNaughton and Vann, 2022).

The subiculum can also interact iteratively with all Papez circuit elements to modify their function. Such modification (if it is based on phenomena like long-term potentiation and depression) must proceed progressively round the loop from the subiculum (see next). There is some evidence that this is the case. As we note when discussing the cingulate cortex in detail in Appendix 3, single units recorded during discriminated active avoidance react differentially to S + and S– during acquisition in both the anteroventral thalamus and the cingulate. Behavioural acquisition of reversal of the task is accompanied by incomplete reversal of unit responses in the thalamic neurones (which are closest to the subiculum) and by little change in the discriminative responses in the cingulate cortex. Thus, the hippocampal system does not eliminate previously formed associations, but alters their capacity to control behaviour.

10.3.3 The special case of repulsors

If simple detection of conflict between alternative courses of action, independent of type, were the basis for hippocampal function, then perhaps direct input of information about those courses of action to the subiculum would be all that is required. However, our theory requires us to treat presentation of an aversive consequence differently from an appetitive one. The theory requires that the omission of an expected punisher is equivalent to an unexpected reward; and vice versa. We propose that differing treatments are accorded to conflicts of different types as a result of the operation of a series of gates between the different hippocampal subfields. The anatomy suggests that essentially the same neural messages, representing the animal's current plans, can be sent through all the nodes in the hippocampal circuit to the subicular area, as well as directly by way of the entorhinal-subicular projection (Van Hoesen et al., 1979). We propose that these inputs interact with gates (Fig. 10.3) so that, in some cases, the subiculum will receive only a direct input from the entorhinal cortex, while in others it will receive parallel input both from the entorhinal cortex and, as a result of specific gates being open, from the hippocampus proper.

10.3.4 Information filtering

It is in the four synapses of the, superficially unnecessary, unidirectional loop through the hippocampus proper (Fig. 10.3) that Vinogradova (1975) places her proposed basic comparator function. The single-unit evidence, both her own and that of others, as well as the research which has followed evoked potentials round the hippocampal circuit (Appendix 5), gives strong support to her hypothesis that this hippocampal circuitry can show habituation to, or preserve from habituation (depending on the importance of the message), signals emanating from the entorhinal cortex and destined for the subicular area. The main purpose of this circuitry (we propose) is to filter information destined for the subiculum, so that the latter receives only those items of information that need to be assessed for conflict value. As detailed in Appendix 5, there appears to be a logical gate located between the dentate gyrus and CA3. This passes on activity when stimuli are novel (i.e. when there is no coincidence between septal and entorhinal input), but not when they are both familiar and lacking in behavioural significance (Vinogradova, 1975). However, as a result of the operations of the ascending monoamine systems (Chapter 6; Appendix 10), activity is also passed on if stimuli have been associated (by classical conditioning) with events of primary biological importance, or if they are of conflicting significance. Segal's (1977a; Segal, 1977b) experiments illustrate this point well: with the parameters of electrical stimulation on the entorhinal side of the dentate-CA3 gate set so that responses on the other side rapidly habituated, both concurrent presentation of environmental CSs associated with punishment and direct stimulation of the locus coeruleus prevented this habituation (see also Seo et al., 2021 for effects on contextual generalization).

We talked earlier about 'activity' being passed on because Vinogradova's experiments make it very clear that any 'information' processed in CA3 is of a very non-specific kind. As she puts it 'the neuronal reactions in CA3 do not code (and consequently cannot transmit) information about the quality of their sensory input. Their activity appears to be a strong generalized regulatory signal, which may possibly exert modulatory effects on the output structures' (Vinogradova, 1975, p. 10). The dentate-CA3 gate must work, therefore, in parallel with the direct pathway from the entorhinal area to the subiculum. Thus, specific information is sent continuously to the subiculum, but it only affects processing in the loops connecting the subiculum with other areas if it receives an 'enabling signal' from CA1. This enabling signal is sent only in connection with combinations of inputs that signify conflict, otherwise they are filtered out during their passage through the dentate-CA3 gate. Thus, direct input from the entorhinal area to the subiculum describes the state of the world, while the input relayed via the other subfields of the hippocampus, utilizing the gating capacities illustrated in Fig. 10.3, determines the precise kind of comparison that is carried out, depending on the way in which the stimuli are important to the animal.

10.3.5 Entorhinal cortex—the information funnel

If one views the SHS in this way, then the known effect upon it of monoamine inputs (Chapters 6, 9) could be phrased in English as a tag 'the current entorhinal input is important, it needs checking'. The entorhinal area is a major funnel for *cortical* information (Fig. 10.2) arriving in the subiculum, and appears to be the only major source of cortical information for other areas of the SHS in non-primates. It also appears to gate amygdala information (Roesler and McGaugh, 2022).

However, in primates there are inputs to subiculum, as well as to other parts of the hippocampus proper, directly from prefrontal cortex, parietal cortex, temporal cortex, and cingulate cortex. Such direct input likely fulfils the same general functions as that normally relayed by the entorhinal cortex. While we have talked specifically of entorhinal cortex (and in the absence of much further data should continue to be so), the same ideas apply, with no functional distortion, to any route by which cortical information reaches the SHS.

10.3.6 Entorhinal-septal interactions

Here, we should recall that input to the SHS via the septum is far too modest to code highly specific information of the type needed for conflict resolution—with simple restoration of RSA/'theta' rhythmicity, *per se*, restoring function (McNaughton et al., 2006b). Likewise, cellular responses in area CA3 likely code 'goals' in general terms; but are too broad to code for the external stimulus features of the world that the subiculum will require for conflict resolution. We see CA3 as providing a crude signal that then determines whether or not the subiculum processes information. Septal input could flag, for example, 'importance'; and other routes identify the specifics of the goal giving rise to this alerting signal. This separation is in keeping with both the reticular origin of the septal information and the indiscriminate integration of activity apparently carried out by the theta-frequency-coding supramammillary nucleus and the theta-gating ascending cholinergic system (Fig. 10.3; Appendix 5 and 10). Thus, the input from the septum can be seen as classifying information as important in the same general way as do the monoamine inputs (a view consistent with the similar effects of acetylcholine, dopamine, noradrenaline, and 5HT on neuronal signal-to-noise ratios), but on a dimension of potential response intensity rather than the dimensions

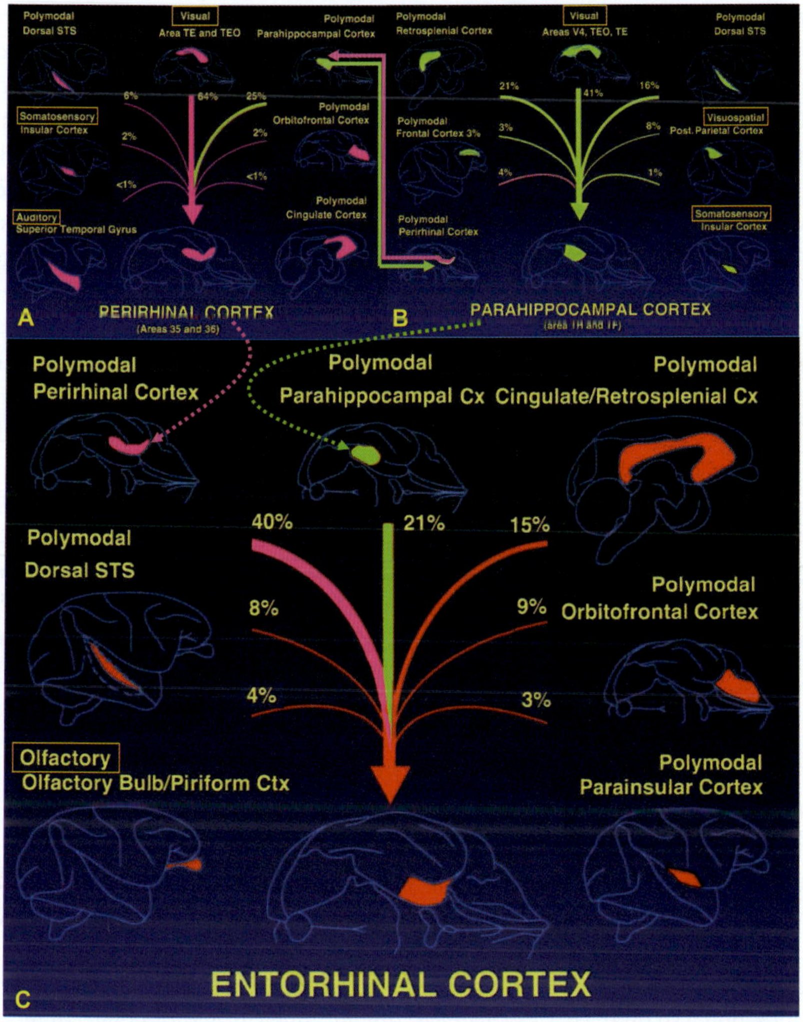

Fig. 10.2 The perirhinal (A) and parahippocampal (B) cortices largely relay cortical inputs to the entorhinal cortex (C). The density of connections is given as a percentage and indicated by width of arrows. Modalities of unimodal cortex are shown in an orange box. Figure is adapted from originals supplied by W.A. Suzuki, who summarized the data from Suzuki and Amaral (1994) and Insausti, Amaral and Cowan (1987).

of response quality (determined by the nature of reinforcement) signalled by the monoamine inputs.

It is this input from the septum that makes habituation of hippocampal responses an active rather than a passive process (Vinogradova, 1975). As described in Appendix 6, disruption of either the entorhinal or the septal input to CA3 prevents habituation of the neuronal responses in this region. From this evidence it can be deduced that hippocampal habituation depends on some kind of matching of these two inputs in CA3. If we consider Vinogradova's findings in more detail, it seems that the changes which give rise to hippocampal habituation take place on both the septal and entorhinal sides of CA3, but in rather different ways.

On the entorhinal side, there is a gradual build-up of responses to repeated, unimportant stimuli in both the dentate gyrus and the entorhinal cortex itself. The build-up of response in these regions takes about the same number of stimulus presentations (2–12 in the entorhinal area, 15–20 in the dentate gyrus) as does habituation in CA3 (8–15). This is consistent with the fact that long-term potentiation of the entorhinal input to the dentate gyrus blocks sensory responses within the SHS. Thus, long-term potentiation of this kind has an effect (loss of response in CA3) that is equivalent to instant habituation of responses to most neutral stimuli simultaneously. In parallel with the spread of incremental responses from entorhinal cortex to dentate, culminating in habituation in CA3, there is a spread of incremental responses progressively from CA1 to mammillary bodies to anteroventral thalamus to cingulate cortex (Fig. 10.4), with maximal augmentation being obtained in the cingulate in 8–15 trials, concurrent with habituation in CA3. In line with our arguments earlier, the cingulate could then be viewed as holding at least a partial model of the occurrence of the stimulus.

This formulation places the burden of hippocampal habituation on the entorhinal side of the CA3 gate. However, the septal area also plays an active role in the process. Unit responses in the medial septal area neither augment nor show much habituation. Lateral septal unit responses undergo habituation, which appears shortly after habituation of CA3 neurones, and so is more likely to be a consequence than a cause of CA3 habituation. Sectioning the fornix–fimbria disrupts normal habituation of CA3 responses and replaces it with augmentation (Vinogradova, 1975; Vinogradova and Brazhnik, 1978).

10.3.7 Septal and aminergic influences on signal-to-noise ratio

This pattern of effects suggests that what we are seeing is not what is conventionally thought of as habituation at all (remember that hippocampal lesions do not interfere with the habituation of behavioural orienting responses to the stimuli used in these experiments). Rather, like the aminergic inputs from the subcortex, the septal input increases signal-to-noise ratios, doing so on the basis of average stimulus intensity across a range of modalities. This is consistent with the fact that theta frequency increases with increasing midbrain activation essentially independently of the way in which that activation is produced, with the supramammillary nucleus functioning as a simple integrator.

The phasic input from the septum to CA3 differs from the aminergic inputs, however, in the precise way in which it alters signal-to-noise ratios. The septal input is predominantly GABAergic and inhibitory, depressing presynaptic release of neurotransmitter in many terminals at the same time that the excitability of the cells is increased by other (e.g. cholinergic) inputs. Thus, the septal GABAergic input changes signal-to-noise ratio largely by suppressing noise.[5] In the absence of the septal input, depolarization may be sufficient to induce long-term potentiation, particularly under conditions that produce hippocampal sharp waves; these, according to Buzsáki and Haas (1988; see Appendix 5), promote long-term potentiation (theta having the opposing effect). However, in the presence of the septal input, the majority of other concurrent inputs will be taken below the critical depolarization threshold and undergo long-term depression. In contrast, in cases in which there is significant input from

[5] This fact may be particular important for the role of theta in REM sleep see Chapter 8, particularly §8.5.

the monoamine systems, signal-to-noise ratio is increased largely by an increase in signal, and the capacity for long-term potentiation, at least of the most active concurrent inputs, is restored.

Thus, the SHS consists of a cascade of logical gates, each of which can, but need not, produce functional output. The interaction of these gates, and their modulation by ascending aminergic inputs, then allows, not only for the distinct modes of operation of the system ('just checking', 'control'), but also for quite different logical combinations of simple stimuli and quite different resulting states of the goal processing systems of the brain, all nonetheless to be treated as sharing the higher order property of 'goal conflict'.

10.4 Some scenarios

To see how this theory (including the major assumptions detailed earlier; and principles detailed in Chapter 9) applies to the available data, we must first distinguish between four different general scenarios.

Scenario 1—novelty You are in a totally, or significantly, new environment, and so have no ongoing plans being executed. Novelty will activate your subcortex and cause septal input to your CA3 comparator that is not matched by a predictive cortical model of the environment via the entorhinal cortex. This *mismatch* flags conflict between different goals (and so choices of action). So, your SHS will assume direct behavioural control; inhibit output from all prepotent goals; and then elicit information gathering (particularly risk assessment) that should update your view of the world and allow one goal to be chosen or an absence of any significant goal to be registered. Stimuli not linked to important consequences will update to 'familiar-ignore' with a 'null' motor program.

Scenario 2—just checking You are going about your normal routines. Your continuously updated (entorhinal) action expectations are continuously matched to current (septal) events. Your CA3 comparator fails to detect a subcortical-cortical mismatch. CA3 cell firing signals that expectations have been met and this actively prevents the final elements of the SHS from producing functional output.

Scenario 3—conflict Your normal routines are unexpectedly interrupted. Your continuously updated (entorhinal) action expectations *mismatch* to current (septal) events. This interruption includes when some predicted event *fails* to occur. Both unexpected presence and unexpected omission can be seen as special variants of ***Scenario 1*** (unexpected occurrence); and so, the SHS assumes direct behavioural control, activating information gathering to resolve the expectation-outcome discrepancy. However, unlike ***Scenario 1***, there is a currently executing motor program that the SHS must tag as '*faulty needs checking*' – causing both current and future stopping or slowing of execution. Here, appetitive and aversive stimuli will receive different treatment. Aversive interruptions will require more extensive motor program modification. As in ***Scenario 1***, whenever the interrupting stimulus (including omission of reward and other affectively loaded stimuli) is unrelated to subsequent reinforcement, the stimulus will eventually be tagged as 'familiar-ignore', and the initial 'faulty' tag will be removed. (This gives rise, among other things, to latent inhibition and the partial reinforcement extinction effect; see Appendix 9.)

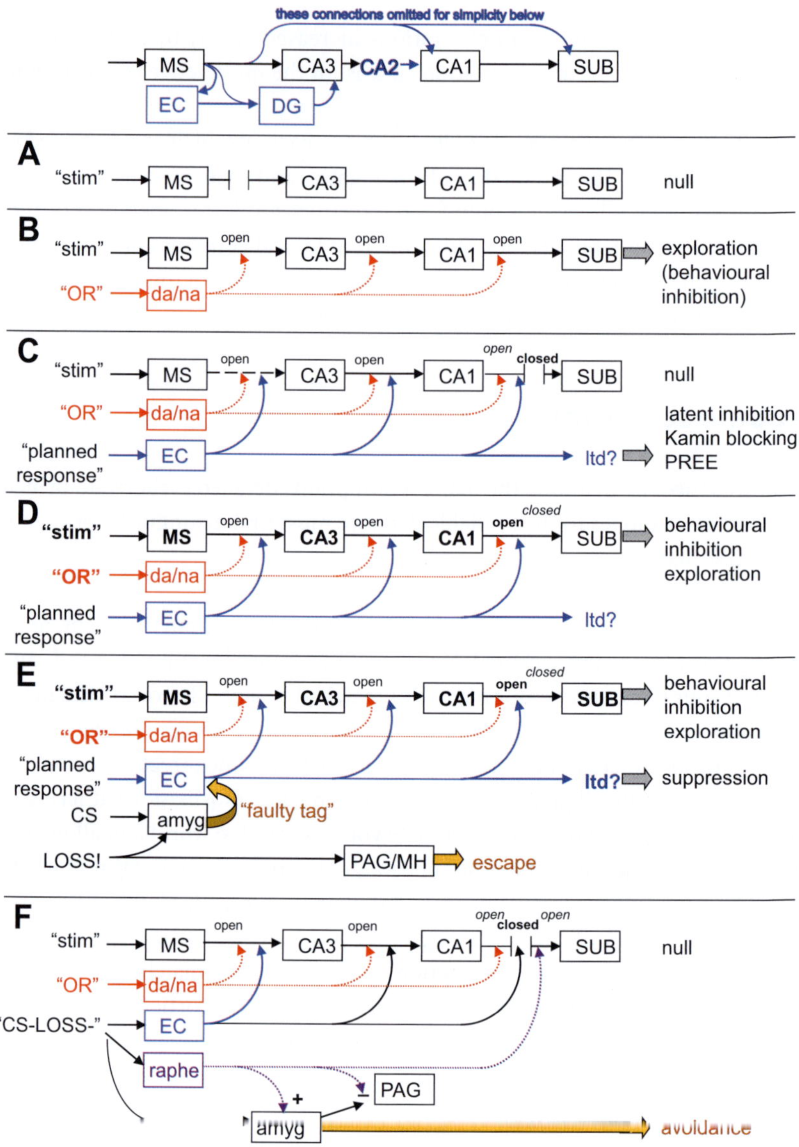

Fig. 10.3 The key goal-conflict detection components of the SHS; and simplified illustrations (A-H) of their role in conflict resolution (see also Figs. 9.8, 10.4). For details see text, particularly §10.4. *Abbreviations:* amyg, amygdala; CA1, CA3 = subfields of hippocampus; da/na = dopaminergic/noradrenergic 'salience' inputs; EC = entorhinal cortex; LS = lateral septum; ltd = long-term depression; MB = mammillary body; MS medial septum/diagonal band complex; "OR" = orienting-eliciting stimulus input; PAG = periaqueductal grey; "stim" = sensory stimulus; SUB = subiculum. For definitions of learning theory elements (e.g., CS-LOSS) see Chapter 3. See opposite page for panels G, H.

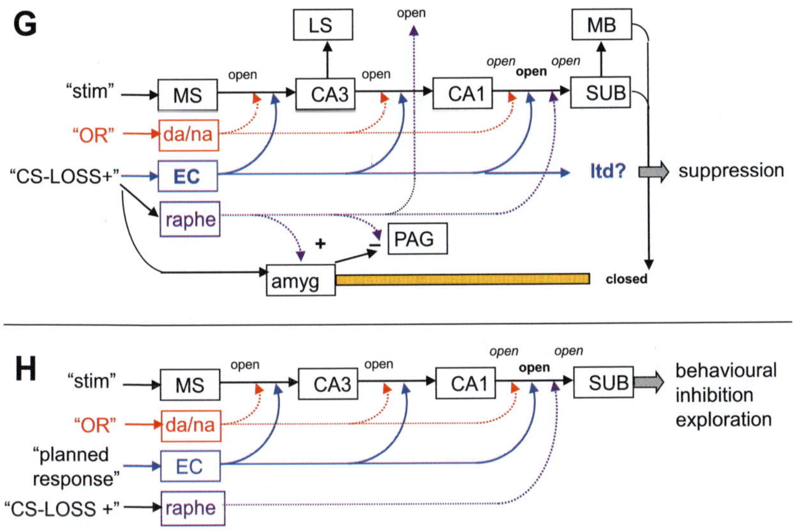

Fig. 10.3 Continued

Scenario 4—disengagement After a discrepancy has been resolved, behavioural control passes back to other systems, which may receive updated information as a result of SHS activity.

We now consider the machinery involved, and these scenarios, in more detail.

10.4.1 Basic circuits and gating

Diagrams of the key operations of the components of the SHS for goal-conflict resolution are shown in Fig. 10.3 and briefly summarized in the current section. More detailed consideration of each is provided next.

The diagrams in Fig. 10.3 are hugely simplified and intended only to illustrate the general types of operation performed by the circuits involved. In terms of the basic circuits within the SHS, as shown at the top, in blue, we have omitted a number of key elements that would normally be considered (as well as the even greater circuit detail covered in Chapter 9). Key inputs flagging salience/novelty (§6.11, 6.12) are summarized as da/na (for detailed circuits controlling 'seeking behaviour' see Kesner et al., 2022). We have also (with a minor exception in panel G) shown only the primary output from subiculum, and ignored the hierarchy of parallel Papez-like circuits that connect CA3, CA1, subiculum, and retrosplenial cortex to the mamillary bodies, thalamus, and then various levels of frontal (including cingulate) cortex (Fig. 9.9; McNaughton and Vann, 2022). We have also omitted, until later in this chapter, consideration of the differences between the septal/dorsal/posterior and temporal/ventral/anterior hippocampus. This difference can be thought of as orthogonal to Fig. 10.3, which essentially describes how any transverse slice from the hippocampus works independent of septo-temporal location.

10.4.2 Scenario 1: novelty

We treat this scenario (see Fig. 10.3B) first because it represents the first step in any dealings with any particular stimulus. With an adult animal, however, ***Scenario 2*** can be viewed as being the 'normal or 'baseline' situation.

We have already noted that simple orienting responses or their habituation do not change after septal or hippocampal lesions. Bar motor disinhibition in novel environments, the few reports of a slight retardation in habituation or of a reduction in the galvanic skin response in lesioned animals (Appendix 8) do not reflect a fundamental disruption in the intake of information about novel stimuli, as required by Vinogradova's original hypothesis. There is no need for an entire organ of the brain to support habituation. In simple organisms, such as *Aplysia californica,* habituation, sensitization and association can all occur within monosynaptic reflex arcs (see Pinel, 1997, p. 390). Nonetheless, electroencephalography (EEG) and single-unit data (Appendix 6) show that the SHS is engaged at such times in registering novel events and, if they have no special significance, in registering this lack of significance as well, by habituating the responses they evoke.

This largely 'hands-off' reaction to novel, and then less novel, information can be better understood if we recall the details of eyeblink conditioning. Single-unit changes during conditioning show that association is reflected in changes in hippocampal unit activity. But lesions show that the SHS plays no part in the acquisition of the conditioned nictitating response—which occurs in cerebellar circuitry.

Thus, the SHS receives *efference copies* from circuits that control simple associative learning; but the hippocampal cells themselves cannot (and need not) distinguish easily between the areas supplying these efference copies, and only take control of behaviour under conditions that these basic circuits cannot handle. As noted in Chapter 6, a similar hierarchical organization appears to be present in the threat system. It is parsimonious, therefore, to presume that the same principles operate in relation to habituation to simple novel stimuli; where again we can suppose that the key circuits are extra-hippocampal. As with simple eyeblink conditioning, then, the SHS is not totally unconcerned about novel stimuli; nor functionally involved in habituation of orienting; nor does it store the neural models that underpin habituation. But, the changes in its unit responses (in e.g. delayed conditioning) are important parts of the role it plays in more complex tasks (in e.g. trace conditioning).

That the SHS does not store specific information (nor code this in its output) fits the rapidity with which hippocampal units picked out at random by the experimenter's electrode respond to stimuli in a totally new environment (Chapter 7 and Appendix 6). This could not happen if the units were already coding specific information; rather, the SHS continuously integrates information arriving from other cortical (and subcortical, Janacsek et al., 2022) areas.

That said, SHS lesions *do* change behaviour in novel situations; particularly, reducing patterning and flexibility of active exploration of spatially extended environments (more study of non-spatial would be useful). Rearing is a major risk-analysis behaviour in response to threat anticipation (Chapter 2); and, in a novel environment, is likely a reaction (even without threat) to multiple conflicting stimuli; and appears critical for forming spatial representations (Shan et al., 2023). Its loss clearly reduces environmental assessment and hippocampal inactivation during rearing reduces spatial memory accuracy with delayed win-shift (Layfield et al., 2023).

Some novel environments involve an implicit approach-avoidance conflict, of the kind that is central to our analysis of anxiety (see Fig. 10.3C, D). The approach component is based on the advantages attached to exploration (such as discovery of new food sources); the avoidance component is based on the potential threat from as yet undiscovered environmental dangers (such as predators). In our view, the SHS is not involved in dealing with novelty or its habituation *per se*, but it does take control of behaviour when a novel environment elicits conflict between a high degree of activation of approach and a simultaneously high degree of activation of avoidance. Even in a spatial environment, by the way, it is not the case, as O'Keefe and Nadel (1978, p. 242) suggest, that 'in the absence of the SHS all forms of exploratory behaviour . . . disappear from the animal's repertoire'. The lesioned animal still explores and (in a straight alley for example) learns its way about and identifies the location of significant stimuli. The chief difference from normal behaviour is that the pattern of exploration is less flexible, less well adapted to ensuring that all parts of the environment are visited. We shall consider how these effects can be explained within the present theory later (see ***Scenario 3***).

In sum, during processing of novelty, the SHS is not *directly* involved with the construction of predictive models of the stimulus situation, nor *directly* with production and habituation of the orienting reaction. Rather, it receives subcortical input that reflects the presence of important stimuli (potential goals). If the SHS does not at the same time receive a matching cortical input (i.e. the goals are novel), it determines the relative strength of the novel goal and of any prepotent goal; and, if there is goal conflict (i.e. neither is sufficiently greater than the other), then its output inhibits the prepotent goals and permits orienting and exploratory programmes to function properly. Importantly, intermediate cases are possible—slowed response execution alternating with modest exploration.

10.4.3 Scenario 2: just checking

In this scenario (see Fig. 10.3A, C, F), the cortex and subcortex provide continuous information about present goals and plans (future goals). There are two possibilities. *First*, the animal is doing little; and change, or lack of change, in the environment simply lives up to expectation (e.g. towards the end of habituation or classical conditioning).[6] *Second*, the animal is doing something: e.g. a rat running in an alley for a food reward on a simple continuous reinforcement schedule.

In this second case, the SHS is active, with continuous high-frequency theta while the rat runs to the food cup; single units will fire in their 'place fields' (O'Keefe and Nadel, 1978, but see Chapter 7); predicting upcoming choices; and determined by the available goals[7] (see Chapter 7). But the rat without a septal area (and so RSA/'theta'), or without a hippocampus, still runs efficiently—or, in an operant chamber *increases* its motor actions. So, the SHS is 'just checking'; receiving and integrating much information; but with its logical gates blocking the functional output that would increase arousal and generate inhibition. Any output will reflect minor discrepancies that result in inhibition and exploration; and it is the loss of these interruptions that sometimes 'improve' learning after SHS lesions. But what is 'checking'?

The hippocampal formation (particularly the entorhinal cortex, Fig. 10.2) receives a mass of goal-related efference copies (even of 'reflexive' eye blinks) and related complex stimulus

[6] This is the natural end-point of the cortical model building elicited during ***Scenario 1***.

[7] Or 'subgoals', if you wish to restrict the meaning of the term 'goal' to the food cup. But this should be avoided, experimenters assume they know and define the rat's goals, via the paradigm. But the rat itself determines what is or is not a goal, which must then be discovered by the experimenter.

information that comes from, e.g. the cerebellum, amygdala, anterior and posterior cingulate cortices, dorsal and ventral trends of prefrontal cortex, and from a wide variety of sensory areas, particularly polymodal association cortex (Fig. 10.2; Appendix 4).

The SHS compares this mass of goal-related data to determine the degree of conflict, i.e. how far different areas are co-activated. Given the operation of ion channels and variations in membrane potential, any instantaneous comparison could be affected as much by small recent events as by large less recent events. So, in both just checking mode and critically in control mode (§10.4.4), precise calculations within the hippocampal circuitry and around Papez-like loops (McNaughton and Vann, 2022) are aided by temporal quantization, i.e. theta activity.

In the simplest case, the inputs need only differentiate sources rather than detailed information content. The SHS compares their relative strengths, ignores the weak (which are not a problem for a 'winner takes all' goal selection mechanism) and determines if there is only one strong 'winner'. If so, no conflict is detected and 'just checking' continues. If there is more than one strong potential 'winner' we move to ***Scenario 3.***

In relation to the subicular conflict detector, Vinogradova's CA3 comparator serves an auxiliary role, passing novel stimuli along for particular attention and filtering out familiar stimuli. Filtering out can be overcome if the monoamines (dopamine, noradrenaline, serotonin) flag importance. Important, familiar, stimuli and novel stimuli are both passed on for further action, but they provoke different actions. Important, familiar, stimuli are simply sent forward for checking. But important novel stimuli take us back to ***Scenario 1***: there is a mismatch between expected and actual events and the SHS must take direct control if information gathering is to occur.

10.4.4 Scenario 3: conflict

This scenario (see Fig. 10.3D, E, H) has four different flavours. Entorhinal input initially provides a '*familiar-ignore*' signal: a motor program will deal with current predicted events, or no motor program is needed. But, absent the predicted event (signalled by medial septal input), entorhinal input flags an *unexpected absence*. Conversely, the medial septal input flags an event (somewhat differently than do the amine inputs); and, absent matching entorhinal input, flags an *unexpected presence*. So, conflict can arise when:

(1) a stimulus event, flagged as significant/salient by an amine input (acetylcholine, dopamine, noradrenaline or serotonin) is not matched by a cortical or subcortical motor signal (which would have meant appropriate action to deal with the event); or
(2) a cortical model is activated but not matched by the expected significant event; or,
(3) in the special case of punishment, an expected but aversive stimulus is predicted or observed concurrently with an expected or observed appetitive stimulus; or,
(4) more generally, multiple cortical representations of incompatible goals are activated. (This can involve different responses to the same stimulus or different stimuli requiring the same response.)

In all cases, this conflict involves concurrently activated goals requiring output from distinct response programming systems. But this can be of two major types.

First, motivation-motivation: the incompatible goals differ primarily in terms of motivation (e.g. approach the box versus avoid the box). Thus, in the presence of two co-localized goals (e.g. food and threat) that elicit competing response tendencies, both approach and avoidance motor program areas will be activated concurrently (at this stage neither can take control over behaviour and their activation represents potential responding). Each sends input to the hippocampal formation, which determines by integration and comparison of the level of input: (a) that more than one goal is present (an attractor and a repulsor); and (b) that activation of these is roughly equivalent. The output from the SHS is required most when the two tendencies are most equal. The subicular output, then, feeds back the signal of conflict to the relevant goals with an iterative (within and between trials) increase in negative affective associations (generating, e.g. risk aversion).

Second, situation-situation: the incompatible goals differ primarily in terms of situation (e.g. approach left arm versus approach right arm); as in concurrent discriminations, delayed matching and similar tasks. In these cases, essentially the same response (e.g. a lever press) must be made in all cases, but a choice is required between two stimuli. Here, we believe that the entorhinal cortex (and its connections with polymodal association cortex) is a key structure. In essence, the entorhinal cortex will receive two separate inputs, to both of which it can produce a '*familiar-ignore*' output given that an existing motor programme can deal with the situation. These will be passed to the hippocampus, which will detect an excess of input, and hence conflict and, produce output to the entorhinal area that then returns directly to the input areas that generated the problem. Like the normal hippocampal output (assumed to increase negative bias in the associative links of the motivationally distinct systems to which it is connected), the output from the entorhinal cortex would increase, in the neocortex, the values of the negative associations of the two competing stimuli and hence normally allow the appropriate stimulus to control behaviour. Even in this stimulus-oriented case, then, the output from the hippocampal formation can be viewed as supplying a form of goal inhibition.

There is a third obvious type, where both situation and motivation differ. We will leave discussion of this to §10.5.

We have examined the various conditions which cause the subiculum and entorhinal cortex to detect conflict. Such detection is identical with the requirement for action. What then ensues? In this context, it is important to recall that the postulated outputs of the SHS/GIS go well beyond simple goal inhibition and, at least in the case of information gathering behaviour ('risk analysis'), can involve the release of active behaviours. We consider the common consequences of these different types of conflict in §10.6.

10.4.5 Scenario 4: disengagement

Conflict engages the SHS. Absent pathology, one would think that it must eventually disengage. What then? We consider four cases.

Scenario 4a—mismatch is unimportant, as in experiments on habituation (Vinogradova, 1975) that we have already analysed. Here, entorhinal input shuts SHS gates with '*familiar-ignore*' (Fig. 10.3 C, D, F); likewise with exploration of a novel environment—the SHS inhibits prepotent responses and habituation of SHS responses releases this inhibition. Neither habituation of the response initially elicited by the stimulus itself nor the orienting reflex are controlled by the SHS. Latent inhibition (see section A9.8 in Appendix 9), here, can be viewed as broadly similar but with little or no initial reaction to the habituated stimulus. The partial reinforcement effect can be viewed as similar to latent inhibition, but where the habituated stimulus is the internal autonomic response, or the memorial representation of the omission of an expected reward, and processing depends on noradrenergic as well as more specific inputs. An important point to note about latent inhibition and the partial reinforcement extinction effect is that the '*familiar-ignore*' signal, while no doubt affecting the hippocampus proper, has its most obvious subsequent behavioural effects through the direct connection between the entorhinal cortex and the nucleus accumbens.

Scenario 4b—mismatch is important and continued performance of the current plan is the problem. Here, the subicular comparator will slow the 'faulty' program, elicit information update, and vary behaviour trying for a more effective program. Any alternative response strategies (e.g. taking a different turn in a maze) will be promoted. This sounds sophisticated. But the subicular signal is simple with complex output controlled by its target structures. The '*faulty*' subicular tag merely decreases *output* from, not activation of, the prepotent goal representation. With a novel stimulus, this inhibition allows exploration (likely via the nucleus accumbens not directly). Likewise with a weak prepotent response, and absent strong general exploration, any familiar stimuli in the environment can control behaviour. So, the 'instruction' to try alternatives is an *indirect* consequence of the suppression of the prepotent actions. If new choice leads to success, diversification will cease, and we will typically engage in unlearned alternatives (e.g. grooming, sleeping); with the SHS '*just checking*'.

Scenario 4c—you must make new, and more complex, distinctions between environmental stimuli, particularly with relational discriminations[8] (e.g. Hirsh, 1974; Cohen and Eichenbaum, 1993; Chapter 8). Like Hirsh, we think the SHS discriminates the contexts of competing responses and causes tagging outside the SHS of a 'contextual label'; this prevents competing responses interfering.[9] Like Cohen and Eichenbaum, we see the relational aspect as critical but have an opposite, simpler, view of SHS function (including the retrosplenial cortex, Smith et al., 2022)—it eliminates incorrect simple connections; it does not directly create complex ones. The simple associative rules of long-term potentiation create problems for associative memory systems (McNaughton and Wickens, 2003), particularly catastrophic forgetting. The SHS solves these by suppressing conflicting goals initially and by adding a 'faulty' tag (essentially long-term depression) to the association that generated the behaviour. Ultimately, long-term potentiation of the correct (e.g. A-B-C) relation and long-term depression of an incorrect (e.g. A-C) link will lead to permanent changes so that A-C no longer tends to elicit any response. At this point only one response tendency (appropriate to A-B-C) is elicited, there is no conflict, and the SHS reverts to '*just checking*'. Thus, again, apparently complex results of hippocampal output (the formation of relations; the addition of contextual tags) are simply a consequence of the way other systems react to receipt of interrupting *mismatch* SHS input (particularly with its increase in affectively negative associations). There is no need for complex cognitive processing by the SHS—accounting for its phylogenetic

[8] While this literature may appear archaic, it is worth noting that it is currently being ignored rather than resolved. Modern views are very much 'my picture of a small part of the data is . . . '. Older views were often thought through in more depth. Modern theories are all cut by Occam's Razor. Except, of course, ours!

[9] Note that distributed (reinstatement) training can also make memories SHS-independent, likely also because interference is reduced in and/or controlled by areas such as perirhinal and anterior cingulate cortex (Shepherd et al., 2021).

failure to expand as fast as neocortex. Taking the brain as a whole 'relational' (and other complex) processing is a simple extension of normal associative processes (Hebb, 1949). This general upside-down relational argument also applies to the role of the SHS in generalization (Zeithamova and Bowman, 2020), item-place-time binding, and so symbolic processing (Do and Hasselmo, 2021); and to the specific case where, superficially, 'the hippocampal formation binds event content and the self's position (and viewpoint in primates) to construct spatially coherent event representations over time ... [and] to facilitate the discrimination of certain moments in event[/episodic] memory' (Ross and Easton, 2022, p. 184).

Scenario 4d—is not a case of disengagement but rather permanent failure of disengagement; where the SHS can never disengage without disrupting performance. If the SHS is promoting strong memories of appropriate associations (by weakening competing, inappropriate ones), it should ultimately be able to disengage. But some deficits produced by SHS damage are apparently absolute, with little sign of recovery even over prolonged periods of testing (Olton et al., 1979a). These tasks use an ever-changing list from which the animal must choose the correct alternative, itself ever-changing. The best examples of tasks of this kind come from Olton's work with the radial-arm maze (Olton et al., 1979a; Olton et al., 1978b) and Gaffan's (1977b; 1977d) experiments on recognition memory (see Chapter 8). Here, even the context cannot be specified in absolute terms. Compare a conditional discrimination with Gaffan's (1977b) experiment where monkeys responded to the *second* appearance of each of a list of 25 pictures (Chapter 8). With conditional discrimination, you can label the correct responses once and for all: for example, go left if the walls of the maze are white, go right if they are black. But in Gaffan's experiment only the general rule (respond always to the second appearance of a slide) can be stored permanently, and this is useless as a guide to action unless the particular list of pictures to be responded to is also constructed afresh each time they occur.

Our analysis, here, has much in common with Olton's (1978a) in terms of working memory:

> The system begins with a sensory input that enters into a temporary register. A comparison process attempts to match the contents of the temporary register with each of the items in working memory. A match indicates that the choice in question (of one of the arms of the maze) has already been made and should not be repeated; information in the temporary register is deleted, a decision made as to whether to reset working memory, a search is initiated for a new choice, and new sensory input is obtained. A failure to match the contents of the temporary register and some item in working memory indicates the choice in question has not been made previously and ought to be made now. Running down the arm produces reward. The information defining the choice which was in the temporary register is stored in working memory so that the choice will not be repeated, the temporary register is cleared, the reset decision is made, a search for another choice is initiated, and new sensory input is obtained.
>
> (Olton, 1978a, pp. 363–364)

We accept the widespread view that pure working memory depends on prefrontal-posterior cortex interactions (Chapter 11; Fig. 11.3; Appendix 3); not the SHS. With novel, discriminable stimuli in, e.g. a simple delayed match to sample task, the recent association of the target stimulus with its secondarily rewarding sample context will make it clearly distinguishable from the comparison stimulus. The two stimuli will have quite distinct values and only the target will be treated as a goal. However, as discussed in greater detail in Chapter 8, previous association of a stimulus with reward, especially if combined with some factor that makes stimuli less discriminable, will allow secondary rewarding value to accrue to the comparison stimulus either by prior conditioning or by generalization. The approach and avoidance tendencies inherent in the choice will then be more evenly balanced, there will be conflict, and the SHS will be required to boost negative associations and hence prevent the incorrect choice from being made. In tasks of this kind, the problem of interference becomes worse rather than better with experience of the stimuli, and so the SHS can never disengage once it has been involved.

10.4.6 Avoiding the experimenter's perspective

Finally, in discussing scenarios, we must emphasize once more a feature of our analysis that will make it unpalatable to those who like sweeping paradigmatic generalizations and who prefer theories that can be reduced to a single sentence or adjective.[10] In all cases, 'conflict' results when the *subject/participant* perceives two or more incompatible goals. These goals are internal to them and not always obvious to the experimenter.

Conflict will not be absolutely predictable from the official (learning/cognitive) paradigm. So, there are virtually no cases in our original review of the lesion literature (Gray and McNaughton, 1983) where there are completely consistent results for any specific nominal paradigm. That said, the exceptions can be shown to involve special features (e.g. the use of olfactory stimuli in simultaneous and successive discriminations) that can be understood *post hoc*, but are not readily predictable in advance. As we note in Chapter 8 when discussing similar problems with the concept of interference, the present version of the theory (and likely any version of any theory) cannot specify exactly where in a range of parametric variations a paradigm will become hippocampal sensitive.

The theory is, nonetheless, readily tested. It makes the unequivocal prediction that, whatever the official nature of a paradigm (e.g. procedural versus declarative memory), it will be possible to create a version sensitive to SHS damage. All that is needed is any one of a variety of manipulations that introduce goal competition, particularly in the form of interference.

This claim fits the many cases in which we know it already to be true. But we are equally certain that any paradigm (except cases in *Scenario 4d)* can be produced in a form which is *insensitive* to SHS damage if we first determine the nature of, and then remove, inherent sources of goal competition. This may not be easy, since competition can come from unobvious species-typical responses (as in the case of Cohen and Eichenbaum's analysis of simultaneous olfactory discrimination; Chapter 8). Further, as with our discussion of interference, it is not the presence of the competition, alone, that makes a task SHS sensitive—controls must be able to suppress the competing response (see Chapter 8 for a relevant experimental demonstration).

A final word should be said here about passive avoidance. This might be thought to be the quintessential paradigm in which the GIS should be involved. We could expect it to always require a SHS. This is not, however, the case. In all our examples so far, it has been

[10] Our thanks go to Ray Kesner for pointing out the necessity to make this clear; and for the many hours he spent constructing thought experiments to challenge our theory.

the conflict between two *equally balanced* ***strong*** tendencies that has required SHS resolution. While often true for acquisition of some passive avoidance, this is not a logically necessity. Consistent with this view, our analysis of the data in Appendix 8 shows that the size of effect of SHS lesions in passive avoidance tasks directly relates to whether approach tendencies (accidentally or intentionally elicited by the procedure) have been as strongly activated as the avoidance tendencies. Balanced conflict is more fundamental than inhibition of behaviour.

10.5 Cortical and hippocampal trends

We have focussed on a general circuit present in any transverse slice from anywhere along the length of the hippocampus. Here we will focus on its length and connections with the dorsal and ventral trends (Yeterian et al., 2012) of neocortex (Fig. 10.4). We view a goal as being a representation (cell assembly) that combines situation (e.g. a place, a definable time, a specific complex of nonspatial stimuli) with motivation (expectation of food delivery when hungry, expectation of pain).

However, goals are distributed representations in the cortex with, for example, 'where' information activating dorsal trend cortex and 'what' information activating ventral trend cortex. This does not fit our everyday assumptions; hence our surprise at 'The Man Who Mistook His Wife for a Hat' (Sacks, 1985).

Dorsal-ventral topography extends into the SHS. Inputs to the SHS have similar topographic mapping (Fig. 10.4, right hand side) to its outputs (Fig. 9.5). The temporal/ventral/anterior hippocampus processes more the ventral cortical trend (amygdala, infralimbic cortex—and vice versa, Cohen and Meyer, 2020), and more dorsal parts process more the dorsal trend. This links to functional hippocampal differences where dorsal control appears more to do with memory/space and ventral control more to do with anxiety/goal inhibition (Bannerman et al., 2004b) and this appears to be matched by appropriate variations in human gene expression (Ayhan et al., 2021).

However, the longitudinal and commissural connections of the hippocampus proper then allow combining dorsal and ventral trend information to create conjunctive activations (Zhao et al., 2022) and determine the true level of goal conflict (e.g. with ventral hippocampus signalling novelty that gates dorsal hippocampal memory processing; Fredes and Shigemoto, 2021). Note also that, despite less direct connections, theta frequency coherence of medial prefrontal (prelimbic) cortex is stronger with dorsal than with ventral hippocampus (Dickson et al., 2022). Matching this mixing in hippocampus proper, medial and lateral entorhinal cortex receive 'where' and 'what' biased information but

> the connectivity matrix [Fig. 10.5] emphasizes the potential of substantial integration of cortical information through interactions between the two entorhinal subdivisions and between the perirhinal and postrhinal/parahippocampal cortices, but most importantly through a new observation that the postrhinal/parahippocampal cortex projects to both lateral and medial entorhinal cortex.
>
> (Nilssen et al., 2019, p. 1238)

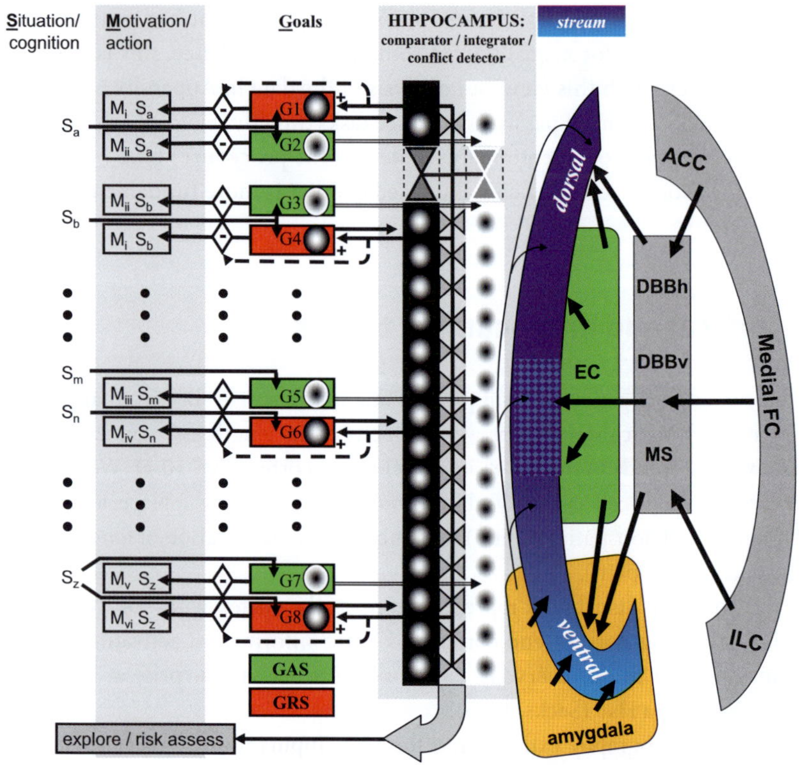

Fig. 10.4 Dorsal-ventral topography of the primary connections of the hippocampus. Attractors (GAS, green) and repulsors (GRS, red) are activated by situations ($S_a \ldots S_z$) and send output that can generate specific motor programs guided by the situation ($M_iS_a \ldots M_{vi}S_z$) with efference copies to the hippocampus. The dorsal trend of frontal cortex (e.g., ACC in medial frontal cortex) carries primarily situational information to dorsal hippocampus; while ventral frontal cortex (e.g., ILC in medial frontal cortex) carries primarily motivational information—with the goal representation distributed between the trends both in cortex and hippocampus. For cortical connections relayed by EC, see Fig. 10.2. The dorsal trend detects conflict that depends more on situation (go left/go right) than motivation; and the ventral detects conflict that depends more on motivation (food/shock) than situation. The middle portion of the hippocampus processes conflicts where both situation and motivation differ between the goals. The 3 parts are not equal and there may be others. Based on figure 1 in Moser and Moser (1998); (see also Strange et al., 2014). Note: internal connections of dorsal and ventral hippocampus can differ (Houser et al., 2021). *Abbreviations:* DBBh/v = Diagonal Band of Broca, horizontal/vertical; EC = entorhinal cortex; GAS = Goal Attraction System; GRS = Goal Repulsion System; MS = medial septum; ACC = anterior cingulate cortex; ILC = infralimbic cortex.

This organization is important for our conclusions about types of conflict (§10.4.4). It is not the case, in neural terms, that a single simple entity mixes situation with motivation, which must be disentangled when assessing conflict. Instead the cell assembly coding the goal is distributed between dorsal and ventral trends in neocortex; and so situation and motivation arrive separately in the SHS (and in humans may be associated with high and low frequency theta, respectively, Goyal et al., 2020); and situation:situation conflict is

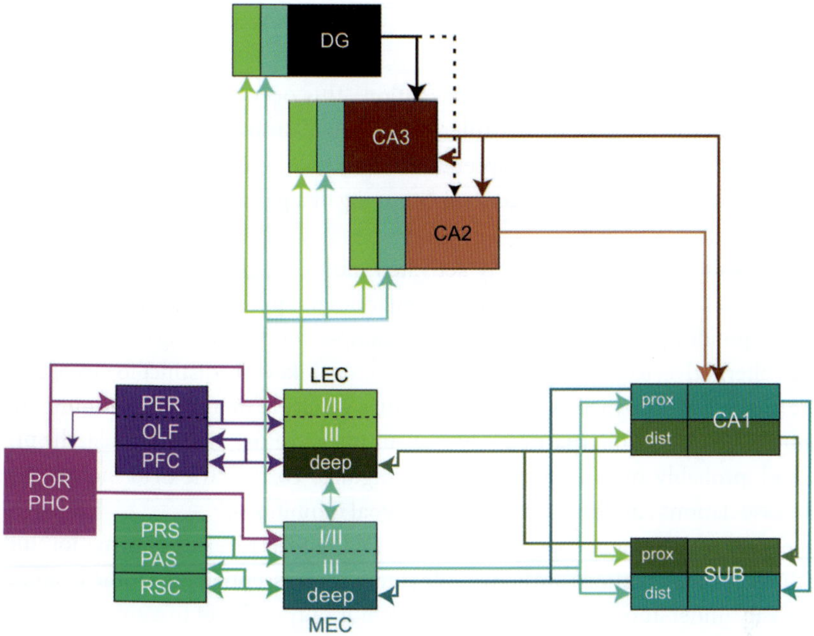

Fig. 10.5 Schematic representation of the proposed updated version of the wiring scheme of the parahippocampal-hippocampal system. The lateral and medial entorhinal cortex mediate parallel input streams, conveying integrated representations of two complementary sets of cortical inputs to the hippocampus. The lateral entorhinal cortex (LEC) receives strong inputs from perirhinal (PER), orbitofrontal, medial prefrontal and insular cortices (PFC), and olfactory structures (OLF) including the olfactory bulb and the olfactory or piriform cortex. In contrast, MEC receives main inputs from presubiculum (PRS), parasubiculum (PAS), and retrosplenial cortex (RSC). The postrhinal/parahippocampal cortex (POR/PHC) provides inputs to both MEC and LEC as well as to PER. Dashed dividers in boxes imply that incoming projections distribute to both components of the box. CA3, CA2, CA1, subfields of the hippocampus proper; DG, dentate gyrus; dist, distal part; prox, proximal part. Figure and legend taken from Nilssen et al. (2019) with permission.

detected in dorsal hippocampus, motivation:motivation in ventral hippocampus (Bryant and Barker, 2020; Abivardi et al., 2020), and conflict of both detected in the middle (Fig. 10.4).

10.6 The nature of SHS output

To a first approximation, *why* conflict has been detected is irrelevant to GIS output. Goal conflict of all types requires increases in: goal inhibition; arousal; attention; and information gathering. The amygdala (and insula, Chapter 11) controls arousal and pure increased attention. Here we look at SHS output: goal inhibition; the '*faulty*' tag; and exploratory/investigative behaviour.

10.6.1 Goal inhibition

Often, conflict blocks motor program execution. This occurs at the level of goal-subgoal execution of motor programmes (Miller et al., 1960; Brooks, 1979), not of acts and actions.[11] Thus, a CS-LOSS+ (see Chapter 3 for terminology), or the odour of a cat, will reduce food gathering behaviour in general. Stopping of a particular action is something else (see Chapter 11).

But, only some of the concurrently activated motor programs will be inhibited; not all motor responses. In complex mazes, SHS output does not prevent responding—it suppresses *incorrect* responding. Large reductions in, for example, food gathering can result from selection of an alternative, e.g. freezing motor programme. Likewise, distinct forms of goal inhibition are mediated through SHS interactions with a variety of motor programming structures for example the cerebellum (particularly nucleus interpositus), the amygdala, the prefrontal cortex and, probably most importantly, the cingulate cortex. The SHS increases affective negative associations (increasing any observed goal inhibition).[12]

At the start of its iterative operations (§10.3.1), the SHS receives information indicating that excessive representations are active. What follows is essentially the same in all cases, but is most easily understood in terms of a single motor output direct to a single target that can result in both an attractor and a repulsor.

Let us consider environmental stimuli that concurrently activate both an old established attractor and a recent repulsor (i.e. an approach-avoidance conflict, Fig. 10.3I). The SHS (receiving concurrent input from two separate and incompatible representations) detects conflict and circulates information between itself and both of the concurrently activated goals. SHS output will have two effects. First, the initially prepotent (attractor) program will be slower and more easily interrupted by hesitations for exploratory behaviour. Second, the representations will be successively altered reducing their impact on working memory. An initial, near equal, activation will thus be iteratively modified until that which may have been originally marginally stronger, but has a larger number of negative associations, is sufficiently weakened to prevent the control of output; while that which was originally marginally weaker will take control. The more equal the original representations, the longer will be the time taken to resolve the conflict and the more slowly the prepotent programme will be executed. Note that, while the conflict is being resolved, prepotent output may be temporarily blocked and replaced with information gathering (which could resolve the conflict) or even displacement activity (Anselme, 2008).

Where the conflict results from concurrent activation of two incompatible stimulus representations (as in relational processing), essentially the same processes occur. Environmental stimuli activate two (or more) incompatible memory representations. The SHS detects this concurrent activation and iteratively feeds back inhibitory signals that eliminate the marginally more negative representations in favour of the most positive (but

[11] See Chapter 11 for goal inhibition versus act/action stopping.

[12] Note that, from an interference point of view, the interfering response *can only be inhibited if it has relatively greater negative associations*. Hence, in several tasks where the controls *show* the effects of interference (and *ex hypothesi* are not suppressing it), hippocampal lesions have little effect. After further training, the controls may show evidence of suppressing the interference, and it is at this point that the hippocampal lesioned subjects will show their lack of capacity to produce this suppression (Chapter 8).

see also next). Critically here, incorrect choice of a nominally positive alternative leads to aversive frustration.

10.6.2 The 'faulty' tag

Any stimulus representation, in control of behaviour when conflict is detected, receives a tag that in English might read '*faulty, needs checking*'. Given long-term potentiation and long-term depression (and metaplasticity Abraham and Bear, 1996), the 'faulty' tag could be no more than the synaptic consequence of goal inhibition, requiring no special machinery. The faulty tag has two consequences.

(i) On future occasions goal output is executed with greater restraint. The SHS could alter once and for all stimulus connections; or itself inhibit the tagged motor program. The latter alternative is more plausible (see next). Such tagging must produce effects in advance of the point at which conflict was detected. Hippocampal long-term potentiation could be the means of providing this tag, but plasticity is much more like modifying the running program than like data storage. The '*faulty needs checking*' tag must logically be independent of the stimulus and response associations that it is qualifying.

(ii) The tagged stimulus receives enhanced attention by the subicular and entorhinal conflict detectors. This scrutiny of faulty goals is a key function we attribute to the SHS—applying the full power of the subicular (and parallel) conflict resolution circuits. Analysis of stimuli (particularly those linked to conflict) ranges over as many dimensions as possible (e.g. brightness, hue, position, size, relation to other stimuli, repetition rate,etc.). Action-outcome dependencies receive similar multidimensional analysis (is a turn in a maze left-going, white-approaching, etc.?). While internal, this analysis is linked to the initiation and execution of exploratory behaviours (§10.6.3), as in Cohen and Eichenbaum's (1993) relational theory (Chapter 8).

Internal scrutiny coupled with exploration adds up to hypothesis generation and testing (Kimble, 1975). Their combined efficiency depends on the capacity and flexibility of the dentate-CA3 gate; producing 'instructed habituation' (Kamin, 1968) and 'instructed dishabituation' (see discussion of Kamin blocking in section A9.8 of Appendix 9). The dentate selectively gates stimuli, their attributes (often originating in the cortex), and response attributes (often originating subcortically) so that, *in effect*, the SHS examines alternative descriptions of conflicting situations (or alternative routes within an environment, Wilmerding et al., 2023) and the response alternatives to resolve them.

This internal scrutiny can be prospective or retrospective. The first, prospective, case is simple—when conflict is detected, the situation is tagged faulty (likely via the simple signal that interrupts ongoing behaviour). Enhanced analysis (as well as slow execution and concomitant information gathering behaviour) then commences only on the next occasion that the tagged program is initiated. The second, retrospective, case may seem more problematic. But it is more fundamental to the operation of the whole system – and particularly important in relation to anxiety. It requires that, when conflict is detected, the ongoing motor program and stimuli associated with it (both predicted and actual) should be 'replayed'[13] by the loops between SHS and the source of efference copies. So enhanced analysis commences immediately (outside the SHS but triggered by it), re-evaluating previous affectively negative associations.

This seems close to 'rehearsal'—most obvious in the verbal case as in Baddeley's (1986) 'articulatory loop' (likely iterative interaction between Broca's and Wernicke's areas). To this phonological loop we can add (Fig. 11.6, see also Fig. 1.8) the (non-human compatible) visuo-spatial scratch pad, central executive, and episodic buffer (Baddeley, 2011). Indeed, Wagner (1978) had considerable success using 'rehearsal' to account for a range of animal learning. Clearly there is non-linguistic rehearsal in non-humans. Rehearsal circulates round a loop. There are loops a-plenty in the SHS and the structures to which it is connected (e.g. Fig. 9.9) with parallel anterodorsal, anteroventral, and anteromedial thalamic relays; also, as originally noted by Parmeggiani et al. (1974), there are loops through the midline and intralaminar thalamic nuclei.

Merely recycling the same information (as in the horizontal circuits of Fig. 1.8) would simply strengthen whatever stimulus representations are current, both appropriate and inappropriate. We presume, in contrast, that the *iterative processing* of the available representations would progressively alter them in roughly the same way as in the global stereopsis example of Chapter 1 (Fig. 1.6, see also Kovács, 2020). We have already assumed that one result of such recursion would be a more extreme separation of 'figure' from 'ground'. However, to retire the faulty motor or stimulus representation as swiftly as possible and replace it with the new, more appropriate one, we assume that iteration increases the weight of affectively negative information (via the vertical Papez circuits of Fig. 1.8; see also Fig. 9.9. In contrast to such flexible iteration, blanket inhibition could eliminate the correct as well as incorrect traces. With iteration, negative bias can be fine-tuned to the amount of residual conflict—affecting consolidation during sleep (Appendix 7; Lerner et al., 2021) as well as during waking.

This bias towards increased negative evaluations will be of particular interest when we transfer our theory of the SHS to one of anxiety disorders (Chapters 13, 14).

10.6.3 Exploratory-investigative behaviour

As well as inhibition of prepotent responses, the SHS initiates positive action when conflict is detected: exploration and investigation designed to gain additional information that can resolve the conflict. In a sense this is an external variation of an internal process of rumination/worry. Conversely, some forms of rumination/worry can be viewed as an exploration of internal information structures (past or projected into the future, respectively) so as to develop plans that can resolve the conflict (§1.14).

As we saw in ***Scenario 1***, during initial exploration of a new environment, stimulus representations and response-stimulus relations are analysed and stored for future use in the cortex and related areas. If we limit ourselves to spatially extended environments, this information gathering is as postulated by O'Keefe and Nadel (1978, p. 242); they described this as construction of a spatial map. With conflict, the novel (or unexpectedly missing) element

[13] Ditto for consolidation in general and sleep in particular (Skaggs and McNaughton, 1996).

(or its context) must be explored. Unlike O'Keefe and Nadel (1978), we do not assume that a 'map' is necessary to initiate such exploration nor that spatial conflicts are resolved differently from other kinds. We think that the SHS reacts to goal conflict in all modalities in the same way.

There are three types of situations where the resulting exploratory behaviour can help solve an animal's problems. First, conflict can be generated by a novel stimulus element without totally disrupting the current motor program. Here, exploration can re-establish familiarity by updating the current stimulus representation (as in ***Scenario 1***). Second, conflict can be inherent in the current motor program being no longer adaptive (e.g. during extinction of a previously rewarded response). Here, exploration increases the probability of detecting a reinforcer that has been relocated in space, has new schedule conditions, or is in an otherwise altered situation. With successive failures to find any reward, the original response chain will be broken for exploration earlier and earlier, resulting, in the runway case, in the familiar pattern of extinction occurring soonest in the goal and then chaining progressively back to the run and start sections. Third, environmental outcomes can be ambiguous. Here, the subicular conflict resolution process (§10.6.2) poses specific questions that can be resolved by means of exploratory and investigative behaviour. For example, the output from this process may be consistent with a situation in which the walls of a T maze are bright on occasions on which left-turning leads to food and dim on occasions on which it does not. To gain further information on this point, the subiculum would command appropriate exploratory behaviour (concerned with the brightness of the walls and the direction of the animal's turn) coupled with appropriate sensory selection. This view is essentially the same as Kimble's (1975) proposal that the SHS is concerned with testing the animal's hypotheses.

Especially given the small relative size of the human hippocampus, it is important to note that the SHS does not contain the programs for exploration. Nor do we propose that the SHS gathers and stores the information made available by exploration. Instead, for all its apparent complex functions, it releases programmes or enables storage maintained by other structures.

In the simplest case of exploratory behaviour, blanket inhibition of prepotent responses could be *all* that is necessary to release exploration. The SHS blocks response output but not goal activation and so not arousal. This high level of arousal could then release adaptive exploration in the same way as stress can release less-adaptive displacement activities (Anselme, 2008). That said, it is likely that the subicular area provides direct excitation to systems that control exploratory behaviour (locomotion, eye-movements, vibrissal movements, etc.) via, e.g. its projection to the cingulate cortex (Meibach and Siegel, 1977). This active promotion of exploration would match the cingulate control of a variety of innate checking programs, possibly originating in the striatum, and its role in obsessive-compulsive disorder (Chapters 13, 14). Excitation of exploration systems could also occur via the subicular projection to the nucleus accumbens and thence to superior colliculus, the mesencephalic motor area and thalamocortical sensory pathways (Gray et al., 1991).

The same simple, indirect, control exists for information storage. In the absence of the SHS, the animal learns simple discriminations as effectively as controls (e.g. in terms of trials to criterion). Thus, the power of extra-hippocampal systems to store the relevant CS+: GAIN and CS–: LOSS associations is intact. But, without an SHS, there is no switching between sampling of the CS+ and the CS–. So, each of the positive and negative associations is formed (as originally noticed by Kimble) in very long runs of similar choice trials. So, in the more complex cases with SHS deficits, the relevant simple associations can probably be formed as easily as before, but the sampling of multiple alternatives is impaired by the failure to inhibit incorrect choices. Conversely, if switching is not required, then there can be errorless acquisition of spatial navigation despite SHS lesions (Appendix 8).

10.7 The 'theta rhythm'/RSA

We must now incorporate RSA/'theta'. The systems that control RSA/'theta' are still unclear (§9.2.1, §9.2.2, §9.2.5). It has also been argued that human SHS 'theta' (i.e. RSA) occurs only at a lower (1–4 Hz) frequency than other species (Jacobs, 2014) but this may only be true for anterior hippocampus with posterior showing higher frequencies during virtual movement (Goyal et al., 2020). (Anterior is substantially larger and so likely more sampled in many studies.) However, a clear 2–7 Hz band (with both iEEG in patients and MEG in healthy participants) has been identified during associative memory encoding, suggesting a similar spread to rodent theta but a downshift of about 3 Hz (Joensen et al., 2023).

Even at the synaptic level much remains to be resolved (§9.2.3, §9.2.4), with completely new models being suggested recently (Colgin, 2013; Grossberg, 2021; Kocsis et al., 2022). The same is true of 'the multifaceted role of [RSA/'theta'] in cognitive functions, including spatial coding, time coding and memory, exploratory locomotion and anxiety-related behaviors' (Korotkova et al., 2018, p. 65). Its supposed functions include: '[to enhance] performance in memory tasks . . . by a shift in network function between an encoding phase [trough] and a retrieval phase [peak] within each cycle of the [RSA/'theta']' (Hasselmo, 2006, p. 712); 'to package related information within individual [RSA/'theta'] cycles for more efficient spatial memory processing' (Colgin, 2013, p. 295); that 'cycle-to-cycle variability of theta-nested spectral components [e.g. gamma] allow[ing] parsing of [RSA/'theta'] oscillations into transient operating modes with complementary mnemonic roles [learning/recall]' (Lopes-dos-Santos et al., 2018, p. 940); and, even, as in our theory, that it supports 'conflict resolution [so as] to inhibit responses to conflicting stimuli [even] during non-spatial stimulus discrimination tasks' (Sakimoto and Sakata, 2020, p. 92) and varies in optimal frequency with the demands of cognitive control (Formica et al., 2022; Senoussi et al., 2022). With overlapping event picture pairs and instructions to imagine, as vividly as possible, the pairs were found interacting meaningfully '[RSA/'theta'] power [2–7 Hz] in the hippocampus increased during encoding, and that this increase differed as a function of subsequent memory, with greater [RSA/'theta'] activity for pairs that were successfully retrieved in their entirety compared with those that were not remembered' (Joensen et al., 2023, p. 1).

These recent complex suggestions are similar to the common view (e.g. Vinogradova, 1975; O'Keefe and Nadel, 1978) that RSA/'theta' is involved in timing, quantizing and indexing information; or, more strictly, that when RSA/'theta' is observed in the EEG it reflects the phase locking of large numbers of hippocampal cells, and this phase locking is important if these functions are to be achieved. We retain this view in a weak form and with a focus on circuit-based iteration. We consider the various strong forms of this hypothesis, first, and give our reasons for rejecting them.

In the O'Keefe and Nadel (1978, p. 220) model (treated as a paradigm case for many more recent ones), RSA/'theta' is critical for determining which neurones store the information that constitutes a spatial map; and subsequently in retrieving this information when it is needed. Clearly information arriving at maximum depolarization of the intracellular RSA/'theta' cycle is more likely to undergo long-term potentiation and conversely for long-term depression (at the trough and peak, respectively of the inhibition-related extracellular rhythm, see Figure 2 in Hasselmo, 2006, see also Appendix 5). This will be true wherever in the brain there are phasic bursting cells. But, the more specifically RSA/'theta', *per se*, is impaired, the less we see of the entire SHS syndrome. A specific reduction in RSA/'theta' frequency (which should grossly impair, e.g. indexing) has only weak effects on spatial navigation (Pan and McNaughton, 1997); although supramammillary injection of a benzodiazepine has a similar effect to systemic injection on both RSA/'theta' and fixed interval behaviour. That said, blocking and then 'bypass' reinstatement of theta, blocks and reinstates water maze learning (McNaughton et al., 2006b).

An equally interesting view is that different RSA/'theta' frequencies may determine which loops in the system achieve priority in iterative processing, by matching the period of the RSA/'theta' wave to the time taken for information to circulate in a particular loop (Parmeggiani et al., 1974).

Miller (1991) provides a detailed justification for the idea that specific RSA/'theta' frequencies act to select contexts for the storage and retrieval of information:

> The total conduction delay time round each one of these patterns of loops is envisaged to correspond to the [RSA/'theta'] period. Such resonance between SHS and cortex is envisaged to have an important functional role in the registration and retrieval of information in the cortex. Each pattern of resonant loops will raise the activation of specific collections of cells which are widely dispersed across the cortical mantle.
>
> Miller (1991, p. 159)

Thus resonance, during storage of information, would cause stimulus information to be stored in a particular (frequency specific) context (i.e. cortical area). Similarly, the same resonance during retrieval would reinstate the original context and hence enhance retrieval. 'The hippocampus thus acts in some ways as an "index" to memories, the cortex being, as it were, the "book" to which this index refers' (Miller, 1991).

This is a very attractive idea, especially with information storage in the cortex rather than the SHS. But, we reject, not just its specifics, but also the principle of circuit selection by frequency encoding, for two reasons. First, information retrieval is as dependent on the frequency of RSA/'theta' as its storage. It cannot handle the data on interference and intrusion errors or intact retrograde memory after hippocampal damage. Second, comparing the relationship of RSA/'theta' to behaviour with the required accuracy of tuning of different loops make it virtually impossible that the model (or any circuit selection variant) could work. RSA/'theta' frequency varies with an animal's level of arousal rather than with the context in which it finds itself. High-frequency RSA/'theta' can be obtained when the animal is freezing hard or running hard. Low frequency RSA/'theta' can be obtained when the animal is still or producing modest movements. RSA/'theta' frequency is highest at the initiation of movement and then settles down to a frequency that is essentially constant during the remainder of a trajectory. In none of these respects can frequency provide an unambiguous or reliable context, and in probably no case will RSA/'theta' frequency be the same during learning occasions or recall occasions of a particular piece of information. Finally, 'frequency' varies markedly from wave to wave driven by chaotic not harmonic dynamics.

We have, then, rejected any overall accurate timing function for RSA/'theta' (although timing is not irrelevant), but what of quantization? Parmeggiani et al. (1971) found the conduction time round the subiculum-mammillary body-anteroventral thalamus-cingulate-subiculum loop was about 50–60 ms. Miller (1991) argued that many subiculo-cortical loops took 100–200 ms. So, simple iterative calculations in several of these loops at once would face major spread and drift. So, we see RSA/'theta' activity (i.e. phase locking of cell firing, not a noticeable local field rhythm) as the exact opposite of 'circuit selection'—that is RSA/'theta' activity maintains the discreteness of individual cycles of iterative calculation *independent* of differences in circuit conduction time. 'If hippocampal output manages to temporally bias the firing patterns of distant cortical sites ... well-timed messages from those same cortical areas will be treated preferentially by the hippocampus' (Buzsáki, 2006, p. 342). So (with some limits) inputs from all the different loops are dealt with by the various hippocampal comparators at functionally the same time on a coarse quantized basis. Like can be compared with like without confusion from timing differences.

One possible example of such synchronization is that between RSA/'theta' and vibrissal movements (Komisaruk, 1970; Macrides et al., 1981). These sometimes are phase locked for short periods; with the vibrissae entrained to theta, not *vice versa*. This phase locking would ensure that chunks of information from the vibrissae, or olfactory channels closely coupled to the vibrissae, are optimally packaged for analysis. Likewise, important stimuli reset the phase of RSA/'theta' (Givens, 1996b)—and this inhibition of ongoing activity would clear the system ready for processing of interrupting items (Park et al., 2021).

Importantly, RSA/'theta' would be expected in both 'just checking' and 'control' modes, as it would quantize both the *receipt* and *comparison* of information[14] by the SHS independent of match/mismatch. So, theta, and indeed hippocampal activation as such, can occur independently of conflict detection. But, theta-coded *output* from the SHS would only occur in control mode (i.e. when iterative processing is required).

10.8 Conclusion

This is our SHS theory. The key circuits are summarized in Fig. 10.6 (c.f. Fig. 9.8). It accounts for much of the data, being based on them. In the first edition we said that 'only future experimental test will tell whether it has any real merit'. Forty years later this remains the case, except relative to other theories that have not lasted the distance or that lack the breadth. As with the second edition, we have altered emphasis and minor details of mechanism. *But the basic theory is unchanged.* We see it as a strength that it retains the early data that memory theories have largely ignored. Critically, if we see science as predictive, it has withstood four decades of challenge—despite data largely biased by those focusing on memory (or, separately, place).

Is the theory our own? We borrow much from others. This is science. It would be a disaster if none of the insights of earlier workers could be preserved. But we have selected our

[14] 'Information' here is intended to include nested gamma cycles and the possibility of resultant multiplexing where 'coupled envelope oscillators may be particularly useful for encoding neuronal messages because they can generate high-dimensional patterns' (Buzsáki, 2006, p. 358) p. 358. We have omitted discussion of gamma and, e.g. sharp-wave-ripples, for simplicity.

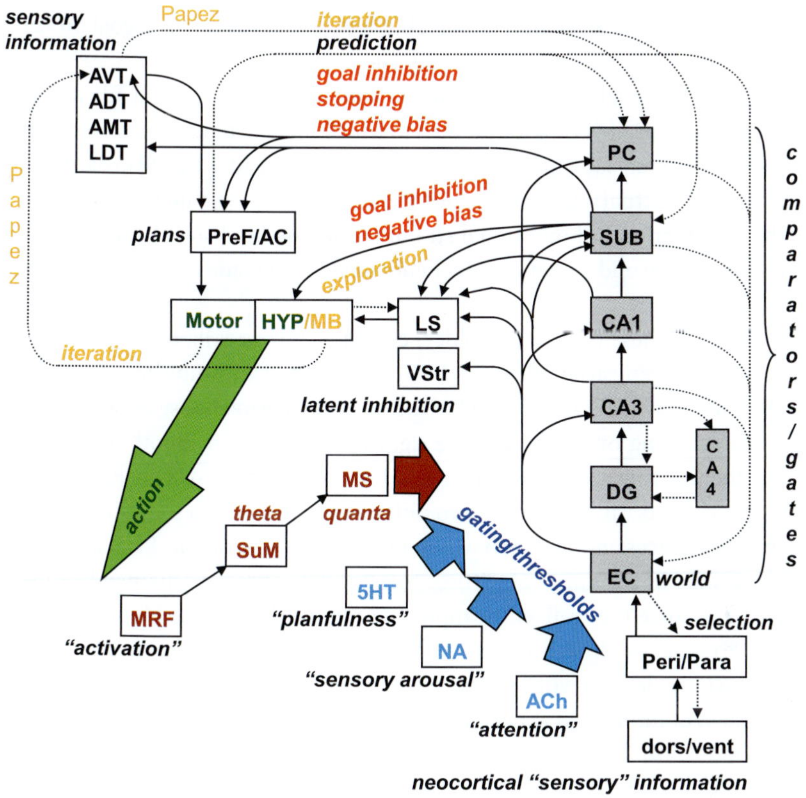

Fig. 10.6 A summary of the SHS circuitry subserving the goal inhibition and attentional outputs of the BIS. The circuits presumed to deal with perception and action have been simplified from Fig. 9.8 and Fig. 11.2 and those controlling RSA/'theta' have been simplified from Fig. 9.3, 9.5, 10.3. For the detailed workings of the system see the earlier parts of chapter 10. The arousal output of the BIS is held to be mediated independently by the amygdala and insula; and has been omitted.

borrowings, and felt free to alter them without the original authors' approval. In all the selections we have attempted to produce a consistent theory that encompasses *all the data* at *all levels of analysis*. Many will dislike how we have put our borrowings together—seeing a patchwork quilt, no stronger than its patches and the weaker for the seams. We see the integration as stronger than its elements. Critically, it should be judged against an equivalent theory that covers all the same data (memorial, innate, emotional, etc.). So far, other theories claim to be competitive (or often stay silent on the comparison) by restricting themselves to a much narrower data set (they never make a direct comparison, over all the data with our theory). They often also provide new explanations, related to new data, while our explanation remains fundamentally the same.

Our central idea is that the SHS is a conflict detector. It contains comparators (c.f., Vinogradova, 1975; O'Keefe and Nadel, 1978; Olton, 1978a; a fact surprisingly ignored, recently). The current edition sees this multiple comparator function as more general, more goal-oriented, and at more different points in SHS circuitry; but in essence the same as our earlier ideas. Likewise, we accept (Kimble, 1975) that the SHS output results in generation and testing of hypotheses given uncertainty; but we see this as release of goal processing systems outside the SHS by a simple '*faulty, needs checking*' flag.

The interaction of goal processing systems with the SHS is critical for its comparator functions—as with Kimble's view for the data to which this can be applied. From Hirsh (1974) we have taken contextual labelling; from Winocur (1981) the idea that SHS damage produces dependence on contextual cues; and melded these two positions. Butters and Cermak (1975) provide the idea that multidimensional stimulus analysis (and so the linguistic channel in humans) is important; and Cohen and Eichenbaum (1993) made clear the importance of relational analysis.

We owe much to these (now much older) concepts, but we still, unashamedly, hark back to and incorporate even earlier views of the SHS as key to the inhibition of maladaptive behaviour (McCleary, 1966; Douglas, 1967). One used to have to choose between the SHS analysing stimuli or acting on responses (see e.g. the discussion in Elliott and Whelan, 1978, p. 306; and the disavowal of non-mnemonic functions of the SHS in Eichenbaum et al., 1994). But this distorts the problem in two different ways. First, on the view developed here, the information-processing and behaviour-inhibitory roles of the SHS are, functionally speaking, two sides of the same coin. These roles are, of course, discharged by different particular neurones, since they reflect the input and output sides of the hippocampal circuitry, respectively. To separate these functions and ask which of them is carried out by the SHS is to forget that we are dealing with a level of the nervous system where perception (detection of a specific class of input) and action (production of a particular class of output) are essentially synonymous. Our frequent emphasis on this equation is again borrowed, this time from MacKay (1987). Second, we have also emphasized the fact that the SHS deals with goals and plans and that it acts to enable representations held in other areas such as neocortex (Esteves et al., 2021). A goal has both stimulus/situation and response/motivation properties. To attempt to remove the stimulus properties from a goal will destroy its qualities just as assuredly as attempting to remove the implied action tendency (Fig. 1.7).

In our treatment of external structures related to the SHS we have also borrowed wholesale. Our view of the defence system is an amalgam of the views of Graeff, LeDoux, and Davis. Our view of the organization of frontal cortex is based largely on Pandya and Barbas. Our view of working memory is a blend of Baddeley, Goldman-Rakic, and Petrides; and our view of the basic nature and different types of memory owes much to Fuster and Hebb. Our view of cingulate cortex combines the views of Vogt and Rapoport. Our view of the eyeblink conditioning circuit is essentially that of Thompson but updated via Berry. In all these cases we have made only minor alterations to make the different authors' views fit each other, and occasionally to bring specific details into line with our overall theory. Thus, however idiosyncratic our views of the SHS itself, our views of the structures to which it is connected are largely those of the current literature.

Since the theory is a blend, we have not provided a detailed analysis of all the findings summarized in the other chapters and appendices to see how well it can account for them. Some of the findings have been used explicitly to develop the theory and to produce its recent modifications. Others are discussed fully elsewhere in the book in terms of the particular theoretical ingredients to which they pertain. The bulk have contributed to the interim conclusions of the various chapters; and it is these conclusions that have supplied the fundamental building blocks of the theory. An important feature of the theory, however, is that its integration of the different data areas provides strong support for the conclusions arrived at in the individual chapters. The overall theory, then, often accommodates recalcitrant data more easily than do the individual hypotheses that tie it together.

This, then, is our basic theory of SHS function. Is it also a theory of anxiety? This step is not yet warranted; it will be addressed in the next three chapters. Chapter 11 provides a new detailed picture of the interaction of the SHS with frontal cortex; Chapter 12 provides a view of the anxious personality; and Chapter 13 converts all the previous material into a picture of disorders of defence (including fear and anxiety) and describes recent development, from the SHS theory, of the first specific anxiety disorder biomarker.

11
The neurology of anxiety—planning circuits

11.1 Treatment of 'anxiety' with prefrontal and cingulate lesions

We have now dealt with the central operations of the septo-hippocampal system (SHS) and must return to our more general focus—*anxiety*.[1] As we ascended the survival circuit 'defence hierarchy' to the SHS (Chapter 6), with conserved simple processes and expansion only at the highest level, we found a progressively better fit of the effects of systemic anxiolytic treatment to those of specific lesions. For the SHS alone, the (partial) fit was truly remarkable—given crude lesions and crude drugs.

However, there are two cortical areas where clinical evidence from gross damage suggests a specific role in anxiety: prefrontal and cingulate (briefly mentioned in Chapter 6). Damage to either of these regions served successfully, in the past, as a treatment of last resort for chronic, severe and disabling states of anxiety or fear (Marks, 1969; Powell, 1979), particularly those characterized by obsessive-compulsive symptoms (which we believe reflect fear not anxiety, §6.7). We would need in any case to consider the prefrontal and cingulate cortices even when focusing on the hippocampus and amygdala, since they are all strongly interconnected, and prefrontal and cingulate outputs match those of the hippocampus much more than do those of any other neocortical areas.

The therapeutic use of prefrontal lesions (prefrontal lobotomy, or the fibre-cutting operation known as 'leucotomy') has a long, rich, and alarming history. It was first used for schizophrenia and, many thousands of gratuitous operations later, found to be of absolutely no use (Willett, 1960). Nonetheless, it (and cingulate lesions) did alleviate symptoms of anxiety, obsession and depression (Marks, 1969; Kelly et al., 1972; Tan et al., 1971; Ström-Olsen and Carlisle, 1971).

With frontal lesions anxiety symptom reduction comes at a heavy price. Swayze (1995) noted that patients' families said that the lesions 'destroyed the soul': the patients 'are described by the nurses and the doctors, over and over, as dull, apathetic, listless, without drive or initiative, flat, lethargic, placid and unconcerned, childlike, docile, needing pushing, passive, lacking in spontaneity, without aim or purpose, preoccupied and dependent' (Hoffman, cited by Swayze, 1995, p. 507; see also Brown, 1985). Cingulate lesions had the advantage that they lacked these major side effects.

The clinical data offer some evidence for a role of prefrontal cortex (PFC) in 'anxiety' (as classified in clinical manuals). Indeed, in the original formulation of the BIS/GIS, prior to the first edition of this book, we (Gray, 1970b) located its cortical representation in the orbital PFC. But a *predominant* role does not fit easily with either the newer versions of our theory

[1] As a reminder, 'anxiety' is for us, that which is affected by anxiolytic drugs that are not also panicolytic drugs; so excluding panic, obsession, etc.

The Neuropsychology of Anxiety, Third Edition. Neil McNaughton and Jeffrey A. Gray, Oxford University Press.
 DOI: 10.1093/oso/9780198843313.003.0011

or global views of the PFC (which emphasize e.g. working memory, which is largely intact in humans treated with anxiolytics). Thus, the 'loss of soul', described by Hoffman, may make an anxious patient more tractable without forcing us to conclude that frontal cortex is the primary source of the pathological anxiety.

11.2 General issues with analysis of prefrontal and cingulate lesions

In dealing with these clinically-sourced problems we will employ three main stratagems: 1) wholesale borrowing and simplification of existing views of PFC; 2) the general acceptance of homology across species (treating monkeys as a paradigm intermediate case between rats and humans)—following the principle that the general parcellation and function of the brain as a whole is homologous (Swanson, 1995); 3) the assumption that the frontal cortex, like posterior cortex, is organized in terms of a succession of levels of processing, each higher than the last, but of essentially the same kind. There are two points to note in support of these assertions.

First, cytoarchitectonics and functional organization provide quite detailed homologies between human and macaque frontal cortex (compare figures 5 and 6 in Petrides and Pandya, 1994) and between primate and rat frontal cortex (see Kolb et al., 1994) with 'a prefrontal region whose general functions appear to be generally similar across a wide variety of mammalian species' (Kolb et al., 1994, p. 678; see also Kolb, 2010). Homology does not entail an exact match. 'While the extent to which regions are homologous across humans and other primates, such as macaques, is relatively clear, correspondences between primates and rodents are more contentious and unlikely to be one-to-one in nature' (Klein-Flügge et al., 2022, p. 2744; but, for a recent direct human to rat prefrontal functional translation, see Banstola et al., 2022). Likewise, comparison of areas 9 and 46 with area 8, shows the same double dissociation between self-ordered working memory and conditional association learning in monkey as in humans (Petrides and Pandya, 1994). A comparison of rat, macaque, and human medial and orbital frontal cortex is shown in Fig. 11.1.

Second, early apparent variations between rat, monkey and human lesion data can be attributed to a failure to involve precisely the same cytoarchitectonic fields and to substantial variation in the physical location of a functional area; with, e.g. rat orbital frontal cortex homologous to human right inferior frontal gyrus (Eagle and Baunez, 2010). That said, some differences in detailed behavioural effects are likely to arise because of variations in sensory input to, and cognitive capacity of, PFC across species. Likewise, 'the anatomical parcellation of subareas is significantly different across species, and it is likely that as the functional properties of the subareas are explored there will be significant interspecies differences in the details of prefrontal organization' (Kolb et al., 1994; see also Kolb, 2010). This matches the fact that, in humans, there are significant individual differences in precise parcellation, so variations 'among the classical maps of Brodman, von Economo and Kiskinas, and Sarkissov, and others may have been due to normal variation among the brains they analysed. Such variations may underlie individual differences in the visuospatial and cognitive capacities subserved by these areas' (Rajkowska and Goldman-Rakic, 1995b, p.323; see also Rajkowska and Goldman-Rakic, 1995a).

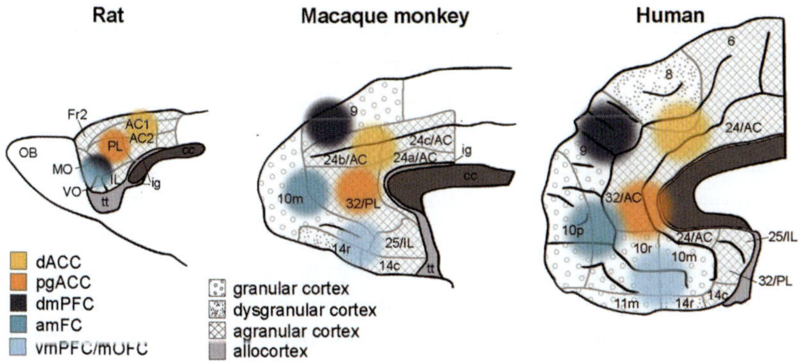

Fig. 11.1 Medial and orbital frontal cortex in rodents, macaques, and humans. Five functional regions, dorsal anterior cingulate cortex (dACC), perigenual anterior cingulate cortex (pgACC), dorsomedial prefrontal cortex (dmPFC), anterior medial frontal cortex (amFC), and ventromedial prefrontal cortex/medial orbitofrontal cortex (vmPFC/mOFC) are shown in relation to cytoarchitectonic maps of rat (left), macaque (center), and human (right) medial and orbital frontal cortex (based on Wise, 2008). All five regions are identifiable in humans and macaques. The color scheme indicates that the orbital region of rodents has some functional features shared with primate dmPFC, amFC, and vmPFC/mOFC but that it does not correspond in a simple way to any of them. Thus, while the extent to which regions are homologous across humans and other primates, such as macaques, is relatively clear, correspondences between primates and rodents are more contentious and unlikely to be one-to-one in nature. This is important to bear in mind when evaluating evidence from different species about the regions' functional contributions. Figure and legend from Klein-Flügge et al. (2022) with permission.

Variation in specific function between individuals or species does not entail lack of common design. We would argue that there are consistent global functions subserved by the dorsal (medial) and ventral (lateral) trends in PFC across species. However, the expansion of cortex that produces Broca's and Wernicke's areas in human brains must entail large differences in the precise organization of PFC between people and monkeys, not to mention between people and rats. Nonetheless, we can see Broca's and Wernicke's areas as each functioning, within the linguistic domain, in a fashion similar to the non-linguistic functioning of their respective surrounding cortices. Our analysis of PFC, therefore, has concentrated on the non-human primate data as a paradigm case. These are more tractable than the equivalent human and rat data. Given the enormous expansion of the human frontal cortex relative to other primates, the non-human primate can, in a sense, be viewed as representing an approximate half-way point between rat and human.

Let us now look at the contribution of frontal (and cingulate) cortex to defence in general and anxiety in particular. It will be useful to take an evolutionary view of this.

11.3 Evolution of the frontal cortex and the defence hierarchy

Simplifying, we can account for the bulk of the results if we identify fear (aversion without conflict, anxiolytic insensitive) with the central and medial amygdala and hypothalamus; and anxiety (where there is goal conflict, typically approach-avoidance, anxiolytic sensitive) with the SHS and basolateral amygdala. But, the full picture is more symmetric and includes different (fear/anxiety) parts of each of the periaqueductal grey (PAG) (Fig. 6.2; Silva and McNaughton, 2019), hypothalamus, amygdala, and cingulate cortex.

To some extent, we now find the trend reversing to a progressively poorer fit, with the archicortical SHS at the functional apex of both neocortical and subcortical systems. For cortex, this reversal of fit arises from phylogeny. Ever more laminated isocortex was added, functionally below, progressively older allocortex. In unimodal sensory systems, the most recent, most anatomically sophisticated, neural architecture is *closest* to the sensory receptors. Likewise, the motor strip, closest to subcortical output, is the most elaborated isocortex in cytoarchitectonic terms. Each new isocortical layer adds extra, *peripheral*, filtering modules to existing more central ancient executive allocortical systems. Deeper/older sensory modules are progressively more multimodal—the evolution of superficial modules adds progressively more sophisticated 'cognitive' filters (e.g. colour vision). Expansion changes increases the quality/resolution of input for solution of the *same* phylogenetically-basic problems. Likewise, deeper (older) motor modules are progressively more plan-like[2]—the evolution of superficial modules permits progressively more sophisticated 'routines'—allowing increased sophistication in the achievement of the *same* ultimate phylogenetic goals.

This reversal is a developmental necessity (ontogenetic and phylogenetic). Cortical expansion must refine rather than replace the function of older structures.[3] Each addition must, while it is evolving, leave earlier (highest order, multimodal) mechanisms, at least initially, unaffected so that they can continue to deal with those problems that they were originally capable of solving. In that sense the subcortex/cortex boundary involves a phase transition. As a result, the highest-level 'emotional'/goal control functions in PFC are executed by ancient conserved allocortex not more recent isocortex. Thus, disparate and distributed peripheral changes increase the computational level of processing in deep, conserved, primordial, multimodal areas—at the cortical-subcortical interface.

This enrichment feature of phylogeny allows us to present a wholistic species-general account of function and even neural organization (with monkeys as a paradigm case). Particularly with PFC this may seem to ignore differences between the species. But we see these as quantitative, species-specific, and relating to the depth of cortical filtering of information. From the lamprey onwards fundamental functional organization remains largely conserved, as is the superficial control of rhythms (Grillner and Robertson, 2016; Loonen and Ivanova, 2018a; Loonen and Ivanova, 2015; Loonen and Ivanova, 2018b; Loonen and Ivanova, 2019; Suryanarayana et al., 2020; Rocchi et al., 2021; Buzsáki, 2006).

This perspective suggests that, while the SHS is the central structure on which the processing of anxiety depends (as the superior colliculus and lateral geniculate are key structures on which vision depends), there will be cortical areas that carry out more sophisticated control of the same forms of anxiety (or *mutatis mutandis* vision). Trivially, all neocortical sensory systems (and ascending non-cortical sensory systems) must be involved in anxiety: they provide the sensory input and cognitive evaluation on which assessment of threat is based.

[2] Note that even the motor strip includes inter-effector segments between its 'homuncular' components that 'coordinate with each other and with the [cingulo-opercular network] to accomplish holistic, whole-body functions in the service of performing actions' (Gordon et al., 2023, p. 356).

[3] This is true, even where there has been encephalization. The human tectum cannot perform, in the absence of the cortex, the kinds of task that are undertaken by the frog tectum. But the cortico-tectal complex retains the original tectal functionality despite physical separation of its upper and lower modules. This resembles the geographic retention of, e.g. marsupials despite separation of the tectonic plates on which they live.

This is the role that we (following LeDoux) have already assigned to them in relation to the conditioning of fear: sensory input is sent monosynaptically from different levels of the sensory systems to the amygdala, where it functions to provide neutral conditioned stimuli (CSs) until long-term potentiation (or some other form of plasticity) produces a functionally active connection of the input to defensive systems. These sensory areas must also provide the basis for the detection of, as opposed to reaction to, innate fear and innate anxiety stimuli (including complex social stimuli). Similarly, all neocortical efferent systems (and descending non-cortical motor systems) may sometimes control behavioural output. However, like the primary sensory systems, this motor involvement is not specific to anxiety and can be linked to the motoric requirements of a specific situation rather than to its defensive aspects.

With the bulk of the cortex, then, lesion evidence provides us with little reason to suppose a primary involvement in anxiety. For example, after lesions of visual cortex, one can demonstrate that anxiety is intact, provided we use a different intact non-visual modality to present significant stimuli; whereas all responses to visual stimuli, anxiogenic or not, are equally degraded. Similarly, one can show with lesions of, e.g. motor cortex that there is a general loss of both non-anxious and anxious responses of some specific type, independent of eliciting stimuli. However (§11.1), prefrontal and cingulate cortex clearly have a role in defence in general and, potentially, anxiety in particular—even while they have related roles in other emotions. We will need the bulk of this chapter to discuss this—and the interlinked role of the insula with both frontal and cingulate areas (§11.7).

11.4 Frontal cortex anatomy

Taken together, the prefrontal and cingulate cortex involve a huge part of the cortical mantle; have a mass of subdivisions; and have received fine-grain functional assessment only recently. Therefore, we start here (see also Appendix 3) with neuroanatomy as a guide to function.

11.4.1 The dorsal and ventral trends

The increasing cytoarchitectonic differentiation that occurs during evolution and development provides an important rostro caudal basis for simplifying and understanding the anatomical connections and functions of the frontal cortex. Orthogonal to this is a division into a part with a 'hippocampal' origin and one with an 'olfactory' origin. Thus, one can see an evolutionary, cytoarchitectural, connectional, and functional 'dorsal trend'(see Barbas and Pandya, 1987; Barbas and Pandya, 1991) originating in hippocampal allocortex and progressing frontally through pyramidal regions until it reaches area 8 (see next). This dorsal trend is mirrored by an equivalent 'ventral trend' originating in olfactory allocortex and progressing frontally through granular regions until it too reaches area 8 (Fig. 11.2). There have been related progressive changes in the basal ganglia (Grillner and Robertson, 2016).

The dorsal and ventral trends in frontal cortex are matched by, and primarily connected to, separate dorsal and ventral trends in each of the unimodal sensory cortices. Put crudely, the ventral trend in both frontal and posterior cortex deals with 'what' stimulus is (or may be) present; the dorsal trend deals with 'where' the stimulus is or may be (Gross, 1994); and, we argue next, that the cingulate and insula are a mesial trend that deals with 'why' we should

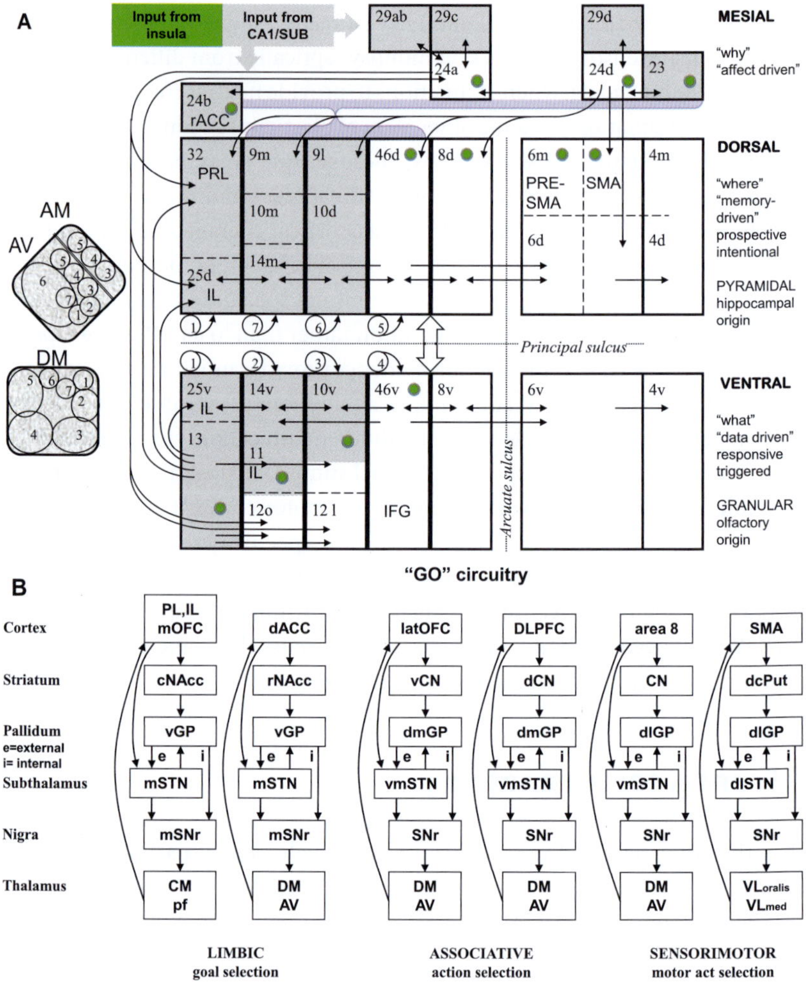

Fig. 11.2 A simplified hierarchical view of frontal cortex. A. Frontal and cingulate cortex represented as modules (areas of boxes do not reflect actual amount of cortex—compare Fig. 11.4B). This is organized in terms of three separate 'trends': dorsal, ventral and mesial (i.e., cingulate cortex and insular cortex, §11.7). Numbers refer to Brodmann Areas (in prefrontal cortex: d = dorsal; l = lateral; m = medial; o = orbital; v = ventral; in cingulate cortex a,b,c,d are conventional subdivisions). The dorsal and ventral trends are shown to some extent as mirror images of each other with the progression of levels from 4m through 32/25d and from 4v through 25v/13 representing a steady increase in the level of essentially the same kind of processing (see text). Shaded areas show input from subiculum and/or area CA1 of the hippocampus; green dots show input from the anterior (and other) insula. The numerals 1-7 in small circles represent the topographically organized input from the antero-ventral (AV), anteromedial (AM) and dorsomedial thalamus (DM), each segment of which innervates an entire level of dorsal or ventral trend. IL = infralimbic cortex; IFG = inferior frontal gyrus; ISO, isocortex; PERI = periallocortex; PRL = prelimbic cortex; PRO = proiscortex; SMA = supplementary motor area. Adapted from Gray and McNaughton (2000) Fig. 1.9; with additional data from Nachev et al. (2008); Price (2006); Cavada et al. (2000); Goldman-Rakic and Porrino (1985); Vogt (2009). **B.** Topographic organization of connections of frontal cortex to subcortical "Go" motor control circuits (for "Stop" see Fig. 11.10). Note the fundamentally similar organization of the parallel topographic units. These are arranged from left to right to match the levels in A. Adapted from Haegelen et al. (2009); with additional data from Jacobson and Trojanowski (1977); Chambers et al. (2009); Humphries and Prescott (2010); Haber and Calzavara (2009); Grillner and Robertson (2016); and (Peng et al., 2018).

worry about the stimulus. Each of these areas is distinguished by its specific thalamic and sensory cortical connections. The dorsal trend receives largely external sensory input, while the ventral trend, then the cingulate, then the insula have inputs that are progressively more weighted towards (but not exclusively devoted to) interoceptive/motivational inputs including those originating in the hypothalamus.

11.4.2 The mesial trend

Cingulate cortex can be viewed as originating from approximately the same allocortical primordium as the dorsal (hippocampal) trend in frontal cortex. However, it is functionally and connectionally more akin to the ventral (olfactory) trend in frontal cortex. In many respects, together with the insula (see §11.7), it represents a quite distinct mesial trend. The anterior cingulate, while being physically located in frontal cortex (defined as cortex anterior to the central sulcus), has none of the posterior sensory cortical connectivity that distinguishes the adjacent dorsal trend. Its sensory input (much modified and largely interoceptive) is provided by the insula. Nonetheless, it terminates (as do the other two prefrontal trends) at the border of area 6, with connections to area 6 and so indirectly to area 4; and we shall argue that it is at least homologous with the dorsal and ventral trends in its relations to motor control. Indeed, one can view the cingulate motor cortex as providing access to the motor system for a large number of limbic areas (Fig. 11.3) in much the same way that frontal cortex provides access for sensory cortical areas. The posterior cingulate is located behind the central sulcus and, we shall argue, is homologous with the posterior sensory cortices, and particularly with the posterior insula, temporal cortex, and archicortex. Nonetheless, its thalamic connectivity is more akin to that of frontal cortex. Thus, cingulate as a whole can be viewed as quite distinct from both frontal and posterior cortex.

11.5 Dorsal and ventral trend processing ('external planning')

Our functional picture (see also Appendix 3) amalgamates two apparently separate views (see, e.g. Passingham, 1993, pp. 208–209): 1) PFC is the apex of the motor system—the highest, executive, level of a hierarchically organized motor programming network that 'is concerned with the process by which new decisions are taken as to what to do' (*op. cit.*, p. 209). 2) PFC subserves working memory (e.g. Goldman-Rakic, 1992), receiving information from many cortical areas for use in current processing—the highest level of a hierarchically organized perceptual analysis network (Fig. 11.4).

11.5.1 The perception-action cycle

While these two proposals sound quite distinct, they are not incompatible. Indeed, if we accept MacKay's (1987) view that perception and action must often involve the *same* neural circuitry, amalgamation of these points of view is not only easy but almost tautologous. Thus, Fuster (1995) argued for the more general term 'active memory' as the key

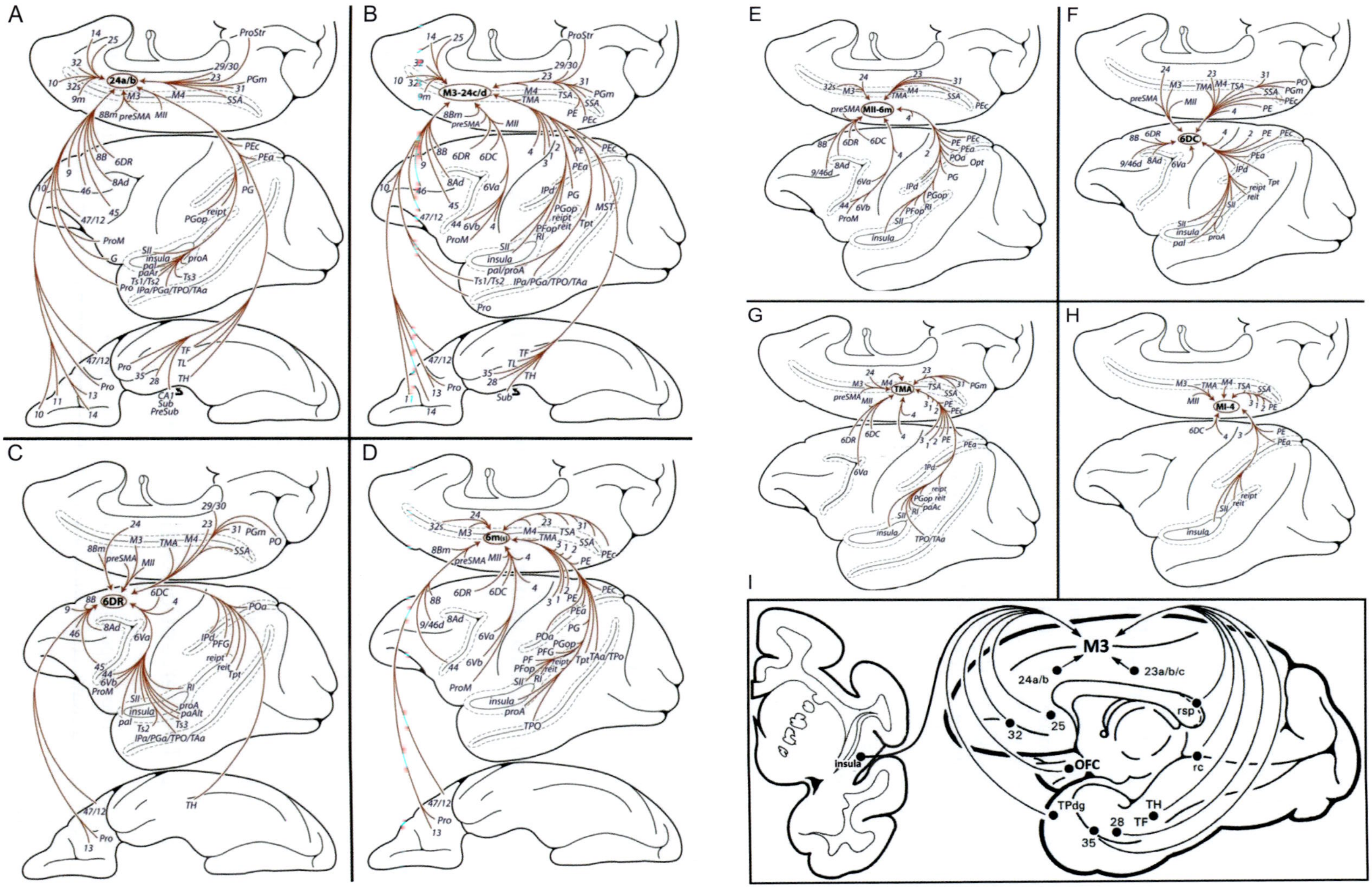

A
24a/b
B
M3-24c/d
C
6DR
D
6m
E
MII-6m
F
6DC
G
TMA
H
MI-4
I
M3
24a/b
23a/b/c
25
32
rsp
rc
OFC
TPdg
TH
TF
28
35
insula

Fig. 11.3 Summary diagrams showing the cortical afferents to supracallosal areas 24a/b (A), mid-levels of M3 or area 24c and d (B), area 6DR (C), sulcal(s) area 6m (D), arm region of area 6m (MII) (E), area 6DC (F), the TMA (G), medial area 4 (H) and a simple overview (I). *Abbreviations:* ac, anterior commissure; amy, amygdala; as, arcuate sulcus; ca, caudate nucleus; cc, corpus callosum; ccg, genu of corpus callosum; ccs, splenium of corpus callosum; cf, calcarine fissure; cgs, cingulate sulcus; cl, claustrum; cs, central sulcus; G, gustatory cortex; gp, globus pallidus; hf, hippocampal fissure; hp, hippocampus; Iag, agranular sector of insula; ic, internal capsule; Idg, dysgranular sector of insula; IG, granular sector of insula; ilas, inferior limb of arcuate sulcus; ios, inferior occipital sulcus; ips, intraparietal sulcus; KA, auditory koniocortex; lf, lateral fissure; los, lateral orbital sulcus; ls, lunate sulcus; MI, primary motor cortex; MII, supplementary motor cortex; M3, rostral cingulate motor cortex; M4, caudal cingulate motor cortex; mos, medial orbital sulcus; OFC, orbitofrontal cortex; ot, optic tract; ots, occipital temporal sulcus; paAc, para-auditory cortex caudal; paAlt, para-auditory cortex lateral; paAr, para-auditory cortex rostral; paI, parainsular cortex; ParaSub, parasubiculum; poms, medial parieto-occipital sulcus; preSMA, presupplementary motor cortex; PreSub, presubiculum; Pro, proisocortex; proA, proauditory cortex; ProM, proisocortical motor cortex; ProStr, prostriata; ProSub, prosubiculum; ps, principle sulcus; pu, putamen; rc, retrocalcarine; reipt, retroinsular parietal temporal cortex; reit, retroinsular temporal cortex; rf, rhinal fissure; RI, retroinsular cortex; ros, rostral sulcus; rsp, retrosplenial, SII, secondary somatosensory cortex; slas, superior limb of arcuate sulcus; spocs, superior postcentral sulcus; sts, superior temporal sulcus; Sub, subiculum; th, thalamus; TH/TF/TP, temperopolar; TMA, transitional motor area; TSA, transitional sensory area; v, ventricle. Figures and legend adapted from Morecraft et al. (2012) and Morecraft and Van Hoesen (1998) with permission.

short-term memory process within the 'perception-action cycle' (Fuster, 1990); and retains this view: 'Insofar as the content of working memory consists largely of updated long-term memory, working memory can [still] be legitimately called *active memory*' (Fuster, 2015, p. 395). Most obviously, if goals reflect the combination of situation and motivation, they will be an amalgam of perception and action.

'1. The entirety of the cortex of the frontal lobe is devoted to the representation and production of action at all levels of biological and behavioural complexity, including language.
2. The neuronal substrate for the representation of any action in the cortex is identical to the substrate for the production of that action.
3. That substrate for action consists of a complex array of widely distributed, partly overlapping and interactive neuronal networks of the frontal lobe, some of which extend into posterior cortex.
4. Networks in the dorsolateral convexity of the frontal lobe are chiefly in charge of the cognitive aspects of action; networks in the ventral (orbital) and medial frontal cortex are in charge of its emotional (affective and reward-related) aspects.
5. Frontal cognitive networks interact with other cortical networks in the frontal lobe and in other cortices; cognitive and emotional networks interact with one another in ventromedial prefrontal cortex.
6. All goal-directed actions, especially if they are new and complex, are processed in the perception—action cycle, the adaptive biocybernetic interface between the cortex and the environment. Two parallel components of that cycle, one cognitive and the other emotional, interact with each other in ventromedial prefrontal cortex.
7. Cognitive networks, as well as the cortical levels of the perception—action cycle, are hierarchically organized, from the most concrete to the most abstract adaptive action: simple actions in lower levels (motor cortex and striatum) and global actions and plans in the prefrontal cortex.'

(Fuster, 2015, p. 376; see also Graziano, 2023; Gordon et al., 2023, on action and motor cortex)

11.5.2 Working/active memory mechanisms

For working/active memory to occur, long-term memories (LTM) and current percepts originating in primary and association sensory areas (including, for example, spatial information stored in the parietal cortex) must be loaded, by direct topographic connections from these areas, into PFC (Fig. 11.4). If we combine Hebb's (1949) view of perceptual cell assemblies and Fuster's (2022) view of Cognits with Baddeley's (2011; detailed in §11.5.3) view of the central executive, phonological loop, visuo-spatial scratch pad, and episodic buffer then we see that working/active memory must be iterative. Mirror image topographic mapping could then support planning by producing activity that arises in a specific area of frontal cortex, in the absence of specific environmental stimuli, initiating the activation of the appropriate part of a specific posterior cortical system (hence providing a basis for imagery).

Working/active memory information is an integral part of the control of ongoing motor acts. This is particularly true where working/active memory keeps a percept active during a

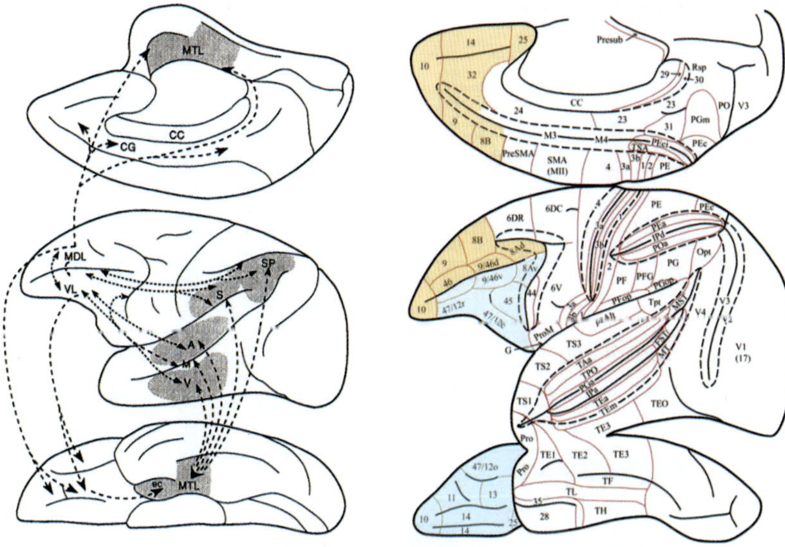

Fig. 11.4 Frontal-sensory cortical connections that may subserve working/active memory. **A.** The reciprocal connections could subserve the transfer of information from the sensory to the frontal cortex or could allow frontal cortex to refresh and keep active circuits encoding particular types of information in sensory cortex. From Petrides (1994) with permission. **B.** Schematic representations of the medial, lateral, and ventral surfaces of the cerebral cortex of the rhesus monkey (Macaca mulatta) according to Petrides and Pandya (Petrides and Pandya, 2007; Petrides and Pandya, 1994). The architectonic areas depicted in these diagrams are based on the findings of several investigators [see original source for citations]. Areas of the dorsal prefrontal (archicortical) architectonic trend are shown in orange, and those of the ventral prefrontal (paleocortical) architectonic trend are shown in blue. From Yeterian et al. (2012) with permission.

delay at the end of which, according to Goldman-Rakic (1992), a '*go*' command terminates the delay firing, which is then read out as a target for the response system (Fig. 11.5).

11.5.3 Planning and the multicomponent approach

Fig. 11.5 involves both extremely simple stimuli (dots that vary in position) and a very simple motor act (moving the eyes). But it is easy to expand the ideas and fundamental architecture both to cases where there is no memory requirement and to cases where the memory requirement is complex. In the first case, absent an explicit '*stop*' signal, the same basic circuit can generate an immediate 'commanded' response of the form ultimately generated as the delayed response. They key in both cases is a gate, opening of which releases the response from inhibition. In the second case, the simple (almost single neuron pair) cell assembly of Fig. 11.5 is replaced by whatever complex cluster of cell assemblies is normally required for detection of the relevant perceptual/cognitive construct. Note also that the figure involves an implicit role for LTM. Both the required response (eye movement) to the target and the nature of the '*go*' stimulus must be learned and made available when needed.

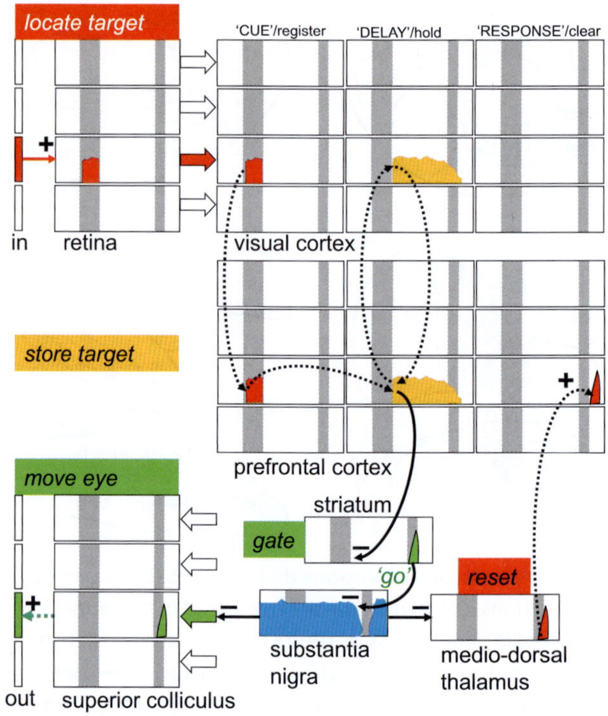

Fig. 11.5 A schematic diagram showing the likely neural architecture underlying responses in a simple working/active memory task in which the monkey must fixate the centre of a screen, remember the position of an offset dot during a delay, and then on presentation of an end-of-delay (***'go'***) signal move its eyes to the position at which the dot was previously displayed. Presentation of a dot at specific point in visual space (red bar at top left) activates the retina topographically (red fill). The retinal input to visual cortex produces topographically mapped activity in two classes of cell `cue' (red) and `delay' (amber). Any tendency to respond to the cue is stopped. Because of the significance of this input for the *upcoming* motor response, activity in the 'cue' cell produces topographically mapped activity in prefrontal cortex 'cue' cells (red) and hence continuous activity in prefrontal 'delay' cells (amber) because of their iterative interaction with visual cortex 'delay' cells, which maintains the visual information during the delay. On presentation of the 'go' signal there is a release of inhibition of motor circuits that allows the animal to move its eye to the position maintained by the activity in the prefrontal-visual cortical loop. There is a feedback signal, via the medio-dorsal thalamus, which resets the working memory system (Adapted from Goldman-Rakic, 1992).

More generally,

> incoming information is processed by systems that themselves are influenced by LTM. I see [working/active memory] as a complex interactive system that is able to provide an interface between cognition and action, an interface that is capable of handling information in a range of modalities and stages of processing.
>
> (Baddeley, 2011, p.18)

This complexity involves variation in modalities and in levels of processing. Most critically, using Fig. 11.5 as a paradigm model, we must be prepared for working/active memory to be a

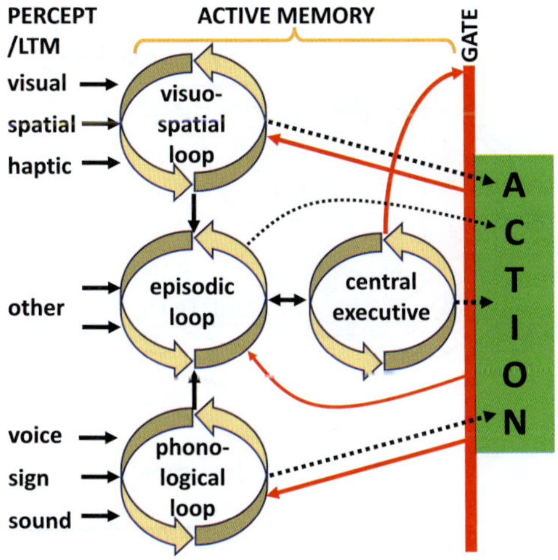

Fig. 11.6 The links between perception/LTM, active memory, and action derived from Baddeley (2011) and Fig. 11.5. 'Crystallised' LTM can only influence behaviour by activating perceptual/cognitive cell assemblies. It, and perception, can then influence behaviour; and the cell assembly retain its activity (or a key part thereof) via one or more loops that act as active 'fluid' memory buffers. Delay activity is maintained while actions are blocked by a command gate. Selective release of a specific action also produces feedback cancelling loop iteration.

property of a set of neural circuits (e.g. visual↔prefrontal) not of a single structure. Fig. 11.6 provides a picture of the systems involved, derived from Baddeley (2011).

As noted already, it is best in this connection to blur the distinction between prefrontal and motor areas (and also to take a spectrum perspective, blurring area boundaries, John et al., 2022). As we progress from the most differentiated areas of frontal cortex to the least (e.g. 4 6 8 46 10 14 25; Fig. 11.7; for a different perspective see Figure 2 in Ben Shalom, 2022), we appear to deal with progressively more anticipatory aspects of motor control (motor →pre-motor →visual attention →working/active memory →planning). Working/active memory appears to acquire its 'working' aspects from the iterative interconnections of the principal sulcus with other frontal areas (more motor in the case of the more differentiated areas of posterior frontal cortex, more planning in the case of the less differentiated areas of anterior and ventral PFC), and its 'memory' aspects from the iterative interconnections of the principal sulcus with posterior cortical areas.

On this view, working/active memory generally would function in an analogous fashion to the 'phonological loop' that supports the subvocal rehearsal of verbal material (Baddeley, 2011; Chapter 5 of Baddeley, 1986; Fig. 11.6). Although we lack a specific psychological terminology for the processes involved in each of the less differentiated levels of PFC, as we move from gaze control to working/active memory to these less differentiated levels it appears likely that the fundamental architecture is the same. The links to the same architectonic level of posterior cortex provide the primary sensory information required, and the links to more and less architectonically differentiated levels of frontal cortex provide coordination between more and less anticipatory levels of pre-motor control (Fig. 11.2A).

This largely matches the view that 'the whole prefrontal cortex is premotor cortex.... the canonical function of orbital frontal cortex (OFC) is optimization of

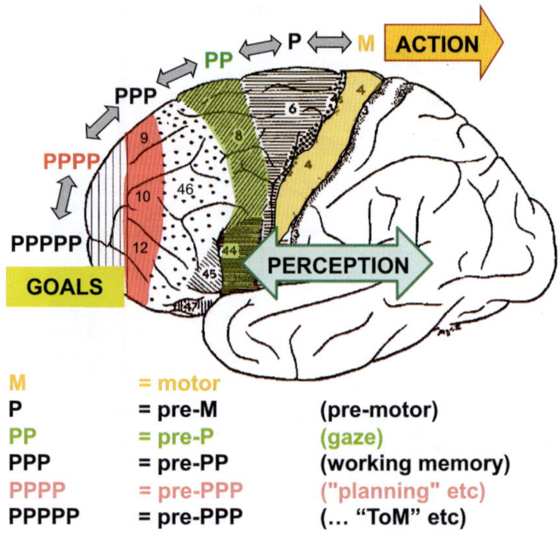

Fig. 11.7 Planning as hierarchical active memory of motor action. The motor strip (Brodman area 4) controls action that has been passed to it from the pre^1-motor area (6). In terms of Fig. 11.5, the frontal eye fields (8) move the eyes, but for many motor acts such fixation is required before the final steps of an action can be carried out, and so the area can be viewed as pre^2-pre^1-motor cortex. During the delay period, the upcoming eye movement is held in what can be viewed as working/active memory cortex (46), i.e., pre^3-pre^2-pre^1-motor cortex. In turn, active memory, holding in advance the intended contents of upcoming working memory, the subgoal level of planning cortex (9, 10, 12), i.e., pre^4-pre^3-pre^2-pre^1-motor cortex; and ever higher levels, i.e., pre^5-pre^4-pre^3-pre^2-pre^1-motor and above, holding in mind current goals both of self and others (via Theory of Mind/ToM). Note that this neurological perspective gives an evolutionarily smooth, hierarchical, perspective of processes to which psychologists apply a range of categorically distinct labels. Note also the highest levels of computational abstraction occur in the oldest, most architectonically simple, cortex. The integration of the senses into a single point of view and ultimate goal of current actions is something, then, that we share with non-humans—allowing them to provide simple models of our fundamental mental processes—and their disorders.

goal-selection policies . . . [being] at the top and most abstract portion of the prefrontal hierarchy. . . . The selection of goals through their own policy optimization ([by] OFC) is hierarchically higher than rule-based policy abstraction. . . . Goals sit hierarchically above rules [but leave a] role of the dorsal frontal cortex in rule policy abstraction, it contextualizes the process of how agents might optimize different rule policies based on which goals have been selected' (Fine and Hayden, 2022, p. 1, p. 6).

11.5.4 Inhibition of actions and goals

Implicit in this picture of planning, and explicit in the execution of delay tasks (Fig. 11.5, 11.6), is the importance of inhibiting planned action until it is appropriate. Here a single goal is involved and subgoals need ordering in time but not cancelling. These operations can easily be undertaken by the push-down-stack architecture of Fig. 11.7.

However, when conditions change, planned actions and goals can also require complete cancellation. With actions this is usually referred to as stopping and with goals as behavioural inhibition (or better, we have argued, goal inhibition). This cancellation involves quite distinct machinery from the working/active memory circuits we have discussed so far—and the circuits involved appear to differ depending on urgency (Fig. 11.8, which see for abbreviations). Maximally fast 'acts' are stopped with a simple, general, 'kill switch'; 'actions' that allow some anticipatory slowing are stopped via a more nuanced, more selective, stopping system; and not-yet-started actions aimed at specific goals (e.g. in go/no-go paradigms) are cancelled by the goal inhibition system.

Consistent with Fig. 11.8, stopping in the simple stop signal task (SST; for details see quote to follow) is impaired by lesions in preSMA and SMA when anticipatory slowing is not available (Floden and Stuss, 2006) and by lesions in rIFG when behaviour can be more flexible (Aron et al., 2003; Aron et al., 2004). Neuroimaging (fMRI) has also identified several neural networks activated during such stopping of an already initiated response—involving rIFG, middle frontal gyrus (dorsolateral prefrontal cortex; areas 91, 101, and 46; DLPFC), medial frontal gyrus (MFG, areas 8m and 9m), basal ganglia (Verbruggen and Logan, 2008; Rubia et al., 2003; Li et al., 2006; Aron, 2007; Chambers et al., 2009; Aron, 2011; Aron et al., 2014a; Aron et al., 2014b) and superior frontal gyrus (Rae et al., 2015).

Importantly, this fast action stopping (unlike the slow goal cancelling that is an output from the GIS) is not affected by anxiolytic drugs (McNaughton et al., 2013; Shadli et al., 2015). Despite this, we found evidence for activation of the GIS when go and stop are in maximal conflict.

> From the goal conflict aspect of the [GIS] theory (McNaughton, 2018; Gray and McNaughton, 2000), and from our 'theta' anxiolytic model (McNaughton et al., 2007), we have developed a human scalp EEG anxiety-process biomarker. Hippocampal 'theta' itself cannot be recorded from the scalp; but we showed in rats that, during risk assessment, it becomes phase locked with anterior frontal and cingulate cortex (Young and McNaughton, 2009). So, for our previous human translation work, 'our primary hypothesis . . . was that conflict should be a source of avoidance, separate from simple aversion. To assess the unique influence of conflict on neural activation and behavior, we manipulated dollar gains and losses in a simple choice task. We predicted that when the potential amounts of gain and loss for a response were equal (generating approach-avoidance conflict), this should increase right frontal . . . theta spectral power more than either net gain (greater approach tendency) or net loss (greater avoidance tendency). . . . [As predicted,] in the first half of the pre-response period, theta power peaked in CONFLICT trials at the right frontal site F8' (Neo and McNaughton, 2011, pp. 396, 398–399).
>
> We then attempted to confirm the role in conflict of right frontal areas in general and F8 in particular, using the SST (Aron et al., 2003) (SST). In the SST, the participant normally makes a left or right mouse click ('go') in response to a left (<=) or right (=>) arrow. However, if a tone is presented, they must withhold responding ('stop'). Variation of the delay of a 'stop' signal can result in approach ('go', short delay), avoidance ('stop', long delay), or a conflict between the two when the theoretically independent (Aron et al., 2003) approach and avoidance tendencies are balanced and there is about 50% correct stopping.

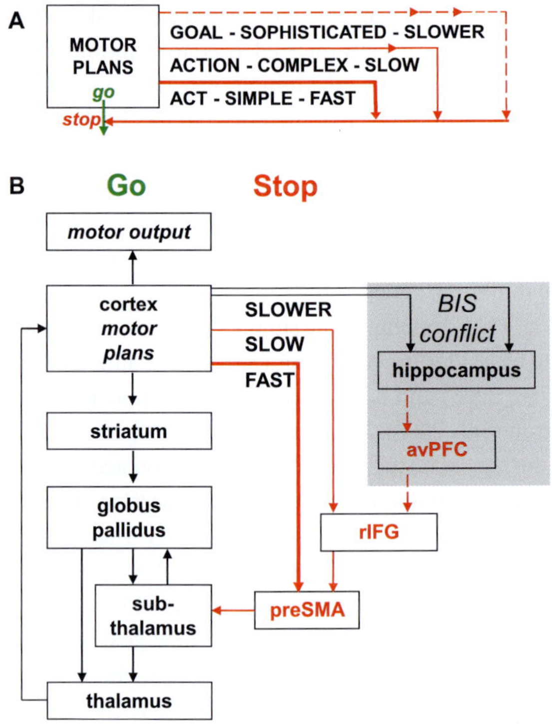

Fig. 11.8 Postulated neural control of going and stopping. **A:** general organisation of motor stopping cicuits. Different types of response output, determined by required speed of response, engage different circuits. **B:** Neural pathways involved in going and stopping in the SST. Motor inhibition uses both fast and slow routes (Nachev et al., 2008) to modulate the Go circuit (Nachev et al., 2005; Nachev et al., 2007). For the fastest stopping preSMA and this output bypasses rIFG acting as a 'kill-switch' type of inhibitory control (Floden and Stuss, 2006). We propose goal inhibition involves, in addition, the Behavioural[/Goal] Inhibition System (BIS, Gray and McNaughton, 2000). **avPFC** = anteroventral prefrontal cortex, precise area not known; **rIFG** = right inferior frontal gyrus; **preSMA** = pre-supplementary motor area. Connections have been simplified and circuits and structures in the BIS, other than the hippocampus, are not shown (e.g., the Papez circuit is omitted). Adapted from Neo et al. (2011) with permission. For more detailed circuitry, see Fig. 11.10.

'To test for stop-specific increases in EEG spectral power within the 4- to 12-Hz range at Fz, F4, and F8 in trials with intermediate delays, as compared to those with either short or long delays. If goal conflict was detected, we predicted that it would be processed as an aversive signal, and so individuals with high trait anxiety and/or neuroticism should show higher goal-conflict-specific EEG power' (Neo and McNaughton, 2011, p. 486).

As predicted, we found a right-frontal goal-conflict-specific EEG rhythmicity (GCSR) that was: a) in the rodent hippocampal 'theta' frequency range (4–12 Hz); b) positively correlated with neuroticism and trait anxiety (Neo et al., 2011); and, c) reduced by all key (non-panicolytic) classes of anxiolytic drugs (McNaughton et al., 2013; Shadli et al., 2015; Shadli et al., 2020a). Note that 'theta' recorded from the human dorsal hippocampus in a virtual reality model of a standard rodent test appears to have a power band of 5–11 Hz with a peak at 8 Hz (Goyal et al., 2020)[[4]], similar to both rat dorsal hippocampus 'theta' and our anxiety process biomarker. . . .

Here we show elevated GCSR in student volunteers divided, after testing, on their STAI-T scores into low, medium, and high (typical of clinical anxiety) groups. We then tested anxiety disorder patients (meeting diagnostic criteria) and similar controls recruited separately from the community. The patient group had higher average GCSR than their controls—with a mixture of high and low GCSR that varied with, but cut across, conventional disorder diagnosis. Consequently, GCSR scores should provide the first theoretically based biomarker that could help diagnose, and so redefine, a psychiatric disorder.

(Shadli et al., 2021a, p. 2, p. 1; see Chapter 13 for clinical details)

In terms of the circuits of Fig. 11.6B these results are consistent with our previous proposal that

efficient and accurate information processing in the [GIS] requires recursive processing—that is, signals carrying information circulate the relevant network for multiple cycles (see Gray & McNaughton, 2000, pp. 24–27). SSRT was approximately 200 ms in the present study. It takes about 430 ms to complete three cycles of a 7-Hz rhythm. If the 7–8 Hz intermediate-delay rhythmic power observed here represented even as few as three recursive cycles of goal-conflict processing by the [GIS], it would have continued after stopping was generated by at least 230 ms—probably too late to affect inhibition. *This could explain the lack of a correlation between the 7–8 Hz power and SSRT.* This suggests that a simple motor inhibition task like the SST, which is expected to recruit relatively fast motor processing, may also activate slower and/or longer lasting recursive motivational processes induced by goal conflict, which would have increased behavioural inhibition in tasks involving slower responses.

(Neo et al., 2011, p. 491—emphasis added)

In sum, for the simple SST, where act/action is already initiated, direct/hyperdirect circuits control stopping with SSRTs in the region of 200–250 ms. Balanced go/stop (attraction/repulsion) conflict generates anxiolytic-sensitive right frontal theta rhythmicity. But SSRT does not correlate with theta and is not sensitive to anxiolytics.

The theta (which the drugs define as an effect of GIS activation) must involve other circuits that in Fig. 11.6 are hypothesized to be limbic and which are so slow that they cannot affect responding in the speeded SST.

Which are these circuits? Fig. 11.6 speculates but gives no guarantee that hippocampal rather than PFC processing detects conflict; and is essentially agnostic as to how the hippocampus influences the tentative target (based on stop control) of rIFG, with 'avPFC' translating as anywhere that has a direct CA1/subiculum input and projects to rIFG.

[4] For rodent-compatible hippocampal RSA/'theta' in humans, see also Ekstrom et al. (2005); Jacobs et al. (2010); Miller (1991).

11.5.5 Circuits for Goal-Conflict-Specific Rhythmicity elicited during action stopping

The somewhat convoluted title of this section is based on the fact that, in our theory, *anywhere* that processes goals (including the cerebellar nuclei for eye blinks) should show functional theta activity when that area is interacting with the hippocampus to resolve conflict. The bulk of both anterior and posterior cortex show concurrent hippocampal theta synchrony during the conflict implied by risk assessment behaviour (Young and McNaughton, 2009).

The beauty (and curse) of the SST is that it is incredibly simple (go/stop, that's it) and has no external sources of motivation (an advantage for clinical use). A key advantage is that its *stopping* circuitry is very well defined (see Fig. 11.10 for an expanded version of Fig. 11.6) but, as we have noted, not functionally impacted by goal conflict because of its speeded responding. Here, therefore, we will talk about only a first, and particularly localized, case of goal processing about which we can ask which circuits control its conflict-related theta against a background of known attraction and repulsion control systems.

You should view the SST as a paradigm not a representative example. You should also view all the data in this section as exploratory and tentative—low N and much unpublished, or only recently, at the time of writing. Note also that the SST is likely not the best paradigm to answer the key circuit questions (see, e.g. McNaughton, 2019; Fung et al., 2019; Qi et al., 2018; Mobbs et al., 2018; Wehrli et al., 2022; Zorowitz et al., 2019; Korn and Bach, 2019). We anticipate publishing better examples soon. A complete picture will take decades.

Our first port of call is not a simple SST but a selective stopping task: go left-AND-right; then stop-left, stop-right, or stop-both. This takes us well beyond the kill switch and clearly into selected action stopping.

> [stop left] produced right frontal 5–12 Hz GCSR that, as in the SST: significantly correlated with trait anxiety and neuroticism; and was sensitive to pregabalin (75 mg), buspirone (10 mg), and perhaps triazolam (0.25 mg). [stop right] and [stop both] produced faster stopping and only 9–10 Hz GCSR, which did not correlate significantly with trait anxiety or neuroticism and was sensitive to pregabalin and buspirone but not triazolam.
>
> (Shadli et al., 2020, p. 547)

These three different sorts of stopping varied both in their stop reaction times and in per cent correction stopping; with stop-both being fastest (224 ms) and most correct, stop-left next (370 ms), and stop-right slowest (526 ms) and least correct. Consistent with the variation of stopping circuitry with stopping speed, the location of GCSR power varied with rIFG most clearly involved with the slowest stopping (Fig. 11.9). Similar variation was seen in the location of GCSR power within simple SST experiments from block to block of testing; and between SST experiments that varied in their stopping reaction times (Shadli et al., unpublished).

> Stopping can be controlled by a range of structures including rIFG, medial frontal gyrus (MFG, areas 8m and 9m), dorsolateral prefrontal cortex (DLPFC, areas 91, 101, and 46), and superior frontal gyrus. As shown in Table [11.1], there is variation both across and within experiments as to which (and how many) of these areas are sources of GCSR—and to what

relative extent they are activated when they are involved. The area most *consistently* as opposed to strongly activated is rIFG, matching the consistency of F8 activation across our previous experiments. The next most consistent is rMFG. For both IFG and MFG left-side activation can also occur but does not seem to occur alone (see also Shadli et al., 2021b). In contrast, there is one case where left DLPFC shows GCSR but right DLPFC does not....

Our data are consistent with evidence for at least two different neural networks that can generate stopping in the SST; involving rIFG (Aron et al., 2003; Verbruggen and Logan, 2008; Aron et al., 2014a) and MFG (Nachev et al., 2008; Nachev et al., 2007; Johansen-Berg et al., 2004), respectively. We also found a GCSR source in the superior frontal gyrus, consistent with fMRI studies of stopping (Rae et al., 2015). During executing stopping action, there is evidence of activations of multiple neural networks using direct, indirect and hyperdirect pathways (Nambua et al., 2002; Rae et al., 2015; Wiecki and Frank, 2013). Our results suggest that goal conflict can interact with all of the areas that control stopping.

(Shadli et al., submitted)

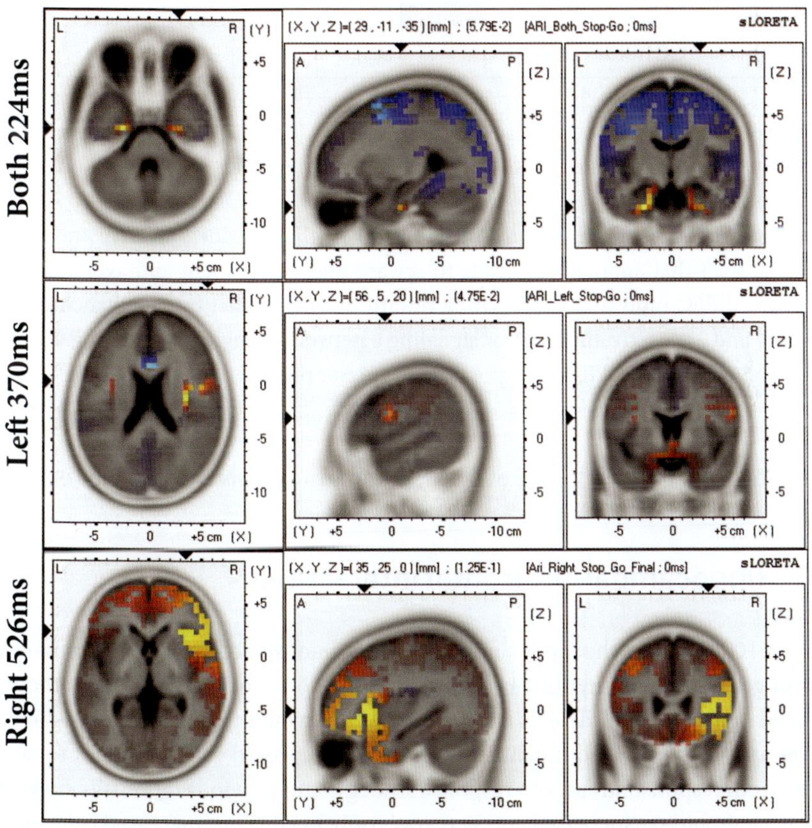

Fig. 11.9 Anatomical locations of GCSR activation estimated by source localization with low-resolution electro-magnetic tomography (sLORETA) The upper panel is for [stop left], the middle for [stop both], and the lower for [stop right]. [X, Y, Z]: coordinates of maximum activated voxel in standard MNI152 space. From Shadli et al. (2020) with permission. From Shadli et al. (submitted) with permission.

Table 11.1 Summary of significant activations seen in key frontal structures across a range of experiments: * (Shadli et al., 2020); 1–2 as reported. Paradigm includes stop condition for the selective stopping task (SG = stop left only; SS = stop both; GS = stop right) and block for the stop signal task. Contrast is as defined in methods. Method identifies sLORETA as low/high depending on resolution (32/256 channels). Previously defined sites of interest are identified as R/L for right/left with IFG = inferior frontal gyrus, MFG = medial frontal gyrus, DLPFC = dorsolateral prefrontal cortex. Additional single site results are reported in the text. Yellow = high activation; brown = moderate activation; salmon = weak/restricted activation. Table and legend adapted from Shadli et al. (submitted) with permission

Expt.	Paradigm	Contrast	Method	R-IFG	R-MFG	L-IFG	L-MFG	R-DLPFC	L-DLPFC
*	Selective SG	GCSR	Low	[yellow]		[brown]			
*	Selective SS	GCSR	Low		[brown]		[brown]		
*	Selective GS	GCSR	Low	[yellow]	[brown]			[brown]	[brown]
1	SST B1	GCSR	Low	[brown]	[yellow]		[brown]		
1	SST B3	GCSR	Low	[yellow]	[brown]	[yellow]	[brown]		
2	SST B1	GCSR	High	[brown]	[yellow]				
2	SST B3	GCSR	High	[salmon]					[yellow]

These conclusions are consistent with the more general view that

> Approach-avoidance conflict arises from decisions with embedded positive and negative outcomes, such that approaching leads to reward and punishment and avoiding to neither.... the dlPFC motivates approaching reward during conflict by 1) enhancing reward sensitivity and 2) coactivating with or signaling a network of regions (including the cingulate, medial/orbital/lateral PFC, temporal, and superior parietal).
>
> (Rolle et al., 2021, p. 1, 14)

It remains for us to consider the role of the hippocampus in suppression of approaching.

11.5.6 Hippocampal-prefrontal interactions

> In the [GIS] theory, the hippocampus can continuously receive goal information (and generate theta rhythm) in 'just checking' mode and only produces theta-paced output when it detects conflict. Its output would then impact on whichever areas had provided the initial input and these would vary from task to task and from response strategy to response strategy. Our previous rat results suggest that we should see increased conflict *power* only in rIFG but increased *coherence* between frontal cortex and hippocampus (Banstola et al., 2022) when a gate is opened by conflict (and particularly risk assessment, Young and McNaughton, 2009). The control of stopping itself is thought (Aron et al., 2014a) to be centred on area 44 (pars opercularis of rIFG).... The widespread distribution of 4–7 Hz GCSR with EEG is consistent with the rodent coherence changes....

> In terms of Fig. [11.8], our . . . results leave open the question of the area labelled avPFC that is presumed to relay information from hippocampus to rIFG. This was included in the figure because there is no direct hippocampal input to area 46 or other areas posterior to it. One possibility is that hippocampal output (occurring from the subiculum only when conflict is detected) engages MFG (area 9).... Area 9 would then relay to area 46 in a way that caused its power to increase (Banstola et al., 2022).
>
> (Shadli et al., unpublished)

The key elements of this proposal are presented in Fig. 11.10, which should be read in conjunction with Fig. 11.2 (showing a more extended version of the 'go' circuits), Fig. 9.9 (showing a more extended version of the Papez circuit) and Fig. 9.7, 9.8 (providing more hippocampal detail). As shown in Fig. 11.2, CA1 and subiculum output directly to a range of more anterior frontal areas (labelled antPFC in Fig. 11.10, note change from avPFC in Fig. 11.8, to include dorsal as well as ventral aspects). Of these, our current data (not shown and preliminary) suggest that the MFG (BA9, BA10) most likely receives coherent theta rhythmicity, sometimes detected by GCSR in the EEG, monosynaptically from the hippocampus, but with insufficient increased activation to be detected by fMRI (except in relation to general stopping rather than conflict *per se*). BA9, BA10 then transfer this monosynaptically to the junction point of BA45, 46, and 47 in the right DLPFC, where increased activity can be detected by fMRI as well as GCSR. This conflict-processing area can then affect area 44 (pars opercularis of rIFG in VLPFC), the main centre for the control of adaptable (as opposed to kill-switch) stopping. In the SST these latter effects are too slow to alter stopping but would be expected to be functionally effective in, for example, go/no-go tasks. The other circuit elements would function as generally accepted (see citations within figure legends). A parallel role for the insula is suggested in §11.7.4.

11.5.7 What do frontal and prefrontal cortex do?

Our picture amalgamates many current and older (reviewed by Grafman, 1995) views of prefrontal function. Some we ascribe to a particular level of frontal cortex (Fig. 11.7); some we blend (e.g. working/active memory) by taking two apparently distinct views (memory versus planning) as simultaneously correct, some we borrow wholesale (Fuster, 2022; Fuster, 2015).

Grafman complained that most older views deny frontal circuits 'any special cognitive status/role other than that they manipulate knowledge that is primarily stored in posterior regions of the cerebral cortex' (*op. cit.*, p. 344). We plead 'guilty' but with extenuating circumstances. Like Hebb (1949), we locate perception, active memory, and recall of long-term memory for any particular cognitive entity all in the same cell assembly—activated by external input, iteratively by frontal cortex, or via associations supported by long-term potentiation, respectively. Further, like Fuster we see these functions intertwined.

> Persistent activity during [a] delay is [not] caused exclusively by the retention of the sensory cue.... The neural substrate of working memory is an array of long-term memory networks, that is, of cognitive networks (*cognits*), updated and orderly activated for the attainment of a behavioral goal.
>
> (Fuster, 2022, p. 1)

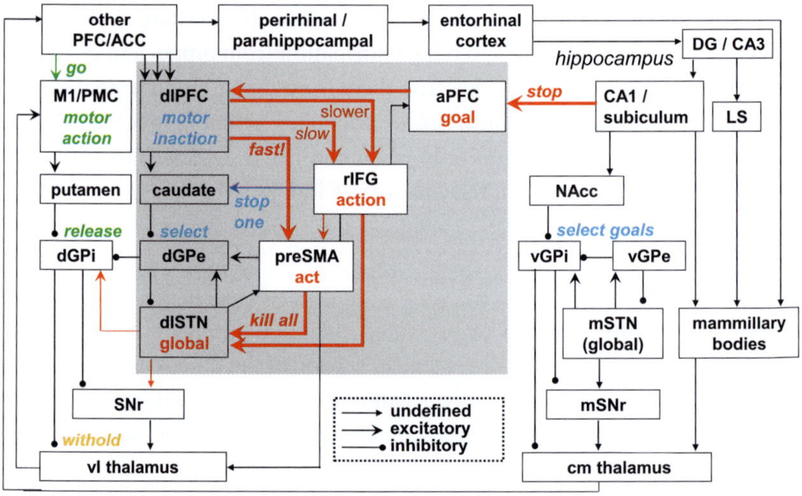

Fig. 11.10 Interaction of going and stopping in frontal circuits. This is simplified in that each element of the diagram stands for a set of parallel circuits—see Fig. 11.2 and Fig. 9.7–9.9 for expansions. "Going" (green/blue, left hand side) is intended to include choices where selected (blue) action alternatives are inhibited and where the executed action is released from inhibition. Action choice is thus often inhibition of inhibition. Thus, available stimuli can 'prime' a range of actions and plans, with execution requiring only release. "Stopping" (red, grey background) includes kill switch, selective stopping, action choice, and goal inhibition. Goal inhibition is generated as one ("stop") output from the Goal Inhibition System (*hippocampus)* that is distinct from its (right hand side) arousal and attention outputs and from its role in goal section. Immediate goal inhibition/stopping (red arrow) of the competing outputs directed towards positive and negative goals (attractors/repulsors) allows sophisticated forms of conflict resolution to occur without interference. Data integrated from (Aron, 2011; Haegelen et al., 2009; Chambers et al., 2009; Johansen-Berg et al., 2004; Nachev et al., 2008; Aron et al., 2007; Duann et al., 2009; Floden and Stuss, 2006; Gray and McNaughton, 2000). *Lowercase abbreviations:* a = anterior c = central, d = dorsal, e = pars externalis, i = pars internalis, l = lateral, m = medial, r = right, v = ventral. *Uppercase abbreviations:* ACC = anterior cingulate cortex, DG = dentate gyrus, GP = globus pallidus, IFG = inferior frontal gyrus, LS = lateral septum, M1 = primary motor cortex, PFC = prefrontal cortex, PMC = premotor cortex, SNr = substantia nigra pars reticulata, SMA = supplementary motor area, STN = subthalamic nucleus.

However, our view of 'planning' and 'intention' imply that frontal cortex should also contain its own cognitive representations. So, we agree with Grafman (e.g. 1995, p. 360) that frontal cortex can store plans, scripts, schemata, themes, or mental models. But we see these nominally higher order constructs as results of the basic capacity to order or relate items that are stored elsewhere. Thus, the *knowledge* embodied in a 'plan' ('What will I see?') would be distributed outside the frontal cortex but, without sequencing information stored in the frontal cortex ('What will I do?'), it could not be integrated into a *plan*. Consistent with Fuster's formulation, the information encoded by DLPFC during a delay often appears to represent the anticipated upcoming goal rather than the stimulus that signalled that goal (Watanabe, 1996). This is consistent with proposed mechanisms where 'temporal coordination dynamically binds prefrontal neurons into functional ensembles' (Hanganu-Opatz et al., 2023, p. 1020).

The loss of behavioural spontaneity after lesions to the dorsal trend of frontal cortex, on this view, is due to the disconnection from the motor system of the capacity to predict in advance critical temporal or spatial aspects of the world. Working/active memory, in this case, can be thought of, not so much as storing information *per se*, but as predicting where an upcoming, delayed, response must be made (e.g. Funahashi et al., 1993; see also Fig. 11.5). Dorsal prefrontal lesions, thus, remove the capacity to initiate action under conditions in which a degree of anticipation is required to achieve particular goals (the 'where' function). They leave intact, however, posterior cortical mechanisms that allow fairly direct reactions to stimuli. Even in the supplementary motor area (area 6, medial premotor cortex), the primary function appears to be the selection of responses on the basis of internal cues, with the result that the provision of external cues, or instructions, can eliminate the problem with motor control resulting from lesions to this region (Chen et al., 1995; Thaler et al., 1995; Viallet et al., 1995).

By contrast, the release of behaviour by lesions to the ventral trend of frontal cortex would, on this view, be due to the disconnection from the motor system (and from the dorsal trend of PFC) of the capacity to predict in advance emotionally significant aspects of the world (the 'what' function). A dysfunction of this kind is likely to be of greatest importance in relation to affectively negative aspects of the world. With a properly functioning ventral trend, prediction of upcoming aversive events can inhibit the more immediate responsive initiation of action by posterior cortex, as well as the less immediate initiation of action by the dorsal trend of PFC. Note that, in this respect the function of the ventral trend of PFC conforms to that proposed for the GIS, and hence potentially to a role in anxiety. However, we qualify this idea next.

On this view, it is the necessity of predicting events of significance by the ventral trend of PFC that requires it to receive input from olfactory cortex. Olfaction is one of the phylogenetically oldest sources of warning of upcoming events; indeed, the simple detection of a specific odour, with no additional analysis, can provide a warning. Likewise, it is the affective loading of predictions by the ventral trend of PFC that requires it to receive similar thalamic information to that received by cingulate, and to receive input from the cingulate cortex itself. But if this is the role of the ventral trend of frontal cortex, what is the role of cingulate cortex?

11.6 Mesial trend processing ('internal planning')

Given what we have just said, why is cingulate cortex necessary at all? To answer this question, we must remember the tendency of the brain to produce parallel structures for related functions (e.g. the dorsal and ventral trends for 'where' and 'what', and the multiple topographic representations of visual space for the extraction of form, movement, and colour). The data we have considered above-link PFC with 'external planning': the anticipatory control of motor programs controlled largely by external percepts or their memories coded by posterior cortex. In a complementary fashion, they (see §9.6 and Appendix 3) link cingulate cortex with 'internal planning' the anticipatory control of motor programs, the steps of which are controlled largely by internal events coded as somatosensory input (e.g. nociception) or as hypothalamic input.

We can now see why, on a small scale, anterior cingulate appears to mirror PFC. It undertakes the same general tasks but with largely 'innate' as opposed to 'acquired' motor plans (this does not mean, however, that the stimuli that elicit the plans cannot be learned). Anterior cingulate presumably adds greater range and anticipatory character to the initiation of, for example, the simple (UCS-UCR) active avoidance reactions that can be generated via the amygdala. (In particular it is likely to operate in an anticipatory fashion, for example, when there is no explicit CS or UCS to elicit the UCR.) Similarly, posterior cingulate may add greater range and anticipatory character to the inhibition of ongoing behaviour and the elicitation of risk analysis which can be generated via the hippocampus. Obsessions, then, can be viewed as the activation (pathological or non-pathological) of largely innate affective motor plans within the cingulate cortex (which could involve the placing of an item into the working/active memory areas of PFC). At least one source of *pathological* obsessions could then be a failure to provide to the cingulate a 'task completed' feedback signal from the motor system analogous to the reset of working/active memory (Fig. 11.5). As with the ventral trend in frontal cortex, then, posterior cingulate has functions that conform to our description of the GIS and could, then, be involved in anxiety; in particular, we now include retrosplenial cortex as an SHS module (McNaughton and Vann, 2022, Fig. 9.9); again, we qualify this inference to some extent next.

Given their parallel functions, it is not surprising that the operation of cingulate cortex is likely to be modified by output from the PFC (Pandya et al., 1971). Reciprocal interconnections between these areas would be necessary to coordinate their distinct roles in the control of ongoing behaviour. There are also close connections between the PFC and the SHS. In monkeys there are prefrontal projections to the entorhinal cortex (Van Hoesen et al., 1972; Van Hoesen et al., 1975; Van Hoesen and Pandya, 1975), to the hippocampus (Leichnetz and Astruc, 1976), to the septal area (Johnson et al., 1968; Tanaka and Goldman, 1976) and to the mammillary bodies (Jacobson et al., 1978). All of these components of the SHS can influence the cingulate cortex fairly directly. Similarly, all areas of cingulate cortex project to entorhinal cortex (Suzuki and Amaral, 1994) and hence can influence the PFC indirectly. Note, however, that, while there is good evidence for homologous functions of rat prefrontal and primate PFC, there is, as yet, no evidence that the descending connections just described for the monkey are present in the rat. Thus, while the possible link between PFC and anxiety that is indicated here is likely to be phylogenetically old, the role of cortical structures in anxiety appears to have greatly expanded at the primate level. We shall argue later, however, that this expansion is purely quantitative and does not change the general qualitative principles of operation of the networks controlling anxiety.

We have so far taken the mesial trend of PFC to equate with anterior cingulate cortex. However, it should be noted that in Fig. 10.4 (where we outline connections to and from the hippocampus) anterior cingulate appears, connectionally, as a dorsal trend component of medial prefrontal cortex—with the infralimbic cortex representing the ventral trend component and prelimbic cortex occupying the middle ground. This raises the possibility that Fig. 11.2 should be redrawn to show BA24b (rostral ACC), BA32, BA25, and perhaps BA13 as a coherent mesial strip (consistent with the rat medial frontal strip and its production of theta, Fig. 11.11, and impact on hippocampus-sensitive tasks; Kolb et al., 1994). This strip receives direct input from area CA1 and the subiculum and input from retrosplenial cortex (which we treat as adjacent to subiculum in the hippocampal formation) via a Papez circuit (Fig. 9.9).

But, also potentially part of a mesial trend, and not discussed in previous editions, is the insula.

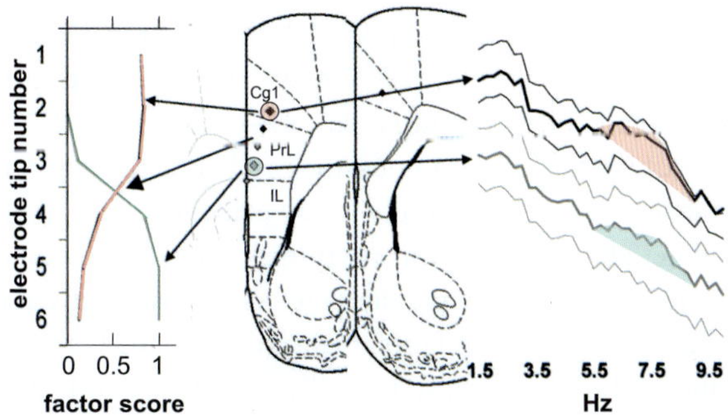

Fig. 11.11 Source localisation of theta rhythm in medial frontal cortex. recordings from a single six-electrode array in a single rat were separated into two separate profiles. The graph on the right shows two lines representing the change in partial coherence (x-axis, factor score) across the six recording tips (y-axis). The pink line corresponds to a single factor that electrodes 1, 2 and 3 shared that was significantly different from the single factor shared by electrodes 4, 5 and 6 (green line). The single electrodes with the largest scores on their respective actor were designated (tips circled) as the "source" electrode, representing the field activity of the given area. Power spectra (right hand side) from each electrode were also used to corroborate the designation of "source" electrodes by both the shapes of the spectra and the power. Note the departure (highlighted) from simple 1/f decay in the region of 5.5-9.5Hz (theta). Both sources show clear theta but the dorsal (cingulate, Cg1) and more ventral (prelimbic, PrL/infralimbic, IL) are distinct in terms of their coherence. Figure and legend adapted from Young and McNaughton (2009) with permission.

11.7 Insula ('internal monitoring')

What is the role, if any, of the insula (aka insular cortex) in anxiety? Before answering this, it is important to remind you that we see anxiety (mediated by the GIS) as distinct from fear/panic/phobia/obsession/depression. Anxiety, but not the other states/disorders, is sensitive to anxiolytics, while panicolytics affect panic, phobia, fear, obsession (all GRS) *and* anxiety (GIS). Despite its diagnostic separation by DSM (as opposed to ICD) 'panicolytics' also affect depression. Likewise, we link anxiety to hippocampal function. From this point of view, it turns out there is strong reason to link the insula to the GIS.

11.7.1 Linking the insula to the GIS

An important initial fact, is that the anxiolytic lorazepam produces a dose-dependent reduction in the activation of both the amygdala and insula during emotional face processing; but does not change activation of medial prefrontal cortex or visual cortex (Paulus et al., 2005). Similar effects are obtained with pregabalin (Aupperle et al., 2012). Consistent with these results being due to an action directly on $GABA_A$ receptors in the insula, PTSD patients show significantly reduced flumazenil binding potential in the insula (and many other areas including amygdala and hippocampus, Geuze et al., 2007; Cameron et al., 2007). In rats $5HT1_A$ activation in the agranular insula impairs consolidation of passive avoidance (Souza et al., 2001).

There are also parallels with the hippocampus. Like hippocampal lesions, and anxiolytics, lesions of the insula affect passive avoidance (Kaada et al., 1962) and spatial learning in the Morris Water Maze (Nerad, 1997; Nerad et al., 1996) as does NMDA receptor blockade (Gutiérrez et al., 1999). Like the hippocampus, the insula is activated by mental route navigation in humans (Ghaem et al., 1997). There is also evidence for local insula theta activity, at least in slices (Saito et al., 2012), but this rhythmicity may not be functionally linked to hippocampal RSA. These hippocampal parallels are not surprising given the important role of interoceptive stimuli for spatial orientation (Teaford et al., 2022) and the vestibular input to both the insular and the hippocampal systems (Evrard, 2019; Smith, 2017) with its links to theta rhythmicity (Russell et al., 2006). More directly, functional connectivity between right hippocampus and left insula is negatively related to risk taking and positively to trait anxiety (Huo et al., 2020).

The key questions to ask, then, are: what specific contributions does the insula make to anxiety; and to what extent is it involved more generally in other, particularly emotional, functions? The fast answer to this latter question is that the insula has been implicated in a vast array of functions, is likely the only area where interoceptive stimuli of all types are processed (§11.7.2), and is one of the areas that has been proposed as key for consciousness and perception of self. There is good reason to see it as limbic sensory cortex, paired bidirectionally with the anterior cingulate as limbic motor cortex (Craig, 2002; Craig, 2009); but also as an emotional command centre with direct, unidirectional, output to pontine nuclei (§11.7.3). It is also seen as a key source of control of the salience, executive, and default mode cortical networks (§11.7.6). To understand this plethora of possibilities, we first need to have a clear picture of its distinctive functional anatomy.

11.7.2 Functional divisions of the insula

The insula is an infolded region, like the hippocampus but occupying an opposite boundary of the temporal lobe (Fig. 11.12C). It is also immediately adjacent to the piriform cortex (which can be viewed as olfactory association cortex, Johnson et al., 2000) and its input connections make it part of the 'rhinencephalon'. 'Smell brain' is factually incorrect, and outdated, but we think usefully identifies older brain areas located synaptically close to the olfactory system (Gastaut and Lammers, 1961). Critically, the rhinencephalic areas of interest have no obvious *olfactory* processing function; but have clear 'cognitive/emotional' processing links with homologues in reptilian cortex (Laurent et al., 2016). In evolutionary terms, this is likely because an odour can identify a predator directly and so does not require the higher-order processing of other sensory inputs; while the odour is the earliest and simplest signal of an impending predator.

The insula also appears to be a site of convergence of frontal, limbic, autonomic, and other sensory inputs (see §11.7.3). Its efferent targets include frontal, parietal, temporal, cingulate, and olfactory cortex; as well as subcortical areas such as the hippocampus and amygdala—with anterior insula (of which more next) more strongly linked to frontal areas and posterior insula more linked to cingulate and parietal areas. Right anterior insula, in particular, appears to control executive function by gating various frontal functional networks (Molnar-Szakacs and Uddin, 2022). That said, as we will see, the anterior insula also plays a key role in the control of the most basic emotional functions.

> Long perceived as a primitive and poorly differentiated brain structure, the primate insular cortex recently emerged as a highly evolved, organized and richly connected cortical hub interfacing bodily states with sensorimotor, environmental, and limbic activities. This insular interface likely substantiates emotional embodiment and has the potential to have a key role in the interoceptive shaping of cognitive processes, including perceptual awareness. [If so] interoceptive afferents that represent the ongoing physiological status of all . . . organs of the body [will] receive [input to] the granular dorsal fundus of the insula or 'primary interoceptive cortex' [process this in] dysgranular polymodal 'insular stripes', and . . . anterior agranular areas . . . as an additional sensory platform for visceral functions and as an output stage for efferent autonomic regulation. One of the agranular areas hosts the specialized von Economo and Fork neurons [as does the anterior cingulate cortex], which could provide a decisive evolutionary advantage for the role of the anterior insula in the autonomic and emotional binding inherent to subjective awareness. . . . Although both human and non-human primates have an anterior agranular sector, the disproportionate expansion of [anterior insular cortex] in humans . . . suggests that it might host more refined and diversified representations of complex and abstract embodied functions.
>
> (Evrard, 2019, p. 1, p. 16; see Fig. 11.12; see also Evrard, 2022)

Evrard (2019) sees the insula as encapsulating three different axes: sensory-motor; spinocranial; and cognition-emotion. Primary interoceptive (*including vestibular and auditory*) information flows (Fig. 11.12F) from dorsal-posterior-granular (i.e. cytoarchitectonically like primary somatosensory cortex) to ventral-anterior agranular (i.e. cytoarchitectonically like motor and premotor cortex.

> One dimension that needs to be added to the sensory-motor axis relates to the anatomical sympathetic and parasympathetic autonomic branches of the autonomic nervous system. The dorsal fundus of the insula is topographically organized with a posterior-to-anterior representation of spinal (foot-to-hand), trigeminal (head/face), and vagal (taste/viscera) inputs. . . . [Essentially orthogonal to the sensory-motor axis is a] continuous dorsoventral 'division', which shifts from ego-/allo-centric, posteriorly, to cognition/emotion, anteriorly, suggests a mechanistic relationship that, if true, could prove insightful for our understanding of the neurobiological correlate of cognition and emotion.
>
> (Evrard, 2019, p. 16; see Fig. 11.12)

One phenomenon that straddles this sensory/motor/cognition/emotion territory is alexithymia. This involves difficulty in labelling feelings and in separating feelings from bodily sensations and can be linked to (particularly anterior) insular dysfunction: reduced size, reduced functional coherence, damage, and reduced activation in emotional challenge tasks (Ben Shalom, 2022). But there is reason to emphasize higher-order, cognitive, aspects.

Output from the most anterior insula (which is very substantially expanded in humans and includes specialized 'von Economo' neurons/VENs) appears to involve functions as complicated as self-recognition. Note that VENs are most obvious in primates, occur in only one insular area in the macaque but occupy a range of distinct areas in the much-expanded human

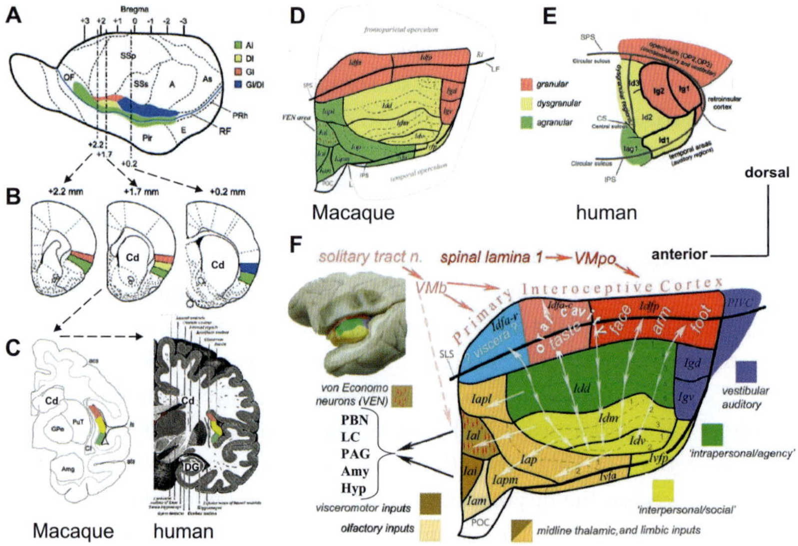

Fig. 11.12 Gross anatomy of the insula in rat, monkey, and human. Its location is most easily understood in the rat. **A.** The coloured area represents the location of the insula on the cortical surface of the rat. Note that it is immediately below somatosensory and auditory primary and secondary cortex, and immediately above piriform cortex (which can be viewed as olfactory association cortex, Johnson et al., 2000). **B.** It has three main cytoarchitectonic areas (agranular, AI; dysgranular, DI; and granular, GI) and a mixed GI/DI area. *(A, B adapted, with permission from Saito et al., 2012.)* **C.** As the neocortex expands in phylogeny, the insula becomes embedded progressively deeper under the adjacent 'opercular' cortices. Thus, it and the dentate gyrus (DG) can be viewed as opposite sides of the temporal cortical sheet, buried within neocortex in the same way as other parts of the 'rhinencephalon'. *(Macaque adapted, with permission, from Gallay et al., 2011; human adapted from https://commons.wikimedia.org/wiki/File:Gray717.png - Henry Vandyke Carter, Public domain, via Wikimedia Commons)* **D, E.** Flat maps of the Macaque and human insula, respectively, when compared with panel A, show a relative decrease in the more anterior and ventral agranular insula; and a relative increase in the more central dysgranular insula and dorsal and posterior granular insula. **F.** A functional map for the areas shown in D, shows that primary interoceptive input (including a parallel pain input to that sent to anterior cingulate cortex) as well as vestibular and auditory input arrives in the dorsal and posterior granular areas. 'intrapersonal/agency' information (from S1, S2, SMA, PCC, BA44, BA46vc-c, BA12r, PMv, dorsal striatum, . . .) and 'interpersonal/social' information (from pre-SMA, mirror neuron PMv, BA45a, BA46vc-r, BA7a, lateral amygdala, ventral striatum . . .) arrive in the more dorsal and ventral, respectively, dysgranular insula. Visceromotor, olfactory, and midline thalamic and limbic inputs arrive in the agranular area. This also receives direct internal inputs from the dysgranular insula, which in turn receives inputs from the granular insula. *(D, E, F adapted, with permission, from Evrard, 2019.)* *Abbreviations:* A, Auditory cortex; Amg, amygdala; As, association cortex; Cd, caudate nucleus; DG, dentate gyrus; E, entorhinal cortex; GPe globus pallidus—external; Hyp, hypothalamus; LC, locus coeruleus; OF, orbitofrontal cortex; PAG, periaqueductal grey; PBN, parabrachial nucleus; Pir, piriform cortex; PRh, perirhinal cortex; PuT, putamen; SSp, primary somatosensory cortex; SSs, secondary somatosensory cortex; VMb, VMpo, basal and posterior parts of the ventral medial nucleus of the thalamus, respectively.

anterior insula, and also occur throughout anterior cingulate cortex (Allman et al., 2011). 'VENs are particularly vulnerable in neuropsychiatric conditions characterized by deficits in social and emotional functioning, autonomic control, and decision-making, which, when considered in the context of the functional role of the cortical regions that host them, points to a likely role in executive functioning' (Molnar-Szakacs and Uddin, 2022, p. 10). Activation-likelihood-estimation meta-analysis finds that the anterior-dorsal insula is the only brain area participating in all of emotion, empathy, olfaction, gustation, interception, pain, attention, language, speech, working memory, and memory; but not somatosensation or motion (Kurth et al., 2010). Likewise, it has been proposed that the anterior insula is a gatekeeper of executive control (Molnar-Szakacs and Uddin, 2022).

In contrast to these ultra-high-level functions, the key direct outputs from the anterior insula listed in Fig. 11.12 include the parabrachial area, locus coeruleus, PAG, amygdala, and hypothalamus. The posterior insular cortex contacts neurons of the central amygdala that, in turn, send an output stream to the lateral hypothalamus, more than to the bed nucleus of the stria terminalis (Ponserre et al., 2020). All these directly targeted subcortical areas are key to emotional control. Interestingly, 'as with orbital [cortex] projections, cells from the insular cortices terminate strongly in the VLPAG and DR, with no registered projections aimed at the dorsal parts of the PAG .... Both the dorsal and ventral divisions of the agranular insular cortex project to the PAG/DR. [The same pattern is seen with PAG/DR projections to the insula.]' (Silva et al., 2022, p. 36, p. 40). These latter connectional data suggest a particularly strong link at the PAG level between the insula and conflict processing as compared to simple approach or withdrawal (see Fig. 6.2). But, in this context, conflict processing must be seen as a higher-order executive function.

11.7.3 Network connections of the insula

Fig. 11.13C is a diagram of the general pattern of connections of the insula (see also 11.12F). It has a mass of bidirectional connections with frontal, limbic, and parietal cortices and unidirectional outputs (primarily from the anterior insula) to monoamine systems and the striatum. It has extensive interconnections with the defence hierarchy (anterior cingulate, amygdala, hypothalamus); but only the anterior insula connects (unidirectionally) to PAG. Its amygdala connections (Fig. 11.13A, B) appear topographically organized to the lateral, basolateral, centrolateral, and centromedial nuclei with only anterior insula connecting to the centromedial amygdala. The organization of the prefrontal connections is shown in Fig. 11.14

> It participates with the caudal orbitofrontal cortex in the formation of an 'orbital network', involved in the analysis and integration of food-related information. The insula receives afferents from the primary somatosensory cortex SI, the somatosensory association areas 5 and 7b, the primary vestibular areas 3a and 2v, as well as from the auditory association areas surrounding the primary auditory cortex. All of these sensory cortical areas project to the posterosuperior portion of the insula, which may hence be characterized as the insular somatic association cortex (ISAC). Some high-order association areas, including the anterior

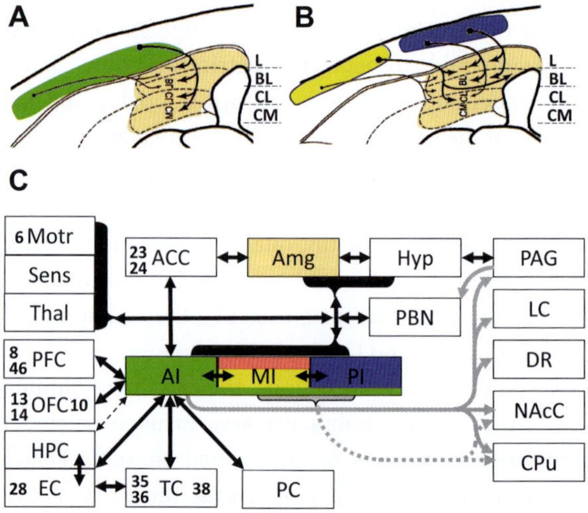

Fig. 11.13 Connections of the insula, see also Fig. 11.2A, Fig. 11.12F, Fig. 11.14. **A.** Connections of anterior and posterior agranular insula to the amygdala. The posterior agranular connections include all of the L, BL, CL, and CM amygdala. **B.** Connections of middle dysgranular (yellow) and posterior dysgranular (blue) insula to the amygdala. Again, posterior connections are more extensive, but do not include CM. A, B are adapted from Shi and Cassell (1998) with permission. **C.** Overview of the connections of the insula with simplified connections. Gray arrows show largely unidirectional outputs, black show bidirectional connections. Based on Paulus and Stein (2006) and Gehrlach et al. (2020) see also Nieuwenhuys (2012). For detailed weights and excitatory/inhibitory nature of connections see Gehrlach et al. (2020) and (Reynolds and Zahm, 2005). *Abbreviations:* ACC, anterior cingulate cortex; AI, anterior and other agranular insula; Amg, amygdala; CPu, caudate/putamen (dorsal striatum); EC, entorhinal cortex; HPC, hippocampus proper; Hyp, hypothalamus; LC, locus coeruleus; MI, middle insula (granular and dysgranular, colour coding as in Fig. 11.12); Motr, supplementary and presupplementary motor cortex; NAcC, nucleus accumbens, core (ventral striatum); PI, posterior (mixed granular and dysgranular) insula; OFC, orbital frontal cortex; PAG, periaqueductal grey; PBN, parabrachial nucleus; PC, parietal cortex. Sens, sensor-motor cortex; TC, temporal cortex; Thal, thalamus

> orbitofrontal cortex (area 11), the prefrontal cortex (areas 45, 46), and the polymodal association cortex occupying the banks of the superior temporal sulcus, are also known to be connected with the insula. Limbic structures, including the entorhinal (area 28), perirhinal (areas 35, 36), posterior orbitofrontal (areas 13, 14), temporopolar (area 38), and cingulate (areas 23, 24) cortices, as well as the amygdaloid complex, are strongly and reciprocally connected with the anterobasal sector of the insula. I designate this sector as the insular limbic cortex (ILC).... ISAC and the ILC may represent way stations in a somatolimbic projection . . . for interrelating events in the extrapersonal world with relevant motivational states. Finally, it may be mentioned that the insula projects to the supplementary and presupplementary motor areas forming part of the medial premotor cortex (area 6), as well as to the ventral and dorsal striatum.
>
> Nieuwenhuys (2012, p. 126–, for which see citations)

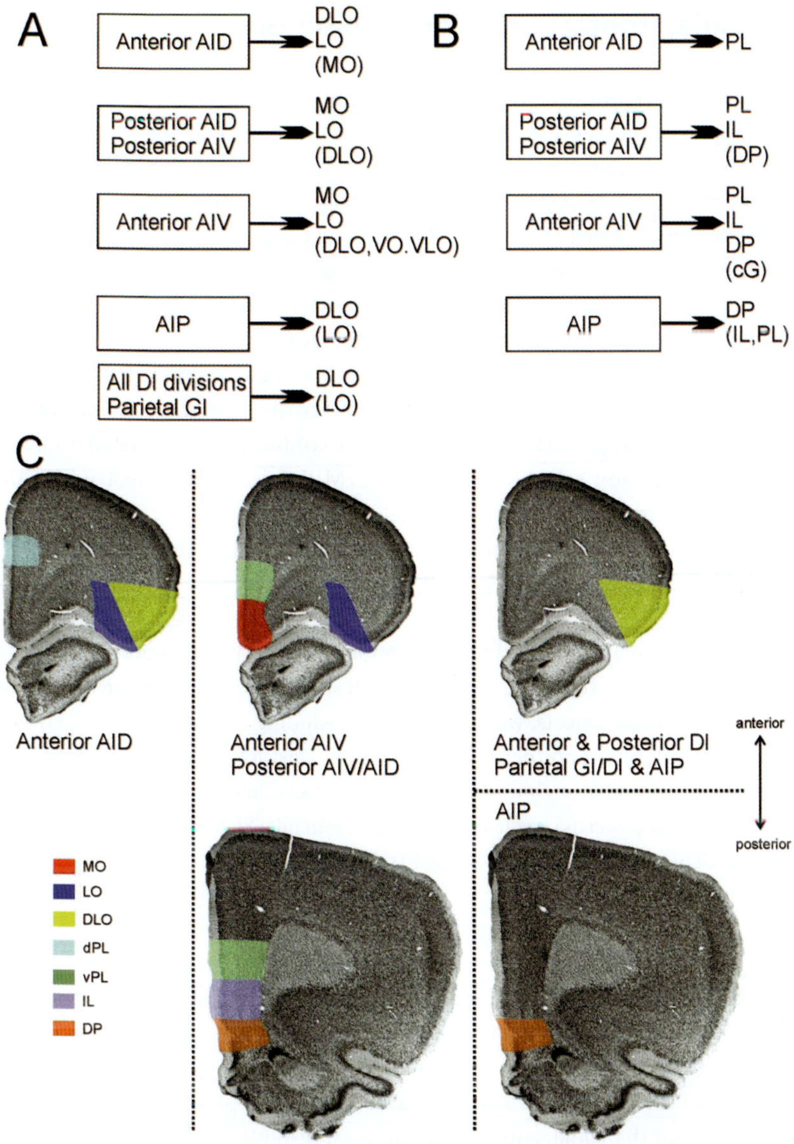

Fig. 11.14 Main patterns of projections from insular cortex to orbitofrontal and medial prefrontal cortex. (A) Schematic diagram summarizing projections from distinct insular fields to the orbitofrontal cortex. (B) Schematic diagram summarizing projections from distinct insular fields to the medial prefrontal cortex. In both A and B, weaker projections are listed within brackets. (C) Visualization of the projections to orbitofrontal and medial prefrontal cortices, including the more detailed dorso-ventral and anterior—posterior organization of projections to the medial prefrontal areas. Termination of insular fiber pathways in the orbitofrontal and medial prefrontal cortex are indicated by a specific color for each orbital field that receives dense projections (shown in A,B). The anterior dorsal agranular insular field (anterior AID) targets the dorsolateral (DLO) and lateral (LO) orbital fields as well as the dorsal portion of the prelimbic cortex (dPL), specifically at rostral levels. The anterior ventral agranular field (anterior AIV), in contrast, targets lateral orbital (LO), medial orbital (MO), ventral prelimbic (vPL) anteriorly, and vPL, infralimbic (IL), and dorsal peduncular cortex (DP) at more posterior levels.

(Contd.)

11.7.4 Insula, frontal cortex, and inhibition

Smith and Lane (2015) proposed 'An integrative multi-hierarchical model of embodied emotion' where appraisal, perception, and regulation of an emotional episode are processed in parallel systems—each hierarchical (as in Fig. 6.5B). The body/emotion perception hierarchy represents: at the lowest level (Stage 1) discrete body parts with posterior insula acting as primary interoceptive cortex (Fig. 11.12F); at the next level (Stage 2) whole-body patterns 'through a conjunctive integration over stage 1 representations within the mid- and anterior insula, and these representations correspond to phenomenologically distinguishable bodily feelings when such feelings are conscious' (p. 16); finally (Stage 3) these are integrated into an emotion category representation within rostral anterior cingulate cortex (rACC), medial prefrontal cortex (MPFC), and lateral anterior temporal cortex. 'On this model, while VMPFC is involved in high-level appraisal of a stimulus-in-a-context (and associated influences over autonomic activity, action selection, etc.), rACC/MPFC is instead involved in high-level evaluation of the emotional meaning of one's felt body state' (p. 16).

Ben Shalom (2022, pp. 1–2) combines this view with earlier suggestions (Ben Shalom, 2009; Ronel, 2018; Ben Shalom and Bonneh, 2019) to a picture of

> four streams of information, from dorsal to ventral (motor [BA 8], emotion [BA 9], memory [BA 10/46], and sensory [BA 11/47]). Within each stream, the medial prefrontal cortex integrates basic cognitive objects, while the lateral [including orbital] prefrontal cortex performs selection/inhibition on these objects [with] at least four consecutive stations: Stage 1 (discrete body features), such as in the posterior insula, and presumably the amygdala; Stage 2 (whole body patterns), such as in the anterior insula; Stage 3 (integration of emotion concepts) such as medial BA 9; and Stage 4 (selection/inhibition of emotion concepts), in lateral BA 9.

In terms of Fig. 11.2A, these streams (re-ordered: BA 8; BA 10/46; BA 9; BA 11/47) form a diagonal. Inhibition is more caudal in the dorsal trend and more rostral in the ventral.

Interestingly, the caudal boundary for SHS input is linked to inhibition (in Ben Shalom's terms). But the CA1/SUB input *also* characterizes 'integration' and does *not* occur in areas like BA 6 and BA 4 that are classically treated as separate from prefrontal cortex and linked to act and action, rather than goal, control. The simplest resolution of these results is to see goal inhibition, goal choice, and planning as fundamentally similar but on different time scales. For Ben Shalom, there is a transition from integration to inhibition/choice. For us, there is

---

Fig. 11.14 *(continued)*

These same areas are receiving inputs from both posterior agranular fields (posterior AIV/AID) The agranular parietal insular field (AIP) targets more specifically the dorsolateral (DLO) field and the dorsal peduncular cortex (DP). Finally, all the dysgranular portions, as well as the parietal granular field, provide a projection that is restricted to the dorsolateral field (DLO), avoiding mPFC regions. Figure and legend from Mathiasen et al. (2023) © 2023 Mathiasen, Aggleton and Witter. This is an open-access article distributed under the terms of the Creative Commons Attribution License (CC BY 4.0) [http://creativecommons.org/licenses/by/4.0/] and with permission from the authors.

a spectrum of nuanced inhibition (planning) through more direct inhibition (choice) to simple single goal inhibition ('inhibition', not to be confused with action inhibition).

Perhaps more interestingly, there is input from the anterior insula to areas that either are at or just caudal to the termination of SHS input (green dots, Fig. 11.2A). This insular input appears to form a boundary strip, with integration rostral to an 'inhibition' strip rostral to an insular strip rostral to primary action/act control. The insula also has input to the presupplementary motor area and supplementary motor area. This suggests that insula output is tightly linked, but not identical, to goal inhibition. That said, right inferior frontal cortex function is dissociable from insular. Right anterior insula (rAI) and right inferior frontal cortex (rIFC)

> have distinct patterns of intrinsic functional connectivity.... The rAI has stronger intrinsic functional connectivity with the ACC [while] the rIFC [has] stronger connectivity with key nodes of the dorsolateral frontoparietal network . . . part of a 'central executive' network implicated in allocating attentional resources for selectively enhancing task-relevant information, maintaining information online, and facilitating appropriate behavioral responses. In contrast, the AI and ACC constitute key nodes of the salience network, a system that facilitates detection of, and attention to, salient events, such as stop signals and errors. [Thus] rAI and rIFC interact with distinct intrinsically connected brain systems during inhibitory control and . . . play different roles in implementing this process. Activation of the rAI . . . is likely related to detection of . . . unexpected and salient stop signals [and] increase with stimulus saliency [being] causally involved in the detection of infrequent, unexpected, events embedded in a stream of frequent events [or] related to error processing.... [rAI appears to play] an important and dissociable role in detection and processing of behaviorally relevant salient stop signals, an essential process in inhibitory control. In contrast, . . . the rIFC is more involved in the early, initiation stages of implementing the stop process . . . highlighting the significant and differential roles of the rAI and rIFC in inhibitory control.
>
> (Cai et al., 2014, p. 14665)

11.7.5 'An insular view of [trait] anxiety'

> We propose a general hypothesis that integrates affective and cognitive processing with neuroanatomy to explain anxiety proneness. The premise is that individuals who are *prone to anxiety* show an altered interoceptive prediction signal, i.e. manifest augmented detection of the difference between the observed and expected body state. As a consequence, the increased prediction signal of a prospective aversive body state triggers an increase in anxious affect, worrisome thoughts and other avoidance behaviors. The anterior insula is proposed to play a key role in this process. Further testing of this model—which should include investigation of genetic and environmental influences—may lead to the development of novel treatments that attenuate this altered interoceptive prediction signal in patients with anxiety disorders.
>
> Paulus and Stein (2006, p. 383; our emphasis)

The 'anxiety' resulting from this *proneness* is broadly defined. It essentially includes all the neurotic disorders. But this breadth does not appear to be the result of a broad single action. Rather, a patchwork of functions includes not only anxiety (GIS) and fear (GRS) but also extends to positive affect (GAS).

> Neuroimaging studies suggest that the insula plays a critical role in the pathophysiology of [neurotic] disorders [with] increased insular activity . . . in patients suffering from generalized anxiety, panic disorders, phobias, OCD and PTSD . . . and decreased in response to effective treatment.... *The role of the insula in anxiety per se remains unclear.* A handful of studies in humans suggest that the insula may have a role in anxiety; anxiety may modulate insula recruitment; the severity of anxiety may be positively correlated with central amygdala-insula functional connectivity; and *lorazepam induces a dose-dependent reduction in the activation of both the amygdala and insula during emotion processing* [(Paulus et al., 2005)]. Hence, insular activation may be considered a common feature among anxiety-related disorders, and it may have a role in anxiety *per se*, in concert with amygdala activation.
>
> (Mendez-Ruette et al., 2019, p. 2, our emphasis)

In §11.7.1, we concluded there was strong reason to treat the insula as part of the GIS. The reduction in its activity produced by anxiolytic drugs can be explained by a direct action on its $GABA_A$ receptors. However its links (including those of the receptors) to 'panic disorders, phobias, OCD and PTSD' clearly extend to neurotic disorders in general; since insula activation mediates the capacity of neuroticism to increase perceived uncertainty (Feinstein et al., 2006).

There is also reason to see the insula as part of the GRS. It has strong connections with the anterior cingulate (Fig. 11.2A); is activated by error monitoring in humans (Bastin et al., 2017); and reflects the emotional component of pain processing (Orenius et al., 2017). The posterior insular cortex is necessary for the consolidation of tone fear conditioning (de Paiva et al., 2021). Interestingly, post-training lesions affect tone but *not* context fear conditioning and neither is affected by pre-training lesions (Brunzell and Kim, 2001).

The insula, therefore, can be included in both GRS and GIS (i.e. controlling active as well as passive avoidance). Pre- and post-synaptic aspects of long-term plasticity in the insula reflect the salience of anxiety and fear stimuli, respectively (Shi et al., 2018); with resultant activity giving rise to feelings of 'anxious anticipation' (Carlson et al., 2011).

The insula also appears to be part of the GAS. It is 'necessary for action selection based on current outcome value' (Parkes et al., 2018, p. 2313); and appears to encode the incentive value assigned to outcomes that produce food (Balleine and Dickinson, 2000) and water (Tsujimoto et al., 1999). The agranular insula is involved in working/active memory for food but, unlike the posterior insula, not for space (Ragozzino and Kesner, 1999).

These results suggest a multi-faceted role where different parts of the insula contribute to somewhat different processes. Its internal connections (Fig. 11.12F) then hold together a patchwork, including not only simple approach, avoidance, and conflict but also—e.g. via its oxytocin receptors, control of social approach and avoidance (Rogers-Carter et al., 2018). This allows us to take an 'insular view of anxiety' (Paulus and Stein, 2006) but also maintain a parallel insular view of fear, hunger, thirst, and social interaction. We must now carefully select the lens through which we obtain these views.

11.7.6 Consciousness/attention/switching/integration/network control

> How do you feel—now? . . . The anterior insular cortex (AIC) is implicated in a wide range of conditions and behaviours, from bowel distension and orgasm, to cigarette craving and maternal love, to decision making and sudden insight. Its function in the re-representation of interoception offers one possible basis for its involvement in all subjective feelings. New findings suggest a fundamental role for the AIC (and the von Economo neurons it contains) in awareness, and thus it needs to be considered as a potential neural correlate of consciousness.
>
> (Craig, 2009, p. 59; see also Medford and Critchley, 2010)

Despite previous 'creeping up on the hard problem' of consciousness (Gray, 2004) and its potential importance for the experience of anxiety (LeDoux, 2021; LeDoux, 2015), we will omit consciousness itself from our discussion of anxiety. We will consider the role of active memory in anxiety disorder in Chapter 13; but see no need to consider the role in this of conscious awareness. Awareness reflects narrow attentional processes and, arguably, acts as a spotlight that illuminates, and allows self-report of, but does not create, objects like fear. Further, the insula appears largely devoted to interoception and the contents of consciousness can also include exteroception—making consciousness itself likely distinct from either form of perception.

As noted (§11.7.1), we can view the insula as limbic sensory cortex, paired bidirectionally with the anterior cingulate as limbic motor cortex (Craig, 2002; Craig, 2009; Medford and Critchley, 2010). However, inspection of Fig. 11.2A shows that AIC and ACC provide overlapping inputs to act/action control areas (BA 6, 8, 46), where there is no hippocampal input; but, with more rostral goal control areas, they provide distinct dorsal trend (ACC) and ventral trend (AIC) inputs that overlap with hippocampal input but not each other. This pattern does not fit with the idea that ACC is acting as a form of relay for AIC, and is much better explained if AIC is integrating interoceptive information to guide motivated action, while ACC (with its parallel direct pain input as well as action-related input from areas like the amygdala) integrates exteroceptive information; with the two collaborating to coordinate acts/actions and providing the parallel dorsal (where) and ventral (what) goal control streams with mesial (why) information derived from exteroception and interoception, respectively.

But the functional differentiation (Kurth et al., 2010) and flow of information in the insula suggests a more complex picture. As shown in Fig. 11.12F the PIC deals more with sensorimotor integration (via connections to premotor, supplementary motor, and hippocampal areas; Cauda et al., 2011; Chang et al., 2013) and the AIC with emotion integration (via connections to temporal and limbic areas; Cauda et al., 2011; Chang et al., 2013) and, in its dorsal part, greatly expanded in humans, cognition (via connections to dACC, dlPFC, dorsal striatum, and temperopolar junction Chang et al., 2013). The central insula is also a key node in the social decision network (Rogers-Carter and Christianson, 2019). However (Fig. 11.12F), these disparate forms of information all appear to converge on the anterior insula (Kurth et al., 2010) and become integrated there (Craig, 2002; Craig, 2009; Evrard, 2019).

> The crucial insight . . . is of the anterior insula as an integral hub [of saliency, switching, attention and control of] dynamic interactions between other large-scale brain networks

> involved in externally oriented attention and internally oriented or self-related cognition.... The anterior insula and the anterior cingulate cortex form a 'salience network' [(see also Uddin, 2015)] that functions to segregate the most relevant among internal and extrapersonal stimuli in order to guide behavior [via]: (1) bottom–up detection of salient events, (2) switching between other large-scale networks to facilitate access to attention and working memory resources when a salient event is detected, (3) interaction of the anterior and posterior insula to modulate autonomic reactivity to salient stimuli, and (4) strong functional coupling with the anterior cingulate cortex that facilitates rapid access to the motor system. In this manner, with the insula as its integral hub, the salience network assists target brain regions in the generation of appropriate behavioral responses to salient stimuli.
>
> Menon and Uddin (2010, p. 655)

This assistance of choice of behaviour (and we would think goals also) clearly goes beyond simple tagging of key goals or actions as salient. Indeed, recently, Molnar-Szakacs and Uddin (2022, p.1, our emphasis) have proposed that:

> Executive control is a complex high-level cognitive function that relies on distributed brain circuitry.... The anterior insular cortex plays an under-appreciated role in executive processes, acting as a gatekeeper to other brain regions and networks by virtue of primacy of action and effective connectivity. The flexible functional profile of the anterior insular subdivision renders it a key hub within the broader midcingulo-insular 'salience network', allowing it to *orchestrate and drive activity of other major functional brain networks* including the medial frontoparietal 'default mode network' and lateral frontoparietal 'central executive network'. The microanatomy and large-scale connectivity of the insular cortex positions it to play a critical role in triaging and integrating internal and external multisensory stimuli in the service of initiating higher-order control functions. Multiple lines of evidence scaffold the novel hypothesis that, *as a key hub for integration and a lever of network switching, the anterior insula serves as a critical gatekeeper to executive control.*
>
> On self-awareness, they say (pp. 8–9, our emphasis),

> Alongside salience processing and attention, the insula plays a key role in interoception & self-awareness.... integration of signals from interoception and visceromotion via the AI guides large scale brain network dynamics underlying adaptive behavior, creating a causal pathway for access to executive control. ... the right *AI mediates the incorporation of autonomic nervous signals with conscious thought processing* to represent an individual's subjective and conscious emotional state, as well as the emotive value of external stimuli—such as feeling disgust.... Alexithymia ... could be explained as a direct result of the breakdown of the integration of multisensory information from interoceptive and exteroceptive domains at the level of the AI, reflecting a dis-integration of the experience of selfhood as supported by the AI.... The perception and regulation of interoceptive signals are important components of self-awareness and executive control. It has been theorized that the insula may provide the neural substrate for interoceptive inference, in which predictions regarding interoceptive signals are compared with actual sensory and interoceptive afferent inputs... the *processing of internal bodily signals in the insular cortex modulates exteroceptive awareness.*

Neither in Craig's quoted fundamental role in and correlate of consciousness nor in the above incorporation of interoception into consciousness (and a clear separation from exteroception) do we see an identity of insular activity with consciousness. Critically, to understand the systems of interest, the activity of which is not identical to the current contents of reportable awareness, we see no reason to entangle theories with the labile and fundamentally indeterminate concept of 'consciousness'. Seeing the insula as involved in all subjective feelings (including feelings of anxiety and fear) and as a key integrative centre controlling (via arousal and attention) the salience, default mode, and executive networks (including social decision making) is sufficient and provides a basis for seeing it as contributing to a role for the salience network in 'conscientiousness as a function of variation in neural networks underlying effective prioritization of goals' (Sassenberg et al., 2023, p. 1).

11.8 Frontal cortex and anxiety

11.8.1 Insula, cingulate, and orbital cortex

Our conclusion from §11.7 is that the insula integrates interoceptive information, determining salience, and controlling switching among the salience, executive, and default mode networks. Critically there is good reason to see it as including a cortical component of the GIS—as well as of the GAS and GRS likely via modularity similar to the PAG (Fig. 6.2). Interestingly, the insula projects to GIS, but not other, modules of the PAG; and, also, potentially inputs to all levels of the GIS.

However, there is no strong reason to see the insula as specifically involved in the essentially subtractive (Fig. 5.1) decision between conflicting goals or the blocking of the output from those goals (goal inhibition) that releases, for example, risk assessment. In contrast, there is good reason (Fig. 11.2A) to see the insula as having a broader summative control of actions. At present then, it would seem to be the ideal cortical candidate to fill a blank in our original neurology; being a key route through which, together with the amygdala, attention and arousal (already generated by GAS and GRS and summated) are *amplified* by GIS activation (Fig. 1.2, Fig. 3.1, Fig. 5.1); including by, for example, the transfer from the insula of pain information to the amygdala to enable fear potentiated startle (Davis, 2006).

In contrast to the interoception-focused 'why' of the insula, the cingulate cortex provides an exteroception-focused 'why'. The posterior cingulate cortex appears to be involved in what could be called innate anxiety plans (inhibiting action)[5]; and the anterior cingulate in the generation of (potentially obsessive) fear plans (largely generating action). The 'anterior' cingulate here includes areas adjacent to and connected with infralimbic and prelimbic cortex and may form part of an anterior midline strip where ACC (BA 24) represents the dorsal trend and IRL (BA 25) the ventral (Fig. 11.1; Fig. 11.2A).

Orbital cortex, in rats, is adjacent to the most anterior agranular portions of the insula, and then protrudes rostrally (Fig. 11.12). It shares with the insula mixed effects of inactivation on passive avoidance (contrasting with strong effects for septum, BL amygdala and ventral hippocampus; and null effects for ACC, PrL, and IRL; Fig. 6.5A). In §11.5 we provided reasons for seeing hippocampal theta-coded output as passing to DLPFC to signal

[5] For a view of posterior cingulate as controlling interoceptive attention see Smith and Lane (2015).

anticipatory goal conflict and, given enough time, generate or enhance stopping. Critically, with high time pressure, stopping itself in the SST (as opposed to go/no-go) is not sensitive to anxiolytic drugs but is associated with anxiolytic-sensitive theta-pattern activation of a region that appears to involve rIFG and/or the insula. Orbital frontal areas have substantial numbers of $GABA_A$ receptors that (like those in the insula) are reduced in panic disorder and generalized anxiety disorder; and 'the anxiolytic effects of [a] benzodiazepine most closely relate to modulation in brain metabolism in insula and orbitofrontal cortex' (Nutt and Malizia, 2001, p. 392). Consistent with this, BA 10, BA 11, and BA 13 are the only frontal areas receiving direct input from both hippocampus and insula (Fig. 11.2A). All these data suggest that orbital cortex processes goal conflict rather than just being a location through which the hippocampus activates goal inhibition but also, given the passive avoidance data, that the central structure of the GIS is the hippocampus. This conflict processing can be seen as part of a wider role for orbital cortex in optimization of goal-selection policies (Fine and Hayden, 2022) linked to its coding of reward value and resultant effects on, for example, navigation and consolidation (Rolls, 2023).

11.8.2 Dorsal and ventral prefrontal cortex

At one remove, in terms of emotion and motivation, the dorsal and ventral PFC maintain the working/active memory and motor programming functions required for acquired anxiety plans but also for, e.g. action stopping that is not sensitive to anxiolytic drugs (§11.5.4). This raises two questions. First, can this more caudal part of PFC be seen as the principal seat of anxiety (LeDoux, 2012; LeDoux, 2015; LeDoux, 2021)? Second, is it likely to be a principal site of action of anxiolytic drugs? Critically, *we* define anxiety via anxiolytics—and this determines our psychological descriptions, not the other way round. We thus exclude panic, phobia, and obsession grouping them as aspects of fear not anxiety.

Certainly, there are superficial parallels between the anxiolytic/SHS syndrome and the effects of prefrontal lesions as a whole. In rats (which have been the main species used to define the anxiolytic/SHS syndrome, but where it is hard to identify the homologues of human orbital and dorsolateral frontal cortex), prefrontal lesions impair water maze performance, radial arm maze performance, Lashley III maze performance, delayed response, delayed alternation, spontaneous alternation, and delayed non-matching to sample, but not matching to sample. They also impair discrimination reversal, performance on a DRL schedule, and extinction. Consistent with the idea that changes in the delayed non-matching task reflect a loss of working/active memory, and that different areas code for different types of working/active memory, there appears to be some differentiation between deficits in visual working/active memory produced by more medial prefrontal lesions and deficits in olfactory working/active memory produced by more orbital regions (for all of the above, see Kolb, 1984). Further, frontal deficits appear to be selective for working/active as opposed to reference memory and are strongly affected by interference (Granon et al., 1994).

In monkeys (Kolb, 1984), there appears to be a substantial separation between orbital deficits (response inhibition, odour discrimination, feeding, social aggression, and *increased* activity) and dorsolateral deficits (opening of puzzles, temporal ordering, spatial orientation, associative learning, *increased* social aggression, *hyper*-reactivity). In both human beings and rats, there appear to be a number of other dissociations, some of which may be related. For example, item recognition and order recognition are both impaired by hippocampal lesions, but only order recognition is impaired by prefrontal lesions (Kesner et al., 1994b; for a lack of effect in monkeys see Colombo et al., 1993). Successive odour discrimination is impaired by frontal but not hippocampal lesions (Eichenbaum et al., 1980; Cohen and Eichenbaum, 1993), as is the temporal order function in paired associate learning (Kesner, 1993). It also appears that, in at least some cases of conditional and non-conditional matching to sample, prefrontal lesions produce delay-independent and hippocampal lesions delay-dependent impairments (Winocur, 1992; Pigott and Milner, 1994; Chao and Knight, 1995). Hippocampal but not frontal lesions impair recall of incidentally-learned locations (Smith and Milner, 1984). Prefrontal but not hippocampal lesions produce impairments on the Wisconsin card sorting test, while the reverse is found with face recognition, recall of spatial location and 'on various perceptual and memory tests that have proved difficult for patients with left or right temporal lobe lesion' (Milner, 1995, p. 69).

There are thus positive and negative discrepancies between the effects of prefrontal and SHS lesions and between orbital and dorsolateral prefrontal lesions. Overall, lesions of the SHS have effects more like anxiolytic drugs than do frontal lesions. There is also good reason to see orbital cortex as part of the GIS and fundamentally linked to goal control (with goal inhibition being anxiolytic-sensitive). Conversely, dorsolateral cortex controls goal-directed behaviour (with action stopping being anxiolytic-insensitive), particularly the control of subgoal scaffolding, and can be seen as fundamentally linked to rules and rule policies (Fine and Hayden, 2022) and cognitive control (Friedman and Robbins, 2022).

We have already commented on the fact that prefrontal and cingulate cortex lesions were used for treating 'anxiety' specifically in those patients who did *not* respond to anxiolytic drugs. There must, therefore, be other structures than frontal and cingulate cortex that contribute to anxiety and on which the drugs normally act (but see also Chapter 14); and, as we have already argued, the SHS seems the most central of these. Equally, the fact that *both* cingulate *and* prefrontal lesions were used to treat 'anxiety' implies that neither region can be the sole seat of even the residual disorder not affected by anxiolytic drugs (see Sachdev and Hay, 1996 for problems identifying the lesions).

11.8.3 Language

So far, we have taken a species-general approach; but there is one additional feature of anxiety in human beings (particularly to its personality and clinical assessment) that is tightly linked to the functions we have described for prefrontal and cingulate cortices: verbal behaviour. In several studies of the effects of prefrontal damage in humans it has been observed that there is a dissociation between, on the one hand, the patient's ability (intact) to describe the requirements or contingencies of the task they are set and, on the other, their ability (impaired) to control their behaviour in accordance with this description (Rosenkilde, 1979). This is similar to the dissociation observed with cingulate damage between reportable pain detection (increased) and affective value (decreased). Note that this dissociation is opposite in sign to that of the amnesic syndrome consequent upon damage to the hippocampus. In the latter, memory can be behaviourally intact despite the patients' incapacity to describe the contingencies that control their behaviour (§8.1.1). Intact verbal report of contingencies with impaired behavioural control in patients with prefrontal lesion has been reported in a go/no-go discrimination (Drewe, 1975a; Drewe, 1975b; Toczek, 1960) and on the Wisconsin card sorting test (Milner, 1963; Milner, 1964). The fact that the patients were able correctly to describe the contingencies of reinforcement operating in these experiments, yet could not use this knowledge to control their behaviour, suggests that in human beings the PFC serves as a way station by which language systems normally *can* contribute to the inhibition of incorrect behaviour. But it also suggests that reportability (and 'consciousness') are not crucial for functional output.

This conclusion implies that frontal cortex could provide an extra layer of inhibitory control, dependent on highly processed cortical information, superimposed on psychologically simpler subcortical and archicortical control. One specific suggestion, is that the performance of prefrontal lesioned patients 'is best explained in terms of an inability to see or resolve a goal-subgoal conflict. This interpretation is compatible with several existing accounts of frontal lobe dysfunction that postulate a failure of inhibition of a prepotent response to explain poor performance on the Wisconsin Card Sorting task, the Stroop task, the Antisaccade task, the A-Not-B task, and the Delayed Alternation task' (Goel and Grafman, 1995). We shall accordingly argue that the similarities and differences between frontal and hippocampal damage arise from the fact that the former is concerned with resolving goal-subgoal conflicts. This includes ordering goals in the correct sequence (Funahashi et al., 1993; Sirigu et al., 1995), essentially by inhibiting actions that have been completed (Kolb, 1984) as well as those that are not yet required. By contrast (see Lee et al., 2023, for a direct within-subject comparison), the hippocampus is concerned with resolving goal/goal conflicts; and, at the next level down, the motor system is concerned with resolving action/action and act/act conflicts of the sort that arise in, e.g. mirror drawing or action/no action conflicts of the sort that arise in the stop-signal task.

Such a development would make good evolutionary sense. The hierarchical defensive systems described earlier have at their subcortical (survival circuit) apex the hippocampal formation, whose function we characterized as that of indirectly correcting motor programs by directly generating 'hesitation and doubt' when things go wrong. This is the sort of problem on which, typically, human beings bring to bear their full powers of verbal analysis. Thus, it would not be surprising if, in the human brain, some sort of liaison were established between the language systems of the temporal and frontal cortex (Lenneberg, 1967) and the SHS, so as to arrange, as it were, mutual cooperation. This could take place by way of SHS activation of appropriate language circuits, by way of descending cortical control over the SHS, or both. The fact that prefrontal lesions leave verbal descriptions of behavioural contingencies intact, while the behaviour itself fails, suggests that the PFC is in the second of these routes.

The notion that prefrontal lesions disconnect the SHS from the language system is supported by Homskaya (1964), who showed that, in normal subjects or patients with other brain lesions, the galvanic skin response and vasomotor orienting response (Sokolov, 1960) appear and disappear rapidly in response to verbal instructions (e.g. the patient is told that a stimulus will, or will no longer, be followed by pain). But these responses to *verbal* stimuli are absent in patients with prefrontal damage. Conditioning and extinction of the galvanic skin response and vasomotor response to *non-verbal* stimuli, while not entirely normal, did take place in prefrontal lesioned patients. Thus, the disturbance produced by prefrontal lesions was relatively selective to verbal control of orienting responses.

These observations suggest an explanation of the powerful effects of prefrontal lesions on human anxiety. For this we require the assumption that the circuit connecting, by way of the PFC, language mechanisms and the SHS permits activation of the latter by verbally coded description of threats. These pathways would constitute an alternative alarm bell acting instead of, or in tandem with, the phylogenetically older systems that activate the amygdala and SHS. If so, one would expect the 'cortical alarm bell' to be relatively unimportant in the anxiety elicited by innate anxiety stimuli or innate fear stimuli (Seligman, 1971) such as snakes or spiders (Chapter 12). Conversely, the cortical system would play a relatively large role in anxious, phobic or compulsive behaviour that depends heavily on such processes as semantic generalization (Razran, 1971), verbal self-description of potential threats, or the perception of situations as threatening only in virtue of their verbal description (e.g. the possibility that one will fail to meet a self-imposed deadline at work). These considerations are *consistent* with—but the argument is too tenuous to permit a stronger term (see also caveats in Chapter 14)—the type of patient who in the past was supposed to benefit (but see §11.1 and §13.5) from psychosurgery: extreme neurotic introverts displaying obsessional symptoms, widely generalized phobic behaviour or anxiety states (Marks et al., 1966; Tan et al., 1971; Powell, 1979).

This view is also consistent with the impressive success of cognitive restructuring and related psychological methods in treating anxiety disorders (Dalgleish and Power, 1999; see Chapter 14). Whether the disorder *originates* in the prefrontal area, language area, or lower parts of the defence system, it is clear that appropriate alterations to the language system would be expected to influence the PFC and through it the cingulate, hippocampus, and amygdala. It should also be noted that other high-order cognitive abstractions, akin to language and similarly dependent on cortical processing, could well take the same route. This also fits with our general defence system hierarchy, where lower levels are 'primed' and will also receive an anticipatory output-blocking signal that indicates when a higher level will take over control.

Our hypothesis of a descending cortical alarm mechanism travelling by way of the PFC does not eliminate the possibility that there is also traffic in the other, corticopetal direction. For example, the subiculum (an output station of the SHS) could influence much of the PFC via its projections to the prefrontal and cingulate cortex (Fig. 11.2A) as well as via its more limited direct projections to the temporal lobe.

If we are correct, the role of cortical structures in anxiety has become *relatively* greater in humans; almost a truism. However, PFC controls much more than linguistics (see e.g. Fig. 11.5). If working/active memory and its more sophisticated relatives are, as seems likely, as much part and parcel of threat processing as they are of motor control, then we would expect the PFC to play a role in non-humans comparable to that which it plays in humans, with a quantitative rather than qualitative increase in its influence as its relative size increases. Indeed, it has been suggested that our linguistic capacities are simply an evolutionary elaboration of the pre-existing properties of frontal networks in other primates (which are themselves unusually elaborate; Aboitiz, 1995).

11.9 Final summary—2D planning and survival systems

We have now ascended the hierarchical defence system to its top. We started with the PAG, which controls the simplest, undirected, responses to the most immediate threats, and have reached cortical systems that control the most complex, directed, anticipatory plans for future threats. The multiple neural levels we have traversed essentially map functionally to the defensive distance with which they deal (see Calhoon and Tye, 2015, for a more input-output layered perspective). For all levels we have distinguished defensive direction (active avoidance versus passive avoidance; defensive repulsion versus defensive attraction, with its related risk assessment).

The match between the effects of lesions of a structure on goal inhibition and those of anxiolytic drugs (Chapter 4) is greatest in the case of the SHS. This is partly because anxiolytics act on structures (locus coeruleus, raphe nuclei, supramammillary nucleus, amygdala) that project to the SHS; with lesions of each providing a separate component of the overall anxiolytic/SHS syndrome (e.g. McNaughton and Mason, 1980). But direct manipulations of the SHS, or of inputs to it (Woodnorth and McNaughton, 2002; McNaughton et al., 2006b), show the hippocampus itself is key.

This match with the SHS fails with the 'increase arousal' and 'increase attention' outputs of the GIS. These are clearly separately controlled by the amygdala and insula. With part of the insula clearly included in the GIS (§11.7.1), and the insula as a whole contributing generally to arousal, attention, and network control, we propose that the insula contains GAS and GRS modules as well as GIS. In this context it is the apex of a parallel (additive) hierarchy to the (subtractive) ones controlling goal selection. In that sense, the insula can be seen as a structural inclusion similar to the hippocampus but at the opposite border of the temporal lobe; and acting, together with the posterior cingulate, as emotional sensory cortex in parallel with the ACC as emotional motor cortex.

The organization of these decision and arousal control hierarchies (for GAS, GRS, and GIS) are shown in Fig. 11.15. It should be noted that the mathematical distinction between decision (based on a subtractive comparison of the alternatives) and attention/arousal (based on additive summation of the alternatives) requires distinct networks for the calculations. However, decision and arousal must be combined to generate motor commands: decision determines to what goal response sequences are made, and arousal determines how energetic is the execution of those responses (Gray and Smith, 1969).

The GAS, GRS, and GIS are also all impacted by diffuse modulatory systems as detailed in Chapter 6. These modulators are often biased to specific systems (serotonin to avoidance, dopamine to approach, etc). However, as discussed in more detail in the next chapter, we believe it is better to see the modulators as each controlling a high-level factor that impacts on all three systems but with effects that may be more salient to the experimenter for one or another of them.

In sum, we conclude (with only minor caveats) that anxiolytics act directly or indirectly to impair the functions of the SHS and related structures. The SHS is the core of the GIS. But both subcortical and frontal areas also contribute. We leave for chapters 13 and 14 how far the SHS is directly or indirectly involved in the various 'anxiety disorders' as categorized by DSM-IIIR, IV, 5 (American Psychiatric Association, 1987; American Psychiatric Association, 1994; American Psychiatric Association, 2013; see Chapter 11) and will argue that ICD-11 (Iacovides et al., 2002; Slade and Watson, 2006; World Health Organization, 2021) may

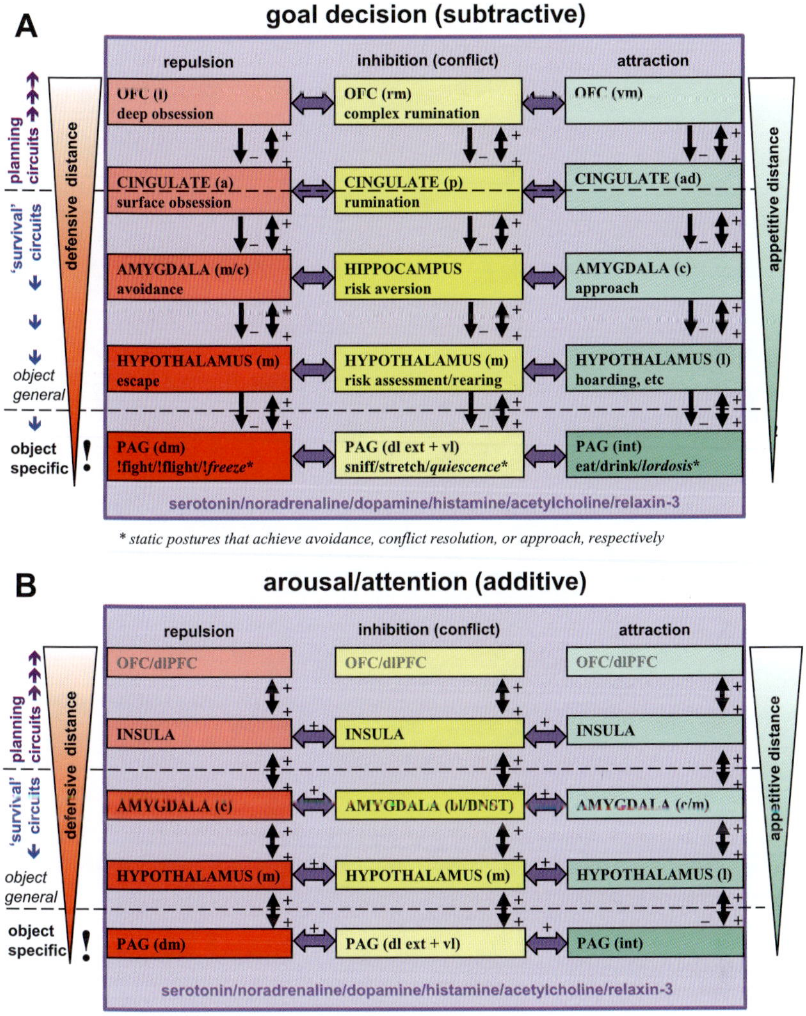

Fig. 11.15 Hierarchical organisation of goal control by the GRS (repulsion), GIS (conflict), and GAS (attraction) systems. For details of survival circuits, see Chapter 6; for planning circuits, see Chapter 11. Control of subgoal sequences, and conversion of goals to rules, actions, and acts is carried out by non-orbital frontal cortex (§11.8.2; see also Fine and Hayden, 2022). **A.** Decision circuits—where effects of attraction and repulsion subtract from each other; and where conflict can block the output from both and replace goal direction with risk assessment. **B.** Arousal/attention circuits—where adding attraction to repulsion, or vice-versa can result in a more energetic goal-directed output; and where conflict (essentially equal attraction and repulsion) increases arousal further.

provide a clearer view. However, Chapter 12 must first make clear how the model of Fig. 11.15 translates to human personality and particularly to the Reinforcement Sensitivity Theory built (see Corr, 2008b) on the models of the first and second editions. This provides a necessary bedrock for Chapter 13, which presents a picture of disorder that has a similar hierarchical trait perspective (as with The Hierarchical Taxonomy of Psychopathology, HiTOP, Kotov et al., 2017).

12
Anxiety and personality

The previous chapters presented a theory of the GIS based in ethology and behaviour analysis, coupled to a detailed picture of the neural system involved. Throughout, the common foundation has been an unusual, tight, definition of 'anxiety' as whatever is affected similarly by anxiolytic drugs that are not also panicolytic ('selective anxiolytics'; Table 4.1); including their effects on healthy non-human and human brain and behaviour (Chapter 4).

Chapter 13 extends this theory to a theory of the defensive disorders—anxiety disorder (anxiolytic-sensitive) in particular and other neurotic/internalizing disorders including depression (panicolytic/antidepressant sensitive) more generally. Anxiety (depending on the GIS), as defined by the theory, can be adaptive or pathological. However, the extreme nature and chronic course of disorder requires additional processes. In particular, I[1] will treat neuroticism and worry as common factors contributing to all the defensive disorders, not solely disorders of the GIS (for more detail on worry see §2.8).

The key assumption for this extension is that psychiatric syndromes and their treatments exist at extremes within a space defined by dimensions of *healthy* personality (Eysenck and Eysenck, 1969). In this context, I will discuss lacunae in the mapping of contemporary personality perspectives to GIS theory. Given that Reinforcement Sensitivity Theory (RST) was nominally founded on the original 'anxiolytic' neuropsychology (and particularly on Gray, 1970a), I will comment on appetitive aspects of RST as well as defensive ones. Where appropriate (as with neuroticism), I will also comment on elements of the Big 5 and various stand-alone scales (e.g. the Penn State Worry Questionnaire). It should be noted that Chapter 13 describes distinct *syndromes* (with different neural trait extremes) that would have very similar *symptom* patterns and so likely be conflated into a single nominal trait with surface-level item analysis or incorrectly grouped into a single disorder category by current diagnostic systems.

Much of the chapter, then, focuses on how far existing scales reflect the neuropsychology of the theory in its current extended form, accommodating two additional decades of data. The remainder considers how far the neuropsychology can be used to assess personality either by direct neural measurement or via neurally derived scales or by assessing existing scales. Along the way I provide recommendations based on my analysis. Being data-based, and still incomplete, albeit predictive, it seems likely that the theory will continue to require a new edition every ~20 years.

[1] Jeffrey Gray was essentially the sole author of the personality chapter in the 2nd edition. As the current sole author, rewriting it in the light of new data and critique, I have changed much of the content and many of his conclusions. So, in contrast to the other chapters, I have used 'I' rather than 'we' to make clear that changes have been made to his original position with which he might not have agreed. I thank Luke Smillie, Philip Corr, and Colin DeYoung for their careful reading of the entire text of various drafts, extensive comment, detailed textual corrections, and directional advice; and apologize for my departures from their suggestions.

The Neuropsychology of Anxiety, Third Edition. Neil McNaughton and Jeffrey A. Gray, Oxford University Press.
 DOI: 10.1093/oso/9780198843313.003.0012

12.1 Mapping personality to neuropsychology

12.1.1 The problem of word meanings

'Anxiety' means many different things to many different people (§1.4, Fig. 1.1), including whether it is seen as automatically maladaptive or not. Most current usage does not conform with the GIS theory. So, in the past, the translation between its neuropsychology and personality traits and thence to clinical disorder has been plagued by linguistic problems. So has discussion of 'anxiety' more generally.

A particularly serious problem has always been that anxiety, as defined by the selective anxiolytics, has a much more restricted meaning than 'anxiety' in DSM-5 (American Psychiatric Association, 2013), or ICD-10 (World Health Organization, 2010), or in current 'Trait Anxiety' scales. To avoid future confusion, I suggest that 'trait GIS sensitivity' should be used when selective-anxiolytic-sensitive anxiety is intended and has been demonstrated. Likewise, I will argue (§12.5) that 'neuroticism' (or more precisely Neurotic Introversion) should be seen as a key factor (potentially together with worry) *common to* what DSM would now call '[fear] + anxiety + obsession + depression', ICD calls 'neurotic, stress-related, and somatoform disorders', and the Hierarchical Taxonomy of Psychopathology (HiTOP, Kotov et al., 2017) calls 'internalizing disorders'. For this reason, I have placed 'trait anxiety' in quotes if it appears below and refer to Taylor's Manifest Anxiety Scale (TMAS; Taylor, 1953), and Spielberger's State-Trait Anxiety Inventory (STAI, Spielberger et al., 1983), which has state (STAI-S) and trait (STAI-T) scales, with their acronyms rather than full names two avoid use of the word 'Anxiety'. Like neuroticism, these 'Trait Anxiety' scales all relate to the whole gamut of neurotic/internalizing disorders (including depression) rather than to just anxiety as defined via the GIS (see also Chapter 13).

A particularly challenging problem has been the ambiguity of key motivational terms in the neuropsychological exposition—with 'punishment' a long-term offender (§12.8.1; McNaughton and Corr, 2019b) and 'fight' a more recent one (§12.14). Within contemporary RST, there is also the problem of varying mappings to the neuropsychology, which is compounded by different scales having been nominally based on different versions of the core neuropsychological architecture with resultant changes in concrete referents. I will distinguish these versions via the number of factors nominally involved. RST2 (based on Gray, 1970a; Gray, 1982; 'old RST'); RST3 (based on Gray and McNaughton, 2000; 'revised RST'); and RST5 based on the neuropsychology presented in this edition (see also Corr and McNaughton, 2012), which I will combine with a novel neuropsychology for RST2 that better conforms to Gray's original labelling but not his detailed exposition. These problems of meaning for the experimenter are all in addition to whether the participant understands the questions in the way the experimenter intended.

A related issue is the use of words like 'worry' (see also §12.9.3); it is hard to translate this into a form where one can easily determine if a nonhuman is in the same state. The same is true of neuroticism as a trait. 'Emotionality' has been defined in terms of rat breeding models (see §12.9.3) but may not then match the way this term is used within, for example, the Big 5. Such terms will require additional work in determining the nature of the underlying constructs before the relevant scales can be anchored to the theory (but see §12.9.1).

RECOMMENDATION 1: DO NOT TRUST SCALE/CONSTRUCT NAMES

Whether mapping to the GIS or not, it is important that, with scales intended to assess motivational constructs, existing names are not taken as definitive. This criterion can be applied to old and new items and scales. But in all cases, the first step should be to determine, rather than assume, the theoretical nature of the neuropsychological construct or constructs being assessed by the scale.

Recommendation 1: ensure that you have a clear idea of the scale construct, in terms of the relation of its items to neuropsychological theory, before attempting to link a scale to the neurology.

12.1.2 The evolution and labelling of adaptive systems

I have previously argued that emotions are coherent and nameable if one treats their referent as a specific product of evolution (McNaughton, 1989b). Each emotion can be characterized in terms of its specific evolutionary function (strictly, teleonomy, Pittendrigh, 1958). This fixed, long-term, mostly-general adaptive pressure, given sufficient mutations and polygenic control, explains the usual superficial coherence of the neural and hormonal components of the emotion and allows a surface-level description in approximate functional terms (Table 12.1). Critically, coherence of emotion elements can result from the consistent relation of eliciting stimuli with each other in the environment even when there is no internal control connection between emotion components (McNaughton, 1989a). Also important for this coherence is the fact that simple selection for a single behavioural character can produce widespread changes not only in emotion control systems (§12.9; Broadhurst, 1960; Gray, 1987a), but also peripheral hormonal systems and bodily traits (Trut, 1999; Dugatkin, 2018). I believe that the GAS, GRS, and GIS can be characterized as coherent for such reasons.

Personality is an abstraction used to explain consistency and coherency in an individual's pattern of affects, cognitions, desires and behaviors [ABCDs]' (Revelle, 2007, p. 37). But

Table 12.1 Emotions defined via teleonomic purpose and 'adaptive value'. Note that, for example we would expect love to be strong in albatrosses as a chick needs food supplied by both parents if it is to survive

Emotion	Teleonomic purpose/goal/ function	'Adaptive value'	
Lust	copulation		*offspring*
Fear	repulsion from danger	survive threat	[→offspring]
Anxiety	cautious approach to danger	get food despite threat	[→offspring]
Love	pair bonding	survival, through care, of offspring	*offspring*
etc.	*etc.*	*etc.*	*offspring*

> personality research currently provides more a taxonomy of patterns than theories of fundamental causes. I argue that teleonomic 'purpose' explains the organisation and outputs of conserved brain emotion systems, where high activation is adaptive in specific situations but is otherwise maladaptive. Simple modulators of whole-system sensitivity evolved because the requisite adaptive level can vary across people and time. Sensitivity to a modulator is an abstract predictive personality factor that operates at the neural level but *provides a causal explanation of both coherence and occasional apparent incoherence in ABCD variation*. Neuromodulators impact all levels of the 'personality hierarchy' from metatraits to [facets]: stability appears altered by serotonergic drugs, neuroticism by ketamine, and trait anxiety by simple anxiolytic drugs. Here, the tools of psychiatry transfer to personality research and imply both interaction between levels and oblique factor mappings to ABCD. On this view, much psychopathology reflects extremes of neural-level personality factors [§12.1.3], and we can view much pharmacotherapy as temporarily altering personality. So, particularly for personality factors linked to basic emotions and their disorders, I think we should start with evolutionary biology and look directly at conserved neural-level modulators for our explanatory personality constructs and only invoke higher order, emergent, explanations when neural-level explanation fails.
>
> (McNaughton, 2020, p. 1, emphasis added)

That is, provided care is taken to follow appropriate ethological and experimental analysis (Chapter 2, 3, 4), especially when this is based on human behaviour (Blanchard et al., 2001) and comparisons of homology (Blanchard and Meyza, 2017), it should be possible to design scales *based on reported long-term consistent patterns of* ***behaviour*** and then carefully validate them via neural challenge. Here key questions will be on specificity and sensitivity. Does your supposed GIS scale correlate only with your GIS-specific biomarker but not your GRS-specific biomarker? How do these relate to more system-general serotonergic measures? How sensitive is the scale in comparison with the biomarker in predicting theory-compatible consequences?

Deriving scales from neural measures could also be useful (§12.16) but using neural biomarkers directly is preferable, where possible. It is also clearly appropriate, albeit challenging, to characterize/deconstruct existing scales (whether nominally measures of RST or not) using such neural measures.

RECOMMENDATION 2: FOCUS ON THE ADAPTIVE FUNCTION OF BEHAVIOUR

I will make the case, despite the contrary views of both Smillie and DeYoung quoted below, that scales can be constructed to assess neural *system* sensitivities provided these systems can be characterized by their adaptive function. But a critical proviso is that the theory should expect specific phenotypic expressions reflecting a consistent high-order adaptive requirement. That is, the control of patterns of behaviour has been shaped by evolutionary pressure and can be characterized in terms of their common teleonomy/function (e.g. Table 12.1) with care being taken that the name of the scale correctly identifies the relevant function (§12.13).

Recommendation 2: Focus on the theoretical teleonomy (adaptive function) of the system of interest; then ensure that scale items are objectively diagnostic of this function by capturing the species-typical behaviour linked to it.

RECOMMENDATION 3: CHOOSE OBJECTIVELY DESCRIPTIVE ITEMS

Also, as with *Recommendation 1* for scale names, it will be important that the words of items and the phrasing are assessed carefully. Items for new scales should be chosen both to reduce the spread of their normal meaning and to capture the specific adaptive or neural function intended. The self-report items should be of a type that matches the observational reports of an external observer and be objectively diagnostic of the adaptive phenotype.

The same approach can be taken in assessing the item quality and constructs of existing scales provided these can be directly linked to the neuropsychology[2]. Linking of any scale to a specific neuropsychological construct in the theory would also require biological validation (neural, pharmacological, genetic). This would also be true of dissection of existing scales that might embed multiple constructs (McNaughton, 2020). A key point here is that in all these cases the biological bedrock is important and vagaries of language should be minimized.

Despite these difficulties, my final conclusion (§12.17) will be that, properly carried out, such personality neuroscience is 'an emerging field with bright prospects' (DeYoung et al., 2022; Corr and Mobbs, 2023).

Recommendation 2: Focus where possible on simple words and direct concrete terms that can refer directly to the behaviour or neural activity of the system of interest in both humans and nonhumans. Create new, or retain good quality old, scale items (or entire scales) that are unambiguous equivalents of the report of an external observer.

12.1.3 The need for biomarkers for Reinforcement Sensitivity Theory (RST)

The core of the theory is about goal control by motivational systems that have been highly conserved during evolution (§12.1.2). Its perspective on personality, then, has a clear disconnect from approaches that use the lexical strategy where it is assumed that 'the major dimensions of personality should be represented in the common personality descriptive adjectives of natural languages' (Ashton and Lee, 2005, p.5; which also see for 'a defence of the lexical approach to the study of personality structure').

The prime basis for this disconnect between results of lexical and neurophysiological methods for deriving models of personality is the strong overlay of (or filter provided

[2] With scales such as Neuroticism theory-free neural mapping (§12.15.4) can be a first step to integration.

> by) moral distinctions in personality language. As a result of this overlay, the most compelling organizations of natural-language concepts are perturbed by moral distinctions, and thereby become defined in a manner that, while highly sensible to everyday users of the language, fit rather poorly the aims of the biology-oriented personality researcher. To assess and detect convergence between [lexical approaches] and approaches used in studying animal behaviour-patterns, it will help to employ a set of variables that, while inclusive, focuses on variables that are, relatively, indifferently applicable across many species.
>
> (Saucier, 2018, p. 2)

Existing RST-related scales have been 'rationally' rather than lexically derived. Nonetheless, they generally use linguistically complex questions that are authored by experimenters inspired by higher-level theoretical considerations. While the items are then statistically refined, this has been done without neural or behavioural measures being used directly either to select items or validate the scales during development (see McNaughton, 2020 for a similar criticism of the 'biological' personality theories of Panksepp and Cloninger).

This opens up two language-related problems. First, item content depends on the experimenter's personal understanding, and then linguistic translation, of the neuropsychological theory. If this is faulty then the nominal label of an otherwise 'good' scale may not match the construct actually being assessed by the items (e.g. §12.8.4). This is a special case of the more general problem of determining the place of existing scales within the neuropsychology. Second, if an item is semantically complex and refers to a cognitive construct (e.g. 'worry') instead of being a report of observable behaviour that is as simple as possible (equivalent to that provided by an ethoexperimental study of a rat, Chapter 2) then it is difficult to know what it is in biological terms; and there is also a high risk that participants may interpret the content idiosyncratically.

In this context, I am in sympathy with the view that

> 'Reinforcement sensitivities' are lower-level brain-behaviour parameters and should be measured as such. After doing so, you can then ask questions about whether and how they relate to personality traits (abstract descriptions of what a person is like, such as outgoing, curious, hard-working, and so on), which are reasonable to assess using a self-report questionnaire. You can then answer questions like 'does extraversion relate to this specific proxy for sensitivity to reward (e.g. the ERP reward positivity)?'
>
> But by using a self-report questionnaire to assess reinforcement sensitivity, you're just going to end up measuring (and perhaps mislabelling) some personality trait that likely already exists as a facet within personality taxonomies such as the Big Five . . . . Finding that a questionnaire measure of reward sensitivity is related to extraversion might not tell you much—it could mean you've just unwittingly measured a facet of extraversion and then correlated it with another, broader measure of extraversion. . . . Alternatively, you might try to validate the questionnaire measure of reward sensitivity against some kind of brain-behaviour variable. *But in that case, why not just take the biological marker and relate it to our existing personality scales?*'
>
> Luke Smillie, personal communication, 13 January 2023, emphasis added

A more extreme position could be taken: that it would always be a mistake to use 'surface descriptions' to assess aspects of any neuropsychological theory. Why not apply neural and/or behavioural measures directly with no questionnaires, RST-based or otherwise?

One answer is that all direct measures of the neural basis of RST will have their trait component overlaid with 'error' due to state variations—and so require repeated administration to separate out the trait elements. At present there are few such direct measures; and none have yet been demonstrated to have the appropriate test-retest reliability (but see §12.14.3).

A second answer is that applying a wide range of highly specific neural and behavioural measures, extracted from a battery of carefully constructed (e.g. §11.5.4) tasks, is prohibitively expensive in participant time if nothing else for general experimental use, especially with large N. However, it may be possible in the future to have appropriate tests (e.g. via a computer game linked to a clip-on EEG headset of the type currently available for $100-$1,000; LaRocco et al., 2020).

A third answer, as detailed in §12.1.2, is that the *system* sensitivities that are the core elements of RST result from evolved covariance of a range of system measures (e.g. release of corticosterone, serotonin, and noradrenaline in parallel in response to stress) and also have covariance due to interaction of system control elements and so are best characterized by their teleonomy, which may be accessible via questionnaire (Recommendation 3).

What follows are suggestions as to how, in the current state of knowledge, to approach solutions that vary from direct neural measures through to neurally validated scales.

RECOMMENDATION 4: USE BIOMARKERS TO CHARACTERIZE SCALES

The covariance of neuropsychological measures means, on the one hand, that *no single specific biological measure is likely to be a perfect measure of sensitivity of the whole system*, which is expressed in varying behaviours across repeated occasions and is the key basis for natural selection of the conserved elements of the system. That said, availability of measures like GCSR/Rhythmical Slow Activity (RSA/'theta') that represent a final common path can go a long way to ameliorate this problem (§12.8). Equally, with highly correlated specific biological measures any one of them should provide a reasonable assessment of system sensitivity; and, as with scale items, the average of a suitable set of such measures should be better still.

> *Recommendation 4: As direct measures, or to assess both existing and new scales, choose as 'challenge' biomarkers those that are specific to the system of interest; prefer those that represent a final common path for others; treat individual biomarkers as indicators of a latent variable.*

12.1.4 The problem to solve

My focus is the neuropsychology of anxiety and not personality theory and so I will not look in detail at the currently available personality systems or RST scales. I see my task as trying to deal with the long-term problem that

> there are considerable difficulties . . . in establishing mappings between neural systems and dimensions of mood due to the complexity of the physiological basis for affect . . . [so] it is difficult to find suitable indices of the underlying conceptual neural systems.
>
> (Matthews and Gilliland, 1999, p. 598, p. 587)

This book has attempted to describe the neural systems in a way that reduces this problem. In this chapter, I attempt to link traits to the theory, especially using biomarkers. This linkage continues in Chapter 13, where defensive disorders are presented as extremes of traits—with many requiring extremes of more than one dimension (McNaughton and Glue, 2020). Some of the current chapter is driven in the reverse direction, with my view of traits driven by the picture I will later present of disorder.

This chapter aims to redress the 'mapping' problem by emphasizing the relevant aspects of the theory and by describing recent developments both in neural imaging (§12.8, §12.15) and in the paradigms that can be used to assess the relevant constructs (§12.14). In particular, I next provide a provisional example (§12.8), where I have translated my rodent electrophysiological model of anxiolytic action, via the theoretical construct of goal conflict, to a human biomarker that, like the rodent test, is sensitive to all classes of anxiolytic drug. This biomarker appears to define a new syndrome within the 'anxiety disorders' (Shadli et al., 2021a); and has allowed a challenge, and a consequent re-evaluation, of the Carver and White (1994) Behavioural Inhibition System scale (C&W BIS; §12.8.4). I also discuss the issue of scale assessment/dissection more generally in §12.15 and provide a brief summary of what I see as the key points in §12.17.

In what follows I will look at specific cases of three general types of mapping problem: 1) constructs where neither the underlying psychology nor neurology is yet characterized (§12.5, §12.6 take neuroticism as an example); 2) constructs where the underlying psychology and neurology are characterized but represent additions to existing RST neurology (§12.8 takes reinforcement as an example); and 3) constructs where both underlying psychology and neurology are well characterized in the theory (§12.8 takes goal conflict as an example).

I have tried to focus on how one can solve the general problems of linking traits to motivational system sensitivities, and vice versa. There will be those, like Smillie, who think system sensitivities should be measured directly rather than with scales—and this is definitely preferable where possible. There are those who will want to 'unscramble' (§12.15) old scales in terms of the neurology—this would allow data collected with them to connect to the theory even if the scales are not specific to a neuropsychological construct. There are those who will think that older scales should be replaced completely with purpose-built neurally mapped scales. I suspect a blend of these approaches will be needed—but I am sure that what is currently needed in all cases is neural characterization; and some method of reducing the confusion arising from the plethora of overlapping current scales with theoretically inappropriate titles inconsistent with their item content and often with each other.

12.2 From neural hierarchies to trait hierarchies

There are many lexically or rationally derived scale systems and stand-alone scales used in personality research. But consensus appears to be being achieved on the nature, if not precise number or detailed architecture, of major personality dimensions. In particular, the number and nature of those that define individuals *prone to* defensive disorders as a whole (panic, fear, anxiety, obsession, depression) are generally accepted. My analysis will be fairly coarse, seeing Neuroticism or Extraversion, for example, as mapping to the same basic underlying biology whether in Eysenck's 3-factor model, or the Big 5 (Watson et al., 1994; Eysenck and Eysenck, 1964; Eysenck et al., 1984; McCrae and Costa, 2008; Markon et al., 2005).

Next, I will first take a close look at Eysenck's EPQ-N and EPQ-E (but not EPQ-P). These were the explicit focus of the first two editions and, I would argue, are still relevant.

> Eysenck's three-factor model, N, E, and P, map onto other personality three-factor models well. The domain that most personality psychologists disagree with is P ... 'psychoticism' is really externalizing, but Eysenck argued that extreme levels of EXT transcended thought disorder, which is why he used the psychoticism label. That's the most controversial part. Most would view the model as essentially neuroticism, extraversion, and disinhibition, which is the third-level of most other personality models ... even if you forced a three-factor structure of the Big 5 (N=N; E=E+O; 'P' =A+C) [c.f. Markon et al. (2005) fig 1 and 2].
>
> Martin Sellbom, personal communication, 21 February 2022

Despite the theory's historical association with Eysenck's scales, I will also attempt to map to the theory some facets of a recent presentation of the Big 5 (with a focus on scales derived from NEO-PI-R). I have several reasons for this choice:

1. The EPQ can be seen as reflecting one of two layers of covariance structure between the Big 5 Metatraits (α/β; Stability/Plasticity) and the Big 5 traits (Markon et al., 2005)—and, as noted earlier, maps fairly cleanly with EPQ-N = N, EPQ-E = E + O, EPQ-P = A + C.
2. The Big 5 is thus more comprehensive and also is more used than Eysenck in non-clinical personality research; and more commonly used at present than the 'Big 6' HEXACO.
3. The specific presentation of the Big 5 that I focus on is the Cybernetic Big 5 Theory. This attempts to link the conventional Big 5 to 'goal-directed, adaptive systems' (DeYoung, 2015, p. 33; see also DeYoung and Krueger, 2018 for an extension to psychopathology). Its top-down perspective may be seen as bold, but its approach maps easily to our bottom-up goal-control-based theory. With additional work (and especially additional data) I believe they should at least partially converge. In particular, it provides a mapping of its two metatraits (Stability, Plasticity) to serotonin and dopamine, respectively, in a way that then allows direct mapping to our neurology (e.g. §12.8).
4. The Big 5 model is hierarchical (Fig. 12.1)—allowing approximate mapping to a range of features of our hierarchical neural model (Fig. 11.15). That is, it is intended to capture the major threads of covariation among all traits via dimensions that anchor trait space (as latitude and longitude anchor location on the earth's surface). But its 'Big 5' dimensions (Neuroticism, Agreeableness, Conscientiousness, Extraversion, Openness/Intellect) are not orthogonal and so can also (c.f., Cieciuch and Strus, 2017) be captured by higher order metatraits; while also fractionating into low-level aspects, and even lower-level facets. This non-orthogonality and fractionation will help us understand how scales might map to the interacting systems and structures of our neuropsychology.

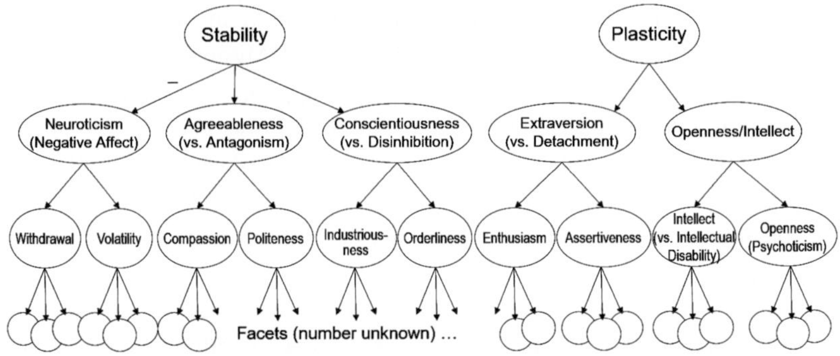

Fig. 12.1 A hierarchical taxonomy of personality traits, with the five major dimensions of psychopathology (plus intellectual disability) indicated in parentheses.

Note. Top level: metatraits. Second level: Big 5. Third level: aspects. Bottom level: facets. (Constructs at every level are traits.) Negative sign indicates inverse association of Neuroticism with Stability. Figure and legend from DeYoung and Krueger (2018) with permission.

The most important thing to note in Fig. 12.1 is that most factors involved are not orthogonal (nor, in practice, are Eysenck's Neuroticism and Extraversion). Stability reflects common variance in Neuroticism, Agreeableness, and Conscientiousness. Neuroticism reflects common variance in Withdrawal and Volatility. Withdrawal represents common variance in a range of facets (including anxiety and depressivity).

In interpreting these relationships (treating lexical constructs as potentially linked to neural reality), one should remember that not only does correlation not imply causation (which could be supplied by an unmeasured common cause) but also that even direct causation can produce weak correlations: with a risk factor 'causing' an outcome only when it combines with additional factors (including events). As a result, there appears to be a single general factor of psychopathology (encompassing internalizing, externalizing, and thought disorder) 'associated with more life impairment, greater familiality, worse developmental histories, and more compromised early-life brain function' (Caspi et al., 2014, p. 119). That is, external environmental factors can produce population-level correlations among the outputs of systems that are fundamentally independent in internal neural terms (c.f. my treatment of 'emotion' in §12.1.2).

In what follows, then, you must be prepared for the fundamental system sensitivities (the causal bedrock of the related neural traits) to be impacted *in concert* by genetic and life factors that cause intercorrelation. The systems of Fig. 11.15 each contain multiple interlinked levels, with each level dependent on a range of polygenes, this allows smooth variation in trait sensitivities within a population. To this, as you shall see, one must add the inherent state interactions between independent system sensitivities, when the systems interact with each other neurally or via the environment at the state level to produce correlated output even when their neural sensitivities are not correlated at the population level.

Critically, each system has been shaped *as a whole* by a specific adaptive pressure so that each of the levels and polygenes within a system has been driven to optimize a function for the phenotype; and so, the system (and related emotion and personality traits) can be characterized in terms of this higher order function rather than the myriad contributing chemicals and synapses (§12.1.2). So, mapping between scales and neuropsychology can be based on the higher-level cognitive and emotional constructs (e.g. 'goal conflict') defined by the neuropsychological theory. That said, it is important that scales intended to map to the theory involve items that remain firmly anchored in the biology of the theory (including behaviour, pharmacology, and neurology) not everyday use of language. Conversely, you will need to ask at what level/s of the personality hierarchy such a specific system sensitivity would express itself.

A crucial final point is that Big 5 scales are derived from correlations among trait descriptors, taken from the dictionary or from existing questionnaires. The same is largely true of the RST scales I will comment on. Given the problems with meanings in general (§12.1.1), the constructs actually measured by the scales are unlikely to match the concept that the scale name elicits in your mind. Critically, the scale names will very often not match the label used to capture the relevant causes of behaviour of a nonhuman under specific ethological circumstances. Great care must be taken in translation and biological validation (which, for me at least, is wanted).

This is not to say that scales are meaningless at the behavioural level. One must take seriously the advice of Colin DeYoung (personal communication, 13 February 2020, emphasis added):

> I think we have to be very careful not to assume that if trait measures assess *behavioral tendencies,* then these are merely 'superficial patterns of verbal behavior'. Rather they are valid measures of behavioral tendencies more generally. I trust (because there is good validity evidence) that people who score high on extraversion do not merely say that they are more gregarious, assertive, talkative, dominant, excitable, enthusiastic, and joyful, but that they really are all of those things in their lives in general. . . . I hate the whole canard about the Big Five being 'lexical'. That is totally irrelevant *as long as they are measuring real, general patterns of behavior. . . .*
>
> [However,] let us not jump to believing that some questionnaire measures a neural sensitivity, or we are foregoing all of the crucial research that would actually allow us to understand the causes of personality! I will never accept that '[BAS] sensitivity' and 'BIS sensitivity' can be adequately measured by a questionnaire, and so I hate that Carver's scale used those labels. Surely, we must have neural measures to determine [BAS] and BIS sensitivity! [Neuroticism] is biological in the sense that it is caused by variation in biology. But again: something is not identical to its causes, and a behavioral tendency is not a neural sensitivity.

In what follows I will try to link our hierarchical neuropsychology to the trait hierarchy approach to personality and then, in Chapter 13, link both to the hierarchical approach to psychopathology. Note that our neuropsychology is doubly hierarchical. It involves hierarchically organized systems to capture motivational distance. But it also has, embedded in it, hierarchical levels of correlation equivalent to Fig. 12.1—serotonin operates on all components of all systems (essentially at the metatrait level), each system operates as an essentially separate whole (essentially at the aspect level), and each structure within a system operates to generate specific classes of behaviour (essentially at the facet level).

But I will not attempt to resolve differences in current questionnaire measurement of RST. It is only once you have directly measured human variation in a clearly defined 'reinforcement sensitivity' that you can then ask how it corresponds to any personality questionnaire—and the field is only at the beginning of that road (§12.8.1). However, as you will see, application of even a few functionally characterized neural measures can drive very clear conclusions about what many scales are *not* measuring. Further, even simple textual analysis can drive very clear conclusions about the degree of overlap of questionnaires; and the existence of overlaps can be detected, *en masse*, by simple statistical analysis (Bainbridge et al., 2022). These are all fundamental initial steps for clarity.

You should note here that with the second edition of this book, it was

> Jeffrey Gray's view that the modifications that I made to the state version of his original theory (Gray, 1982) had shattered its conceptual unity. As he put it in a section heading of the book (p. 282) 'Humpty Dumpty had a great fall'. In his writing of the personality chapter of the book (pp. 333–349), he attempted 'Putting Humpty Dumpty together again'. However, at the neural level, I am convinced that his choice of original analogy was right and that 'All the King's horses and all the King's men [cannot] put Humpty together again'—or, at least, not as an egg. The reverse process is required. 'You can't make a [personality] omelette without breaking [neural] eggs' but, of course, if you break a number of eggs and then follow the right recipe you can produce a largely unitary and highly desirable omelette.
>
> (McNaughton, 2008b, p. 403; see also §12.15)

Overall, then, while one may be able to identify neural elements as *ingredients* of traits within systems such as the Big 5, it will be virtually impossible to unscramble them into causal systems of the type outlined by our neuropsychology. Rather we can bootstrap from them to neural systems and then back to new, related, neurally derived measures.

12.3 Extreme traits or categorical disorders?

People do not all run equal risks of developing phobia, generalized anxiety, obsessive-compulsive behaviour, and so on. In particular, certain kinds of people are much more likely to *develop disorder* with these symptoms than others. Analysis of just *which* people (and which disorder) has, historically, been clouded by the general difference between psychiatry and psychology. There is also clouding by the difficulty, with anxiety, of distinguishing between a predisposing factor (akin to high blood pressure) and disorder (akin to stroke).

The 'medical' model focuses on 'anxiety *disorder*' seeking specific causative agents and aetiological routes. It also seeks specific organs in which to locate primary pathological processes (mirroring our approach in Chapters 6 and 11). Panic disorder (in the purest sense, see Chapter 13) could translate to an 'epileptic' PAG (Dantendorfer et al., 1995a). Even recently, despite early alternative suggestions (e.g. Cloninger et al., 1993), the medical approach has been largely categorical (American Psychiatric Association, 2013; American Psychiatric Association, 2022) but this is changing (Chapter 13).

The 'mental' model, in contrast, sees psychiatric (as opposed to neurological) disorders as extremes of statistical distributions of personality traits. Unlike many physical diseases (such as stroke), there is no dichotomy of 'well' or 'ill'. Individuals who need psychiatric help are simply at an extreme of one or another normal distribution (Eysenck, 1960), like those at an extreme of blood pressure (e.g. hypertension); with different disorders located in different specific parts of a multidimensional trait space.

> Taxometric procedures have been used extensively to investigate whether individual differences in personality and psychopathology are latently dimensional or categorical ('taxonic'). . . . The first meta-analysis of taxometric research . . . [found that results] supporting dimensional models outnumbered those supporting taxonic models five to one. There were systematic differences among 17 construct domains in support for the two models, but psychopathology was no more likely to generate taxonic findings than normal variation (i.e. individual differences in personality, response styles, gender, and sexuality). No content domain showed aggregate support for the taxonic model. Six variables—alcohol use disorder, intermittent explosive disorder, problem gambling, autism, suicide risk, and pedophilia—emerged as the most plausible taxon candidates based on a preponderance of independently replicated findings. . . . Studies that used the [comparative fit] index were 4.88 times more likely to generate dimensional findings than those that did not after controlling for construct domain, implying that many taxonic findings obtained before the popularization of simulation-based techniques are spurious. The meta-analytic findings support the conclusion that *the great majority of psychological differences between people are latently continuous, and that psychopathology is no exception.*
>
> Haslam et al. (2020, p. 1418)

RECOMMENDATION 5: INCLUDE PSYCHOPATHOLOGY

From this perspective, at its simplest, a specific 'disorder' would be an extreme of a single trait. That is, high trait anxiety would translate to anxiety disorder; and high trait panic would translate to panic disorder. Chapter 13 presents a more complicated multidimensional view and argues that single dimensions, even of the HiTOP (Kotov et al., 2017), may not map one-to-one to specific psychiatric disorders. That said, as with EPQ-N (§12.5), a group of disordered individuals can provide an anchor within personality space for linguistically based scales and you should also be prepared for extreme values of biologically based scales to be found in psychiatric disorder, whether alone or in combination with other trait extremes.

> *Recommendation 5: Look to psychopathology both as an anchoring tool for scale construction or evaluation and as a target of healthy personality theory.*

12.4 Trait susceptibility versus defensive disorder

I will start the attempt to link the theory to personality, as such, and thence to pathology by trying to clarify the meaning of 'neuroticism' (following Recommendation 1) and (in §12.5) the semantic relationship between it and 'trait anxiety'. This is a case where there are existing rationally derived scales with nominal constructs of clear relevance to defensive disorders but which have not yet been mapped to the neurology of the theory. I discuss how to achieve such mapping in §12.15.4 and the possible pharmacological basis of neuroticism in Chapter 13.

Within the dimensional framework, excessive defensive symptoms are found predominantly in those in the Neurotic-Introvert portion of the two-dimensional space described by Eysenck and Eysenck (1969); with little contribution from the third, Psychoticism, dimension of Eysenck and Eysenck (1976). Neuroticism is the stronger, with a smaller contribution (§12.5) from Introversion (i.e. those low on the dimension of Extraversion) and a slightly greater contribution from inverted Conscientiousness than inverted Extraversion with the Big 5 (Kotov et al., 2010).[3] Importantly for our understanding of disorder (Chapter 13). Neurotic-Introversion appears to be a risk factor for disorder, not a measure of disorder itself.

Existing 'Trait Anxiety' scales (which do not distinguish between the defensive disorders), such as the TMAS and STAI-T, load about 0.7 on neuroticism and about −0.3 on Extraversion (§12.5). There is also a tendency for one such neurotic disorder to often be followed by a different neurotic disorder (Andrews et al., 1990; Poulton et al., 2023; but see also Caspi et al., 2014) and for neuroticism to be higher when conditions are comorbid (Weinstock and Whisman, 2006). Thus, while neuroticism is important for defensive disorders as a whole, it reflects susceptibility and cannot be equated with trait panic, trait fear, trait anxiety, trait obsession, trait depression, etc.; nor with disorders linked to them.

One partial exception to this general neurotic susceptibility is people with specific phobias, e.g. of small animals. Marks (1969) reported them as occurring anywhere in personality space; but later work suggests they have neuroticism scores that are moderately elevated relative to control but lower than other neurotic disorders (Weinstock and Whisman, 2006; Bienvenu et al., 2007). We will class them as neurotic disorders in Chapter 13.

Specific phobias are likely to depend on specific early experience. 'Genetic factors that influence individual variation in extraversion and neuroticism appear to account entirely for the genetic liability to social phobia and agoraphobia, but not animal phobia' (Bienvenu et al., 2007, p. 1714). There is also no spill-over from specific phobias into other areas of the person's life; and they can usually be easily treated with behavioural methods (see Chapter 13) but not selective anxiolytics (Sartory et al., 1990; Nutt, 2005; Sinclair and Nutt, 2007).

Likewise, a sufficiently extreme event will generate many cases of post-traumatic stress disorder (PTSD), and so inclusion of these cases in a simple cross-sectional analysis can obscure any influence of personality. For example, as many as 30% of the male firefighters of an Australian bush fire had chronic PTSD 29 months later (McFarlane, 1989). Given the long-lasting and pervasive nature of PTSD, it is like a *change* in personality—a persistent increase in the reactivity of the entire defence system (see the discussion of Adamec's experiments in §13.11). In this way, then, severe environmental circumstances in adulthood can exacerbate or even mimic personality traits that, in most cases, are established much earlier in life. That said, despite recruitment criteria for firefighting jobs tending to exclude extremely neurotic individuals, the level of neuroticism was a better predictor of PTSD in the firefighters than the degree of exposure to the disaster itself (see also Ogle et al., 2017; Ogle et al., 2016; Lommen et al., 2014). Likewise, C&W BIS (which we will argue measures worry not sensitivity of the GIS, §12.8.4) predicts increased PTSD-scale scores in response to a 'traumatic' film—though the film would not meet criteria for a traumatic event and the resultant scores remained below the clinical threshold[4] (Kehyayan et al., 2023).

To be a risk factor for defensive (neurotic) disorders in general is clearly not 'trait anxiety' in the sense of trait GIS sensitivity, nor 'trait panic', etc. in terms of sensitivity of the relevant parts of the GRS—nor in terms of clinical scales that assess current psychopathology (see Chapter 13). Instead, neuroticism appears to be a contributing cause of these disorders,

[3] They also found 'that Eysenck's inventories showed weaker associations than NEO-scales' (p. 768).
[4] An obvious requirement for ethics approval!

preceding and outlasting them. I will need to take a more detailed look at traits and their architecture to clarify this; but it is clear that if one can assign cause then one can interpret certain correlations as being between distinct constructs, and so biologically meaningful—and not just an artefact of the overlapping items of mutually redundant scales (e.g. §12.8.4). In particular, I must ask if what has previously been called 'Trait Anxiety' is redundant with neuroticism.

12.5 Neuroticism versus 'trait anxiety'

This is the first of several cases for which the problem is primarily linguistic but where a previous slight unclarity of terms (in this case 'trait anxiety') has led to theoretical problems. I will need to distinguish between trait GIS sensitivity (which, in our usage, would be extreme in anxiolytic-sensitive disorder but not in other neurotic disorders) versus neurotic introversion (which if extreme would increase the probability of other neurotic disorder as well as anxiolytic-sensitive disorder developing in the future).

Eysenck derived his item content from observation of those suffering from defensive disorders *as a whole*. Filtering out their superficial differences in presentation, he tapped into core descriptive commonalities across what DSM would now call '[fear] + anxiety + obsession + depression', ICD calls 'Neurotic, stress-related, and somatoform' disorders, and HiTOP calls 'Internalizing' disorders. As noted earlier, these disorders appear to share a common susceptibility linked to Neuroticism and Introversion but this very commonality means that high scores on Eysenck's dimensions are not restricted to any single disorder as currently diagnosed[5] and so cannot be equated with what the theory defines as anxiety.

Eysenck then used factor analysis, which can establish *how many* factors or dimensions there are in a given space, but not *where* they should be located. His choice of location placed the defensive disorders in the Neurotic–Introvert quadrant (Fig. 12.2). So, seeking dimensional simplicity, Gray (1970a) proposed rotating Eysenck's Neuroticism and Extraversion by 30° (Fig. 12.2) so that, within the same 2D space, one axis runs diagonally from the Neurotic-Introvert quadrant (where defensive disorders cluster) to the Stable-Extravert quadrant. Cingulectomy and prefrontal lesions reduce neuroticism more than introversion (Powell, 1979). This, and the observed correlations (Gray, 1970a; Torrubia and Tobena, 1984) between the Eysenck dimensions and the TMAS (Taylor, 1953) suggested to Gray (1981) that the disorder-related dimension should be rotated closer to Neuroticism than to Introversion. The same can be concluded with the clinic-oriented STAI-T scale (Díaz and Pickering, 1993)[6] and with a comparison of Big 5 Neuroticism and Introversion (inverted Extraversion) scores and groups diagnosed with depressive, anxiety, and substance use disorders (Kotov et al., 2010).

But note that this new dimension within the Eysenck space shares only ~50% of its variance with any scale that assesses the extent of clinical disorder, i.e. no more than EPQ-N does without rotation. Conversely, Neuroticism correlates 0.98 with Internalizing 'suggesting that

[5] I do not see these diagnoses as biologically correct (see Chapter 13) but they are useful descriptors of perceived symptom clusters that one can then use to 'bootstrap' new biomarker-based diagnoses via the selective partial success of, e.g. anxiolytic drugs. There is an at least approximate relationship between DSM symptom clusters and patterns of action of different drugs (Table 4.1).

[6] Thanks to Alan Pickering for help with this section.

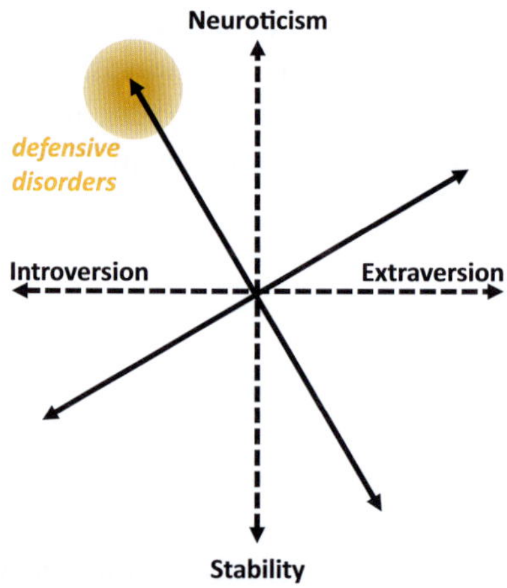

Fig. 12.2 A simplified geometrical representation of relationships between the "rival" personality axis systems of Gray (1970a) and Eysenck. The axis systems lie at a 30° angle to one another. Defensive disorders cluster at the extreme of a pole that Gray labelled 'Trait Anxiety' in a way that matches previous uses of this term (Taylor, 1953; Cattell, 1965; Spielberger et al., 1983; Bainbridge et al., 2022) but that is incorrect in relation to Trait GIS sensitivity. Figure and legend adapted from Pickering et al. (1999) with permission.

neuroticism may be the core of internalizing psychopathology' (Griffith et al., 2010, p. 1125). This breadth is not surprising, as for both Eysenck (1957) and Gray (1970a) the factor/s of interest reflect the likelihood of past or future disorder as much as present and for neither of them was 'disorder' restricted to those that are anxiolytic-sensitive.

This creates a problem with Gray's original (1970a) position on 'Trait Anxiety'—and for conventional perceptions of TMAS and STAI-T. Our current definition of anxiety and the GIS is in terms of goal conflict; and of the action of specific anxiolytic drugs. So, trait GIS sensitivity, in the sense of a trait that will be high in selective-anxiolytic-sensitive disorder, is narrower than, and cannot be equated with, Neurotic Introversion. That is, Neuroticism (for both Eysenck and the Big 5) reflects general sensitivity to negative affect (or perhaps threat imminence, Abend, 2023), whether or not this gives rise to goal conflict and so anxiety.

RECOMMENDATION 6: CARE ABOUT CAUSE

Given the distinct content of Neuroticism versus Introversion (and so Eysenck's choice of this particular axis rotation) it seems preferable (as I did in §12.4) to see Neuroticism as a primary risk factor, with smaller, potentially interacting, contributions from Conscientiousness and Introversion (Kotov et al., 2010). I will discuss in more detail in the next chapter the fact that the STAI-T distinguishes health from disorder to a similar extent across the whole gamut of neurotic diagnoses, including depression.

In my terms, then, STAI-T (which is normed for the general population) measures a trait or combination of traits that is high in defensive disorders, broadly defined. Its weak (~50% of the variance) relation to Neuroticism suggests that STAI-T is not just the result of a 2D or 3D rotation of Neuroticism, Conscientiousness, and Introversion with its low correlation resulting merely from a weak scale. On present evidence (Chapter 13) it seems more likely that STAI-T reflects key multifactorial aspects of defensive disorders *once they have developed*; whereas Neuroticism is a key risk factor prior to development as well as one of the maintaining factors during disorder. As to why the tendency to defensive disorder should be multifactorial, it could be that, e.g. the tendency to experience negative affect interacts with the tendency to turn one's focus inwards to increase 'toxicity'. Note that, in Chapter 13, I will argue that the bulk of current defensive diagnoses of those seeking treatment involve not only extreme Neurotic Introversion but also other trait extremes where disorder requires a kind of 'double hit'.

Recommendation 6: In assessing scale constructs, attempt to determine the causal relationship behind their correlations. With moderately correlated scales attempt to determine whether this is from a biological cause-effect relationship or from partial item overlap.

12.6 Neuroticism as threat sensitivity

So far, I have concluded that, in terms of the theory, Neuroticism is not 'Trait Anxiety'. It is heritable so depends on some underlying biology, which should connect with the theory in some way. Likewise, its linguistic coherence suggests that it should be possible to map it conceptually, if not yet neurally to the theory. What then is it? Where would it fit within Fig. 11.15?

The heritability of both EPQ-N and EPQ-E is about 50% (Floderus-Myhred et al., 1980), which matches the Big 5 (Jang et al., 1996). The scores, on each dimension, are distributed according to a normal Gaussian curve with a number of polygenes, each of relatively small effect, contributing additively to the final phenotype with overlap across disorders (Genetics of Personality Consortium, 2015; Gandal et al., 2018) but, at present, limited capacity to generate useful polygenic risk scores (Bogdan et al., 2018). The defensive disorders themselves are also substantially heritable (estimates range from 30% to 40% for general anxiety and phobic disorders (Kendler et al., 1992a; Kendler et al., 1992b).

Critically, what appears to be inherited with Neuroticism is the *general predisposition to neurotic disorders*, rather than specific symptoms (Andrews et al., 1990; Widiger and Oltmanns, 2017). Thus, comorbidity of generalized anxiety disorder with other conditions, extending even to neurotic depression, is dependent on heritable factors to the same extent (30%) as generalized anxiety disorder itself (Kendler et al., 1992c). The remainder of the reliable variance in individual *susceptibility* to these conditions is largely due to specific within-family environmental factors (that is, life events that happen uniquely to the individual concerned; or group members as a whole, as with the Australian firefighters of §12.4; see also Ogle et al., 2016), the between-family environment (including such socioeconomic factors as class, poverty, access to educational materials, etc.) playing only a minor role.

The best single index of the heritable component of the comorbidity between the neurotic disorders consists in scores on Neuroticism or on similar scales highly correlated with it. One can thus see Neuroticism as a developmentally related factor that *pre-disposes* to the later appearance of defensive disorders (and henceforth I will refer to them, including depression, as 'neurotic disorders'); while not representing a disorder by itself.

On this view, current Neuroticism could combine with other (particularly environmental) factors to lead to future increases in disorder (as with my PTSD example). In Chapter 13, I will make the case that Neuroticism is not just a predisposing factor but also a maintaining factor for such disorders. This opens the possibility that it simply combines with, rather than causing, high levels of disorder-specific traits to generate a specific disorder. As noted earlier, it could be joined in this enabling role to various extents in different cases by Introversion and Conscientiousness.

An additional reason to retain Eysenck's general formulation is that it is essentially retained in the consensus of the Big 5 (§12.2; Fig. 12.1). Critically, this analysis suggests that Neuroticism, whether measured by EPQ-N or not, should be related to threat *sensitivity* (as should rodent emotionality, Broadhurst, 1960; Gray, 1987a) rather than to ongoing negative affect but, like the Big 5, I will also distinguish it (§12.9) from serotonergic rodent emotionality (taken as a homologue of the inverse of Big 5 Stability, i.e. 'the inability to restrain urgent emotional impulses'; DeYoung and Krueger, 2018, p. 131).

RECOMMENDATION 7: CHARACTERIZE ESTABLISHED SCALES

In sum, given that it is not a form of trait GIS sensitivity, there is currently no clear way to fit Neuroticism into the neurology of Fig. 11.15. Neither its psychological construct nor neural basis (§12.15.4; Chapter 13) are yet sufficiently well characterized. But neither should one simply exclude it as unrelated to the theory.

> Neuroticism is the trait disposition to experience negative affects, including anger, anxiety, self-consciousness, irritability, emotional instability, and depression. Persons with elevated levels of neuroticism respond poorly to environmental stress, interpret ordinary situations as threatening, and can experience minor frustrations as hopelessly overwhelming. . . .
>
> Neuroticism is a fundamental domain of personality that has enormous public health implications, impacting a wide array of psychopathological and physical health care concerns. It contributes to the occurrence of many significantly harmful life outcomes, as well as impairing the ability of persons to adequately address them. *It has long been recognized as one of the more important and significant domains of personality and is being increasingly recognized as a fundamental domain of personality disorder and psychopathology more generally.*
>
> Widiger and Oltmanns (2017, p. 144, emphasis added)

Notably, the progression here, has been a kind of bootstrapping from observation of a pool of patients with a range of defensive disorders, through to extraction of an apparently genetically controlled biological factor from questionnaire scores. I will take up the issue of the pharmacological substrate of this factor in the next chapter (concluding that at least seven neurotransmitter systems are involved) and of its neurological substrate in §12.15.4; but note here that with this factor (and with rodent Emotionality) I am more fitting them into the current neuropsychological theory than deriving them predictively from it. The key steps to take then must involve biological analysis of the scale (both in behavioural and, particularly, neural terms) to map its nature into the model of Fig. 11.15—there is no obvious candidate in the existing model from which to derive an equivalent measure.

> *Recommendation 7: Retain and biologically characterize scales* **that have proven utility** *so they can be added to the theory. The resultant mapping should both identify the nature of the scale and identify scales with partial overlap. Neuroticism is a well-established disorder risk factor that appears to reflect a broad (multi-system) 'threat sensitivity'. 'Trait Anxiety' scales may be measuring its consequences—or be measuring a variant of it, coupled with contributions from inverted Conscientiousness and inverted Extraversion (Introversion). Neither they nor Neuroticism can yet be clearly linked to the neurology of Fig. 11.15, but see §12.15.4 and Chapter 13 for initial steps.*

12.7 Dopamine—reinforcement sensitivity

So, Neurotic Introversion, even when rotated (Gray, 1970a), is not specific to the GIS but is much more general capturing underlying factors common to the development of all defensive disorders, including depression. I have left open its exact nature and neurology within the theory. I have also left open the linked issue of 'reinforcement'.

'Reinforcement' needs further consideration. Importantly for personality theory, Gray redefined the *functions* of his rotated axes; identifying them as susceptibility to punishment ('anxiety') and susceptibility to reward ('impulsivity'), respectively (Gray, 1970a). My rejection of his axis rotation implicitly involves a rejection of this re-assignment of axis function; particularly the 'anxiety' and 'impulsivity' labels. Surprisingly, this does not mean one has to reject his more general suggestion that there are personality traits linked to reinforcement sensitivity (positive and negative).

Experimentally, there were extensive efforts to test Gray's original (1970a) model of personality (later termed RST) or subsequent elaborations of it (Gorenstein and Newman, 1969; Fowles, 1980; Newman, 1987; Cloninger et al., 1993). But no clear picture emerged (Pickering et al., 1997; Matthews and Gilliland, 1999). Pickering et al. (1997) noted the 'bewildering array of outcomes' and were tempted 'to abandon it altogether'. But commented that

> one cannot but remain impressed by the sheer frequency with which significant relationships nonetheless do emerge between one or other relevant personality trait and one or other relevant change in behaviour due to reinforcement effects. Somewhere in the human brain there clearly are systems which influence individual differences in sensitivity to reinforcement.
>
> (Pickering et al., 1997, p. 63)

In what follows, I will look carefully at the details of the current theory, and the different meanings that people have assigned to descriptive terms like 'reward' and attempt to resolve some of the remaining bewilderment—mainly by splitting and carefully defining ambiguous terms. In particular, I will provide a critique of Gray's use of the word 'punishment' (§12.7.1) and I will start to draw a strong distinction between reinforc**ement** (which will become the core of RST2 redux) and reinfor**cers** (which are the core of RST3 and RST5).

12.7.1 Old Reinforcement Sensitivity Theory (RST2 = BIS/BAS)

To make the reinfor**cer**/reinforc**ement** distinction clear, I must first critique Gray's original position:

> Gray's 1970 synthesis was unprecedented and fundamentally changed personality psychology. However, his approach had several problems, some of which linger to this day [i.e. 2019]. Most obviously, its theoretical elegance is fraught with complexity. . . .
>
> Gray's detailed exposition also has some specific problems that we discuss here. At the theoretical level, his use of the terms 'punishment' and 'fear' were ambiguous: blurring key points when he shifted between one and the other conceptually. . . .
>
> 'Punishment' (or its alter ego 'frustrative nonreward') can suppress ongoing responding (passive avoidance); generate approach to safety; or elicit escape/ withdrawal. Extraverting drugs reduce only the . . . first of these three effects. For the second case, Gray argued that, for example, shuttle-box avoidance is unimpaired by the drugs because relief rewards avoidance rather than fear punishing non-avoidance. *His paper focused on 'reward' and 'punishment' in the context of conditioning.* He, therefore, did not discuss the third case of escape/withdrawal in any detail. At this time, he distinguished between a learning-related 'punishment mechanism for passive avoidance [and] a separate punishment mechanism for organizing the unconditioned response to a punishment. We shall call this the 'fight/flight' system' (Gray, 1971, p. 194; *note that 'punishment' means three different things within this one quote*). However, it is via fight/flight that he included obsessive-compulsive disorder, with its compulsive rituals and obsessive rumination, within the dysthymic disorders. Gray says the 'symptoms bear all the marks of an *active* avoidance response' (p. 255, our italics) equating this with fear. However, we cannot link this (active avoidance) 'fear' to (passive avoidance) 'punishment' behaviourally; nor do extraverting drugs (like amylobarbitone) treat obsessions or compulsions. . . . Gray notes that Maudsley Reactive rats, taken[7] as a model of introversion, 'show a bigger frustration effect in the ... double runway' (1970a, p. 256) but he *does not note* that he had already shown that amylobarbitone does not reduce the frustration effect (Gray, 1967, p. 601). Gray's 'punishment sensitivity' *as defined by the drugs*, even at the time, was more restricted than neurotic introversion or dysthymia.
>
> (from a detailed critique by McNaughton and Corr, 2019b, pp. 129–130; some emphasis added)

RST was initially a supposedly simple theory of 'reward' sensitivity (equated with the BAS) and 'punishment' sensitivity (equated with the BIS). But, in practice, both 'reward' and 'punishment' confused the anticipatory behavioural and internal reactions to reinfor**cers** (controlled by GAS, GRS, and GIS) with the consequential neural plasticity of reinforc**ement** (controlled elsewhere) that changed future behaviour. Gray's use of 'Punishment', in addition, confused passive avoidance (anxiolytic-sensitive) with active avoidance (anxiolytic insensitive; panicolytic sensitive).

It is unsurprising that testing of the 'simple' (5 concepts confused with 2) theory produced 'bewildering' reactions. In what follows (especially §12.10) I will argue that, when dealing

[7] Rightly or wrongly, see also §12.9.3.

with reinforcers, the *object* labels, reward/punishment, be avoided and replaced with gain/loss or attractor/repulsor as appropriate (Corr and McNaughton, 2012). My original hope was to abolish reward/punishment and their attendant confusions completely. However, this is hard to do without mind-numbing circumlocutions when one comes to discussing the *process* labels for reinforcement. Note also that with positive/negative reinforcement there is no counterpart to the goal conflict that can occur between reinforcers (i.e. attractors, repulsors).

As discussed in Chapter 3 (see also §12.10 and 12.5), both GAIN presentation and LOSS omission can result in the process of positive reinforcement—with LOSS omission, thus, being 'a reward'. Note also that a GAIN does not equate simply to a food pellet or $1 but the responder must be hungry for food or dollars[8], respectively. Note also that positive reinforcement as such is a general result of presentation or omission of quite disparate objects. Likewise, simple GAIN presentation or LOSS omission will not result in reinforcement (and so not change subsequent behaviour) if it is habitually expected (Choi et al., 2005)—it must be unexpected (Bouton et al., 2020). Finally, *unexpected* GAIN presentation and *unexpected* LOSS *omission* are the *cause* of positive reinforcement, and, as objects, *cannot equate with the process of reinforcement* itself. The key event for positive reinforcement is what is usually termed Reward Prediction Error (RPE); that is, the discrepancy between the reward that has occurred and a prediction that it would not (Schultz, 1998; Cooper et al., 2014; Watabe-Uchida et al., 2017).

RECOMMENDATION 8: DISTINGUISH REINFORCEMENT FROM REINFORCERS

The terminology in this area is confusing because a *predicted* GAIN is *not* a reward in the functional sense—reinforcement requires an RPE. In principle, you should start referring to 'GAIN presentation or LOSS omission positive Prediction Error' as generating 'reward' (in the pure sense) and so positive reinforcement but this can only lead to confusion given current usage. So, in the context of positive and negative reinforcement, I feel forced to retain the terms 'reward' and 'punishment' for the relevant precursors while flagging that these are dynamic constructs dependent on prediction error and *should not be used for* ***expected*** *gains and losses*.

> *Recommendation 8: Ensure that trait reinforc****ement*** *sensitivity is kept distinct from trait reinforc****er*** *sensitivity; avoid 'reward'/'punishment' as far as possible and use only in the context of reinforc****ement****.*

12.7.2 New Reinforcement Sensitivity theory (RST2 redux = dopamine)

With neuroticism, neither the psychological construct nor neurology are yet clear. However, with reinforcement, the construct has been well developed (Chapter 3) and has a tight neurology that forces a particular Conceptual Nervous System meaning of the term. However, in

[8] Our Student Job Search participants volunteer for available jobs at close to the minimum wage.

contrast with much prior usage, this meaning does not map the key construct uniquely to the GAS.

Typical mammalian reinforc**ement** (both positive and negative; and in contrast to Hebbian association) depends on dopamine. In instrumental learning, dopamine presence engages long-term potentiation and dopamine absence engages long-term depression (Reynolds et al., 2001; Reynolds and Wickens, 2002; Wickens et al., 2003; Redgrave et al., 2011). In §6.12, I saw dopamine as contributing to: 1) positive reinforc**ement** by encoding 'Reward Prediction Error' (Schultz, 2002; Schultz, 2016); and 2) negative reinforc**ement** when it is suppressed by habenula input (Sosa et al., 2021). I can now call on this prior neurology (developed independently of the theory) to assess the role of dopamine in personality, particularly traits of reinforc**ement** sensitivity (*not* reinfor**cer** sensitivity) and Extraversion (§12.7.3).

In terms of Fig. 11.15 one would expect system-specific modulators, like benzodiazepines or RSA/'theta', to underlie any trait specific to the GIS. However, the monoamine systems send out collaterals that diffusely innervate all three of GAS, GRS, and GIS (and the neocortex in general) and so should underlie traits with a more general character. But what is the nature of those traits? I will look at dopamine in the context of RST here, dopamine in the context of the Big 5 in §12.7.3, and serotonin in §12.9.

A crucial point is that dopamine release or inhibition is the result of positive or negative RPE, respectively.

> 'In-depth analysis of dopamine cell firing in animals (Bromberg-Martin et al., 2010; Fiorillo, 2013; Matsumoto and Hikosaka, 2009) suggests that release of dopamine primarily signals [RPE]. The RPE is operationalized by observations that dopamine cell activation increases with unexpected reward, and decreases (from baseline) with omission of an expected reward (Schultz et al., 1997). Importantly, current animal work (Redgrave and Gurney, 2006; Schultz, 2016; Schultz et al., 2017) reports two RPE signals: an early (70–100 ms) 'salience' component; and a later (200–300 ms) 'valuation' component. The early component detects, and orients us to, the occurrence of any unpredicted event (Redgrave and Gurney, 2006). The late [increase or decrease] component, as emphasized by Schultz (2016), codes the subjective motivational value [positive or negative, respectively] of the unpredicted event (Schultz, 2016; Schultz et al., 2017). . . .
>
> Here, we evaluated the validity of evoked electroencephalography responses to unexpected reward in a monetary gain/loss task . . . over the 0–400 ms period in which feedback on the outcome was presented, responses evoked by unexpected reward contributed to all theoretically relevant approach motivation trait domains (*disinhibition*, *extraversion* and the *behavioural activation system*); and did so only at times when dopamine responses normally peak and reportedly code salience (70–100 ms) and valuation (200–300 ms)'[9].
>
> (Neo et al., 2021, p. 2, p. 1; emphasis added)

Reward in the sense of *unexpected* GAIN presentation or LOSS omission should, against a null background, produce orienting (GIS); and if consistently following a particular response it should increase response probability (GAS). Punishment in the sense of *unexpected*

[9] 'Some evidence suggests it is less about early vs late as about different populations of DA neurons with different functions. Plus it's important not to equate DA function with learning exclusively, since it triggers approach/exploratory behavior in the immediate as well as producing learning that will affect future decisions' (Colin DeYoung, personal communication, 23 February 2023).

LOSS presentation or GAIN omission should produce similar orienting but suppress the response. Thus, a dopamine signal as such is not identical to pure reinforc**ement** since the early salience component (producing orienting) is valence-independent and more linked to orienting and exploration. Nor can the dopamine system as such be specifically equated with either positive or negative reinforc**ement** since it can generate either depending on its direction of the late component change relative to baseline. But, under typical test conditions (i.e. presentation but not explicit omission), it is reasonable to equate the extent of late (200–300 ms) dopamine release (positive or negative) with reinforc**ement** (positive or negative). Note that behaviourally there will be distinct reward and punishment sensitivities (the latter mediated by variation in, e.g. habenula input to the VTA) but these will be correlated with each other *and with exploration, etc.*, via shared changes in the dopamine system (§12.7.3).

On this view, the Gray (1970a) BIS/BAS traits, phrased in terms of reinforc**ement**, are distinct from reinfor**cer**-related traits such as gain sensitivity, loss sensitivity (with loss/gain assessed via 'loss aversion'), attractor sensitivity, repulsor sensitivity, and conflict sensitivity. Critically, the dopamine systems innervate *all three* of the GAS, GRS, and GIS. This range of output targets allows for differing effects of, and so sensitivities to, the different forms of dopamine release. With the late dopamine signal, which discriminates motivational direction, not only will positive and negative reinforc**ement** have opposing effects on a particular goal (with positive increasing an attractor, and negative decreasing) but they will have opposite effects on opposite types of goal (with negative reinforc**ement** increasing a repulsor). This would allow reinforc**ement** sensitivities whether positive or negative to have different values determined by their targets (or by habenular input), while nonetheless being at least partially correlated because of their common dependence on dopamine.

On this view, at least some components of the C&W 'BAS' scale may, as designed, reflect reward in the sense of positive reinforc**ement** (Neo et al., 2021). But other components may be more linked to gain/loss or attractors/repulsors. Conversely, a negative RPE will reflect the *outcome* conflict between actual outcome and expectation (i.e. error monitoring rather than anticipatory goal conflict, Botvinick, 2007) with *GRS*-related effects (e.g. escape from frustration; Adelman and Maatsch, 1956) mediated by, e.g. anterior cingulate cortex (Botvinick et al., 1999; Botvinick et al., 2004). But note that I conclude in §12.8.4 that this is not what is being measured by C&W 'BIS' and assessing punishment prediction sensitivity (in the sense used here) would need a different scale.

RECOMMENDATION 9: USE ALL THE NEUROPSYCHOLOGY AVAILABLE

Reinforc**ement** is just one example of a range of Conceptual Nervous System constructs where there has been extensive electrophysiological analysis of state processes (from the single neuron to scalp EEG) that should be able to be repurposed to answer trait questions. In turn this can fine-tune cognitive level labels (e.g. reward prediction error) for constructs that are tied to defined neural processes (e.g. dopamine release). Critically, once a neural substrate is known, this can be linked to other such substrates and so other constructs. Dopamine and its neural targets are already included in Fig. 11.15 at the neural level. The analysis of the current section can therefore be transplanted directly into the body of the theory.

Recommendation 9: In challenging motivational traits use all the prior neuropsychological analysis you can get, whether neurally focused (as with dopamine, §12.7.2) or theoretically focused (as with GCSR, §12.8). It should all ultimately connect to the theory.

12.7.3 Big 5 (Extraversion/Plasticity = dopamine)

Within the Big 5, dopamine has been linked to the trait (similar to that in the EPQ) of

> extraversion, the broad tendency toward assertiveness, sociability, activity, and high-energy positive emotions. One influential theory posited that extraversion is at least partly driven by sensitivity to incentive reward governed by dopaminergic function (Depue and Collins, 1999) . . . [M]oderation of the effects of dopaminergic drugs by extraversion . . . provides evidence that extraversion is related to variation in dopaminergic function. Additional evidence [is] that extraversion is positively correlated with the magnitude of [the reward positivity (§12.7.1)] that appears to reflect dopaminergic signaling . . . . Thus, we have reasonably good evidence to support the dopaminergic reward sensitivity theory of extraversion. In fact, the amount of neurobiological evidence that extraversion reflects reward sensitivity is currently greater than the amount of evidence from direct behavioral tests of reward sensitivity (judging by the number of reasonably powered studies reporting significant results of each type), a striking example of the value of neuroscience for personality theory.
>
> (DeYoung et al., 2022, p.7)

There is a complication for interpretation here.

> Dopamine neurons come in multiple types that are connected with distinct brain networks and have distinct roles in motivational control. Some dopamine neurons encode motivational value, supporting brain networks for seeking, evaluation, and value learning. Others encode motivational salience, supporting brain networks for orienting, cognition, and general motivation. *Both types of dopamine neurons are augmented by an alerting signal involved in rapid detection of potentially important sensory cues.* We hypothesize that these dopaminergic pathways for value, salience, and alerting cooperate to support adaptive behavior.
>
> (Bromberg-Martin et al., 2010, p. 815, added emphasis)

'The broad tendency toward assertiveness, sociability, activity, and high-energy positive emotions' (DeYoung et al., 2022, p.7) seems likely to be an effect of more than a simple positive RPE. In addition to its role in reinforc**ement**, §6.12 saw dopamine as contributing to novelty seeking and to novelty-induced approach-avoidance conflict (DeYoung, 2013; Tapper and Molas, 2020). Thus, Extraversion could be linked to shared dopaminergic variation in *positive* reinforc**ement** (e.g. positive RPE, 200–300 ms, see Smillie et al., 2019)[10] and exploration (e.g. salience RPE, 70–100 ms, Neo et al., 2021); while the positive and negative reinforc**ement** sensitivities (positive and negative RPE, 200–300 ms) would be detected as separate entities at the facet level in the hierarchy of Fig. 12.1. Similar arguments

[10] Their Figure 4 suggests that the effect may have been proportionally larger at the earlier 'salience' peak.

can account for the apparent correlations between RPE and measures of openness/intellect (Smillie et al., 2019).

RECOMMENDATION 10: ASSESS CAUSAL SPREAD

At a yet higher-level of combination, it is reasonable to see dopamine (early + late positive + late negative) as supporting both reinforc**ement** and novelty seeking, combined in the metatrait of Plasticity (DeYoung et al., 2002; DeYoung, 2010), which represents the shared variance of Extraversion and Openness. Note here, that the early dopamine 'salience' signal could act via the dopamine input to the hippocampus to affect orienting, exploration, and the information gathering required by risk assessment—with 'salience' thus filling in the gap between positive and negative reinforc**ement** when mapping dopamine to goal control systems. Critically, the correlational nature of the Big 5 makes a possible direct role for dopamine in 'Plasticity' difficult to separate from its equally possible direct effects on intercorrelated facets that then interact with experience to generate complex but consistent patterns of ABCD.

Recommendation 10: You must be prepared for trait-level causes to generate correlations at the facet level (as with Neuroticism) and vice versa (as likely with Extraversion) and further interactions in both directions; in all three cases as a result of their long-term interaction with experience. You should attempt to assess these relationships; with this recommendation being a corollary of Recommendation 6. The goal should be neural bedrock with adjustment of names and content of trait constructs where necessary.

12.8 Rhythmic slow activity—goal conflict sensitivity

12.8.1 The phylogeny of trait anxiety

In this section I will make my first direct link to personality from the theory expounded over the previous 11 chapters. I start with the trait component of elicitation of 4–12 Hz RSA/'theta') that has provided us with a perfect predictive rodent model of anxiolytic action. The control of RSA/'theta' involves multiple nuclei but these operate in concert maintaining synchrony and operating in a summative manner. RSA provides input to the GIS as a whole—affecting all the structures from the PAG up to the insula in a largely synchronous fashion over the whole GIS—and providing one common path for anxiolytic drug action on the GIS. I will use this to obtain a neural biomarker of trait GIS sensitivity.

The primary anchor for both the neural and psychological aspects of the theory of *state* anxiety has been triangulating the actions of specifically anxiolytic drugs and so eliminating side effects that vary across their radically different primary pharmacological and neural targets. To retain this meaning (following Recommendation 7), *trait* anxiety should map to the reactivity (sensitivity to normal functional input) of the same systems (e.g. receptor density, ligand synthesis). The low-anxious person should act, relative to the high, as if chronically treated with a 'consensus' anxiolytic (consensus anxiogenics are not yet obviously available). In this sense, trait anxiety will be highly conserved—with the relevant systems being present in fish (Mathuru and Jesuthasan, 2013; Soares et al., 2018; Costa de Melo et al., 2019; see special issue editorial by Lages and McNaughton, 2022).

A key point here is that fundamental functions will be subject to equally fundamental modulation. Taking 'fear' to mean the simple adaptive response to a repulsor, it will be important to set appropriate levels of 'fearfulness'—too much and you will remain in your burrow and starve, too little and you will leave too early and be eaten. But note that in this sense 'fearfulness' (i.e. repulsor sensitivity) relates to defensive distance, changes in which affect the whole GRS (see also Abend, 2023).

Both hormonal and neuromodulatory control will tend to expand as systems evolve (with enlarged structures splitting and migrating taking modulation with them). For this view of the GIS, one should focus on the now well-studied benzodiazepine receptor system (Fig. 4.3). This is highly conserved, includes key anxiolytic functions, and does not include more extended neurotic disorder functions. There are aspects (e.g. muscle relaxation) that are phylogenetically important but that are not included within the anxiolytic envelope as defined by $5HT1_A$ and calcium channel systems.

Given benzodiazepine control of the primordial PAG, expansion of the primitive motivational systems within it (attraction, repulsion, conflict) would have retained[11] benzodiazepine receptors and so benzodiazepine sensitivity in the relevant functional modules. Critically, here, I assume that the endogenous benzodiazepines (plural) are circulating hormone-like compounds, but have argued that the synaptic connections of the diffuse monoamine neuromodulatory systems will have evolved in a similar fashion (McNaughton, 2020).

12.8.2 From non-human to human

But how does one translate such a phylogenetic neurology into the normal parlance of those studying human personality? The genes for the anxiolytic-like micro-level control systems were retained by functional pressure *on the whole organism* (§12.1.2) to optimize the reactions of the GIS. Their functional effect, then, will be to alter levels of state anxiety (as I have defined it) and so they will represent trait anxiety (as this equates with sensitivity of the GIS). That is, the resultant trait GIS sensitivity will be of goal conflict sensitivity. By pharmacological definition, this is narrower than Neuroticism and I will discuss in Chapter 13 how these two factors could interact to produce anxiety disorder.

RECOMMENDATION 11: USE COMPLEX CONTRASTS FOR BIOMARKERS

As described in Chapter 11, I developed (§11.5.4) a biomarker—goal-conflict-specific rhythmicity (GCSR)—for GIS activation that fits my proposed GIS neurology (§11.5.5). Critically, this development started theoretically with goal conflict as a means of eliciting theta rhythmicity in humans; and then validated the result with the consensus set of anxiolytic drugs. Specificity to goal conflict was achieved by taking six trial types (stop-go × short | medium |

[11] Unless there was negative selection.

long delay) and applying a contrast (linear × quadratic) that reduced them to a single value (Shadli et al., 2015)—and so eliminated the effects of a range of potential confounding factors.

Importantly, this GCSR increased in power on average with increasing STAI-T scores—demonstrating a trait component (Shadli et al., 2021a). But it also had somewhat different average values for different DSM-defined 'anxiety disorders'; whereas, STAI-T values strongly separated DSM disorders from healthy but not from each other (see Fig. 13.1). So, trait GIS sensitivity as indexed by this *anxiolytic-validated* biomarker can be identified with a sensitivity to goal conflict and is involved for a *subset* of those patients conventionally diagnosed with neurotic disorders (or people with subclinical neurotic-related 'trait anxiety').

I argue that the use of such complex contrasts within carefully designed tasks is a key to imaging of RST-related constructs and, indeed, any constructs intended to be linked to a known background neurology (e.g. the use of the RPE contrast with the Feedback Related Negativity in §12.7.2).

Recommendation 11: For each theoretical construct of interest, where no biomarker is available from existing paradigms, create a biomarker by first designing a paradigm that will provide a pure measure by subtraction, via appropriate contrasts, of all other confounding constructs. Then challenge the resultant measure neurally or pharmacologically to ensure specificity.

12.8.3 From biomarker to scale challenge

These results represent proof-of-concept for measurement of a GIS personality trait based on goal-conflict sensitivity. Unfortunately, the existing form of the biomarker does not have the sensitivity or stability for work with individuals or repeat testing. But it is sufficient to answer interesting questions when larger numbers of participants are being tested at a single time point (§12.8.4) or cross-sectionally as diagnostic groups in the clinic (Chapter 13).

The development of a better biomarker is discussed later in the context of GAS and GRS measures, as is the potential to use these biomarkers to challenge scales (with scales being much easier to administer than the biomarkers themselves). I must also add two warnings as to how both the neurology and psychology of the GIS should be interpreted.

Warning 1: multiple correlated causes. In neurological terms, I have used a benzodiazepine-sensitive measure and in Fig. 4.3 benzodiazepines as an example. However, the consistent patterns that one can identify as changes in state GIS or as determined by trait GIS sensitivity (and mediated by RSA/'theta') are also produced, *through independent primary mechanisms*, via $5HT1_A$ receptors. Part of the behavioural pattern of the anxiolytics can also be produced via the dorsal ascending noradrenergic bundle system via somewhat different changes in RSA control. *Normally all these systems act in concert* to deliver 'conflict sensitivity' and if that is the adaptive function being selected by a current environment then they will all (given appropriate mutations) co-evolve in the direction of optimality. In addition to there being these multiple, linked, substrates for trait GIS sensitivity, there will in each case be a host of polygenes affecting the function of each substrate (via synthesis, receptors, uptake systems, degradation). This apparent complexity leads to a simple idea: *Trait GIS sensitivity can be viewed as polygenic, with multiple quite different types of change all converging on the same adaptive outcome across a population* *experiencing a particular selection pressure and interpretable in terms of the phenotypic target of that pressure (e.g. tameness, emotionality; see §12.9).*

Warning 2: A goal is not an action. In psychological terms, I have focused on goal conflict as a source of goal inhibition. However, this should not be equated with what many might call 'behavioural inhibition'. As discussed in §11.5.4 the inhibition of simple acts and actions (which are easier to equate with 'behaviour' than are goals) is *not* sensitive to anxiolytic drugs and so not controlled directly by the GIS. There may be some minor involvement of the GIS (as indexed by my biomarker) in disorders like ADHD (in the inattentive but not combined subtype; Sadeghi et al., 2018) but this does not explain their deficits in *action* stopping.

12.8.4 Does Carver & White (C&W) 'BIS' assess the GIS?

The selective relation of GCSR to DSM neurotic disorders (and its dissimilarity to the more general neurotic relation of STAI-T; Shadli et al., 2021a) suggests that any scale truly measuring GIS should have a higher correlation with GCSR than do either EPQ-N or STAI-T. One immediately obvious first use of my GCSR biomarker, then, is to use it to challenge C&W 'BIS'.

RECOMMENDATION 12: COMPARE SCALES VIA BIOMARKERS

Fig. 12.3 shows a very preliminary[12] comparison of correlations with GCSR for EPQ-N, STAI-T, and C&W BIS. At least in this small sample, C&W BIS is not more strongly related to GCSR than the other two scales and 'stepwise multiple regression detected a significant relation of GCSR only with neuroticism at 7 Hz in block 1 ($r = 0.264$, $F_{change} = 4.254$, $df = 1/57$, $P<0.05$)' (Shadli et al., 2015, p. 5). A forced enter multiple regression (not reported in the paper) showed that, in block 1, GCSR (averaged over all the frequencies) was uniquely positively correlated with neuroticism (4%), if anything uniquely *negatively* correlated with C&W BIS (0.1%), and with a small positive shared variance (1%). In block 3 the only correlation of the GCSR average was with neuroticism.

> *Recommendation 12: Compare related scales by challenge with available biomarkers for key theoretical constructs.*

12.8.5 What does Carver & White 'BIS' assess?

This, albeit preliminary, result made me directly inspect the C&W BIS scale items—and find that its similarity to EPQ-N and STAI-T is not surprising. The items of the C&W 'BIS' scale ***do not*** *relate to behavioural inhibition*, nor to punishment as a source of passive avoidance, nor to goal conflict. Instead, they focus on worry (40%), anticipatory fear (30%), and stress

[12] We are currently following this up with larger N and development of a stronger biomarker variant.

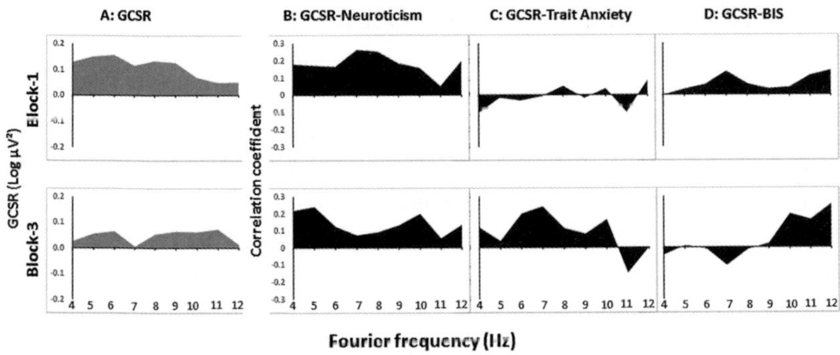

Fig. 12.3 (a) Variation in GCSR power with frequency at F8, averaged across all the participants. The value plotted was obtained by first subtracting power at the matching point in the preceding Go trial from power in the Stop trial and then taking this value for medium SSD trials and subtracting the average Stop—Go value for the short and long SSD trials. (b) Correlation between GCSR at F8 and neuroticism scores (EPQ-R). (c) Correlation between GCSR at F8 and trait anxiety scores. (d) Correlation between GCSR at F8 and BIS scores. BIS, behavioural inhibition system; GCSR, goal-conflict-specific rhythmicity; SSD, stop-signal delay. Figure and legend from Shadli et al. (2015) with permission.

(15%). These are essentially the same proportions as for the NEO-PI-R 'Anxiety' facet (as measured by the IPIP) and scores on the two measures correlate 0.90, i.e. 80% shared variance, while NEO-PI-R Anxiety and Penn State Worry correlate 0.98, i.e. 96% shared variance (Bainbridge et al., 2022, Table 3, p. 17). In an unpublished data set (N>300) I found that EPQ-N was a stronger predictor of C&W 'BIS' (12% unique, 25% shared with STAI-T, $p<0.001$) than was STAI-T (1% unique, $p = 0.019$). But note that the 37% overlap of C&W BIS with EPQ-N is well short of its 90% overlap with NEO-PI-R Anxiety. C&W 'BIS', NEO-PI-R Anxiety, and Penn State Worry may, then, all be largely assessing worry.

But what is 'worry'? It has been shown to cause general distress (McLaughlin et al., 2007) and may constitute a risk factor that works in parallel with Neuroticism to generate internalizing disorders in general (Griffith et al., 2010) rather than GIS-related anxiety in particular (see also §2.8). This would be consistent with the finding (Johnson et al., 2003) of univariate (but not multivariate) links between C&W 'BIS' and both 'anxiety disorders' (= GAD, panic disorder, social anxiety, and PTSD; $p<0.001$) *and* 'depressive disorders' (major depression, dysthymia; $p<0.01$). The bulk of these are insensitive to selective anxiolytic drugs.

That is, C&W 'BIS' appears related to the whole gamut of neurotic disorders. In this context the transdiagnostic character of worry and its comorbidity with obsession (Besharat et al., 2019) and rumination (Nolen-Hoeksema et al., 2008) could link to a more fundamental factor that controls working memory directly and emotion only indirectly (and, particularly when coupled with Neuroticism, to generate negative affect). On this view the difference between the processes would be that rumination would be about the past, obsession about the present, and worry about the future (see also §2.8). But, in all cases, without an additional source of goal conflict (e.g. blocking the compulsion linked to an obsession), no anxiety (anxiolytic-sensitive GIS activation) would be generated (see discussion of obsession in Chapter 13).

RECOMMENDATION 13: CHECK FOR REDUNDANCY AND CONTENT

For someone like me, entering the field from outside, redundance of scales with different names is a serious problem. It generates confusion and so difficulties for neuropsychological translation. I have argued that behavioural inhibition (as measured by the Carver and White, 1994 scale), Anxiety (as measured by the IPIP version of the NEO-PI-R, Bainbridge et al., 2022), and Worry (as measured by the Penn State Worry Questionnaire, Meyer et al., 1990) measure an essentially identical 'Worry'.

One solution to the problems created by this equivalence of the scales is the suggestion that the Big 5 can 'serve as an organizing framework for a sizable majority of stand-alone psychological trait scales . . . where reliable, valid scales are located within the Big Five . . . [so] construct proliferation may be abated' (Bainbridge et al., 2022, p. 1). But this raises a question. If the Big 5 is used as the framework and NEO-PI-R Anxiety is statistically >95% Penn State Worry, then should one rename the NEO-PI-R facet scale from 'Anxiety' to 'Worry'? Indeed, should 'Worry' be formally included as a Big 5 facet construct to create the required pigeon hole in which to house the three scales and others like them?

Given the costs of biomarker analysis, prior detection and flagging of such redundancy should be a major part of any attempt to link a scale to the neuropsychology of the theory, whether in part or in whole. Given that motivation-related variables in any system must depend on the same fundamental evolutionarily conserved neurology, I believe that the neural architecture and neuropsychology of the theory will be useful as a concrete anchor for all personality systems (including for any organizing framework of lexical origin, like the Big 5); and can provide an objective framework for any attempt to see functional parallels or identities/redundancies between scales or systems. That is, whether or not earlier statistical analysis has detected redundance, functionally similar scales will necessarily become attached to the same brain locus, system, or process as each other—unlike scales that do not share that function.

Recommendation 13: An important first step in neuropsychological mapping should be scale reduction to avoid redundant biomarker testing. This can be achieved without assumptions about content (e.g. by facet intercorrelation, see Bainbridge et al., 2022, Table 3, p. 17). Where redundance is detected assessing common content is likely to help identify the common construct being assessed.

12.9 Serotonin—Stability/Emotionality

Continuing with traits/metatraits linked to diffuse multi-system modulators, I will now look at serotonin. Low serotonin can be linked to emotionality, impulsiveness, aggression, and to the whole range of neurotic disorders (and so GRS and GIS) as well as appetitive problems such as anorexia nervosa (and so GAS). Mirroring this, high serotonin can be linked to the metatrait of Stability (DeYoung et al., 2002; DeYoung, 2010) but this may be a non-linear relationship appearing only with the highest Stability levels (Wright et al., 2019).

One simple way to describe serotonin's effects is as an increasing of motivational distance (both aversive/defensive and appetitive). This fits with, for example, the fact that it has opposite effects on anxiety/fear versus panic—enhancing higher-level integrated processing and suppressing lower-level reflexive output (Fig. 6.8). That is, it is not directly related to threat reactivity—but, for *both* aversive *and* appetitive stimuli, it alters the neural (and so cognitive) level at which behavioural output is controlled. In more cognitive terms, its effects can be seen as a shift (Carver et al., 2008) from the automatic System 1 to the effortful System 2 of Kahneman (2011), i.e. from the lowest level survival circuits (Chapter 6) to progressively higher order, particularly planning, circuits (Chapter 11). These ideas are discussed in detail in §6.10. Critically, here, I will link serotonin to rat emotional reactivity and distinguish that from threat sensitivity and so from Neuroticism.

12.9.1 The Maudsley model

Of interest in this context was the selection at the Maudsley Hospital of emotional reactive (MR) and non-reactive (MNR) strains—using only open field defecation as the selection criterion. The Maudsley strains were shown to differ on many behavioural and physiological parameters (for reviews see Broadhurst, 1960; Blizard, 1981; Gray, 1987a; Blizard et al., 2023). Importantly for the current section, the Maudsley strains differ in the concentration of serotonin in the limbic system (Maas, 1963; but did not differ in dorsal raphe activity, Verbanac et al., 1995); and selection also led to differences in gonadal and thyroid function, central noradrenaline (see also next), and in responses to a wide range of drugs.

Consistent with the change in serotonin, the MR and MNR lines differ in a broad range of emotional reactions. Relative to the MNR strain, the high-defecating and low-active MR animals explore less (take longer to emerge from a familiar to a novel environment in an emergence test, show less rearing behaviour), show higher heart rate, especially in response to stress, have lower food and water intake under threat, show a greater frustration effect to food omission in Amsel and Roussel's double-runway, greater conditioned suppression of bar pressing, greater passive avoidance, faster escape from shock and from immersion in water, and poorer shuttlebox avoidance (Broadhurst, 1975; Gray, 1987a).

In many cases, these differences parallel the effects of anxiolytic drugs (especially benzodiazepines) in unselected animals. Anxiolytics match the MR strain in: reduced emergence time, increased rearing in a high stress open field (McNaughton et al., 1984), decreased conditioned suppression and passive avoidance, and improved shuttlebox avoidance. But, importantly, the differences between the Maudsley strains also extend beyond the effects of anxiolytics and extends to effects of SSRI antidepressants: most notably defecation in the open field itself, open field activity, escape from shock, the double-runway frustration effect, and to an animal model of depression (Commissaris et al., 1996).

RECOMMENDATION 14: USE ANIMAL MODELS

The pattern of difference between the Maudsley strains suggests a general change in sensitivity to threatening stimuli, which would affect the functioning of *both* the GIS *and* the GRS (Gray, 1987a, pp. 266–268); i.e. both the SHS and the primary defence structures (see Chapter 6). Consistent with GIS changes, septal driving of RSA/'theta' in MNR rats resembles unselected rats treated with anxiolytic drugs (Drewett et al., 1977), as do their dorsal ascending noradrenergic bundle changes (Blizard and Liang, 1979; Sara et al., 1993; Verbanac et al., 1994). The involvement of the GRS is suggested by the strain differences in autonomic reactivity (defecation, heart rate), shock escape, and the double-runway frustration effect; thus, e.g. defecation is reduced by lesions of the PAG (Liebman et al., 1970) and the frustration effect by lesions of the amygdala (Henke, 1977), but neither of these is changed by SHS lesions (Appendix 8).

Recommendation 14: Use animal models to select for trait patterns that can then be experimentally analysed genetically and neurally in detail gaining insight into homologous human traits.

12.9.2 Selection for homology

There is a long early history of experimental tests of a Neuroticism/Emotional Reactivity trait in animals, and evidence of substantial heritability (Broadhurst, 1960; Gray, 1987a). Starting with Hall's (Hall, 1951) selective breeding studies in the rat in the 1930s, replicated by Broadhurst at the Institute of Psychiatry (Maudsley Hospital), London, in the 1960s (see Gray, 1987a). As noted earlier, selection was simple: for defecation (number of faecal boli) in an open field, under bright lights and white noise, high scorers being brother–sister mated with high scorers, and low with low, over successive generations to produce the two (MR, MNR) inbred lines.

Choice of defecation as a measure of fear (Broadhurst, 1960) *was based on human experience*, as formally documented in World War II, where the strain of battle resulted in involuntary excretion in >20% of the sample studied (Stouffer et al., 1949; for a table of the data, and citations to functionally similar emotional defecation in dogs, pigs, monkeys, and chickens, see McNaughton, 1989b, p. 155; Note that defecation is a measure of fear not anxiety since it is not affected by anxiolytic drugs.). As with the famous Silver Fox Experiment (where with selection for willingnes to approach the experimenter not only many behaviours became 'domesticated' but also physical appearance changed to more dog-like, Trut, 1999; Dugatkin, 2018), selection for *a single simple behavioural response to a specific challenge* resulted in quite widespread changes attributable to a high-level personality trait or metatrait.

The Maudsley strains of rats were maintained continuously (for over 35 years) after selection (Broadhurst, 1960) and were intensively studied. The size of the difference between the strain averages, as measured by *t*-test, was about $t = 6–7$ each generation at the time of the second edition. The strain difference in open field defecation is not a simple metabolic effect, since the difference in home cage defecation is the opposite (MNR defecating more; Broadhurst, 1960). Broadhurst ruled out effects of both post-natal (by cross-fostering) and pre-natal (by reciprocal cross) maternal environment as factors in the observed strain differences. He also reported a correlated response to selection for defecation on activity measures in the open field, MR being less active than MNR. This difference, too, was reliable across 35 years ($t = 7$). The persistence over the years of these strain differences was in spite of vicissitudes in the breeding programme; and remained also across sub-lines of the original Maudsley populations, based upon founders exported at various times from London (Blizard, 1981). Broadhurst (1960) derived estimates of the narrow heritability of open-field defecation and activity from a 6 × 6 diallel cross, including the MR and MNR strains; these were 46% and 68% respectively. These figures are, however, somewhat inflated since they refer to the heritability between litter means; inspection of Broadhurst's published results suggests true heritabilities nearer one-half these figures.

RECOMMENDATION 15: EXPECT PHENOTYPIC CONSISTENCE

The Broadhurst selection for open field defecation chose a human-homologous innate selection criterion. Interestingly, it appears that a very similar behavioural phenotype can be obtained with selection for avoidance learning. Each of these simple criteria affects inheritance of a number of additional forms of behaviour. This alternative behaviour includes in each case the alternative selection criterion. Broadhurst selected for defecation and got changes in shuttlebox avoidance. Selection for performance in the shuttlebox avoidance task (Bignami, 1965; Brush et al., 1985) led to correlated changes in open field defecation and locomotor activity that mirror the Maudsley rat strains. In both selection programmes, poor shuttlebox performance is associated with high defecation and low activity. These data reinforce the impression of a unified system, manifest in a variety of tests of emotional behaviour, some (e.g. shuttlebox avoidance) sensitive to anxiolytic drugs and some (open field defecation) not. This encourages us to believe that individual biomarkers can track systems where the nature of the system can be understood in terms of adaptive function (§12.1.2). (See Cruz et al., 2023, for an equivalent generalized anxiety model.)

Recommendation 15: A simple selection criterion produces consistent patterns of widespread changes; expect the result to be similar when selecting for other elements of this consistent pattern.

12.9.3 The Maudsley perspective on serotonin: Neuroticism versus Emotional Reactivity

I have several reasons for suggesting that the Emotional Reactivity selected for here is not a homologue of human Neuroticism. First is the link to serotonin. In Chapter 13 I will argue that changes in serotonin produce changes in Stability that are distinct from (slower and weaker than) changes in threat reactivity. Second is an interesting study of the nature of the MR-MNR difference.

> 'Broadhurst (1957) carried out an experiment to test the Yerkes-Dodson Law . . . that optimum motivation for performance of a response decreases with increasing task difficulty . . . in an underwater [Y] maze . . . detaining the animals underwater for different lengths of time before they could start swimming. . . . Task difficulty was manipulated by adjusting the brightness of the dimmer arm to make it more or less like the correct arm.
>
> The critical results are presented diagrammatically in [Fig. 12.4]. If the genetic difference between the MR and MNR groups was simply one of the extent to which any fear-inducing condition actually produced fear, then all that should be needed to make an MNR rat like an MR rat is to increase its motivation [Fig. 12.4A]. In fact, the data show that an increase

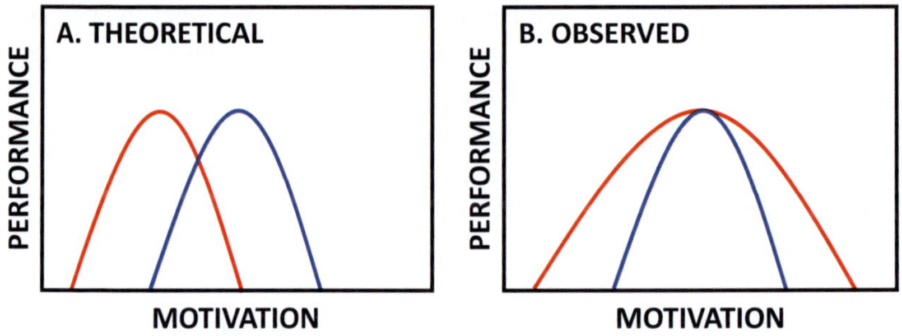

Fig. 12.4 Diagrammatic representation of the conclusions to be drawn from Broadhurst's analysis of the effects on performance of increasing levels of motivation in MR and MNR rats. The original theoretical position was that MR and MNR differ in terms of fearfulness. **A.** The THEORETICAL graph shows one inverted U, Yerkes-Dodson, function for the relation between PERFORMANCE and MOTIVATION (... minutes of imposed air deprivation ...) for the MR and MNR animals. The curves are identical except that the curve for the MNR (blue) is shifted to the right because of the lower level of fear ... engendered by any specific amount of air deprivation. **B.** The OBSERVED curve represents, diagrammatically, the conclusion of the experiment: that rather than differing terms of fearfulness the MR rats have an equivalent peak of the performance-motivation curve and show better performance and both higher and lower levels of motivation. Figure and legend adapted from (McNaughton, 1989b) with permission.

> in emotionality is not entirely equivalent to an increase in fear [but more like an increase of dynamic range]'
>
> McNaughton (1989b, pp.156–157; our figure number)

It remains to be seen precisely where the Maudsley rats fit into the neuropsychology. However, these results, and the neural analysis described in 12.9.1, clearly distinguish their trait (and so serotonergic input to the GAS, GRS, and GIS) from simple threat sensitivity (i.e. Neuroticism) and bring it close to the more general control of motivational distance that shifts behaviour from control by System 1 to System 2 (Kahneman, 2011).

12.10 Reinfor<u>cer</u> Sensitivity Theory (RST5)—system level

I now turn to the traits with which one needs to be concerned in relation to the operation of the GAS, GRS, and GIS, themselves. As noted already I think it is important to avoid the words 'reward' and 'punishment' here and replace them (as in Chapter 3 and §12.7) with GAIN/LOSS and attractor/repulsor. An important complication is that normally one sees a GAIN as automatically generating an attractor (hence the desire to use the word 'reward'). But a single class of motivational stimulus can create opposite goals depending on the contingencies. This led us (see Fig. 3.1) to an RST5 that has five major (likely aspect level) traits as well as a range of more specific (likely facet level) traits (e.g. obsessiveness, panic proneness). (This excludes RST2, §12.7.2, where there are positive and negative reinforce**<u>ment</u>** sensitivities that involve more general systems.) Note that existing scales are likely to already cover key elements here (e.g. gain *versus* loss would be assessed by any existing measure of loss aversion) and may not need alteration (e.g. a suitably designed approach/attractor, avoidance/repulsor scale that is not contaminated by gain/loss).

While tedious, the separation of gain/loss from attraction/repulsion is fairly straight forward. Hall et al. (2011, p. 243, 246; emphasis added)

> administered a task in which human participants received all four of the [valence × contingency] conditions illustrated in Fig. [3.1].
>
> In one phase of the experiment, participants started with zero dollars and gain was pitted against loss: clicking on a target resulted in a 50:50 chance of gaining money or losing money. Nonresponding resulted in no gain or loss. People responded more on trials with net gain than those with net loss and so the final amount earned was always positive. *The gain and loss values were fixed and known within a block of trials. [So, no reinforcement was involved.]* Across blocks, gain and loss values were changed. Gain and loss each had the same set of possible values and all possible combinations of these gain and loss values were tested in combination. The response to be made was modelled on rat runway experiments and involved moving the mouse cursor a fixed distance to a target and clicking on the target. The overall speed of responding was measured. Speed was used as a measure rather than simple choice as it gives a numerical measure of motivation on each trial and is the measure usually used in the animal experiments on which RST is based.
>
> In a second phase, all details were the same except that participants started with a set number of dollars and each click prevented the loss of money but with a 50:50 risk of preventing the gain of money. That is, they received the [⊘] consequences of Fig. [3.1]. (Note that from a 'rational economic' perspective, there is no difference between this second set of phases and the first. A gain of $1 and prevention of loss of $1 have identical consequences on take-home amount. The click response differs only in whether it is against a background of starting the experiment with nothing or with something.)
>
> Across these conditions, we then analysed sensitivity to dollar consequences either: (1) with respect to approach and avoidance (averaging across gain and loss); or (2) with respect to the difference between gain and loss (averaging across approach and avoidance). . . .
>
> The main findings of the present experiment are: (1) approach and avoidance tendencies have different strengths for a range of given external dollar values when averaged across gain and loss omission or loss and gain omission, respectively; and, (2) at least with higher values, the loss aversion typically reported in the literature is obtained when averaging across approach and avoidance tendencies. . . .
>
> We can, therefore, take the fact that approach was greater than avoidance as being inconsistent with the control of avoidance being identical to the control of loss (given our demonstration of loss aversion); and, of course, any effect of loss *per se* was averaged out before fitting the approach-avoidance curves.

With this method, while gain/loss can be separated from attraction/repulsion each of these is represented as a ratio and so for gain and loss, or attraction and repulsion, to be separated, additional conditions would be required to allow the simultaneous equations involved to be solved completely. This may not be necessary if selective imaging methods are used to assess the systems.

RECOMMENDATION 16: SEPARATE REINFORCEMENT, VALUATION, AND MOTIVATION

The most important conclusion here is that positive reinforcement sensitivity, gain sensitivity, and attraction sensitivity are independent and separable at the neural level—scales like the C&W BAS are likely to conflate them; especially where the neural measures have common variance in the population. The same is true for negative reinforcement sensitivity, loss sensitivity (loss aversion when relative to gain sensitivity), and repulsion sensitivity.

> *Recommendation 16: Ensure both in scale assessment and construction that reinforcement (learning), valuation, and motivation are kept distinct as far as possible. With valuation and motivation, separation can be achieved by including an omission contingency, and applying appropriate contrasts.*

12.11 Reinforcer Sensitivity Theory (RST5)—structure level

Simpler to deal with, and largely unchanged over time, the neuropsychology implies not only system-level sensitivities that will map to broader traits but also structure-level sensitivities that will map to more specific traits lower in the trait hierarchy. I will deal with these more specifically in Chapter 13 but, here, note some general issues in translating the neurology into trait space.

First is the necessity of trait overlap. This follows the hierarchical model of Fig. 12.1 where a metatrait will share variance with a trait or facet. Serotonin provides input to both the anterior cingulate cortex and the PAG. Changes in it will, therefore, alter both obsessionality and panic proneness. Such changes will necessarily be correlated. However, obsessionality will also be changed by local changes in the serotonin re-uptake system (which is clomipramine- but not imipramine-sensitive; §4.3.4) of a type not shared with the PAG (where re-uptake is sensitive to both drugs); while panic proneness will be selectively changed via the CCK system (Wang et al., 1998), which, throughout the PAG, appears to selectively control flight as opposed to freezing (La-Vu et al., 2022) and, in the dorsal pre-mammillary nucleus, versatile flight (Wang et al., 2021). Because of this, GAD and panic share only about half of their genetic control, each having a distinct other half (Scherrer et al., 2000). One would thus expect 'trait panic' (as I would define it) to be obliquely rotated with respect to Stability or to Trait GRS and neither perfectly nor zero correlated with either.

Second is the polygenetics of phenotypic selection (with epigenetics also playing a role in non-human personality, van Oers et al., 2023). Part of this is good news: the phenotype (which carries the genes) is selected in relation to achievement of an adaptive function (goal-conflict resolution) not of a particular chemical (benzodiazepine). I expect the resultant trait, therefore, to make sense at the level of emergent properties (McNaughton, 2020; §12.1.2). But part of this represents causal overlap. Even if the $GABA_A$ receptor were the only means of controlling anxiety systems, it has a large number of distinct sites for a range of ligands—including an atypical benzodiazepine site through which ethanol achieves its anxiolytic effect on RSA/'theta' (Coop et al., 1990). Likewise, I already noted that the Maudsley rats differ in both their serotonin and noradrenaline systems (with these, and the dopamine system, being involved in parallel in the response to stress). One cannot, then, make a simple identification of a trait with a neuromodulator but, as you will see with my comparison of Neuroticism and Stability in Chapter 13, careful mapping to neuromodulators can be helpful in refining the concepts of traits and of their relationships with each other.

Finally, and fairly obviously, 'RST' = RST2 + RST5 (reinforc**ement** + reinfor**cer**) may have expanded conceptually since its birth but this has largely been a matter of dissection and fractionation of the cognitive concepts that were blurred and confounded in the original trait exposition (McNaughton and Corr, 2019b). I have presented in Fig. 3.1 a more detailed and nuanced view of, for example, why a male rat decides to press a lever to obtain a chocolate button or a receptive female rat presses a lever to obtain a male rat; Bermant, 1961a; Bermant, 1961b) or why a human undertakes any homologous goal-oriented activity. But what I have presented in relation to anxiety is just one strand of Reinfor**cer**-related Sensitivity Theory, and will only occupy a moderate space within Fig. 12.1 as a facet of Neuroticism, with a minor contribution from Introversion; and will be distinct from the NEO-PI-R Anxiety facet (i.e. Worry).

12.12 RST personality questionnaires

12.12.1 The mapping problem

The half-century since Gray (1970a) has seen a large mass of work developing, analysing, and querying personality questionnaires nominally based on his (binary, RST2) constructs. The early work was bedevilled by his derivation of a 2-factor trait theory from what, even then, was a 3-factor state theory—by nominally (but not actually) focusing on conditioned, and rejecting unconditioned, responses while confounding reinforc**ement** with reinfor**cers**. But, worse, there were serious ambiguities and, in retrospect, objective confusions in the expression of the 2-factor trait theory (McNaughton and Corr, 2019b).

On top of this are problems with item content (Recommendations 2 & 3).

> Gray's own Gray–Wilson Personality Questionnaire was largely [rationally] derived but ... was designed to assess human reactions to the equivalent of six key animal behaviour paradigms: approach, active avoidance, passive avoidance, extinction, fight and flight (Wilson et al., 1989; Wilson et al., 1990). Questions ... were not linked to simple behaviours and included 'Are you inclined to curse audibly when things go wrong?'; 'Do you visit the doctor for regular check-ups?'; 'If a fight broke out in a bar where you were drinking, would you leave as fast as possible?'. However, rather than coalescing into his three key theoretical systems (which at that time were activation/approach + active avoidance, inhibition/passive avoidance + extinction and fight/flight = fight + flight) analysis extracted six factors and the conclusion that 'the sources of individual variation that emerge as salient in human society may draw upon complex mixtures of biological systems' (Wilson et al., 1990, p. 1041).
>
> (McNaughton, 2020, p. 6)

Likewise, I have already implied that from a theoretical point of view, the misnamed original C&W BIS/BAS questionnaires (Carver and White, 1994) do not relate to the RST3 (revised) goal control systems or to gain/loss; nor in any simply way to the RST2 (original) reinforc**ement** constructs. In terms of links to dopamine, C&W BAS could also reflect MMPI impulsivity (Table 12.2)—but I will leave to others the deconstruction of the BAS subscales (see Smillie et al., 2006). Nor have I asked how far the C&W BIS scale (or its potentially separable parts, Corr and McNaughton, 2008; Heym et al., 2008; Espinoza Oyarce et al., 2021; Beck et al., 2009; Poythress et al., 2008; Chen et al., 2023) relates to negative reinforcement, versus repulsion, versus conflict—although I believe the evidence points to it being more a measure of worry than any of these (§12.8.4). Indeed, the equation of C&W BIS with NEO-PI-R Anxiety (as a 'worry' facet of neuroticism) goes far towards explaining its value and so persistent use while destroying its supposed conceptual foundations.

A similar approach to elements of the Big 5 should clarify their nature (with careful lower-level renaming, e.g. 'worry', being important). For example,

> Integrative, structural analyses have demonstrated that measures of extraversion and BAS tap a single latent factor. [They share] three factors associated with approach—assertiveness, enthusiasm, and sensation seeking—[that] map onto the manifestations of BAS proposed by Carver and White (1994)—namely, Drive, Reward Responsiveness, and Fun Seeking—and onto the three conceptualizations of Extraversion described by Depue and Collins (1999)—agency, affiliation, and impulsivity.
>
> (Quilty et al., 2014, p. 87, 92)

Faced with this situation, the temptation is to wipe the slate and start with fresh scales. But, with RST, this has not so far resulted in a unique solution but rather a creation of a new set of similar problems (§12.12.3). Further, many existing scales (notably MMPI) have been designed for quite different purposes with no intention to have neural anchors. These new RST systems and older non-RST systems are unlikely to be given up by their current users. I believe the way to go, under these circumstances, is to use appropriate biomarkers to categorize and assess the existing scales and so determine their degree of linkage to the neuropsychology. Again, we should treat neuropsychology as bedrock; determine the neural ingredients of the scales; and rename or reconstruct the scales where appropriate.

RECOMMENDATION 17: NEURALLY MAP EXISTING SCALES

I next discuss the issues relating to using biomarkers instead of scales and to generating new scales. My immediate advice is to first challenge existing apparently relevant scales with the neural tools available before increasing the number of scales needing such analysis. Indeed, as with the purely linguistic Recommendation 13, the goal should be to reduce the number of redundant scales by identifying that, when mapped neurally, A = B = C (or, for some scales, A = B + C). This neural bedrock should provide a basis for choosing scales to match proposed usage even when there is considerable overlap (an intended design feature with the MMPI system).

> *Recommendation 17: Before creating new scales, one should check if a biomarker can be used directly instead; and, if not, then neurally map existing scales in whole or as dissected parts—potentially linking several scales to a single neural entity and so showing their redundancy if this has not already been detected statistically (Recommendation 13).*

12.12.2 Revised RST scales (RST3)

A number of newer questionnaires have been built with the nominal intent to match the neuropsychology of the second edition (essentially RST-3, ignoring the gain/loss versus positive/negative reinforcement confound resolved by RST-5). While these have been 'rationally' derived, item content often has no clear theoretical basis. Also, to my knowledge, they have not usually been assessed *during construction* via neural or behavioural measures (c.f., §12.8; but see §12.15). Indeed, there appears to be no consensus neural theory among them. This may be why new scales are generated more than old scales analysed (§12.13). The bulk of these have been trait 'sensitivity' scales but an attempt has also been made to produce a state 'activation' set of BAS, BIS and FFFS scales (Franchina et al., 2023, NB: correlations with the matching trait RST-PQ measures were surprising).

However, all scales whether stand-alone or within a system, can be neurally assessed, deconstructed, invalidated, or integrated *post-hoc*; and that is what I believe should be done (see also discussion in Leue et al., 2022). One surely does not need yet more RST scales for the same few primary neural entities especially if existing scales are largely redundant across the different systems at least at the facet level. What is needed is a determination of which scales have clear constructs (e.g. reward prediction error) that map to the neuropsychology (e.g. dopamine release). Where no scale exists to capture a key construct then one can consider building a new one.

Such assessment is important, not only from a theoretical point of view but from the practical perspective. Unless they can be perfectly mapped to each other without neural anchors (due to sheer linguistic redundance as with worry), a choice must ultimately be made between the existing scales. Otherwise, you are asking how many angels can fit on the head of the needle (while concurrently trying to remember that the eye of *that* needle is not a gate into Jerusalem). The problem is that the newer RST scales are not fully consistent with each other (nor, of course, with the Big 5).

Krupić et al. (2016, p. 19; emphasis added) itemized

> six purpose-built Reinforcement Sensitivity Theory (RST) personality questionnaires currently in use to measure the fight flight-freeze system (FFFS), the behavioural inhibition system (BIS), and the behavioural approach system (BAS). *They differ in their conceptualizations and operational constructs*, and this poses a problem for their differential validity and the generalizability of results, and comparison of results from different studies. . . . The psychometric properties of five of these RST questionnaires . . . (the Croatian translations of [the C&W] BIS/BAS scales, SPSRQ, Jackson-5, RSQ and RST-PQ) . . . were analysed by correlational and confirmatory factor analyses. [The rRST-Q] postdates the collection of data reported. We found some of these questionnaires achieved marginal to adequate fit indices, and they showed ambiguity in terms of convergent validity for all three general behavioural systems. These findings highlight the difficulties with generalization and comparison of results with the use of different RST questionnaires.

Nominal intended structure also varies. For example, the 'Jackson 5' (Jackson, 2009) and RSQ (Smederevac et al., 2014; see Smederevac et al., 2022 for genetic analysis) each contain one 'BAS' scale, one 'BIS' scale, and *three* 'FFFS' scales (essentially one for each of fight, flight, and freezing) with no biological checks. Meanwhile, the RST-PQ (Corr and Cooper,

2016) contains one 'FFFS' scale (with Flight, Freeze, and Active Avoidance subscales; with fight relegated to a *separate* supplementary defensive fight scale), one 'BIS' scale, and *four* 'BAS' scales (Reward Interest, Goal-Drive Persistence, Reward Reactivity, and Impulsivity) that are statistically relatively independent (Corr, personal communication, 15 January 2023); and, again, no biological checks. The Hierarchical Reinforcement Sensitivity Theory of Personality Questionnaire (HRST-PQ) has two BAS subscales, two FFS (Fight excluded) subscales and one BIS scale.

Assessment of construct validity of such systems delivers numerous 'good model fit' solutions with 2 or 4 factors—and can include models with 4 'BIS', 4 'BAS', and no 'FFFS' factors (Leue et al., 2022). They all may be satisfactory in terms of factor analysis, as opposed to neural validity, with

> good to very good psychometric properties and moderate to excellent internal consistencies. . . . with a very good model fit for the first-order, four factor models of the Carver-White BIS/BAS scales, Reinforcement Sensitivity Theory—Personality Questionnaire (RST-PQ), the two-factor model of revised Reinforcement Sensitivity Theory-Questionnaire (rRST-Q) and for the bifactor model of the Conflict Monitoring Questionnaire (CMQ-44) are promising personality questionnaires for the (r)RST trait space with sufficient psychometric properties.
>
> (Leue et al., 2022, p.1, p. 13)

Given this plethora of functional ambiguity, I will use the rRST-Q (Reuter et al., 2015) as a paradigm case to map to the theory since (unlike the others) it has a single scale for each of 'BIS', 'BAS', and 'FFFS'(see Franchina et al., 2023, for a three-factor set of 'state' scales; but see Leue et al., 2022, for a global 2D factor structure); its presentation included comparison with the Carver and White scales; and its 'FFFS' amalgamated only partially distinct fight, flight, and freeze subscales. Both in the original report (Reuter et al., 2015) and a recent validation (Espinoza Oyarce et al., 2023) a 3-factor model produces a good fit but a 5-factor model (BAS, BIS, Fight, Flight, Freeze) gives a better fit. I will next discuss the fact that the rRST-Q 'FFFS' (like the RST-PQ and HRST-PQ) explicitly excluded defensive fight (in my terms, !FIGHT) and the fact that 'fight', with varying meanings, is a major source of variation among the RST scales. I will also comment on their biological challenge of their BIS versus FFFS scales.

12.12.3 Why so many?

RST development has involved a succession of new *questionnaire* systems for the same nominal fundamental *neural* constructs. Each system is implicitly justified by rejection of all the preceding rationally derived systems; while the C&W scales continue to be used and analysed for their structure (Chen et al., 2023). But there has usually been no validation (or questioning of the older systems) via the underlying biology. Each constructor chooses a system that fits with their rational understanding—of their interpretation—of the neuropsychology; and similarly with respect to dialect variations when translating from one language to another. Of course, the plethora of other 'personality' systems from Big 5 through MMPI suffer from the same problem. They all lack neural anchoring bedrock and differ philosophically and philologically as well as in terms of scientific target.

With my paradigm case, Reuter et al. (2015), their original scale development was in German (N = 1,814; with 1,090 also completing the German version of the C&W BIS/BAS). So, they published it together with a tested (N = 299) English translation. As noted earlier, it is distinctive for having one scale to map to each of 'BAS'/GAS, 'BIS'/GIS, 'FFFS'/GRS and including a biological challenge distinguishing 'BIS'/GIS from 'FFFS'/GRS (essentially excluding !FFFS). You would have thought this would gain ready acceptance. However, recently, Espinoza Oyarce et al. (2023, p. 6; emphasis added) complained that

> It has been over 20 years since the revision of the RST, yet contemporary research is still being conducted with the [C&W] BIS/BAS scales despite their limitations in reflecting current neurobiological and theoretical knowledge. . . . *A new measure, the rRSTQ, has shown better construct validity for the FFFS compared to early measures, but limited supporting psychometric data have slowed its adoption favoring the continued use of the [C&W] BIS/BAS scales despite their limitations.*
>
> In the present study, we provide, to our knowledge for the first time, a validation of [the English version of] Reuter and Montag's rRST-Q, a questionnaire designed to assess sensitivities to approach and avoidance behaviors formalized in the revised RST and demonstrate that the constructs estimated are sex invariant. Based on our assessment, we conclude that the rRST-Q is an effective and reliable measure of the revised RST, but future studies are still required for further validation in other populations.

Espinoza Oyarce et al. (2023) compared (N>1,200) the rRST-Q with the C&W BIS/BAS and the EPQ, plus the clinically oriented Goldberg Anxiety and Depression Scales (GADS). (I like the way they think!) The rBAS, rBIS, and rFFFS scales showed sex, age, and longitudinal invariance. The correlation map for the various scales/subscales is shown in Fig. 12.5. Obviously with correlations one cannot tell cause from effect. But I suspect many of the correlations with EPQ-N are due to its measuring a general risk factor (note that N was measured many years earlier, see also Andrews et al., 1990). rBIS and rBAS relate to C&W BIS and C&W BAS, respectively, at ~25% of the variance (matching the estimates of Reuter et al., 2015). But this is no different from their relation to Neuroticism and close to its relation (~15%) to Goldberg anxiety *and* depression. Note that their Fear construct (derived from and representing about 30% of C&W BIS) is similarly related (~15%) to rBIS, rFFFS, and EPQ-N. rBIS has a, theoretically incompatible,[13] somewhat higher correlation with Goldberg Depression (14.5%) than Anxiety (11%) but both are somewhat weaker than for Neuroticism (see also §12.8.4); with FFFS weaker still (7%, 5%). For comparison, the EPQ-N and the general measure of neurotic disorder STAI-T share >50% variance (e.g. Torrubia et al., 2001).

Key questions that arise from this are: 1) what neural anchors are available for the constructs; 2) how can these be used to validate or at least challenge scales; and 3) can one use such anchors to derive scales. Embedded, here, is the issue that the neurally separate system sensitivities are instantiated by outputs that: 1) involve state-level interactions between the specific systems (attraction subtracts from repulsion and vice versa, expression of conflict depends on *where in the trait space* attraction and repulsion are balanced); 2) confound interactions with, e.g. neuroticism; 3) can be similarly influenced, at the population level, by

[13] But expected if, like C&W BIS, it is just a Worry scale.

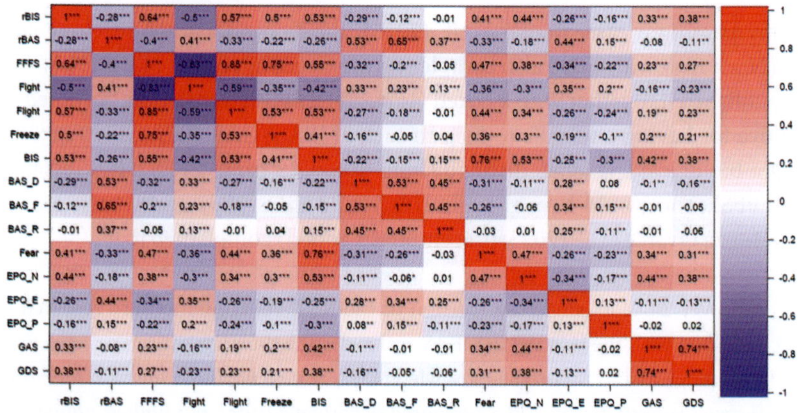

Fig. 12.5 Correlation heat-map of rRST-Q, C&W BIS/BAS, EPQ-R, and GADS scales. Far right bar shows the value of correlation. BAS = behavioral approach/activation system; BIS = behavioral inhibition system; BAS-D = drive; BAS-F = fun-seeking; BAS-R = reward responsiveness; EPQ = Eysenck personality questionnaire; EPQ-E = extraversion; EPQ-N = neuroticism; EPQ-P = psychoticism; Fear = fight—flight–freeze system fear construct; FFFS = fight—flight–freeze system; GAS = Goldberg anxiety; GDS = Goldberg depression; rBAS = revised BAS; rBIS = revised BIS. *p ≤ .05. **p ≤ .01. ***p ≤ .001. Figure and legend adapted from Espinoza Oyarce, D. A., Burns, R. A., Butterworth, P., & Cherbuin, N. (Espinoza Oyarce et al., 2023). A new measure of the Revised Reinforcement Sensitivity Theory. Social Psychology, 53(6), 327-340. https://doi.org/10.1027/1864-9335/a000502. This work is licensed under CC BY 4.0. To view a copy of this license, visit http://creativecommons.org/licenses/by/4.0/

developmental or more recent events linked to trauma. All of these factors will lead to intercorrelation of relevant scales based on observable behaviour.

But first, some linguistic issues.

12.13 Trait translation problems—!FIGHT !FLIGHT !FREEZE

Before considering scale anchors/dissectors as such, I need to highlight a number of translation issues that can, and have, impacted on rational construction. These also have clear implications for choice of anchor for a scale.

I have already discussed the need to:

1) distinguish reinforc**ement** from reinfor**cer**;
2) separate GAIN/LOSS | positive/negative reinforcement | attraction/repulsion;
3) Use 'reward' and 'punishment' only for reinforcement within the confines of reward prediction error and punishment prediction error. (NB: RPE is a signal that gain presentation or loss omission *has* occurred when loss or gain omission was expected—it has positive valence.)

Note that all of these issues arise from neuropsychological considerations and the resultant attempt to provide everyday rational translation. Words are dangerous things (§1.4) and

I would follow Darwin in seeing non-human work as useful because it avoids the danger of substituting a verbal for a behavioural response and then treating the perceived lexical content of the verbal response as more veridical than behaviour itself.

It is quite easy to 'phrase questions' with behavioural answers (via homologous experimental paradigms) similarly for humans and non-humans. Unfortunately, for many people, 'of course' humans *must* (for political not scientific reasons) be different (McNaughton and Corr, 2008). In contrast, I urge you to be scientific and behaviour-oriented not anthropocentric and language-oriented. For fundamental motivational systems, the questionnaire approach should be seen as an economical variant of behaviour analysis (Chapters 2 and 3) with no special scientific status accorded to language itself.

With these as reminders, I will now focus on an important use-of-language problem that arises with the old system label 'FFFS', my translation of it to GRS (with !FFFS embedded), and the meaning common to both old and new system labels—but more restrictive than common usage—of the word 'fight' in particular.

Reuter et al. (2015, p. 5, emphasis added), working with rRST, explicitly say they, in my view correctly, excluded 'fight' during their scale construction because

> in the revised RST *fight behavior is only observable if the distance between predator and prey is close to zero*, leaving no option for flight or freezing. The probability of such situations occurring for human beings is extremely low . . . We would characterize a high trait FFFS individual as high in flight and freezing behavior, but a low scorer on fight behavior. A person who is not willing to fight when being attacked might typically withdraw more quickly from unpleasant situations, compared to a person who is more willing to fight when threatened.

But note that having supposedly excluded !FIGHT they then include 'fight' as an *inverse* factor in what I would call GRS. They also miss the point that (at predator-ground-zero) fight, flight, and freeze are all available but fight only occurs if the others are blocked by the situation. All three are forms of extreme panic (see Chapter 13 for nuances and the possibility of mild panic). Their 'might typically withdraw' involves a non-reflexive choice and so is not flight but rather is escape or avoidance. These occur at non-zero defensive distance and are under non-reflexive directional control; whereas true !FLIGHT is undirected and totally reflexive.

In Table 1.1 and Fig. 11.15 I take this issue into account by flagging (!) the object-specific (immediate ground-zero predator) behaviours as !FIGHT, !FLIGHT and !FREEZE to indicate their urgency. Critically, in *all three* cases the responses are basically automatic and unlike the more flexible behaviours shown at larger defensive distance. As emphasized in the quote, !FIGHT (explosive, screaming, face-directed, bared-teeth) is only elicited when !FREEZE is not an option; and !FREEZE occurs to a ground-zero (as opposed to distant) predator only if !FLIGHT is not available (Fig. 2.2A). These are *all* situation-dependent expressions of *panic* during which, if you were the rat, you would think you were going to die. (The *choice* to escape rather than fight is a quite different thing—panic negates the time required for true choice.) They also involve distinct postures that only appear at high threat levels or with stimulation of the hypothalamus or PAG (§1.6).

The meaning of !FIGHT is worth considering in detail here. The English word 'fight' can be applied to many behaviour patterns that are quite distinct in both their form and their biological function.

!FIGHT in a rat involves an explosive, screaming, leap directed towards the face (and so, paradoxically, teeth) of the predator (see image in Fig. 2.2A). Its sole adaptive function[14] is to make !FLIGHT available (usually behind the blocking predator, which ducks to avoid the explosive attack); other defensive functions would be reflected in different patterns of aggression or other behaviour. !FIGHT is usually *inter*-species when prey of one species (rat/mouse) defensively attacks a predator of another species (cat/rat).

There is likely an intra-species form of !FIGHT, 'reactive aggression [that] refers to aggressive behaviour in response to real or perceived threat, provocation or frustration, and is typically impulsive, immediate, and directed toward the perceived perpetrator' and has also been linked to !FIGHT, !FLIGHT, and !FREEZE but may involve amygdala control as well as hypothalamus and periaqueductal grey (Lickley and Sebastian, 2018, p. 313). This intra-species form is also shown by rats; who will attack a conspecific after receiving a shock to the feet delivered by an experimenter.

'Fight' in the sense of *intra*-species defence, in contrast, is usually defence against social aggression. In rats and humans, it involves boxing and other attempts to protect the back—with no baring of the teeth and, clearly, no expectation of immediate death.[15]

'Fight' in the sense of *social* aggression in rats is undertaken in pursuit or maintenance of social dominance and involves attacks from the side aiming at the opponent's back. Social aggression and *instrumental* aggression in humans appear to be variants of this.

Finally, 'fight' in the sense of intra-species *predatory* aggression (where the rat's purpose is to eat the mouse) can involve quiet stalking. When an attack is launched, bites are aimed at the back of the neck (a common predator target across many phyla).

There are then at least four different meanings of 'fight' that apply to all sexes and ages,[14] each with its own adaptive equation, typical behaviour pattern, and (in rats with homologous variations in humans) specific target of attack behaviour (face, front, side/back, neck).

Here I would depart slightly from the reasoning, but not choice, of Reuter et al. (2015). Their apparent concern is that !FIGHT is low probability and so (implicitly) that it will be hard to sample. But they then say 'a low scorer on fight behavior . . . might typically withdraw more quickly from unpleasant situations'. This involves a contradiction since fight (in the sense of !FIGHT) and withdraw are mutually incompatible. But I see !FIGHT and 'fight' as distinct for a quite different reason. !FFFS fundamentally involves panic and the periaqueductal grey. Importantly, therefore, this is a part of the GRS where there is an additional CCK control of trait input (particularly flight, §12.11). Whatever its low sampling probability in questionnaire items, a more important reason for excluding !FFFS items from GRS questionnaires is that their trait control involves an additional independent factor—and !FFFS is better treated as a distinct facet of GRS.

Failure to take this massive ambiguity into account means that 'fight' is used variously across the RST3 questionnaire systems. This issue has been to some extent pre-empted recently by the exclusion of !FIGHT from the main systems of both rRST-Q and RST-PQ (for further comment on the RST-PQ/HRST-PQ) and fight, see §12.15.5). But it flags the need for a PANIC subscale (potentially with !FIGHT, !FLIGHT, !FREEZE sub-subscale questionnaires but likely better with probes that target the panic state itself, not the stimuli that

14 Leaving maternal aggression as a special case. Note second use of this same footnote later.

15 Yes, I DO mean from a rat's point of view. I don't think anyone verbalizes their thoughts and feelings during a panic attack (I certainly don't) and I think a rat's experience is homologous.

determine the different immediate behaviours that can be elicited by the state). It also raises the question of what is meant by 'freeze' or 'flight' if these have been retained (escape and avoidance are not !FLIGHT); and whether !FREEZE was distinguished from defensive quiescence. (In the rat, they involve distinct postures as well as functional circumstances. Note that lordosis is also freeze-like. See Table 1.1).

In the RST-PQ, there is a separate 'fight' questionnaire (Corr and Cooper, 2016, their Appendix D). Inspection of the items shows that this is clearly linked to *intra*-species *non-acute* defensive aggression as opposed to *inter*-species *acute* defensive aggression (or social acquisitive, or predatory aggression). All the items are related to an open-ended reaction, where 'flight' (or directed escape) is a viable alternative and, as a result, 'fight' and 'freeze' are not required as sole alternatives to 'fight'. In my view, it would best be relabelled 'Intraspecies fight', or it should at least be distinguished in some way from a !FIGHT (acute explosive defensive aggression) questionnaire (as indeed the authors' text seems to do). The problem is with the loose linguistic use in this area of the word 'fight' and a failure to flag which of the many functionally distinct ethological forms of aggression is being measured.

An important cause of this problem is the naming in the second edition which confused what is in fact a !FFFS subsystem, controlling proximal behaviour, with a GRS primary system, controlling repulsion generally (see also Young, 2022, for additional sources of complication). As with my changing of the system names for the current edition, the solution for 'fight' scales seems to be, if possible, to change their labelling by adding the appropriate adjective to match their item content. I can agree with DeYoung (quoted earlier) that self-statement items related to *behaviour* will often provide accurate reports—but one needs then to make sure that the title of a questionnaire (which will often drive interpretation) is an unambiguous and correct label for its behavioural item contents and that the context of the nominal behaviour tightly maps to the ethologically/pharmacologically defined construct (pausing for thought is not !FREEZE). Relabelling should be fairly easy to do in retrospect in cases like 'intraspecies fight' where only an adjective need be added. Importantly, with 'fight'/ !FIGHT scales it should be possible to retain the scale unchanged while only changing the theoretical expectations generated by the scale name—and prompting assessment of equivalence of similarly named scales between systems. That said, it will be important to check that scales so labelled have appropriate behavioural content (Recommendation 2); and do not open the way to linguistic ambiguity (Recommendation 3).

12.14 Developing neural anchors

I have so far provided a brief overview of some currently available questionnaire and biological measures in the context of the neuropsychology of the previous chapters. This has been a patchwork since, so far, scales have not been directly challenged with neural biomarkers; nor have biomarkers been used as trait measures. In what follows, I will look at the issues involved in developing and using neuropsychologically appropriate biomarkers in the future.

An important feature of RST is that, by definition, its trait constructs *must* map back to explicit function-related neural bedrock (e.g. Fig. 11.15, §11.5.4, §11.5.5, §12.8). It is crucial that the biomarkers used for this mapping be derived from appropriately-designed task-related electrophysiological or otherwise biological measures; and then *validated* with appropriate drug or other neural challenges (§11.5.4). It may also be possible to use genetic measures that have been appropriately characterized in animal behaviour test batteries (e.g. Reuter et al., 2015); or use fMRI activation patterns that map the systems themselves directly ($11.5.5). In the reverse direction, as with the dopamine system (§12.7), starting with neural modulators as measures should allow use to identify related traits (Fig. 4.3; §4.5; McNaughton, 2020).

I will argue that, with appropriate contrasts to extract specific signal components, RST biomarkers can be obtained in humans from both ethoexperimental (§12.14.1, c.f. Chapter 2) and operant-style tasks (§12.14.2, c.f. Chapter 3). However, use of such tasks necessarily produces measures that combine both trait and state components. This could be avoided with trait biomarkers (e.g. perhaps, levels of endogenous benzodiazepine receptor ligands). But it should also be possible to extract the trait component via multiple testing (§12.14.3).

12.14.1 Human ethoexperimental tasks

How can we test if humans are like rodents when responding to threats? The clearest view of the nature of, and distinctions between, fear and anxiety in both rats and mice comes from 'ethoexperimental' (Blanchard and Blanchard, 1988; [see also Chapter 2]) exposure to predators, the effects of which we can subject to challenge with anxiolytic and panicolytic drugs (Blanchard et al., 1997b) and translate to people (Blanchard, 2017).

How do we expose people to a real predator in an experiment? Doing so, especially while asking them to remain still in a scanner, sounds tricky. This problem has been solved using virtual worlds that contain 'predators' that deliver real world pain. Fung et al. (2019) used virtual predators that, when contacting the player's avatar, delivered real shock. Korn and Bach (2019) used predators that destroyed previous gains in a complex foraging situation, which pitted nominal starvation against nominal predation. (The 'fear = frustration' hypothesis in rodent work would see the predators in the two studies as functionally equivalent, Gray, 1971.)

Both studies found that semi-urgent/heuristic responding to a predator engaged the amygdala, and the part of the hippocampus ('temporal'/'ventral'/'anterior') close to the amygdala. *Fung et al. (2019) showed that this activation varied with neurotic personality (assessed with the STAI-T).* Although participants were stationary in an fMRI scanner, there is every reason to think the amygdala and hippocampus will be engaged when you (or a rodent) are uncertain as to how to respond to any truly threatening situation such as a predator. In contrast, urgent/reactive responses to virtual predators, engage subcortical 'survival circuits' (LeDoux, 2012), such as the periaqueductal grey (Mobbs et al., 2007). This hierarchy seen in humans is consistent with prior rodent data (McNaughton and Corr, 2004; Graeff, 1994; LeDoux, 1994).

Frontal cortex activation also appeared to depend on the hierarchical level of threat. Fung et al. (2019) show that, with semi-urgent threat ventromedial prefrontal cortex activation (and information flow from the hippocampus to it) increases with trait anxiety. Similarly, Korn and Bach (2019) show that responses based on predator probability (a simple heuristic) activated dorsolateral prefrontal cortex (as well as amygdala and hippocampus). Their ingenious analysis, taking advantage of Markov chain decision processes, showed similar increases when the nature of events became relatively certain at high or low predator probability. However, responses based on a less heuristic, and so even more computationally intensive, optimal policy activated posterior dorsomedial prefrontal cortex but not amygdala or hippocampus. Across the studies, then, increasing depth of processing (linked to decreasing urgency of decision) appears to produce a progressive shift in main locus of processing from anterior ventromedial via more central dorsolateral to more posterior dorsomedial prefrontal cortex.

Taken together these results extend to prefrontal cortex the picture of hierarchical neural systems controlling fear and anxiety where decision urgency (from reactive through heuristic to predictive) determines the level of the hierarchy engaged (McNaughton and Corr, 2004; Graeff, 1994). But they also suggest that at the highest levels of processing—where simple heuristics give way to complex optimizing policies and amygdala/hippocampus cease to be engaged—there may be a functional change from tactical/how to strategic/why processing that means we are no longer dealing with hot emotion but only cold cognition. It may be significant, here, that hippocampal projections are strong in ventromedial and absent in posterior dorsomedial regions (which do not show accompanying hippocampal activation).

(McNaughton, 2019, p. 1. emphasis added)

RECOMMENDATION 18: USE VIRTUAL PREDATOR ETHOEXPERIMENTAL PARADIGMS

Detailed analysis (Fung et al., 2019; Qi et al., 2018; Castegnetti et al., 2020; Bach et al., 2020) can be applied to these data-rich paradigms to assess attraction, repulsion, and conflict—while manipulating pain levels and the sizes of gains and losses. In recent unpublished work my laboratory simplified the code from Qi et al. (2018) to make it more like a rat straight alley task, replaced shock with aversive noise to avoid electrical artefacts, and used EEG to reproduce and drug validate a GCSR biomarker using an early-predator versus late-predator contrast. This is a high-order of 'replication'. The task retained variation in gain ($) level, included periods where gain was earned, where escape was produced, where escape failed with a successful predator attack, etc., and so should have the capacity to assess each of GAS, GRS, GIS and, likely !FFFS via appropriate evoked potentials or (as with GCSR) rhythmic activity. But I have yet to undertake the detailed analysis required to confirm this and to confirm source localization using sLORETA (c.f., §11.5.5). Further work will also be needed to assess its repeatability (in progress), specificity, and sensitivity.

Recommendation 18: One should use both 'foraging' and 'straight alley' paradigms, coupled with sophisticated modelling and imaging, in virtual screen worlds with predator avatars that can deliver pain and prey avatars controlled by the participant, as homologues of rodent ethoexperimental analysis.

12.14.2 Human operant-style tasks

I have already described the development of the first theoretically based GIS/anxiety biomarker (§11.5.4) in a simple operant-style task (the Stop Signal Task) that can be used in both rats and humans (Eagle and Robbins, 2003), discussed its likely biological trait basis with some cautions as to its interpretation (§12.8), and shown that, when extreme, it is linked to different DSM diagnoses to different extents (Shadli et al., 2021a). Related biomarkers for the GRS and for its !FFFS subsystem are needed. As with the GIS biomarker, such new biomarkers can be validated by appropriate drug challenge (but see Perkins et al., 2009; Perkins et al., 2013; and, especially, clarification by Lippold et al., 2020); e.g. a GRS biomarker (particularly !FFFS) should be sensitive to panicolytic but *not* selective anxiolytic drugs.

Alternatively, as with the RPE potential (§12.7), one can take existing measures that link to relevant known biology (the dopamine system for RPE, see Schultz et al., 2017; Schultz, 2016) and then locate them in the existing neural map (Fig. 11.15). This location then provides a basis for interpreting the potential (with RPE/dopamine being expected to be linked to all of GAS, GRS, and GIS; and so potentially linked to plasticity and so extraversion, §12.7). This is RST writ large—even if a neural system is not included in the current version of the theory, it can be added by extension later; which is the history of the three editions.

Importantly, there are a large number of well-characterized evoked potentials and evoked rhythmicities, including tasks with distinct components of electrical responses to gains and losses that allow researchers to 'parse the temporal dynamics of *both anticipatory and consummatory* reward processing components' (Bowyer et al., 2021, p. 1, emphasis added). Thus, a single simple task (that one can test for homology in rodents) can concurrently deliver indices for a range of processes depending on the time window chosen and, particularly, the contrasts applied to sets of different types of trial; and demonstrate relative contributions of different processes to, for example, depression within the same task (Thompson et al., 2023).

RECOMMENDATION 19: USE OPERANT-STYLE TASKS WITH CONTRASTS

The use of simple individual behavioural tests, rather than test batteries, and without tightly focused contrasts (§12.7, §12.8) requires caution (Bach, 2021). For this purpose, operant-style tasks designed with suitable trial differences are ideal, but not the only possibility.

> *Recommendation 19: Use simple operant-style tasks (e.g. Stop Signal Task, Gold Bar Lemon Task, Doors Task)—these allow selective contrasts (see Recommendation 11) and direct rodent comparisons.*

12.14.3 Separating the trait component

As noted, GCSR as measured in the stop signal task is currently too labile (Shadli et al., 2020b) and insensitive to be used as a measure of an individual's trait GIS sensitivity. However, I expect its elicitation with virtual predators to both increase sensitivity and allow repeat testing.

This is not a vain hope as there are already data showing that the reward positivity (RewP; linked to gain, §12.7) and the feedback negativity (FN, linked to loss) show significant test-retest correlations over a one-week interval with acceptable internal consistency within a time point (Levinson et al., 2017). Treated as individual difference measures, then, RewP and FN have good psychometric properties.

Both improvements in task design and the use of repeat testing and averaging should, therefore, allow assessment of the trait component of function-related electrophysiological measures at a level that may allow assessment of individuals. Even the current measures could potentially be used to assess the neuropsychological content of existing scales—and I turn to that next.

12.15 Unscrambling the trait omelette?

As you have seen, the validity of a biomarker can be assessed by a combination of the design of the eliciting paradigm, application of suitable contrasts to remove confounds for the theoretical construct of interest, and appropriate drug validation linked to specific system modulation. A similar approach can be taken with existing questionnaires—but, following my omelette analogy (§12.2), I urge caution as to how far any existing questionnaire can be seen as a measure of a neural system as opposed to being a measure of its behavioural correlates or of their verbal correlates.

12.15.1 Item content

In relation to the design + contrasts aspect of biomarkers, there is a problem with the bulk of RST questionnaires that

> they have not followed a theoretically-driven process in the development of scale items based on the typical human reactions to defensive and approach RST-defined scenarios. The latter point is important because using 'face validity' on its own to develop test items begs the question of the nature of the expressions of the FFFS, BIS and BAS in humans, as measured by questionnaire (Corr, 2013). . . . *[One alternative is] starting with qualitative responses to defensive and approach scenarios modelled on typical rodent ethoexperimental situations.*
>
> Corr and Cooper (2016, p. 1428. emphasis added)

I would see it as important to give primacy to such ethoexperimentally derived, or experimentally derived, items. It is also important to ensure simple phrasing of questions in a form where a non-human could provide the answer behaviourally in a suitable paradigm (§12.13); with appropriate detailed variations to ensure homology (e.g. in rats, boxing is more stereotypical as an intraspecific defence and side-biting as an intraspecific offence and so these are likely not good items for a human scale). For example, in the rRST-Q

> fight is strongly negatively correlated with the FFFS (-.0.78), which may reflect the [surprising] nature of some of the scale content (e.g. 'I am a rather quick-witted person', Q.22)

> which does not seem to reflect defensive fight . . . [and] may relate to a predatory form of psychopathy, which itself is negatively correlated with the FFFS.
>
> (Corr and Cooper, 2016, p. 1428).

This is one example of the fact that current RST questionnaires often include extremely complicated questions where the content departs from behaviour *per se*. Words like 'worry' are clearly hard to map back to non-human behaviour—and likely to generate problems with varying meanings (§1.4) and results—not to mention problems for translation between languages. That said, superficially similar behaviours may not be homologous between humans; and so, it may be better to create new questionnaires that start with a large pool of items and refine these with the biomarker (§12.16).

In this translational context I should note that 'risk assessment behaviour' is characteristic of rodent anxiety, and is

> an evolved, generally adaptive, mechanism comprising focused attention and appraisal of potential threat stimuli and situations. Initially characterized in animal models, it provides a number of behavioral and functional parallels [in humans] to patterns of *rumination, gaze biases, and other forms of affective cognition that appear to be disregulated in depression and anxiety*. Serotonergic mechanisms are involved in these mood disorders, and an emerging body of evidence suggests that they may modulate the affective cognitive changes common to such psychopathologies.
>
> (Blanchard and Meyza, 2017, p. 9)

This is not only a key active output of the GIS when conflict is detected but can be seen as linking cortical processes of cognition and emotion via the Default Mode Network and the Salience Network (Blanchard, 2018; with the latter a potential substrate of Conscientiousness, Sassenberg et al., 2023). Blanchard has thus started to translate the ethoexperimental approach and its detailed analysis wholesale from non-human to human (particularly via scenarios) and has challenged both species with, e.g. serotonergic (particularly $5HT1_A$) drugs. This could provide a means of obtaining behaviourally based scales of, e.g. trait rumination/worry/repetitive thought (§12.8.4).

12.15.2 Modulator challenge—RST scales

Direct drug challenge of a questionnaire response has the problem that chronic administration (as in clinical settings) would be required to change responding to 'trait' questions. However, the reverse approach, screening people into high and low groups[16] on the basis of questionnaire scores and then testing for group differences in drug response, or genetic markers, is, in principle, straightforward. Likewise, one can ask if the difference between the groups in their pattern across a battery of psychological and/or physiological test matches the pattern of change produced by the relevant drugs.

This approach is likely to be most productive with multiple challenge measures coupled with multiple scale measures to generate dissociations. Critically, for RST, two steps are

16 A dimensional design would also be possible but usually higher cost.

required. First, the challenge must be chosen so there is evidence that it is both sensitive for and specific to the RST system (or system component) of interest. Second, drugs must be tested on groups selected for extreme scale scores; while genes must be used to select separate groups that are then tested for scale score differences.

> Further research is warranted to elucidate the trait-neurotransmitter relationship especially for the newly published (r)RST questionnaires (for an example [using COMT and DRD2 polymorphisms] see Reuter et al., 2006). In this respect alternative item-to parcel allocations could be tested in order to disentangle whether a theory-related item-to-parcel allocation results in more precise trait-neurotransmitter relations than more random item-to-parcel allocations which might increase parcel allocation variability. Moreover, studies on the trait-neurotransmitter relation would further our knowledge on the multi-trait-multi-method matrix of (r)RST-related personality questionnaires as would be other studies combining psychometric data and data from the field of personality neuroscience.
>
> (Leue et al., 2022, p. 14)

Clearly, care is required here in the potential equation of the GAS (or even BAS) with dopaminergic markers. With a hierarchical structure (Fig. 12.1) correlations of dopaminergic measures with 'plasticity', 'extraversion', 'BAS' and anything to do with GAS would be expected. But *to equate dopamine* with the GAS (i.e. having excluded higher order plasticity or extraversion, §12.7.3) would be another matter given that the GAS is not its sole target.

Note that there can be multiple challenges to, e.g. the GIS system. As discussed in §12.1.2, §12.8.3, and §12.11, the theory deals with systems where clusters of neural elements, each controlled by clusters of genes have co-evolved to achieve a particular adaptive phenotype. Groups based on extremes of the resultant adaptive dimension should differ on all of the relevant characters. One could, therefore, challenge the GIS with GCSR or benzodiazepine biomarkers or $5HT1_A$ biomarkers. But a key theoretical feature of GCSR (deriving from my analysis of RSA/'theta') is that it reflects a *final common path* for all the different anxiolytic drugs and so should be a more reliable challenge of the GIS system than the other two.

12.15.3 Modulator challenge—Big 5 scales and facets

Since the Big 5 is not derived from a neuropsychological theory it does not have to characterize its modulators or genes in relation to specific target neural entities. Neural analysis can therefore proceed on the basis of simple hypotheses about neurotransmitter systems, such as dopamine, using manipulations based on known pharmacology or genetics. As a paradigm example, I will look here (as earlier) at Extraversion and its links to dopamine.

Early work on dopamine and extraversion suggested (albeit in a small sample) that dopamine delivery and turnover did not differ between introverts and extraverts but that introverts were more sensitive to D_2 receptor challenge than extraverts (see Rammsayer, 1998). Based on an extensive analysis of non-human work Depue and Collins (1999) saw dopamine as *modulating* incentive motivation by (long-term) facilitation—with, e.g. D_2 antagonists impairing self-stimulation reward. They postulated a trait dimension of receptor activation where a low trait activation person will have a smaller response to incentive stimulus than a high trait activation person; who will experience incentive stimuli as more salient—and so, via a range of complex networks innervated by the ventral tegmental area, have the enhanced emotions and motivations that one can see as extraversion. Note that increased post-synaptic effectiveness of dopamine is not the same as having high levels, or high throughput, of dopamine. But the behavioural effects of increased dopamine (via amphetamine or cocaine treatment) would be similar to those of increased receptor sensitivity.

> Extraverts are more enthusiastic and tend to view events more positively; they also are more active, are more talkative, and spend more time with other people. *This entire package* of affect, behavior, and cognition can be parsimoniously explained in terms of higher levels of dopamine causing extraverts to experience positive activation and approach motivation more often and more strongly, leading to the pursuit of all sorts of social and non-social rewards more often and more vigorously (Depue and Collins, 1999).
>
> (Wacker and Smillie, 2015, p. 2, emphasis added)

One way to read these data is that, in addition to driving immediate approach behaviour, frequent strong positive reinforcement (i.e. fundamentally a change in RPE, §12.7) causes widespread plastic changes 'leading to' the resultant extravert profile and related changes picked up as the metatrait of Plasticity (Smillie et al., 2019). Here both the trait and metrait would be seen as fundamentally dependent on the aspect/facet of positive RPE sensitivity producing progressive correlated changes in a range of observed ABCDs.

12.15.4 Electrophysiological challenge

An important advantage of electrophysiology is that its precise timing can separate and identify functional components—and provide clear homologies with non-human data. You have already seen two examples of the use of an electrophysiological anchor in the form of RPE—using its 200–300 ms component to link both reward/punishment sensitivity (§12.7.1) and extraversion (§12.7.3) to dopamine and so the *neural basis* of reinforcement; and its 70–100 ms component to salience. There is also evidence that within the later component it should be possible to separate an early pure valence signal and a later value (signed quantitative prediction error) signal (Stewardson and Sambrook, 2023). Similarly, I used GCSR (based on RSA/'theta' and a time-locked linear × quadratic contrast) to question the basis of the C&W BIS scale and then conclude that it measures worry rather than goal conflict (§12.8.4).

So, even with scales that are not officially linked to RST, I agree that, for example,

> to elucidate the neuroscientific basis of reward-facilitating investment of cognitive demand, individual differences of CMQ-44 cognitive demand and performance monitoring should be experimentally assessed in a study measuring event-related potentials like N2, error related negativity (ERN/Ne), and feedback negativity (FN). The items of the included questionnaires were not developed based on psychopharmacological predictors. *Future research might investigate which of those items are sufficient for correlations with psychopharmacological predictors.*
>
> (Leue et al., 2022, p. 14, added emphasis)

In this context it is worth noting that one needs both further development of RPE paradigms (e.g. via the doors task; Levinson et al., 2017; Bowyer et al., 2021) and proper pharmacological validation of them and their components by manipulations that affect the dopamine system. Full development of similar anchors is required for both the GAS (trait attraction rather than trait positive reinforcement or metatrait plasticity) and GRS (trait repulsion rather than trait negative reinforcement).

Here, GIS is a leader. With a half-century of background work, it has unique pharmacological (anxiolytics as a whole, contrasted with panicolytics that also have anxiolytic properties), neural (reticular and septal theta reduction), and anatomical (SHS) anchors. I believe it is no accident (given the theoretical basis of its construction) that my anxiety process biomarker, GCSR, partially binds but is distinct from DSM (and other definitions) of 'anxiety' (Shadli et al., 2021a; Shadli et al., 2015). That is, the rodent theta results (McNaughton et al., 2007) are not 'just an assay' for anxiolytic action but tap into the primary neural target through which the drugs achieve their effect (McNaughton et al., 2006b; Woodnorth and McNaughton, 2002b). GCSR correlates weakly with STAI-T (which is a better match than GCSR for DSM anxiety in general) and to a similar extent with C&W BIS (which is likely just worry) and to EPQ-N—and preliminary data suggest that these three correlations are functionally somewhat different from each other (Shadli et al., 2015, Fig. 12.3); but there are currently no data on any of the revised (RST3) 'BIS' scales. Before assessing these scales, I think it may be worth developing a more sensitive and stable (Shadli et al., 2020b) biomarker (§12.14) but these present data provide proof-of-concept.

12.15.5 Imaging challenge

Particularly with the paradigms I described in §12.14, there are different phases within a task where the pattern of network activation can be assessed. Changes in particular functional activity can then be linked to particular brain areas predicted by RST (usually assessed via Regions of Interest) as in §11.5.5 (see also Marwood et al., 2022, for a case excluding a role for depression). This can be undertaken with EEG and sLORETA (which allows fine grain time resolution and frequency band selection but does not assess deep structures) and with fMRI (which has coarse time resolution but allows assessment of, e.g. hippocampus). Individual variation in these responses can then be linked to scale scores (e.g. Fung et al., 2019).

When attempting to map a scale where the theory does not yet have a clear neuropsychology for its target construct (e.g. Neuroticism), a 'resting state' approach can be taken. This loses the advantage of using contrasts to obtain a clear functional cause for the observed activity—but potentially lacks the biases that may be introduced by the specific choice of eliciting task and bypasses the difficulty of designing a task intended to specifically assess something as complex as Neuroticism. That said, resting state studies appear to vary with 'differences in sample characteristics, personality measurements, imaging methodologies and statistical analyses' (Lin et al., 2023, p. 2).

In the case of Neuroticism, meta-analysis (Lin et al., 2023) of resting state fMRI has shown positive relations with activity in the middle temporal gyrus (where hyperactivity to negative stimulus may reflect increased conflict and negative affect); in the right hippocampus (where it may mediate the relationship between Neuroticism and subsequent depression through increased contextual fear learning); in the left striatum (where it may result from increased D2 receptor density); and in the subgenual anterior cingulate cortex (where it may mediate overexpression of negative affect). This pattern involves, at least in part, each of GAS, GRS, and GIS and so is similar to but less diffuse than serotonin.

From the trait point of view, simple volumetric MRI, is also attractive. Where there are differences, these cannot be confounded with state variation. This approach has promise. For example,

> To investigate the link between brain and RST systems using measures that additionally assess the FFFS to better understand the neurobiological drivers of behaviour, middle aged adults underwent an MRI brain scan and completed health and personality questionnaires, including the re-structured BIS/BAS/FFFS scales.
>
> Regions of interest (ROI), selected *a priori* based on existing literature and neurobiological function: FFFS: caudal and rostral ACC, amygdala; BAS: nucleus accumbens, caudate, putamen, pallidum; BIS: PCC, hippocampus, entorhinal cortex, amygdala. Positive associations were detected in ROIs: FFFS and left caudal ACC; BAS and right caudate; BIS and right PCC. Laterality analyses showed that BIS was additionally associated with hippocampus.
>
> (Espinoza Oyarce et al., 2021–2022)

12.15.6 What's in a name?

I have noted already that it is important to distinguish supposedly similar (e.g. 'anxiety') scales that come from different systems. I have also discussed, over a whole section (§12.13), the problems with failure to be clear as to which of the many forms of 'fight' is measured by a scale. This has been coupled with a general (although not complete) lack of recognition that, in all versions of the theory, 'fight' has referred solely to !FIGHT, i.e. panic-laden intraspecific explosive attack.

With the alternative fight scales/subscales and C&W BIS, a clear step towards proper naming is careful inspection of the items and determination of their real-world referent (or ambiguous referents) in relation to the neuropsychology. This will be most easy, in the context of the theory, where items specify, or are strongly constrained by, behavioural observation (as with the separate RST-PQ Fight scale).

You have also, with Worry, seen the importance of using item content and high intercorrelation (Bainbridge et al., 2022) to determine construct overlap (lexical or neural) despite dissimilar names (BIS, Anxiety, Worry). In this context, it was somewhat startling to look at the items of the C&W BIS, which has continued in use for three decades, and realize that it never contained any behavioural inhibition items at all (§12.8.4). Indeed, routinely testing for high intercorrelation and then comparing item content would seem advisable before using any scale, and certainly before attempting neural assessment.

The main items that link C&W BIS to 'anxiety' match the separately constructed NEO-PI-R Anxiety scale; and it makes no distinctions within the spectrum of neurotic disorders including 'depression' (Johnson et al., 2003) with no recognition that the BIS theory is restricted to anxiolytic-drug-sensitive entities. 'A rose by any other name . . . ' can cause serious pain with its unexpected thorns. Such misnaming is clearly one reason for the 'bewildering array of outcomes' about which Pickering et al. (1997) complained.

So, one can conclude with considerable certainty (§12.8.4) that C&W BIS is, essentially, a worry scale—albeit raising difficulties if one wants to test for non-human homology or even to know exactly what worry is neurally. Worry (and a high BIS score) is common across the range of neurotic disorders, including ones like depression that are not sensitive to selective anxiolytics. So, whatever Worry is, it is clearly not isomorphic with risk assessment (anxiolytic-sensitive) and is likely linked to obsession (Besharat et al., 2019) and rumination (Nolen-Hoeksema et al., 2008) and so share their links to depression.

So, on the current evidence it might appear preferable to replace BIS within the C&W BIS/BAS questionnaire and Anxiety within the NEO-PI-R with routine use of the Penn State Worry Scale. But knowing they are equivalent and simple referring to them as C&W BIS/Worry, NEO-PI-R-Anxiety/Worry, Penn State/Worry retains comparability of new data with old and, statistically, should deliver essentially similar (>90% shared variance) results when assessing Worry, *per se*, independent of the scale used. A similar construct addendum could be used where the scale name is the same in two systems but the constructs are found to differ.

RECOMMENDATION 20: MAKE CLEAR HOW RST-BASED SCALES HAVE BEEN NEURALLY ASSESSED

This issue of naming is likely to become acute if neural anchors are used—especially if scale items are included or removed to match the anchor. In all these cases it will also be important to make clear the basis for scale construction and the extent of any neural validation.

Where a name change (including simple construct addendum) is prompted by neural analysis, this could prompt reorganization of items into new, more neurally valid, behaviour-oriented, scales or sub-scales. To avoid confusion, I suggest renaming as GIS/GAS/GRS/!FFFS only scales that have been *constructed* to fit with the neurology of this book, *that use behaviour-report items*, and have been *neurally or pharmacologically **derived***—or re-derived in the case of a modified existing scale with deletions and/or addition. This renaming of existing RST scales should occur when, *but not before*, they are neurally re-derived. Thus 'BIS' would be a rationally derived scale nominally based on RST2 (or perhaps also RST3), 'rBIS' would a rationally derived scale nominally based on (revised) RST3, and 'GIS' would be a new, or re-derived old scale based on the current RST5 validated via a specific *selective* link to GCSR or a similar whole-system-specific biological anchor. That is, a GIS scale should be explicitly anchored to global trait GIS sensitivity, as in §12.8, and separated from global Trait GRS sensitivity. Note that its items do not need to match everyday ideas of anxiety any more than do weight and sleep change match everyday ideas of depression. This should also be the method with facets linked to a specific neural structure, e.g. !FFFS would be anchored to PAG sensitivity.

With the new or modified scales, and existing unmodified scales (whether nominally RST or not) that have been neural assessed, it seems to me that the form of validation/assessment should be indicated as, e.g. McN-GIS$_{[GCSR]}$ (a neurally derived scale, that is not yet completely developed), NEO-PI-R-Extraversion$_{[RewP]}$, rRST-rBIS $_{[AVPR1a]}$ (see Reuter et al., 2015 for details on AVPR1a), RST-PQ-BIS$_{[GCSR]}$ (the coding that would be applied after successful GCSR challenge of the existing RST-PQ-BIS). This would allow for variation between biomarkers (e.g. a $BIS_{[GCSR]}$ scale may not have identical properties to a $BIS_{[AVPR1a]}$ scale; and double assessment would be preferred)—but the intent is that a particular scale assesses a particular RST neural entity. Or, with a non-RST scale, one would be interested in the specific mix of RST or other biomarkers that are linked to it.

Recommendation 20: When a scale has been neurally developed or assessed include an indicator of this in the name, e.g. $GIS_{[GCSR]}$; $BIS_{[AVPR1a]}$; $GIS_{[GCSR + AVPR1a]}$

12.16 Can anchors derive scales?

Given that properly validated neural anchors, like GCSR, are available one should first think, as suggested by Smillie (§12.1.1) about using them directly. This could be done with single 'final common path' measures like GCSR, or with latent variables derived from an intercorrelated set. Technical difficulties are receding (the GCSR test could already be delivered via a downloaded app, with the required single channel EEG recorded with a cheap clip-on headset). With such direct use, one could ask about the relation of the personality measure to existing scales (e.g. noting, as I do in Chapter 13, that STAI-T and GCSR are correlated but functionally distinct) but I think the temptation to identify an existing scale with the neural anchor should be avoided.

Unfortunately, state variation contaminates the trait component of the EEG record, as do other sources of noise. As noted, Neuroticism and STAI-T correlate at about + 0.7. For comparison, STAI-T:GCSR is at + 0.2, Neuroticism:GCSR at 0.2 (Shadli et al., 2015), Extraversion:RPE at about + 0.2 and C&W BAS:RPE at 0.17. Substantial effects of drugs on GCSR can be detected with N in the region of 8–12 (McNaughton et al., 2013; Shadli et al., 2015; Shadli et al., 2020a); but, overall, the error variance is not satisfactory for N = 1 scoring. Some ERP measures may be an exception to this (Levinson et al., 2017; Bowyer et al., 2021) but for the present I will assume that current neural measures cannot be used directly to assess traits on an individual single-test basis.

Because of this error variance, current biomarkers also cannot be used for *a priori* scale construction unless very large N are available. That is, if a large weakly selected group of items (e.g. a set generally related to 'bad vibes') is assessed for correlation with GCSR many larger correlations are likely to be due to chance not to a genuine relationship unless very large N is used (Schönbrodt and Perugini, 2013).

> One possibility is that N=400 or 500 should be adequate. One would basically just want to sort the promising from the unpromising items using the correlations and then also consider item content and theoretical matching. Then, once items are aggregated, associations will be higher than for individual items, and one can use an iterative procedure to optimize the scale relative to the biomarker.
>
> Colin DeYoung (personal communication, 16 February 2020)

It will be important also, to show that GCSR correlates with the resultant scale more than with Neuroticism, STAI-T, PSWQ, etc.

One way to proceed is to obtain smaller initial pools of items using a principled theory-based approach (Corr and Cooper, 2016) to create scales that can then be refined and selected between using the chosen biomarker. Or, to allow re-use of existing data, assess the item content of *existing* scales for their match to theoretical 'rodent'/'external observer' optima and either choose between them or refine them or combine them using biomarkers or treat highly correlated scales as equivalent.

12.17 Conclusion

'Personality neuroscience: An emerging field with bright prospects'
(DeYoung et al., 2022; see also Corr and Mobbs, 2023)

I have attempted to make clear the mapping of the theory of the earlier chapters (and of the earlier editions) to anxious personality in particular and to motivational traits more generally. I have argued that care must be taken, during what is in effect translation, to retain the neural, Darwinian, and (rodent-centric) behavioural basis of the theory; and to reduce the risk of linguistic confusions during scale construction and interpretation. Linguistic content *per se* is not a problem (except for lying, or misremembering, when you are asked what you did over the last few years). But questions and answers should as far as possible directly reflect behavioural reality, allowing as little room as possible for political/anthropomorphic/deconstructionist re-interpretation or misunderstanding. 'If a fight broke out in a bar where you were drinking, would you leave as fast as possible?' (Wilson et al., 1989) does not transfer to Islamic culture far less rat behaviour.

I have argued, in particular, that what is needed now is greater *neural* understanding of existing motivation construct scales (including, e.g. Neuroticism). New scales *may* then be needed, either by modifying old scales or creating new ones. I think it likely that where neural data suggest that old scales need alteration or new ones need generating this will best initially involve item selection/sorting of the sort that was undertaken to convert C&W BIS into separate rBIS and rFFFS scales; as well as removal of items that do not fit the theory's neuropsychological criteria. Importantly such re-building can be retrospective, allowing the use (after neural validation) of a mass of old data by item selection. Validating such scales is crucial, and construction of completely new scales may be preferable but I would think this is best left until existing scales (or their modified versions) have proved wanting.

In this it is important to keep clear whether a scale is intended to measure a clearly defined neural sensitivity (as with RST) or whether neural measures are determining the underlying nature of a sensitivity that is defined in terms of the scale itself (as with Big 5). But note that, in the theory, sensitivities will be of systems as a whole and so linked to functional adaptive constructs not specific chemicals or pathways—that is, a specific scale will not be assessing sensitivity of a single neural locus but of a system comprising a large number of polygenically controlled co-evolved loci. In particular, it should be noted that motivational distance emerges from the interaction of all parts of a system.

Importantly, I see the search for neural anchors as being more generally desirable than a focus on RST, *per se*. For example, RPE is quantitatively informative when asking about relationships between scales. As shown in Table 12.2, in one experiment (N = 137; Neo et al.,

Table 12.2 Pearson correlations for reward-prediction-errors (RPE)/unexpected reward (i.e. contrasted with predicted reward). Unless otherwise stated in brackets, traits are MMPI-3 measures. Note that low/negative scores on the blue text traits denote high extraversion (broadly defined) with EPQ extraversion in red. * p < 0.05; ** p < 0.005, one-tailed Pearson correlations, uncorrected. Gray highlight is 0.09 < p < 0.14. Adapted from Neo et al. (2021)

		Salience		Motivation	
RPE interval (ms)	**0–70**	**70–100**	**100–200**	**200–300**	**300–400**
Low positive emotions	−0.02	−0.05	−0.05	−0.04	0.03
Antisocial behaviour	0.03	−0.04	0.05	0.01	−0.01
Social avoidance	−0.12	−0.03	−0.06	0.00	0.05
Disaffiliativeness	−0.05	−0.03	0.07	−0.03	−0.03
Substance abuse	0.01	−0.03	0.01	−0.05	−0.01
Introversion/low positive emotionality	−0.13	−0.02	−0.07	−0.05	0.03
Disconstraint	0.07	0.03	0.03	0.04	0.02
Activation	−0.01	0.08	0.08	0.10	−0.04
Juvenile conduct problems	0.06	0.10	0.10	0.11	0.05
Dominance	−0.06	0.11	0.05	−0.02	−0.06
Hypomanic activation	0.04	0.14 ?	0.08	0.11	0.01
Shyness	−0.06	−0.16 *	−0.06	−0.05	0.07
Extraversion (EPQ-R)	0.10	0.21 **	0.03	0.03	−0.07
Impulsivity	0.12	0.18 *	0.08	0.16 *	0.05
BAS-Drive (C&W)	0.07	0.17 *	0.13	0.15 *	0.01
BAS TOTAL (C&W)	0.07	0.17 *	0.14	0.18 *	0.00
BAS reward responsivity (C&W)	−0.01	0.08	0.10	0.16 *	0.02
BAS fun seeking (C&W)	0.10	0.12	0.08	0.10	−0.02

2021), EPQ Extraversion correlates 0.2[17] with ERP 'Salience' (RPE at 70–100 ms) but does not correlate with 'Motivation' (RPE at 200–300 ms; but see Smillie et al., 2011). MMPI shyness does the same (inverted). But, importantly, MMPI Social Avoidance, Disaffiliativeness, and perhaps Introversion/Low Positive Emotionality do not show this relationship. Note that, in terms of the MMPI labelling, Introversion/low Positive Emotionality essentially blends the inverse of EPQ-E with EPQ-N—with RPE, unsurprisingly, caught in the middle.

I already argued that if RPE is dopamine-related it should link to the trait of Extraversion and the metatrait of Plasticity. These higher order relationships fit with RPE's marginally larger (and definitely more significant) salience (70–100 ms) correlation with Extraversion and the pattern of correlations that are numerically either side of it (with C&W BAS-Drive potentially being an aspect or perhaps facet). Likewise, the motivation (200–300 ms) correlations

[17] You should be beginning to see this correlation as good in this area, for an explanatory model see Pickering and Pesola (2014).

do appear to link to 'reward' (including MMPI Impulsivity) and BAS Fun Seeking is not linked to either salience or motivation.

This example links more to interpretations of RST-2 (ignoring goal control systems). But it uses an extremely simple neural response, which is well-studied at the single unit level in rats, to gain a new view of a large range of questionnaires. The MMPI scales are not intended to link to RST, nor to be distinct from each other. But, arguably, the pattern here makes sense in two dimensions (salience/motivation versus scale content); and may elucidate labelling problems (MMPI-Introversion/Low Positive Emotionality versus EPQ-Introversion/inverted Extraversion). A prime skill (to me as a novice) in this area is the capacity to hold in your head what a scale is really testing while ignoring the label originally applied. As a neuropsychologist, I have suggested renaming of scales as a solution to this—while the name-construct disconnect is something that personality researchers are used to dealing with I suspect it is something that can occasionally lead even them astray; and is certainly a major problem for anyone approaching this area from the outside. Neural anchors are likely to help with this problem since the anchor can stand for its parent construct independent of the scale labels.

Both for RST scales where an explicit mapping is theoretically expected and other scales linked to motivational constructs (like extraversion) where an informative mapping can be observed, I argue for focusing on content that is translatable to the theory's non-human foundations and for neural measures that can then be mapped to its neurology (Fig. 11.15). Here, neuroscience (including behavioural methodologies, pharmacology, etc.) can illuminate not only the nature (and potentially causes) of healthy personality but also the psychopathology that arises from trait extremes. In the next chapter I will apply this approach to the psychopathology of neurotic/internalizing disorders in general and anxiety in particular.

In conclusion,

1) Personality neuroscience must involve challenge of RST questionnaires with neural biomarkers (§12.8.4; §12.7) or carefully characterized genes to determine the extent of match to the theory at the neural as well as functional level.
2) Neural biomarkers can be derived from paradigms that provide, via planned contrasts, a clear functional interpretation (e.g. goal conflict, §12.8.2; reward prediction error, §12.7.1) and can be validated pharmacologically (e.g. via anxiolytic or dopaminergic drugs, respectively).
3) Neural biomarkers can usefully be used to functionally dissect any existing scales whether 'RST' or not.

12.18 Caveat: the role of neuropsychology

This chapter has looked at the implications of the neuropsychology of the previous chapters for anxious personality. I have also commented on the broader RST work that others did based on Gray (1970a) and the first edition; and which was revised in response to the second edition. But, as argued earlier, there is likely to remain a significant divide between current linguistically derived scales and the neuropsychology.

So, I have not tried to solve existing personality problems. My primary goal has been to make clear *how* the 'eggs' of detailed observations and theory (and other neural data) *can* be linked to existing personality theory omelettes. I see the neuropsychology as providing a neural bedrock on which theories (not just RST) can build to account causally for the patterns that emerge at higher levels. I leave to the personality experts the linkage itself, which would require a book larger than this one (c.f., Corr, 2008b). I also made no attempt to resolve the differences between current RST scales (see §12.12). Indeed, I would see the neurally based approach (§12.7; §12.8) as equally useful with approaches such as the Big 5 (§12.7.3) and as, potentially, providing a means of translating between the different personality systems. I also considered how far scales can capture neural system sensitivities; how far such sensitivities can 'validate' scales; whether scales can be constructed based on sensitivities; and, the ultimate ideal, the use of neural measures to assess system sensitivities directly (§12.7).

In Chapter 13, the neuropsychology will also provide a basis for a particular trait-based interpretation of threat-related psychopathologies. While some of this will progress from my anxiety biomarker to novel views of 'trait anxiety'; some will progress from work on neuroticism to a novel view of the neuropsychology of the neurotic disorders; and a potential common neural base for pathology across all the neurotic disorders that is best understood in terms of combined extreme effects of 'healthy' traits.

13
Symptoms and syndromes of anxiety

13.1 Foundations

We have now detailed the actions of the anxiolytic drugs, the functions of the septo-hippocampal system (SHS), the organization of the hierarchical subcortical and cortical defence systems, and their links to anxiety-related personality traits. Here, we consider the implications of these conjoined data for the diagnosis of clinical anxiety and anxiety-related disorders. Throughout we will use current labels (panic, obsession, depression) to refer to symptom clusters and their DSM/ICD related diagnoses. But these should be read as approximations designed to bootstrap to a more syndrome-based reality. As a result, our usage will often appear paradoxical (in our terms pure panic disorder is *not* Panic Disorder as defined by DSM/ICD, which involves additional components and turns out to be plural in any case).

We will start with some foundational concepts. §13.1.1 expands on the idea, presented in Chapter 12, that syndromes are generated by one or more extreme traits—and links this to the National Institute of Health's Research Domain Criteria (RDoC) and Hierarchical Taxonomy of Psychopathology (HiTOP) systems (and more tentatively the Big 5). §13.1.2 provides a clinically oriented recap of the key neural elements of the theory. §13.1.3 emphasizes that our theory of the anxiety defined by the selective anxiolytic drugs encompasses a wide range of neural elements that provide evolved 'Rules of Thumb' that in combination result in a coherent emotion for the surface phenotype that, when extreme, represents dysfunction.

13.1.1 From traits to syndromes

Largely, we will present a picture of disorder resulting from extremes of personality traits (including metatraits, aspects, etc.). But this will not be a direct translation from a single 'trait anxiety' to a matching single 'anxiety disorder'—we will argue that disorders (and their predisposing factors) are more often, but not always, the result of a combination of extremes of two or more traits (e.g. neuroticism + introversion as predisposing and neurotic + introversion + Goal Inhibition System (GIS) as resultant disorder; see §13.2.3). This is close to the view that 'the major dimensions of psychopathology correspond to major trait dimensions of personality, but . . . *extremity on these dimensions is neither necessary nor sufficient* for psychopathology, which requires cybernetic dysfunction' (DeYoung and Krueger, 2018, p. 117, added emphasis). Our emphasis on a common 'neuroticism' component is largely consistent with the view that

> anxiety symptoms could be understood as reflecting the excessive, maladaptive expression of otherwise normative threat-anticipatory defensive responses, and as such could be

The Neuropsychology of Anxiety, Third Edition. Neil McNaughton and Jeffrey A. Gray, Oxford University Press.
 DOI: 10.1093/oso/9780198843313.003.0013

> organized by threat imminence. Such an organization could enhance our theoretical understanding of pathological anxiety by providing a testable framework within which different aspects of symptom presentation and psychobiological correlates are hypothesized to occur and interact.
>
> (Abend, 2023, p. 9)

Importantly, such trait-oriented views implicitly allow true comorbidity (e.g. 'anxiety' *concurrent with* 'depression') via concurrent distinct trait extremes. But we will also describe *apparent* comorbidities at the symptom level ('panic' + 'anxiety') where one pathology indirectly produces symptoms that would also have resulted from the other pathology and so, potentially, there are three types of diagnosis (e.g. panic$^{\rightarrow \text{anxiety}}$, anxiety$^{\rightarrow \text{panic}}$, comorbid panic + anxiety; see §13.5).

With personality (Chapter 12), we emphasized a high-level system-lumping approach seeing Plasticity, Extraversion, and activation-related aspects and facets as all driven to some extent by dopamine; and Stability, Neuroticism, Withdrawal, etc as all driven to some extent by serotonin. With psychopathology we must take a splitting stance, focusing on structures within the systems (e.g. PAG) to account for specific symptoms (e.g. panic). Thus, in the context of Chapter 12, many disorders will map to the facet level (e.g. panic disorder, due to excessive PAG activity) but not all (e.g. generalized anxiety, due to excessive GIS activity, is likely to be at the aspect level) and not serial morbidity (e.g. neurotic disorders where successive presentations are often different nominal disorders; Andrews et al., 1990; and 'sequential comorbidity both inside and external to the family of disorders is the rule not the exception', Poulton et al., 2023, p. 1).

> The main findings [of the longitudinal 'Dunedin Study'] show that the anxiety disorders favour the lumper over the splitter. That is, a general approach to the classification of the anxiety disorders may be warranted. Most Dunedin cohort members with anxiety disorders had histories of prior disorders, and these tended to group around the internalising spectrum, but not exclusively. Some of the specific findings, for example, that specific phobias in adulthood were only associated with prior childhood phobias, but not other disorders in the juvenile years suggest that these disorders may require different classification [see also §13.6.1]. In general, the findings fit well with a hierarchical approach to classification.
>
> (Poulton et al., 2023, p. 3)

The difference between lumping and splitting is just a matter of differing perspectives on a single hierarchical neural reality. We would argue that our hierarchical neural model can also be collapsed into the non-hierarchical perspective of the RDoC (Insel et al., 2010; Carcone and Ruocco, 2017). RdoC can be mapped into the more detailed HiTOP (Kotov et al., 2017; Kotov et al., 2020; Krueger et al., 2021; Watson et al., 2022) and that, in turn, into the Big5 (Fig. 13.1; see also DeYoung and Krueger, 2018, for a matching cybernetic theory of psychopathology).

Note that some lexical translation (and axis rotation) is needed here and we have, in Fig. 13.1, converted[1] HiTOP 'fear' into 'threat' and then placed 'fear' beside rather

1 New terms are underlined.

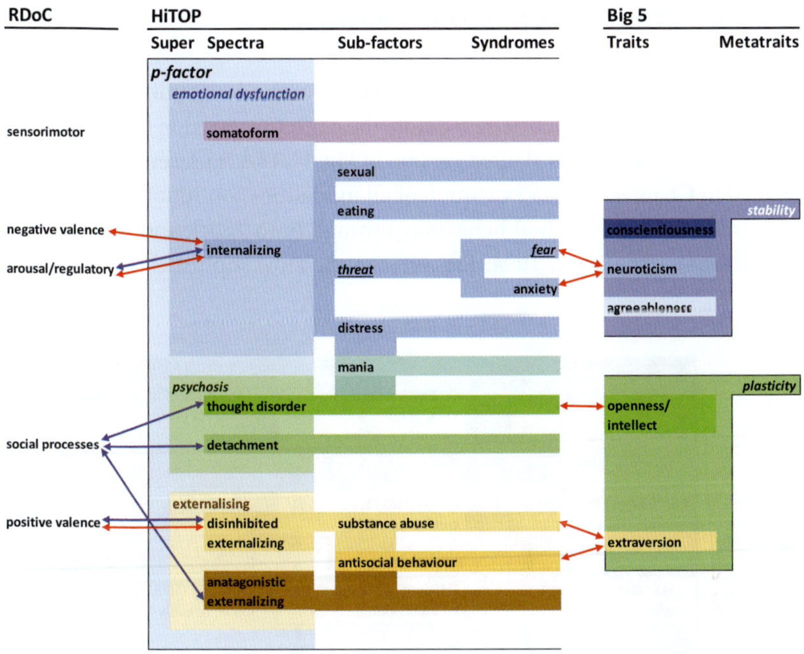

Fig. 13.1 Comparison (based on Michelini et al., 2021; Kotov et al., 2021) of RDoC and HiTOP with addition of a tentative comparison of HiTOP with the Big 5. Note that HiTOP 'fear' has been renamed 'threat' and fear and anxiety included as separate syndromes (matching both RDoC and [Fig. 13.2]). Red arrows represent positive correlations, blue represent negative ones. The mappings of even simple elements are not one-to-one and the systems' structures are different: RDoC has no official hierarchical structure; HiTOP has a single highest order factor (termed a superspectrum and constituting the general factor of psychopathology or p-factor) with 3 embedded superspectra, each reflecting covariance of a pair of spectra; Big 5 has only two separate highest order factors (metatraits). The same conserved neural systems must control the individual trait patterns of affects, behaviors, cognitions and desires (Revelle, 2007) that are meant to be encapsulated by each of these classifications. It should follow that both with animal personality and human classifications their common underlying neuroscience should ultimately provide a foundation for translation between them. (Figure and legend from McNaughton and Corr, 2022, emphasis added).

than above anxiety to conform with both the Big 5 and Fig. 13.2. Note that the original Big 5 'Anxiety' is split into two components (fear/anxiety) and would likely have been better labelled neurotic worry (§12.7.4). Similarly, the factor structure of the MMPI-2-Restructured Form (for review, see Sellbom, 2019) and the MMPI-3 (Sellbom et al., 2021) can be mapped onto HiTOP. When mapping between such systems we should bear in mind that 'the only systematic difference between symptoms and traits in HiTOP is one of time frame. Maladaptive traits are dispositional constructs that describe persistent tendencies to manifest features of psychopathology, whereas symptoms are features of psychopathology as they are manifest during any specific time period' (DeYoung and Krueger, 2018, pp. 20–21). This matches our picture of neural structures delivering much the same behaviour whether this is healthy or pathological with excessive trait sensitivity generating disorder.

13.1.2 From brain to behaviour—a recap

The neurology of the defence system is critical for our understanding of the clinical situation so, in this section, we will briefly reiterate the earlier material in the book from a more clinical perspective. A clinically slanted version of Fig. 11.14A is presented in Fig. 13.2.

As detailed in Chapter 6, sensory stimuli of all modalities continuously bombard the systems responsible for goal-directed behaviour through both 'quick and dirty' and 'slow and sophisticated' routes (LeDoux, 1994; Fig. 6.1). In the slow sophisticated case, the sensory

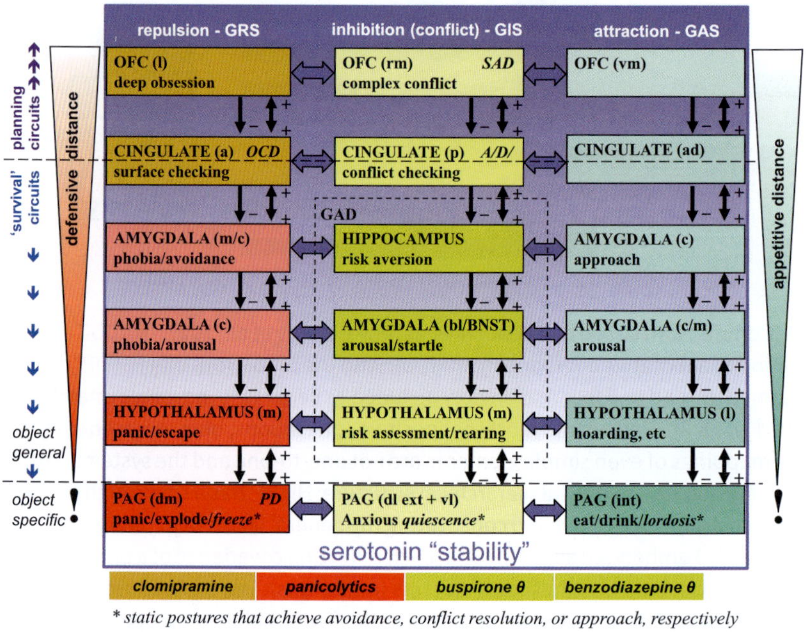

Fig. 13.2 Nosological mapping to hierarchical systems. Goal attraction, goal repulsion, and goal inhibition (activated by conflict between goals) are each controlled by systems in which modules are organized hierarchically in relation to motivational distance (from contacting to distant) and neural location (caudal to rostral). Conservation of modulatory control during phylogeny (McNaughton, 2020; Fig. 12.3) means that hormonal compounds, e.g., benzodiazepine receptor ligands, and neuromodulators, e.g., serotonin, can target all the modules of a specific system (as with benzodiazepines and goal inhibition; yellow highlight) or all the modules of several systems (as with serotonin). Note that in the case of serotonin (most obviously via specific serotonin reuptake inhibitors), its effects (indicated by the gradation of the purple shading) appear to be to shift control from lower to higher levels of the systems (Carver et al., 2008) rather than to increase or decrease activity across an entire system. There is also the capacity for more localized dysfunction and pharmacological specificity, as with obsession (orange highlight) and panic (red highlight). Figure and legend adapted from McNaughton (2022) (based on McNaughton et al., 2016; Silva and McNaughton, 2019; McNaughton, 2020) with permission. a, anterior; b, basal; c, central; d, dorsal; ext, external; int, internal; l, lateral; m, medial; p, posterior v, ventral; A/D/, agoraphobia, fear of the dark, etc; BNST, bed nucleus of the stria terminalis; SAD, Social Anxiety Disorder; OCD, obsessive-compulsive disorder; OFC, orbitofrontal cortex; PAG, periaqueductal gray; PD, Panic Disorder; *θ*, these compounds affect the conflict system as a whole by reducing theta rhythmic input.

input results also in the activation of memory traces that provide additional input to goal-oriented systems. Output from the defence system is also hierarchically organized (Graeff, 1994; Chapter 6). The lowest levels of the system produce the fastest and simplest responses. As one goes to higher and higher levels the speed of response production decreases, but the complexity of responding increases, with the most complex avoidance responses originating in the anterior cingulate and prefrontal cortex. For any individual on any particular occasion faced with a threat, defensive distance is directly related to physical distance from the threat in space or time. But for more, or less, threat-sensitive individuals a particular physical distance represents a lesser or greater, defensive distance, respectively (see Corr & Perkins, 2006).

Concurrent activations of different levels of the defence system (e.g. undirected escape in the PAG, directed avoidance in the amygdala) are resolved by its hierarchical organization. Activation of a higher level sends output (↓-) that prevents the control of behaviour by the lower level, but does not reduce its activation (which can cascade between the levels ⇕+). That said, importantly for clinical phenomena, too great an activation of the lower level (most likely with pathology) can allow it to escape this higher-level control.

Following Graeff, we have argued (Chapter 6; Appendices 2 and 10), that at least part of this hierarchical control results from serotonin release having opposite effects on the PAG versus the amygdala. In a sense, treatments that promote the release of serotonin inform the defence system that a problem is soluble (or, more generally that a situation can be coped with). Note that, in the context of our theory of the SHS (Chapter 10), this suppressive interaction between levels of the defence system does not involve a conflict between goals, does not involve iterative interactions, and requires only simple one-way neural inhibition, the level of which does not have to be adjusted from one occasion to another.

For defence, this hierarchy of structures contains two parallel streams: an active defence system (the Goal Repulsion System/GRS) and a passive defence system (GIS). We have characterized the GIS as detecting goal conflict, inhibiting prepotent behaviour output (whether to an attractor or repulsor), and engaging in processes like risk assessment that can resolve the conflict between concurrent incompatible goals. Importantly for clinical conditions, this inhibition extends to future occurrences of originally prepotent behaviour via SHS output that increases affectively negative associations (diminishing attractors and amplifying repulsors). Equally importantly, the GIS (particularly insula, Chapter 11, not shown in Fig. 13.2) increases existing goal-elicited arousal and attention, and negative affective bias. The arousal, along with activation of the autonomic nervous system, is mediated via the amygdala. Anxiolytic drugs, as a class, impair GIS function.

This theory, then, attributes to the GIS in general and SHS in particular the capacity to increase the valence of affectively negative stimuli (thus, in many cases, increasing perceived threat). It follows that hyperactivity of the GIS should produce a fundamentally cognitive dysfunction—excessive negative bias; see next. The most obvious consequences of this cognitive bias will be affective (i.e. excessive anxiety) through increases in the immediate perception and hence subsequent storage of threatening associations under conditions of conflict with direct control of both aversion and arousal by the amygdala, hypothalamus, and PAG.

On this view, traits involve increased sensitivity to inputs, and this generates hyperactivity that produces the symptoms of disorder. Hyperactivity of structures controlled by RSA/'theta', particularly the SHS, is important for generalized anxiety disorder; and it is through reduction of this hyperactivity that the anxiolytic drugs exert their clinically most important effects. Our hypothesis that hippocampal hyperfunction can lead to anxiety is directly supported by a report that mice with impaired $GABA_A$-receptor function in the hippocampus, parahippocampus and orbitofrontal cortex show increased 'behavioural inhibition ... and an explicit memory bias for threat cues' (Crestani et al., 1999). Similarly, hyperactivity of the amygdala and medial hypothalamus is important for phobia (in the sense of simple active avoidance); and of the PAG is important for panic. However, we argue that, for what is normally seen as *psychiatric* disorder, neuroticism must also be high.

13.1.3 *E pluribus unum*

We must be careful, however, not to fall into the trap of reifying a 'seat of anxiety' (*viz*, the hippocampo–amygdalar circuit). It is better to view anxiety involving many areas (see also LeDoux, 1996; LeDoux, 2012; LeDoux, 2015; LeDoux, 2021). Emotions such as anxiety can derive their apparent coherence, not from the presence in the brain of any single centre coordinating the observed responses, but from the fact that all the observed reactions subserve a common function (or, rather, share a common teleonomy; Pittendrigh, 1958). There can, then, be many separate 'Rules of Thumb' (Krebs et al., 1983; and see Chapter 5, especially §5.5) which have evolved quite independently and which may have no neural overlap (for emotions in general, see McNaughton, 1989b; and anxiety in particular, see §12.1.2), but which are correlated because of environmental regularities and so provide the impression of a seamless, higher order, control system. This appears, in particular, to be the case in relation to the correlated occurrence of, on the one hand, the arousal and autonomic components of activation of the GIS and, on the other, its goal inhibition and attention outputs. For, as we concluded earlier, the former is coordinated in the insula and amygdala, the latter in the SHS; and, at present, we see environmental regularities as a major way in which these two sets of activities are themselves further coordinated. There are two other cases where we must consider parallel controls.

First, as noted in Chapter 9, anxiolytics act on control of RSA/'theta' rhythm in two ways: 1) altering the sensitivity to specific RSA frequencies of the septal input to the hippocampus; 2) reducing the frequency of RSA resulting from a specified intensity of reticular input to the septal area. Only the first of these electrophysiological signatures of anxiolytic drug action reflects dampening of ascending monoaminergic activity; the second, mediated by drug action in the supramammillary nucleus, is a completely independent effect.

Second, we have made much, and justly so, of the fact that the novel anxiolytics have the same behavioural and electrophysiological effects as the classical anxiolytics. However, while this pattern of findings strengthens the case for regarding anxiolytic drug action as an excellent guide to the neurology of anxiety, it simultaneously eliminates enhanced transmission at $GABA_A$ receptors (which the novel anxiolytics do not produce) as a necessary step in such action. So, this receptor cannot play a special role, nor can the allosterically coupled sites upon which the classical anxiolytics act. We need a more complex, neurally realistic, explanation of the role played by the environment in keeping together the congeries of brain structures that must now be included under the rubric of 'the anxiety system'. Co-evolved controls of the RSA/'theta' final common path can account for this.

We can no longer affirm, therefore, that the actions of the anxiolytic drugs that led us to the parsimony of our model of the GIS, at the level of the conceptual nervous system, reflect a single mode of action of these compounds in the real nervous system; and, correspondingly, given the central role that anxiolytic drug action has played in our overall scientific strategy, we can no longer affirm that, in the real nervous system, there exists a neurally unified set of structures that are the GIS. But with an interlinked congeries united by 'Rules of Thumb' (and some evolution of interconnections), we believe that our approach succeeds better than any of its (generally much simpler) rivals in identifying and analysing the set of structures by which the brain handles what we call anxiety.

13.2 Drugs, traits, and defensive syndromes

While we see drugs as an excellent dissecting tool, we do not see them as uniformly effective magic bullets nor as operating in some way separate from cognition nor preferable as a therapy. In the Chapter 14 we will consider them among the various therapy alternatives and combinations thereof for the treatment of defensive disorders. Here we will discuss what can be learned about syndromes from their successful effects (and failures). We will treat drug action as, in effect, a temporary change in a trait or set of traits—where these can also be altered with sufficient psychological treatment.

13.2.1 Pharmacology of panic and anxiety

In §13.4 we will discuss panic and anxiety as both symptoms and syndromes that can have important clinical interactions with each other. Our separation of panic from anxiety assumes that, if there were appropriate differentiation of receptor types, it should be possible to produce drugs that are pure anti-panic agents and others that are pure anxiolytic agents. Some anti-panic drugs would be expected to reduce panic quite generally (by acting on cellular activity in the PAG); others might reduce panic only in a subset of cases of panic disorder (by acting, for example, solely on the terminals that carry an afferent anoxic signal to the PAG), leaving panic attacks undisturbed in cases where panic is a symptom of anxiety or phobic disorder. In practice, receptor differentiation and drug action are not that specific; and, of course, for a psychiatrist, a general anxiolytic/panicolytic drug is more desirable.

That said, currently available selective anxiolytic drugs would be expected to have no effect on the purest cases of panic disorder, to have an ameliorative effect in panic disorder where this is exacerbated by anxiety, and to be fully effective in those cases where a modest incidence of panic attacks is consequent on very high levels of anxiety (§13.3). There are drugs that act differentially on anxiety and panic, justifying for that reason alone a view of panic as separate from anxiety. The same appears to be true of panic and depression (Rosenberg and Jensen, 1994). However, the linkage between anxiety and panic may not be particularly strong. Buspirone has been reported to be ineffective in panic disorder despite its capacity to reduce anxiety and depression (Sheehan et al., 1990; Table 4.1). There are two possibilities here. First, patients selected for test with buspirone may have been of a more purely panic type rather than mixed panic-anxiety. Second, and more likely on our theory, the paradoxical actions of buspirone on 5HT systems or on cortisol levels (Appendix 1) may have produced a counterbalancing direct exacerbation of panic, offsetting any indirect amelioration produced by its anxiolytic action.

13.2.2 Treatment resistance and psychosurgery

However, until very recently there have been two significant problems with any simple interpretation of treatments (both pharmacological and psychological) of panic and other neurotic disorders: 1) they take a long time to show any obvious effect; and 2) a substantial number of patients are treatment resistant. Resistance in the weak sense can simply mean long periods of switching until an effective therapy is found. But treatment resistance (TR) as a category is better defined as when 'after both at least one first-line pharmacological and one psychological treatment failure, provided for an adequate duration (at least 8 weeks) with anxiety severity remaining above a specified threshold' (Bokma et al., 2019, p. 1). In particular, conventional anti-anxiety and anti-depressant medications often target only a subset of neurotic disorders (Muller et al., 2016); and they take months (Muller et al., 2016) to produce their full effects. Worse, 1/3rd of patients are resistant to any conventional treatment (Muller et al., 2016; Nemeroff, 2007), impacting public resources by doubling hospitalizations (Nemeroff, 2007) and suicide attempts; and requiring chronic care.

Before the pharmacological advances of the last 50 years, an 'anxiolytic-insensitive' form of 'anxiety' was recognized, in which clinical benefits were seen, not with administration of a classical anxiolytic drug, but after surgical disruption of descending projections from the cingulate or prefrontal cortex (see §11.1). In the 1970s patients who showed these benefits were described, preoperatively, as having predominantly obsessional symptoms, or widely generalized phobic behaviour (Powell, 1979; Marks et al., 1966; Tan et al., 1971). By the time of our 2nd edition, in clinical practice, obsessive-compulsive disorder (OCD) and major depression (in each case only if TR) were the primary indications for such 'psychosurgery' (Scottish Office, 1996). Fortunately, there are now (Table 4.1) modern drugs, particularly the SSRIs, that appear relatively effective with OCD and major depression. Note that, from our perspective obsession reflects fear, not what we would term anxiety (§6.7).

However, there remains the 30% of TR cases where not only does obsession not predominate, but where other anxiety disorders appear to benefit from psychosurgery to a degree not greatly different from that shown by OCD (Waziri, 1990, Annex D of Scottish Office, 1996). Currently, TR cases of the neurotic disorders are found with diagnoses of panic (PD), generalized anxiety (GAD), social anxiety (SAD), major depression (MDD), post-traumatic stress (PTSD), and OCD.

There are exciting recent developments on this front. A range of psychedelic drugs have been shown to produce essentially immediate improvement in TR neurotic disorders (Rucker et al., 2018), particularly depression: ketamine/K (Walsh et al., 2022); LSD (Varley et al., 2019); MDMA (De Gregorio et al., 2021); mescaline (Vamvakopoulou et al., 2022); and psilocybin (Nutt et al., 2020). In particular, low dose K can treat TR MDD (Lai et al., 2014; George et al., 2017; Machado-Vieira et al., 2008), GAD and SAD (Shadli et al., 2018b; Glue et al., 2011; Glue et al., 2017; Glue et al., 2019), OCD (Rodriguez et al., 2013), SP, and PTSD (Feder et al., 2014a). K acts within hours (Zarate et al., 2013), to reduce symptoms including suicidal ideation and loss of life (DiazGranados et al., 2010). We discuss the implications for treatment further in Chapter 14.

13.2.3 Trait synergy, the double-hit hypothesis

We (McNaughton and Glue, 2020) have recently proposed a 'double-hit' hypothesis of neurotic disorder based on these data. As shown in Fig. 13.3, a range of historical factors can be viewed as promoting a high level of neuroticism that, by itself, does not constitute disorder. This combines with, e.g. high trait panic and environmental trigger factors to generate psychiatric disorder (§13.4.4; note that in this context we treat pure 'irritable heart syndrome' as not constituting a psychiatric disorder). The nature of the neurotic disorder will be determined both by the levels of trait anxiety (in the sense of trait GIS sensitivity), trait panic, trait obsession, and trait depression and by the nature of generally available trigger stimuli.

On this view anxiolytic-sensitive trait GIS sensitivity will interact with current neuroticism to generate a high level of anxious symptoms that can, in a proportion of cases, be reduced with anxiolytic treatment (either selective or with, e.g. SSRIs). The selective anxiolytics and SSRIs act on supporting processes (§13.2.5) that, when reduced, allow the amplification of fear by anxiety (Fig. 5.1) to extinguish over time. Our hypothesis is that ketamine (and likely other psychedelics) acts directly on neuroticism to alter threat perception immediately. We discuss the pharmacology of these effects in Chapter 14.

A similar explanation would apply to the effect of panicolytics (e.g. SSRIs, by reducing trait panic) on panic, and to the effect of non-panicolytic antidepressants (e.g. buspirone, by reducing trait depression) on depression. A key point here is the conventional drugs act on processes that generate and support disorder (potentially initially via aversive memory

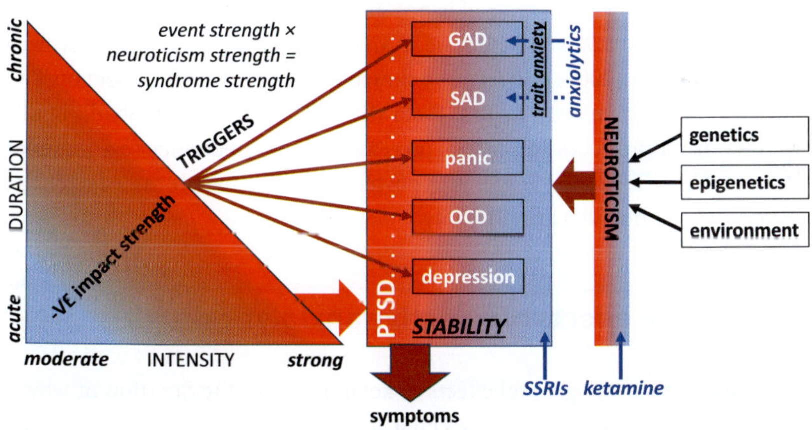

Fig. 13.3 Diagrammatic representation of the 2-hit hypothesis for disorders known to be affected by ketamine. Disorder is held to result when high neuroticism (resulting from genetic, epigenetic, and prior environmental factors) is combined with a high level of a specific trait linked to GAD, SAD, panic, OCD, or depression. High levels of these specific traits can be triggered by moderate chronic or strong acute stress. In the latter case PTSD may result. Specific anxiolytic drugs affect the specific trait linked to GAD and to a lesser extent SAD (see Table [4.1]). SSRIs act on a background higher order trait of 'stability' (DeYoung, 2006), which would not be specific to aversive events (Carver et al., 2008) and which would slowly alter the specific trait levels §12.8.2. Ketamine acts to affect neuroticism §12.5 and so alters the disordered expression of all the specific traits. Figure and legend adapted from McNaughton and Glue (2020) with permission.

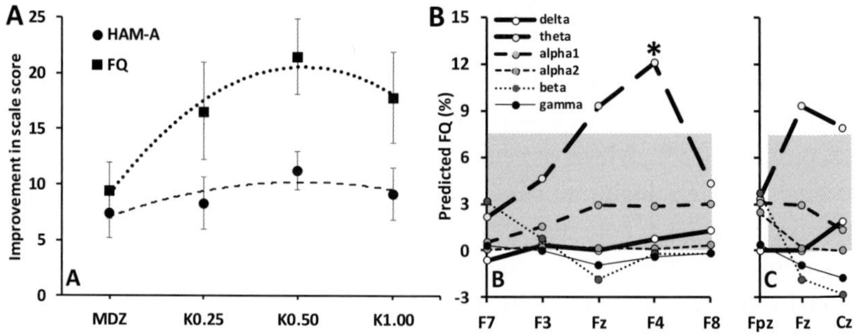

Fig. 13.4 Predose vs postdose improvements in scale scores. (A) Variation with ketamine dose (K, mg) relative to midazolam (MDZ) for Fear (FQ) and Hamilton Anxiety (HAM-A) Questionnaires subjected to separate analyses. Curves are linear + quadratic trend lines (significant for FQ but not HAM-A). Bars are ±SEM and are approximately equal (2.5 vs 2.2, respectively) for the 2 questionnaires in the case of MDZ. (B) Correlation of FQ change with power change in different frequency bands at different electrode sites. Values are signed (±) percent of variance accounted for ($r^2 \times 100$). Height of the grey zone represents the 95% CI uncorrected for multiple comparisons. *Significant effect within stepwise regression ($P < .05$).

formation and subsequently via failed habituation or extinction of aversion) and may be ineffective if support is not required once disorder is generated.

We must also enter a caveat as to ketamine's actions. We can be taken to have implied, with GAD and SAD, that ketamine itself is not 'anxiolytic' in our usual use of the word but, rather, is anti-neurotic. However, ketamine is anxiolytic in our standard reticular-elicited theta model (Engin et al., 2009) and we have shown that its therapeutic effect on TR anxiety is linked to changes only in right frontal theta rhythmicity (Fig. 13.4; Shadli et al., 2018a) despite the fact that it produces substantial increases in high frequency (e.g. gamma) power and decreases in low frequency (e.g. delta) power. This may match the effects of selective anxiolytics on right frontal theta rhythmicity.

13.2.4 Cognitive effects of selective anxiolytic drugs

The immediate and neurotic-general effects of ketamine raise the question of why selective anxiolytics are slow to act and selective. First let us consider the cognitive changes that underlie the effects of the drugs. Then, in the next sections, we will consider their neural effects.

We have already emphasized the fact that the behavioural effects of SHS damage are massively similar to those of the anxiolytics (Appendix 8, Chapters 4 and 6). But there are many tasks (often of most theoretical significance) for which we have data on lesions or drugs but not both. In particular, hippocampal damage in human beings is characterized by amnesia. As we have noted already, anxiety disorder could result from excessive consolidation of fear memories and anxiolytic action could result from enhanced extinction or habituation. But, how far do anxiolytic doses of the drugs affect memory tasks?

High doses of benzodiazepines used as preoperative medication do produce an apparent amnesia but this could be due to sedative or other non-specific effects (McGaughy and Sarter, 1995). Nonetheless, lower doses also suggest that 'the benzodiazepines might simulate, or model, the form of memory dysfunction . . . that is expressed in the typical amnesic patient. . . . [Further,] the sedative and memory impairing effects of benzodiazepines can be dissociated from one another' (Danion et al., 1993, p. 373; Huron et al., 2001; Curran, 1991). These effects appear to be on the capacity to acquire information (Vidailhet et al., 1994). There is also, now, reason to see $5HT_{1A}$ agonists as having amnestic properties (Coray and Quednow, 2022).

In animals, as discussed in Chapter 4, anxiolytics, including buspirone, produce hippocampal-like impairments in the acquisition (but not performance) of the water maze task (McNaughton and Morris, 1987; McNaughton and Morris, 1992). We have also shown that chlordiazepoxide produces a deficit in delayed conditional discrimination (Tan et al., 1990) of the same form as that produced by Alzheimer's disease in delayed matching to sample (Money et al., 1992). $5HT_{1A}$ agonists (unlike classical anxiolytics) do not impair delayed matching to sample (Cole et al., 1994; compare with Cole and Hillmann, 1994), it may be that the amnestic effects of these drugs are more limited even than those of the classical anxiolytics. At least with the benzodiazepines, animal tests suggest 'that the anxiolytic and amnestic effects . . . are closely related' (Graeff et al., 1993, p. 67). However, with long-term, high-dose use, diazepam can have effects on human memory even when its effects on anxiety are no longer evident (Weess et al., 1994).

In sum, anxiolytics produce at least mild hippocampal-like changes in mnemonic function. Consistent with the appearance of theta activity throughout the hippocampal formation and the action of the drugs on theta activity, these effects extend to the more stimulus-oriented tasks which, in the theory, depend more on entorhinal cortex than on hippocampus proper. Thus, the effects of anxiolytic drugs appear to be nearly as 'wide' as those of large SHS lesions, but they are not so 'deep'.

13.2.5 SHS effects of anxiolytic drugs

We have already noted that the action of anxiolytic drugs on the SHS is 'partial' in a quantitative rather than qualitative sense. That is, we see anxiolytic drugs as affecting the SHS through their disruption of the control of theta activity. This disruption will affect all levels of the SHS, since all receive theta input. Indeed, we have defined the SHS as that set of structures which receive this input. However, the disruption cannot be equated with total hippocampal dysfunction. First, anxiolytic drugs do not eliminate theta activity, they merely alter aspects of its control (Appendix 5). Second, even elimination of theta activity does not eliminate all hippocampal processing (Appendix 9). Anxiolytic drug action, therefore, produces a modest, albeit global, dysfunction of the SHS that we view as a reduction in the *acuity* of hippocampal processing. This suggests that one possible source of pathological anxiety is an increase in such acuity, or in some other process which contributes to excessive functional output from the SHS, producing a dysfunctionally high increase in negative cognitive bias.

Inasmuch, then, as the SHS is involved in cognitive and memorial processing (Bannerman et al., 2014; Bannerman et al., 2004b), a consequence of our theory is that *pathological* anxiety itself is likely to result, at least in some cases, from abnormal cognitive and mnemonic processing (McNaughton, 1997). As we consider in more detail shortly, this brings the anxiety aspects of our theory quite close to cognitive theories of generalized anxiety (Mathews, 1993; Eysenck, 1992b; Eysenck et al., 2022). 'Cognitive dysfunction' suggests affective neutrality and a focusing of hippocampal processing on cortical information. But when emergency threatens, the messages received from older structures located in the brainstem take precedence and a fundamentally cognitive dysfunction can have, nonetheless, affective consequences. Importantly, we have argued (§9.9.2) that SHS control of memory depends on parallel 'Papez loops' through the hypothalamus.

> These hypothalamic loops supplement direct hippocampal–cortical connections with iterative reprocessing paced by theta rhythmicity.... recirculation in these loops progressively enhances desired connections, while reducing interference from competing external goals and internal associations. This increases the signal-to-noise ratio in the distributed engrams (neocortical and cerebellar) necessary for complex learning and memory. *The hypothalamic nodes provide key motivational input for engram enhancement during consolidation.*
>
> (McNaughton and Vann, 2022, p. 550; added emphasis)

13.2.6 Anxiolytic action and the amygdala and insula

As detailed in Chapter 6 (and Appendix 8), there is no evidence that SHS lesions, unlike anxiolytics, eliminate the increment in arousal elicited by conditioned aversive stimuli (Dickinson, 1974). With fear-potentiated startle, the anxiolytics (both novel and classical) act directly on the amygdala; while SHS lesions have no effect (McNish et al., 1997). So, the amygdala (and insula, §11.8.1) implements the 'increase arousal' output of the GIS, unlike the 'increase goal inhibition/decision' output produced by the SHS.

On this view, pure fear and pure frustration (the 'purity' arising in each case because of lack of a conflicting approach tendency) would often involve activity in the amygdala (with different patterns of amygdala activity distinguishing these, and all other emotions); resolution of goal conflicts would often involve functional output from the SHS; and anxiety (where pure fear or pure frustration is contaminated with conflict) would equate with activity in the amygdala concurrent with output from the SHS.

Thus, neither SHS nor amygdala/insula output by themselves can be totally identified with anxiety. Indeed, our model is of goal conflict control systems that span from the PAG to the PFC (Fig. 11.14) for the control of both decision and arousal; with a similar organization for the control of attraction and repulsion as well.

13.2.7 Anxiolytic action and the neocortex

We have related a certain type of interaction of the SHS and amygdala/insula to anxiety, but is this type (based on survival circuits) perhaps just one of the rules of thumb contributing to anxiety? This is indeed likely to be the case. We have distinguished 'anxiety' from 'fear' as being the cases where the animal must enter into, as opposed to exit from, a dangerous situation (Chapters 2, 3). Entry clearly involves risk analysis, anticipation, and many other complex processes. Further, anxiety can derive as easily from the anticipation of loss as from the anticipation of pain; and can result simply from the presence of uncertainty. Again, this suggests complex neural organization. Finally, a primary feature of anxiety is the role played by the *anticipation* of both appetitive and aversive events and the need to trade the one off against the other. This suggests that some cases of anxiety could involve the highest levels of the nervous system including computed projections into the future.

Note a key architectural feature of our systems. These are all hierarchically organized with 'quick and dirty' components at the bottom and 'slow and sophisticated' components at the top. We have already included higher areas, such as orbital frontal, posterior cingulate, and insular cortex as involved in anxiety. We know that at least some prefrontal forms of goal conflict processing are affected by anxiolytic drugs (Shadli et al., 2021a) as is arousal in the insula (Paulus et al., 2005), we have now achieved a preliminary prefrontal neurology of anxiety (Fig. 11.14), the finer details of which are determined by our theory of the SHS (Chapter 10).

13.3 Defensive symptom clusters

With current diagnostic systems, symptom clusters are used as the basis for, usually categorical, diagnosis. Particularly in §13.5 we will explain why we think there is only a weak connection between syndromes and symptoms. Our ultimate goal is the equivalent of diagnosing COVID-19 by identifying the SARS-Cov-2 virus, while noting the variability of its symptom presentation and their overlap with the symptoms of a range of corona and influenza viruses. But before testing for COVID-19, you need to have an idea of the symptomatology of these many respiratory viruses. So, here we look at clusters of symptoms and roughly categorize them with the current diagnostic labels.

13.3.1 Behavioural aspects of defensive syndromes

We will describe panic in considerable detail in §13.5. It is not accompanied by any characteristic active behaviour, with most reported symptoms being internal.

Behaviourally, the chief symptom of the phobias is repulsion from the phobic stimulus. If this repulsion is to be classified as pathological, the phobic stimulus should be one that is not objectively dangerous or any avoidance behaviour should be incapacitating.

In a few cases, the phobic stimulus may be idiosyncratic (e.g. cats, a special pattern of wallpaper) and is likely to depend heavily on a specific conditioning history. In many cases, however, the phobic stimulus will evoke fear or anxiety (but not at a level which produces behavioural incapacity) in the healthy population (e.g. spiders, snakes, heights). Here, it can be argued that there is some degree of evolved preparedness (Mineka and Öhman, 2002; Öhman and Mineka, 2001; see McNally, 2016 for recent overview). In most cases of simple phobia, the disorder appears to lie in the unusual magnitude of the fear reaction rather than in any peculiarity of its intrinsic nature or eliciting stimulus.

We argue later that phobia proper should be categorically distinguished from anxiety. In that context, agoraphobia (avoidance of public places) and what used to be termed social phobia are particularly crippling and might seem at first glance to be only extreme and generalized forms of simple phobia.

However, there is now good reason to view 'social phobia' as a quite distinct subtype of anxiety (Mattick, 1990) and, the recent DSM-5-TR, has even removed 'Social Phobia' as an alternate term for 'Social Anxiety' (American Psychiatric Association, 2022; see https://www.psychiatry.org/File Library/Psychiatrists/Practice/DSM/DSM-5-TR/APA-DSM5TR-SocialAnxietyDisorder.pdf).

Similarly, while there are specific place phobias that appear to be simple phobias with a specific place as the phobic object, they should not be confused with generalized agoraphobia. We argue later that agoraphobia, as has happened with 'social phobia', would be better named 'agoranxiety'.

Obsessions (described more fully in the next section) and compulsions appear initially as occasional intrusions into the mental and behavioural life of an individual who perceives them as irrational. The disease is progressive, with an increasing frequency of occurrence of symptoms, and these ultimately become socially incapacitating. In the majority of cases there is a ritual behavioural act ('compulsion') that seems reasonable except in its frequency. The washing of hands to avoid infection is an example: it is the *repetition* for hours on end (to the point sometimes of producing severe dermatitis) that appears unreasonable, not any single act of washing (especially in a COVID environment). It should be emphasized that the compulsive behaviour does not itself constitute anxiety. Indeed, it has been argued (e.g. Rapoport, 1989) that both obsessions and compulsions are the result of a disorder of higher order motor control programs (§6.7), not unlike the disordered simple movements which are symptoms of neurological syndromes such as Huntington's chorea. *Prevention* of the compulsive ritual, however, gives rise to a sharp increase in the subjective experience and physiological signs of anxiety (Röper and Rachman, 1976). Despite the increase in anxiety, response prevention can be used as a behavioural means of controlling compulsive behaviour. But this technique seems much less successful in controlling the associated obsessions. It is a moot point whether the obsessions and compulsions are the result of anxiety, which they effectively decrease, or whether the anxiety is simply the consequence of failure to achieve safety required by the obsession. An everyday ritual such as locking your front door is likely to be performed in a habitual fashion, with no cognitive or bodily signs of anxiety. It is only when you realize that you have forgotten to lock the door (or you are prevented from locking it) that you feel anxious.

13.3.2 Cognitive aspects of defensive syndromes

The cognitive aspects of simple phobias are not dramatic. In practice, they often boil down to the self-report of fear or anxiety, or just a tick in an adjective check list. A problem, here, is that these reports are seldom obtained at the height of an intense attack.

By contrast, OCD has a rich cognitive phenomenology. Obsessions consist of 'intrusive, repetitive thoughts, images or impulses that are unacceptable and/or unwanted and give rise to subjective resistance; the person finds them difficult to dismiss or control' (Rachman, 1978). Given the relative ease with which compulsions can be suppressed and the relatively refractory nature of obsessions, it is possible that the latter constitute the primary aspect of the disorder. Rapoport's (1989) view that the obsessions are a high-level motor disorder is tantamount to the idea that a belief (e.g. that one is dirty) is a high level of motor command. The analogy is with choreic movements. These are spontaneously occurring, isolated elements of normal movements that occur as the result of neurological abnormality in the basal ganglia. In a similar manner, Rapoport views obsessions as the spontaneous occurrence of isolated elements of normal planning, including the accompanying cognitions.

Panic according to DSM-5[2] involves 'an abrupt surge of intense fear or intense discomfort that reaches a peak within minutes' with symptoms including cardiac, autonomic, respiratory, abdominal, and heat sensations; with fear of 'going crazy' or dying. This is covered in more detail in §13.5; with the role of cognition covered particularly in §13.5.7.

Generalized anxiety disorder, in contrast to all of the aforementioned, can be viewed as anxiety, the level of which is out of proportion to the level of any perceived sources of threat. It is, in a sense, anxiety looking for a threat to perceive rather than anxiety resulting from a perceived threat; and 'during the course of the disorder, the focus of worry may shift from one concern to another' (DSM-IV; American Psychiatric Association, 1994, p. 433), p. 433). Earlier suggestions that this involves dysfunction of cognitive, particularly working memory, *systems* (Eysenck and Calvo, 1992; Eysenck, 1992b), or the control of attentional resources (Mathews and MacLeod, 1994; Mathews et al., 2004), evolved into Attentional Control Theory (Eysenck et al., 2007; Eysenck and Derakshan, 2011), which distinguishes between performance effectiveness and processing efficiency. ACT holds

> that high levels of trait anxiety[3] impair processing efficiency more than performance effectiveness, because individuals who experience high levels of anxiety often utilise compensatory strategies or mechanisms to overcome inefficiency caused by non-task processing, without concomitant performance improvement' via an interaction between goal control in the Fronto-Parietal Network and salience control in the Cingular Opercula Network.
>
> (Eysenck et al., 2022, p. 2).

Interestingly, a study of young adults with an extensive neuropsychological battery found that 'despite substantial psychopathological burden, GAD exhibited intact cognitive functioning. These results support the Cognitive Control Theory of Anxiety, suggesting that elevated primary anxiety may not impact 'cold' cognitive functions in the absence of threat or substantial cognitive load' (Leonard and Abramovitch, 2019, p. 1). This fits with the idea that, within ACT, the Default Mode Network (and particularly the posterior cingulate cortex) generates 'perseverative cognition such as worry and rumination, i.e. difficult to control negative thoughts that are a key cognitive component of anxiety' (Eysenck et al., 2022, p. 3)[3]. While the cognitive processes we invoke are different and our use of 'anxiety' more restricted, our theory has much in common with these views, sharing in particular the idea that generalized anxiety is primarily a cognitive disorder that engages emotion-linked circuits (McNaughton and Vann, 2022).

As a final general note on the cognitive front, in all the anxiety-related disorders there is a tendency to attend particularly strongly to environmental stimuli or events that the patient finds particularly threatening. Thus, in panic disorder, the patient is particularly aware of bodily change, e.g. increased heart rate or feelings of breathlessness, which they interpret as signs of impending illness or death; or, in social phobia, patients tend, when anticipating a

[2] https://www.ncbi.nlm.nih.gov/books/NBK519704/table/ch3.t10/

[3] Note that all uses of 'anxiety' by Michael Eysenck are the broader DSM-related meaning not our restricted selective-anxiolytic-sensitive meaning. Note re-use of this footnote below.

social interaction, selectively to 'retrieve negative information about how they may appear to others' (Clark, 1997), especially in the form of negative images of themselves as seen from an outside observer's perspective (Hackmann et al., 1998). This pattern of enhanced attention to threatening stimuli (Mathews and MacLeod, 1994; Mathews and MacLeod, 2005) is, of course, exactly what would be predicted as a consequence of excessive activity in the GIS, since one of the major outputs of this system has just this function. There is evidence that this processing bias is causally related to vulnerability to disorders (Mathews and MacLeod, 2005) and that it can be altered to reduce negative emotion (Hertel and Mathews, 2011).

13.3.3 Physiological aspects of defensive syndromes

In all the defensive syndromes, and with approach-avoidance decisions, there are easily detectable peripheral physiological signs: raised skin conductance with an increased rate of spontaneous fluctuations in conductance level, changed heart rate, increased blood flow, etc. (Lader, 1975; Livermore et al., 2021). When panic attacks are present, there is a chronically raised level of activity in the autonomic nervous system between as well as during attacks (Lader and Wing, 1966; Lader, 1967). Some chronically raised autonomic activity is also seen in social but not simple phobia (Lader, 1967), although in this condition increased responsiveness of the autonomic system to simple physiological challenge may be more important than the increased level of anxiety *per se* (Stein et al., 1994a). There are also parallel changes in autonomic, subjective, and behavioural measures linked to rumination and worry (Cristina, 2018).

13.4 Elements of a theory of defensive disorders

13.4.1 A functional typology for defence

In this section we make explicit the typology of defence, and hence defensive disorders, that has been implicit since our adoption of the Blanchards' analysis of defensive distance, Graeff and Deakin's views on the hierarchical organization of defence systems, and LeDoux's views on the hierarchical organization of the neural systems that detect the adequate stimuli for defence (Chapters 2, 6). We first emphasize the categorical division of threat stimuli, which can be made on purely functional grounds. This is shown in Fig. 13.5 (derived from Fig. 2.3). Threat in general can be divided into two basic types, each with different, indeed in some cases opposed, functional requirements: actual present threat which must be avoided (e.g. the cat in the Blanchards' experiments) and potential threat which must be approached (e.g. the smell of the cat coupled with the smell of cheese). Each of these, in turn, can be divided into two subtypes, with different (and again opposed) functional requirements: avoidable threat and unavoidable threat.

Each of the four resultant categories can be related to different types of required and, in the Blanchards' analysis, actual behaviour. Actual unavoidable threat, for example, can give rise to undirected escape behaviour or explosive attack (!FIGHT). Actual avoidable threat can give rise to directed escape behaviour or active avoidance. Potential avoidable threat can give rise to active risk assessment. Potential unavoidable threat can lead to a suppression of active coping strategies and a conservation of resources. These different functional classes and, to a lesser extent, the behaviour patterns elicited by them, can be mapped as shown in Fig. 13.5, to the emotions of panic, fear, anxiety and depression (though we do not deal with the latter in this book). (For a detailed discussion of the relation between such functional classes and the output of skeletal, autonomic, and hormonal systems, see McNaughton, 1989b). There are two additional categories in the table that can be viewed as special cases of unavoidable actual threat and avoidable potential threat, respectively. First, a weak predator may be definitely present and unavoidable in the sense of flight, but may be perceived as avoidable if attacked. This results in activation of aggression, similar to the attack of an avoidable conspecific when experiencing pain. Second, a potential source of danger (e.g. infection) may be avoidable in the sense that some action can be taken (e.g. hand washing), but there may be no explicit threat stimuli to indicate that the potential danger is present; or, once action has been taken, no explicit safety signals to indicate that it has in fact been avoided. This results in activation of rituals which attempt to anticipate the potential danger.

We see the adaptive emotions of panic, fear, and anxiety as also mapping to the pathological conditions of panic disorder, phobia, and generalized anxiety disorder, respectively. Finally, we attribute the *symptoms* of panic to activity in the PAG, of phobia to activity in the hypothalamus and amygdala, of anxiety to activity in the SHS and amygdala, of obsession to activity in the cingulate cortex, and of compulsion to activity in the basal ganglia. We also attribute what we term below the *primary* disorders of panic, phobia etc to pathological (in the psychological and functional, but not necessarily neurological sense) hyperactivity in these same brain areas. But note that, as explained in §13.5, these latter distinctions do not map neatly onto current clinical classifications.

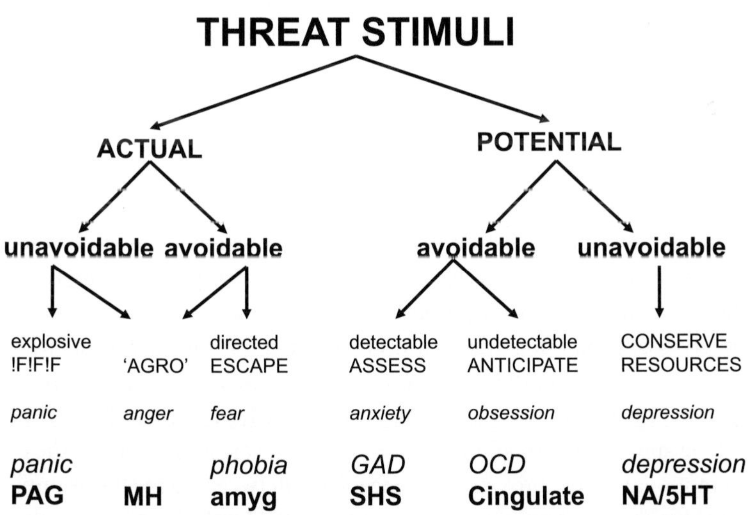

Fig. 13.5 Nature of stimuli (bolded, top three rows) and their relation to function (unbolded capitals), emotion (small italics), psychological disorder (large italics), and principal neural system involved (bottom row).!F!F!F, explosive fight, undirected flight, freezing as opposed to defensive quiescence—all functioning to prevent death/disaster; 'agro', non-explosive aggression; amyg, amygdala; GAD, generalized anxiety disorder; MH, medial hypothalamus; NA, noradrenaline; OCD, obsessive-compulsive disorder; PAG, periaqueductal grey; SHS, septo-hippocampal system; 5HT, 5-hydroxytryptamine. For further details see text.

Now suppose for the moment, that we have to deal with only the specific cases of panic, fear, obsession, and anxiety. There are many who will be happy with the idea of distinguishing between these cases insofar as they refer to symptoms. However, the suggestion that it should be possible to distinguish between them categorically at the syndrome level may seem, especially to clinicians, a gross oversimplification. One further theory-driven step needs to be taken before we can bring this typology into contact with clinical reality. This step will show that the apparent problem arises from the fact that we must distinguish very carefully between symptoms and syndromes. But how can this be, if we identify, as we did in the previous paragraph, *symptoms* with activity in specific brain structures, and *syndromes* with hyperactivity in those same brain structures?

The key, in our opinion, to a deeper understanding of anxiety and other defensive disorders is the recognition that the various neural structures that control defensive behaviour are strongly and recursively interconnected both neurally and through environmental consequences. This property has already been shown to be important in terms of inhibitory interactions, as in the case of Graeff's explanation of relaxation-induced panic as arising from opposite interactions of 5HT systems with amygdala-controlled fear and PAG-controlled panic (Chapter 6). However, it is even more important when we consider the various possible *positive* feedback interactions. In addition to the specific processing that goes with the need to evaluate and react to specific threatening stimuli, activation of any part of the defence system increases overall arousal and activity in the aminergic attentional systems, and hence the sensitivity of all of the elements of the entire distributed network with which we are dealing. This provides a route, for example, for fear or anxiety to produce a level of arousal sufficient to induce a panic attack as a result of the effective decrease in defensive distance (as defined by the Blanchards, see Chapter 2).

The particular cases we consider in most detail next are those in which the prevention of compulsive rituals engenders an anxiety that was not previously evident, and those in which spontaneous panic attacks can elicit anxiety through conditioning. Neural recursive interactions can be presumed to operate similarly in both normal and pathological anxiety. The environmentally mediated ones are likely, however, to be most obtrusive in pathological anxiety. In any case, in most real-life situations, the available stimuli will not in fact be selective for just one of the distinct functional categories we have been considering. The rabbit that sees a fox coming towards it does not necessarily know whether the fox has seen it. Thus, while the presence of the fox is definite and actual, the threat presented by the fox must be treated as having simultaneously the properties of *both* actual *and* potential threat. Thus, *both* fear *and* anxiety goal processing systems will be primed for intense action (with activation of anxiety systems amplifying the activation of fear systems). Likewise, there will be cases (as with a parent and a child in a dangerous situation) where both anxiety and compulsive checking will be appropriate. In all these cases, then, we can see reason for the co-existence of multiple emotional states and for positive feedback between them (for example, the more anxiety-provoking the situation, the greater should be the level of compulsive checking). It is this tendency towards functional co-existence of several adaptive emotional states that, we believe, provides part of the basis for the comorbidity of the different anxiety disorders. The biasing of all these systems by a common underlying personality variable (Chapter 12) provides another part.

These considerations explain the difficulties faced in the diagnosis of anxiety disorders: a specific 'pathological' symptom can arise either because of pathology of its specific controlling centre, or because of changed activity in that centre secondary to pathology in some other part of the distributed defence control network (§13.4). Given that, at least in human beings, display rules can greatly modify the external signs of emotion and that conditioning can alter the internal signs, it follows that pathology in a specific neural centre may give rise to a cluster of symptoms, and that those over which the given neural centre has the most direct control will not necessarily even be the most salient. We consider these possibilities in more detail in relation to individual symptomatological and diagnostic categories next.

A final necessary distinction, before moving on to these diagnostic categories, is that between anxiety itself and the other defensive disorders. To a large extent, we next argue that pathological anxiety is a specific delimited condition to be distinguished from pathological panic, phobia, and obsession. On the other hand, we see it as reasonable to group all these conditions together as neurotic disorders since (i) the symptoms show a high level of co-occurrence, and the syndromes high levels of comorbidity; (ii) in the cases of panic and obsession *comorbid* anxiety is a significant feature of their presentation in the clinic; and (iii) they all respond to ketamine (§13.2.2, §13.2.3).

13.4.2 The theory of anxiety

We began the task of constructing a theory of anxiolytic-sensitive anxiety armed, at the psychological level, with an ethological dissection of defence (Chapter 2). This distinguished immediate from potential threat, the latter mapping onto the learning-theory concept of behavioural inhibition (Chapter 3). The ethological analysis will prove important for the way in which we deal with comorbidity, and also for its functional equation of innate and acquired anxiety stimuli. But it is the learning-theory concept of behavioural inhibition (which we now refer to as goal inhibition to distinguish it from simple stopping) that is fundamental to our view of anxiety as such. This concept was based largely on the results of purely behavioural experiments (Gray, 1975), although the behavioural effects of anxiolytic drugs also played a role in its early development (Gray, 1967; Gray, 1977). Most of this book has been concerned with updating a detailed analysis of the neural structures subserving the various functions allotted to the GIS. But even in this latest edition, it has become necessary to define more sharply and deeply the *psychological* content of the cncepts underlying not only the GIS, but also GRS/!FFFS, and GAS. This fruitful interaction is fundamental to the power of the super-discipline of behavioural neuroscience, where each discipline (psychology, physiology, pharmacology, neurology, anatomy, molecular biology etc.) can force changes, keeping each other honest.

Both the ethological analysis of Chapter 2 and the psychological developments enforced by the neural details of our theory have had the consequence that the original model of the Behavioural Inhibition System (Gray, 1975; 1982) has undergone considerable evolution—although the major postulates that it encapsulated have not been abandoned. This system can still be regarded as responding to stimuli that warn of negative reinforcers, stimuli that warn of omission of positive reinforcers, novel stimuli and innate anxiety stimuli. These form a general functional class of stimuli that warn of potential negative affective events when the organism has some reason to approach them. Importantly, it is the *evaluation* of such stimuli that is critical to their effect, in non-humans as well as humans; and so, we must take into account the highest-level cognitive mechanisms, many of which will show homology across species (see Chapter 8, §8.1.3). Despite this, we can still characterize the outputs of the GIS as increased inhibition of ongoing behaviour, increased attention to environmental stimuli, and increased arousal. To clarify how anxiety constitutes 'activity in the GIS', we must first revisit the theory of the SHS developed in Chapter 10.

As argued there, the SHS compares, quite generally, currently primed goals with each other and with expectations. An individual goal is defined by its situation and motivation and entails a concatenated set of subgoals.

> 'In order to move along the temporo-spatial gradient to the [goal], it is necessary … to engage in sub-goal scaffolding. This process consists of (a) identifying the biological reinforcer, (b) planning behaviour, and (c) executing the plan (i.e., "problem solving") at each stage of the temporo-spatial gradient – this is in accordance with the type of cognitive operations first discussed by Miller et al. (1960)'
>
> (Corr, 2008a, p. 21)

So long as there is no goal conflict, the system does nothing directly to influence ongoing behaviour. But that does not mean it is inactive. On the contrary, it is kept extremely busy, receiving information from a variety of areas primarily concerned with the processing of stimuli, or with the programming of responses, but which all have in common the capacity to direct the upcoming behaviour of the animal. In this comparator or monitoring capacity ('just checking') the GIS is continuously active (as shown by single-cell or slow-wave recording in the hippocampus); but it only produces functionally significant output, and hence controls behaviour, under special conditions. These conditions ('conflict') are those where multiple strongly activated incompatible goals are primed, either because an unpredicted environmental event occurs, or because a predicted event fails to occur, or because there are equal incompatible tendencies (approach/avoidance is the most important for the current chapter, but approach/approach or avoidance/avoidance are also possible).

Conflict between goals causes the GIS to enter 'control mode' and at once interrupts ongoing motor behaviour via its input to the stopping system (Fig. 11.8). This interruption gave rise to the initial concept of the 'Behavioural Inhibition System'. Of particular importance for our understanding of anxiety, not only is behaviour addressed to the current prepotent goal inhibited, but the situation (the stimuli associated with that goal) is tagged 'faulty' and called in for careful inspection (§9.9.2; Fig. 9.9). The 'faulty' tag has the theoretically crucial effect of increasing the negative affective bias of stimulus assessment mechanisms (Fig. 10.4), allowing resolution of the conflict by the resultant inhibition of those positive goals with the greatest negative goal associations. Thus, when the stimuli next occur (and activate the representation of the positive and negative goals), approach behaviour is interrupted so that the system can determine whether alternative programs lead to more satisfactory outcomes. 'Determine' here is used in a distributed sense. In fact, conflict causes the SHS to send very simple feedback signals to the various systems, each of which could potentially take control of behaviour (e.g. Fig. 9.9). These feedback signals increase the valence of affectively negative associations and will reduce the level of activity (priming) in those areas with the greatest negative associations. In many cases this will be sufficient to leave one area with significantly greater priming than the others, and this will then take control. If iterative interaction between the different goal representations and the SHS (§9.9.2) does not fairly swiftly produce a clear winner, the system itself generates exploratory and investigative behaviour (risk analysis), especially checking for sources of environmental threat. As noted in §13.2.6, an important detail is that while the business of the SHS is the resolution of conflict between goals in a decision-making sense, particularly with defensive conflict there will be concurrent activity in both the SHS and amygdala to increase arousal.

A valuable perspective on the clinical situation is provided by the pharmacotherapy of anxiety and defensive disorders (Table 4.1). As we have seen, classical and novel anxiolytics share neither direct receptor actions nor panicolytic main effects nor side effects. Their only common clinical action is on anxiety. Comparison of the effects of these chemically quite different types of drugs gives us, then, a scalpel with which to dissect anxiety from other defensive reactions. Thus, panic disorder proper is not affected by buspirone (despite its anxiolytic and antidepressant actions) and so can no longer be equated with the anxiety that often accompanies it, exacerbates it, or produces it §13.4. Atypical depression (with its anxiety-like somatic symptoms) cannot be equated with anxiety, since it is insensitive to the benzodiazepines; the same is true of major depression since it is insensitive to pregabalin and low potency benzodiazepines (Table 4.1). OCD can be viewed, like panic, as a condition that both gives rise to and is exacerbated by anxiety, but which is nonetheless pharmacologically distinct, as shown by drugs such as clomipramine that are particularly effective at treating it, in contrast to imipramine (Rapoport, 1989). Finally, because they are insensitive to anxiolytic drugs, we can treat specific phobias as being correctly named for pure fear rather than anxiety.

At a more general, psychological level, our analysis leads to the conclusion that, in the core state of anxiety from which panic, phobias, obsessions, and compulsions have been stripped out, the central dysfunction consists in hyperactivity or hyper-re-activity in the GIS, i.e. in the interlinked set of neural structures that mediate the functions of this system, as outlined above. Conversely, disorders of panic, phobias, obsessions, and depression will result from hyperactivity or hyper-re-activity in their own base systems. That said, on the current evidence, we believe that for defensive disorders to be psychiatrically problematic (see discussion of adaptive panic in §13.4) they will also require concurrent high levels of neuroticism and/or worry (§13.2.3; see also §2.8 on rumination, obsession, and worry).

13.4.3 Clinical anxiety and memory

Resolution of conflict, then, is at the core of the theory of the SHS; and defensive conflict is at the core of the application of the GIS theory to anxiety. But we need also to look at the connection between anxiety (where we started the book) and memory (a key destination to which the hippocampal component of the theory took us).

A key fact is that the conventional drugs (selective anxiolytic and panicolytic) do not change the symptoms of pathological anxiety immediately. This appears to be true even of benzodiazepines, which mask the lack of an initial truly anxiolytic effect with muscle relaxant and euphoriant effects (Appendix 1). However, the common effects on the SHS of all classes of drug that have an anxiolytic action in their profile are immediate and show no change with repeated administration (Appendix 5). We conclude from this that the drugs block a mechanism that *creates and maintains* anxious symptomatology, and that the clinical delay results from the time taken to extinguish previously acquired patterns of ABCD. Thus, the 'faulty, needs checking' tag is akin to a memory mechanism consistent with current views of both the functions of the hippocampus (Chapter 8; see, e.g. Kubie et al., 2020; Sadeh and Pertzov, 2020) and of cognitive processes in generalized anxiety disorder (§13.3.2; Eysenck et al., 2022).

As argued in the previous section, anxiety results from overactivity in, or at least excessive functional output from, the SHS. This should lead to both increased risk assessment behaviour and an excessive negative bias in the assessment of goals, via excessive weighting of the negative associations of stimuli, often resulting in excessive tagging of goals as faulty or excessive creation of new negative goals (e.g. via reprocessing during sleep, Inostroza and Born, 2013).

As discussed in §13.3.2, contemporary cognitive theories of generalized anxiety disorder accept that there must be conflict before the relevant cognitive biases are displayed (Leonard and Abramovitch, 2019); and they include in those cognitive biases both increased attention to threatening stimuli and increased magnitude in the level of threat perceived in any particular stimulus that result in reduced processing efficiency via an interaction between goal control in the Fronto-Parietal Network and salience control in the Cingular Opercula Network (Eysenck et al., 2022). We would also emphasize that where a stimulus is ambiguous, having both threatening and nonthreatening aspects, the valence of the former aspects will be increased.

13.5 State, trait, and disorder—panic as an example

Let us now take a closer theoretically driven look at the neurology of Fig. 13.2 using a clinically oriented lens. We will start with the simplest forms of repulsion ('fear') working our way up the GRS to the more complex forms; then distinguish this from complex conflict resolution ('anxiety') and work our way back down the GIS. Anxiety, here, is necessarily more complex than fear, for any given level of the system, since it is generated by a conflict between attractors and the repulsors that engender fear and also has, as one of its outputs, the capacity to enhance repulsion/fear (and possibly reduce attraction).

For each aspect of defence, we will present an argument for a particular structure or group of structures having *activity* that underlies its state output, *re-activity* that underlies its trait sensitivity, and *hyper-re-activity* that (sometimes with other hyper-re-activities) underlies its disorder/s. In this section, we will take panic as the paradigm, simple case, and look in detail at state panic, trait panic, and direct and indirect disorders of panic control.

Following Graeff and others (§6.2) we identify panic attacks *per se* with activity in the PAG—while panic disorder involves additional areas such as the insula (see Graeff and Del-Ben, 2008). That said, the *cognitions reported* in relation to an attack must be mediated cortically, and much of the GRS contributes to full-blown panic disorder as this presents in the psychiatric clinic (Sobanski and Wagner, 2017). Likewise, descending connections from frontal areas provide a basis for complex cognitive processes to elicit an essentially primordial panic response mediated by the dorsomedial PAG. What conclusions does this identification allow us to draw about panic as a symptom and about 'panic disorder'? Further, we now see dorsolateral/external and ventrolateral PAG as generating defensive quiescence, a variant of freezing, that suggests there may be a distinct anxious form of what could still be termed panic §13.5.8. Note that in §13.5.1–13.5.7, wherever we use 'PAG' without qualification this should be read as dorsomedial PAG.

13.5.1 Simple state panic

Panic attacks will occur in healthy individuals under typical ecological circumstances when defensive distance is small and the fear stimulus intense. One particular stimulus, high CO_2 resulting in feelings of being suffocated or trapped,[4] and produces panic attacks in healthy controls with increasing rates at increasing doses (see Rassovsky and Kushner, 2003). This dose relationship and the relatively low number of healthy people experiencing panic under normal living conditions (~10%) suggests a normal distribution of adaptive trait panic in the healthy population. CO_2 has also been used extensively as a challenge to induce panic (at considerably higher rates) in panic disorder patients (see also §13.5.3).

Notably, CO_2 challenge can produce panic attacks and associated reports of 'fear' in humans with bilateral amygdala damage and, in particular, a patient who 'does not condition to aversive stimuli, fails to recognize fearful faces and demonstrates a marked absence of fear during exposure to a variety of fear-provoking stimuli, including life-threatening traumatic events' (Feinstein et al., 2013, p. 270). Thus, CO_2 challenge appears to produce panic attacks by a direct action on the PAG as does electrical stimulation (Iacono and Nashold, 1982).

13.5.2 Symptomatic state panic

There are also individuals whose sensitivity to panic stimuli is normal but who have a concurrent anxiety or phobic disorder and who, because this generates extreme arousal, experience an increased frequency of panic attacks. These individuals will often not be diagnosed as suffering from panic disorder as opposed to anxiety or phobic disorder, for example, but their symptoms would be superficially similar to those with comorbid panic disorder.

Such adaptive panic attacks can occur with apparent morbidity when there is no abnormality within the panic control system itself, but the PAG receives abnormally high input as a result of pathological activity elsewhere (Fig. 13.6; see also Graeff and Del-Ben, 2008). We have supposed that many components of the defensive system can be concurrently activated, and that activity can cascade between levels. Extremely high levels of fear (amygdala) or anxiety (SHS + amygdala) could, then, activate the PAG, breaking through the serotonergic inhibition that would normally keep it in check. Panic could also be elicited or have increased likelihood because of the increase in peripheral arousal produced by anxiety (Fig. 13.6, with effects similar to CO_2 and lactate). Thus, as suggested by Marks (1987), some cases presenting with panic attacks will simply be cases of extreme anxiety not of a disordered panic system. The parallel case in which extreme fear (i.e. repulsion without any conflicting attraction) might result in panic would not often present in the clinic since, under normal circumstances, the pathologically phobic patient will succeed in avoiding or escaping the fear stimulus and so not suffer from panic attacks.

[4] Lactate has similar physiological effects on, for example, pH and is similarly used as a panic challenge.

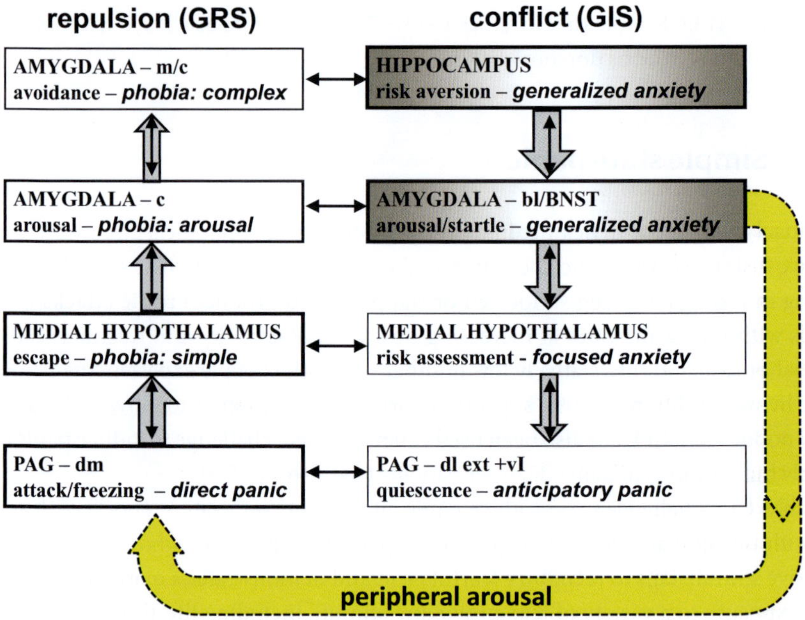

Fig. 13.6 Symptomatic panic with syndromal anxiety disorder. Abbreviations and symbols as in Fig. 13.2. Upper levels of the GIS (top right), show abnormal spontaneous activity (or hyper-reactivity) of the hippocampus, amygdala, or both, generating pathological generalised anxiety. Other aspects of anxiety are increased via existing descending neural connections (solid outline filled grey arrows) of the GIS (and also ascending connections, not shown). Increased peripheral arousal, e.g., levels of adrenaline, activates the PAG (dashed outline filled grey arrow) and generates panic attacks—particularly in panic prone individuals; and also produces a normal spread of neural activity through the GRS. Thus, abnormal anxiety can produce panic and fear that are normal given the level of perceived anticipatory threat generated by the pathological anxiety. Figure modified and updated from (McNaughton and Corr, 2016; McNaughton, 2005).

13.5.3 Trait panic and 'Irritable Heart Syndrome'

Now let us consider trait panic as a disorder representing an extreme of the normal trait (i.e. where there is a high number of panic attacks but not necessarily other symptoms). Note that, given this basis for trait panic disorder, it is theoretically possible for mild panic attacks to occur, despite the fact that 'mild panic' sounds like a contradiction in terms. A weak threat in a pathologically fearful or anxious person will produce an abnormally high input to the PAG and so panic appropriate to the pathological fear or anxiety *experienced* (Goisman et al., 1995). In this, we are close to the view of Marks (1988, p. 127) that a deficiency in DSM-IIIR was that it did not allow for the possibility that 'panics need not be so severe or abrupt in onset as to be called "panic" at the start'. This terminological problem was retained in DSM-5 (American Psychiatric Association, 2013): 'Panic attack—An abrupt surge of *intense fear or intense discomfort* that reaches a peak within minutes' and is unchanged in DSM-5-TR (American Psychiatric Association, 2022).[5]

[5] Extracted from https://www.ncbi.nlm.nih.gov/books/NBK519704/table/ch3.t10/ and https://www.psychiatry.org/psychiatrists/practice/dsm/educational-resources/dsm-5-tr-fact-sheets

Our focusing on the GRS in relation to panic attacks (and trait panic disorder) means that we distinguish (see also Okasha et al., 1994) panic itself (and hence panic disorder) from anxiety (and anxiety disorder). Certainly, the two are not necessarily linked: there are cases of panic attacks that occur only when the patient is asleep, but not when anxiety is experienced in the waking state (Rosenfeld and Furman, 1994); and also indications that panic disorder is associated with autonomic dysfunction (e.g. Yeragani et al., 1994), but no evidence for this with anxiety.

From a neurological point of view pure trait panic (including Marks's mild form) could result from dysfunction of the PAG itself, resulting in spontaneous panic attacks in the absence of any specific fear—or anxiety-provoking stimulus; or when such stimuli are weak. One can imagine two ways in which such trait panic disorder could arise.

First, is the production of spontaneous activity in the PAG via, for example, seizures. These could be focal (Dantendorfer et al., 1995b) or partial and focused in distal structures that then pass activity to the PAG (Alemayehu et al., 1995; Thompson et al., 2000). For example, 'some patients with [temporal lobe epilepsy] have ictal panic, which is often confused with panic attack in panic disorder' (Chang et al., 2022, p. 1). In these cases, the seizures can be treated provided they are detected and so, except for the need for differential diagnosis, such panic attacks can probably be ignored for psychiatric purposes (but see Keck et al., 1993).

Second, is an abnormal sensitivity of the PAG to its normal adequate stimuli, or an abnormal input to it as a result of the occurrence of these stimuli. This would manifest itself as a decreased threshold for panic attacks in a typical provoking situation. Under normal conditions in human society there will be few appropriate external stimuli to demonstrate this sensitivity in any selective fashion. However, suffocation (§13.5.1), is both an adequate stimulus for activation of the PAG and likely to occur, with moderate intensity, under everyday conditions. It could give rise to apparently spontaneous panic attacks; but need not be the only such cause.

Klein (1995 for a brief review, p. 62S) 'proposed the hypothesis that a panic attack may be a suffocation false alarm, that is, patients have a pathologically lowered threshold for estimating suffocation, which would account for the dyspnoea [seen in panic disorder]' (see also Papp et al., 1993; Sinha et al., 1999; for an updated version, see Preter and Klein, 2008). Consistent with Klein's hypothesis, dyspnoea is a common characteristic of patients with a primary diagnosis of panic disorder. Also consistent with Klein, dyspnoea is *not* a characteristic of phobic or obsessional patients (Asmundson and Stein, 1994) *nor* of the adaptive panic provoked by strong environmental stimulation. 'In intense, fearful situations, such as those experienced and recounted by World War II veterans, symptoms of fear include palpitations, trembling, and sweating, but not dyspnoea' (Klein, 1995, p. 62S).

Klein's suffocation hypothesis can also account for the occurrence of panic during dreamless sleep (e.g. Rosenfeld and Furman, 1994); for the cardiac and respiratory abnormalities of patients with panic disorder during sleep (Koenigsberg et al., 1994); for the ease with which respiratory challenges elicit panic; and for the fact that patients with panic disorder terminate breath holding earlier than do those with social anxiety or controls (Asmundson and Stein, 1994). There is also evidence that panic disorder may involve a more pervasive problem with autonomic control (Middleton et al., 1994); or altered central responses to, or levels of, endogenous benzodiazepines (Randall et al., 1995), orexins (Johnson et al., 2010), CCK, or monoamines (Sandford et al., 2000). Thus, some panic patients may be characterized by physical reactions other than dyspnoea.

We have used the term 'panic disorder' in a way that departs from the more overwhelming form classified by DSM-5. But, if we consider the history of panic disorder (Holt, 1990, p. 55), we find that

> during World War I, the symptom complex of palpitation, breathlessness, chest pain, fatigue and digestive disturbance originally identified by Hartshorne (1864) was studied intensively, being called Irritable Heart Syndrome, Disordered Action of the Heart or Da Costa's Syndrome ... However, no evidence of heart disease or heart abnormalities could be found ... Lewis (1919) preferred the term Effort Syndrome ... "because these symptoms and signs are largely, in some cases wholely, the exaggerated physiological response to exercise" ... [but] 76% [of Effort Syndrome patients] reported the involvement of fear in their condition, 70% had attacks at rest (i.e. not after exercise), 50% were depressed and 70% showed evidence that they were anxious.

Thus, it appears that only later was what is now termed panic disorder seen as a particularly psychological condition. It seems possible, also, that there has been some drift in the selection of patients from a group of whom only 70% were anxious to one in which 100% are anxious. Certainly, at the time of our 2nd edition, there was 'little consistency in measures or even types of assessment used to characterize and follow up [panic] patients' (Shear and Maser, 1994, p. 346). So, there were people who were abnormally sensitive to panic stimuli, but who were at the opposite, stable extravert, pole to the neurotic introverted personality that we have argued predisposes to neurotic disorders. In Shear and Maser's (1994, p. 349) words, such patients experience a limited

> physiological, form of panic attack and will have, in our view, the purest form of panic disorder. However, they will not usually present in the psychiatric clinic because the physiological component of the panic attack is not exacerbated by a cognitively-mediated reaction from the defence system—and indeed do not fit with the conventional view that 'anticipatory anxiety is a central symptom of panic disorder'.

Aoki et al. (1994), p. 56), for example, report that in a non-patient population 'panickers seeking help showed a tendency to be less extroverted than those not seeking medical care'. As a result, stable extroverts may either ignore the attack, or seek advice from a heart specialist (who will tell them there is nothing wrong with their heart), and the fear/anxiety components of the attack (already minimal) will extinguish.

13.5.4 Neurotic panic and 'panic disorder'—anxiety as a symptom

But what of Neurotic Introverts? Although our detailed neurology is slightly different from that of Gorman (Gorman et al., 1989; Gorman et al., 2000; see also Lai, 2019), the picture we ultimately paint is consistent with his original view that: 'there are three distinct components of the illness *panic disorder*—the acute panic attack, anticipatory anxiety, and phobic avoidance' (Gorman et al., 1989, p. 149, emphasis added). In particular, our view of what we will call 'neurotic panic disorder' as involving the addition of anticipatory fear and anxiety that can generate phobic avoidance (Fig.13.7) fits with his updated view that

> patients with panic disorder inherit an especially sensitive central nervous system fear mechanism that has at its center the central nucleus of the amygdala and includes the hippocampus, thalamus, and hypothalamus, as well as the PAG region, locus ceruleus, and other brainstem sites. Medications such as SSRIs may reduce panic attacks by decreasing the activity of the amygdala and interfering with its ability to stimulate projection sites in the hypothalamus and brainstem. Once the physiologic/somatic symptoms of anxiety are lessened, there is a secondary reduction in anticipatory anxiety and phobic avoidance. Cognitive behavioral and other effective psychotherapies most likely operate upstream from the amygdala, reducing phobic avoidance by deconditioning contextual fear learned at the level of the hippocampus and decreasing cognitive mis-attributions and abnormal emotional reactions by strengthening the ability of the medial prefrontal cortex to inhibit the amygdala.
>
> (Gorman et al., 2000, p. 503)

Thus, to panic symptomatic of other psychopathology, and high trait panic isolated from other pathology, we can add a third form of problematic panic: high trait panic sensitivity *coupled with* a highly neurotic introvert personality. Such cases develop, through conditioning, concurrent anxiety or phobia that is symptomatic rather than comorbid. This account is consistent with the observation that patients treated with extensive psychological therapy 'were essentially free of panic attacks during the follow up period [of 5 years and] the most significant change, in their view, was that, if an attack did occur, they knew how to deal with it and did not overreact to it, or let it limit their mobility' (Franklin, 1990, p. 89).

13.5.5 Comorbid trait panic and trait anxiety

> It is clear from the extensive overlap in the elements of [Fig. 13.6 and 13.7], that symptomatic comorbidity would be expected to be common and for the primary cause of symptoms of anxiety + panic to be difficult to determine. Coincidence will not always be the case—with both simple panic attacks and pure GAD/agoraphobia/social anxiety occurring, particularly in those who lack a neurotic personality type or a tendency to arousal-elicited panic, respectively. But a combination of symptoms is likely to be common.
>
> A further expectation is that such symptomatic overlap can lead to a true syndromal overlap. Anxiety accompanied by panic is likely to be chronic; anxiety results in the release of stress hormones; and chronic stress is likely to result in a progressive development of sensitivity ('kindling') of the systems involved (Adamec et al., 1997; Adamec, 1997; Adamec et al., 2008; Schmidt et al., 2013). Thus, primary dysfunction of one node (with secondary increases in symptoms mediated by another node) can evolve into primary dysfunction of both nodes and so true syndromal comorbidity.
>
> For related reasons, we would anticipate a considerable level of comorbidity of initial syndromes. Where disorder is generated by chronic stress, this can not only precipitate any one of the neurotic disorders but is likely to precipitate more than one at a time. Similarly, if the source of disorder is a genetic predisposition to anxiety (i.e., [GIS] activation) in general then more than one node of the system (and so more than one form of anxiety disorder) is likely to be involved simultaneously. Likewise, if there is a genetic problem with monoamine systems

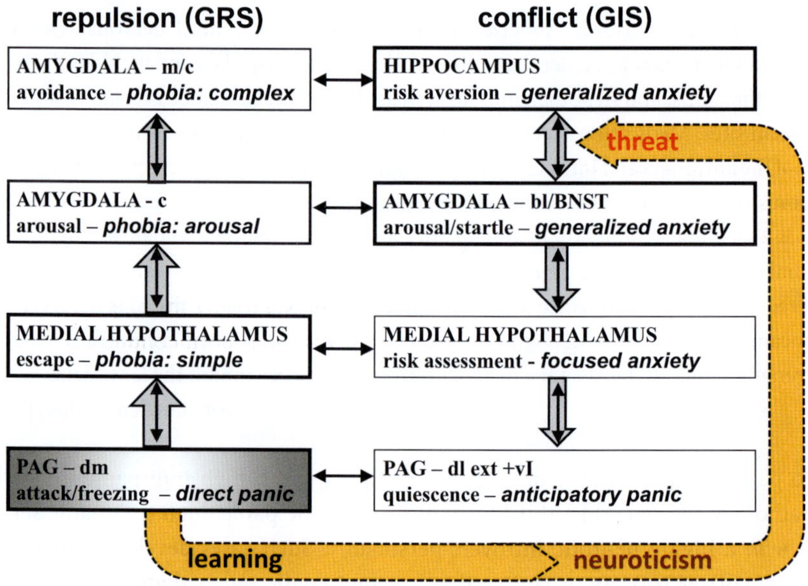

Fig. 13.7 Panic as a syndrome with symptomatic anxiety. Abbreviations and symbols as in Fig. 13.2. Lower levels of the GRS/FFFS) system (bottom left) produce spontaneous activity (or hyper-reactivity) of the PAG generating pathological panic attacks. Active avoidance and arousal are increased via existing ascending neural connections of the FFFS (solid outline filled grey arrows, width indicates degree of activation, simple black double headed arrows show available connections). Coincidence of the occurrence of the panic attack with distinctive or threatening environmental circumstances can result in the learning of anticipatory anxiety (dashed outline filled grey arrow)—particularly in neurotic introverts (filled yellow arrow). This anxiety is mediated by the hippocampus and amygdala, and by the normal spread of neural activity through the GIS. Thus, abnormal panic produces fear and anxiety that are normal given the level of perceived threat generated by the combination of panic with neuroticism. Note that this implies that a treatment such as cognitive behavioural therapy could modify the anxiety, and considerably reduce the incidence and increase the tolerability of panic attacks, while leaving a primary, neurological, incidence of panic intact. Figure modified and updated from (McNaughton and Corr, 2016; McNaughton, 2005).

(potentially expressed as neuroticism or a related trait) then both the FFFS and GIS could contribute multiple disordered nodes.

Whichever of these various routes is involved, our theory accepts that massive apparent comorbidities of its set of proposed symptom clusters will occur with potentially a range of concurrent underlying syndromes. This promiscuity creates the current complex clinical picture and emphasises the difficulty of separating symptom parallels from true syndromal comorbidities. However, while multiple positive feedback loops (Fig. [13.8]) complicate the diagnostic picture, they are also likely to provide some degree of flexibility of treatment. For example, as we have noted already, treating the neurologically normal anxiety that is consequent on abnormal panic will reduce arousal, eliminate avoidance, and reduce, even when it does not eliminate, panic attacks.

(McNaughton and Corr, 2016, p. 1060)

As shown in Fig. 13.8, we would expect positive feedback among these systems. There are several possible ways to achieve this.

First, chronic anxiety is characterized by chronic autonomic arousal; this should increase the probability of panic attacks, given the known capacity of adrenaline infusion to elicit panic (e.g. Veltman et al., 1996; see also Lader and Tyrer, 1975). Such a conditioned increase in arousal is formally equivalent to fear-potentiated startle, and so is likely to be generated by a direct threat input to the amygdala.

Second, the detection of threat itself could activate the PAG and produce panic directly, since even the highest level of the defence system, represented by the cingulate cortex, has a direct input to the PAG (Fig. 6.2). Overlayed on this long-term, conditioning-based, vicious spiral of exacerbation of panic by anxiety, and of anxiety by panic, there could be an acute suppression of panic involving the goal inhibition component of anxiety. It is via this latter, antagonistic relationship (Graeff, 1994) that one can account for the phenomenon of relaxation-induced panic, sometimes to the degree that panic regularly wakes the sufferer

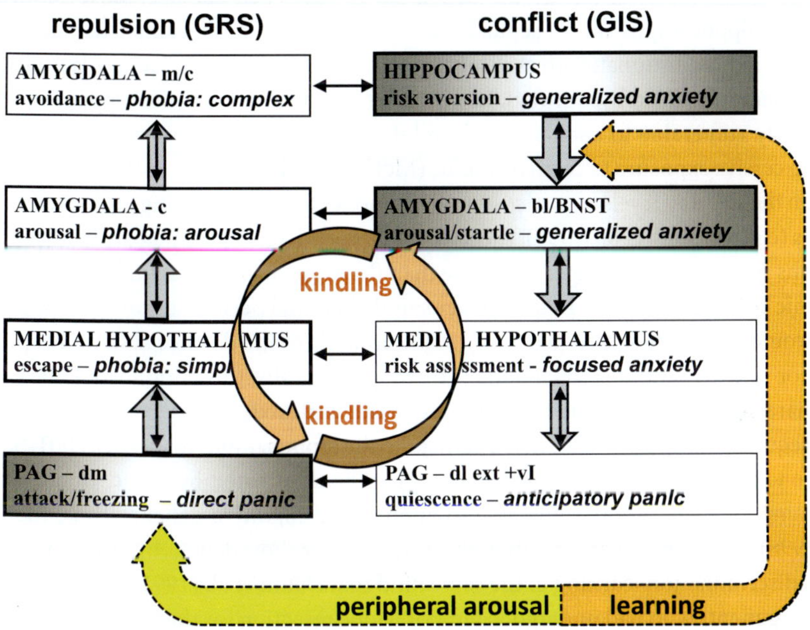

Fig. 13.8 Syndromal comorbidity and positive feedback between anxiety and panic. Abbreviations and symbols as in Fig. 13.2. Genetic and or environmental predisposing factors (particularly those linked to neuroticism) can result in pathological activity in both the PAG, generating panic, and in the hippocampus and amygdala, generating anxiety. These can concurrently reinforce each other through the state feedback mechanisms detailed in Fig. 13.6 and 13.7 (dashed outline filled double headed arrow)—resulting in positive feedback. Repetitive or chronic activation of either or both of the GRS and GIS (and particularly the resultant release of stress hormones) can result in a progressive sensitisation of the other system ('kindling') and this can also generate longer-term trait positive feedback (circular arrows). Not only does this imply that symptomatic comorbidity can result in trait comorbidity but it implies that therapeutic intervention at any one of the main links in these positive feedback circuits can produce some improvement. Figure modified and updated from (McNaughton and Corr, 2016; McNaughton, 2005).

from sleep; although Graeff's account requires the additional, but not implausible, assumption that the descending inhibitory controls from the forebrain are switched off, as relaxation or sleep sets in, prior to the switching off of the lower brain systems that mediate panic symptoms. Given this account, relaxation-induced panic should occur only in patients with primary panic disorder (as defined by, say, CO_2 challenge), not in those whose panic attacks are a consequence of primary anxiety.

As well as the temporary, functional release from forebrain inhibition of lower levels of the defence system which, as noted earlier, appears to underlie relaxation-induced panic, there is also evidence of chronic loss of such inhibitory control due to structural damage in the brain, as assessed by magnetic resonance imaging. Consistent with our overall model, this damage has been localized to the SHS.

Thus, Dantendorfer et al. (1996) first subdivided an initial sample of 120 patients with panic disorder into those with (29%) or without abnormalities (but not sufficient to constitute epilepsy) in conventional scalp electroencephalographic recordings, and then further examined the group showing such abnormalities for structural brain damage. A remarkably high proportion (61%) of this group turned out to have such damage, most frequently affecting the hippocampus and/or septal area. (As we shall see, hippocampal damage has been noted also in post-traumatic stress disorder.) The aetiology of such damage is undoubtedly heterogeneous. Two likely pathways, however, are perinatal anoxia (the hippocampus being particularly vulnerable to anoxic insult) and degeneration in hippocampal pyramidal cells due to excessive exposure to corticosteroids (McEwen et al., 1992).

Given the elevated levels of corticosteroid hormones that occur during prolonged exposure to stress (e.g. Sapolsky et al., 1990), the latter pathway is likely to participate in a second type of vicious spiral, one on a longer time base than the immediate interactions between anxiety and panic considered earlier. In this slower spiral, an initial period of prolonged exposure to stress would involve heightened activity in lower levels of the defence system, coupled with inhibition of their output involving the SHS; psychologically, this period would be expected to be characterized by combined symptoms of panic and anxiety.

Subsequently, after steroid-induced damage to the hippocampus (Sapolsky, 2001; Sapolsky, 2004), one would expect the symptomatology to be dominated by panic. In addition, the hippocampal damage should give rise to appropriate cognitive deficits. Thus, Maierhofer et al. (1998) have shown that patients with panic disorder show deficits in conditional, but not simple, discrimination learning of the same kind that Daum et al. (1991) had previously observed in patients who had undergone temporal lobe resection for the treatment of epilepsy.

13.5.6 Comorbidity and related interactions more generally

If we broaden our focus beyond panic, there are a range of extended pathways that can produce comorbidities. These include ones that extend beyond simple dysfunction of repulsion or conflict to include (e.g. chronic anxiety producing comorbid depression).

Conversely to anxiety producing comorbid depression, SUD can produce comorbid anxiety. (For a more detailed version of the following discussion, see McNaughton, 2008a.) Recreational use of alcohol or the regular use of barbiturates or benzodiazepines as hypnotics results in tolerance, dependence, and addiction. Tolerance, in particular, then leads

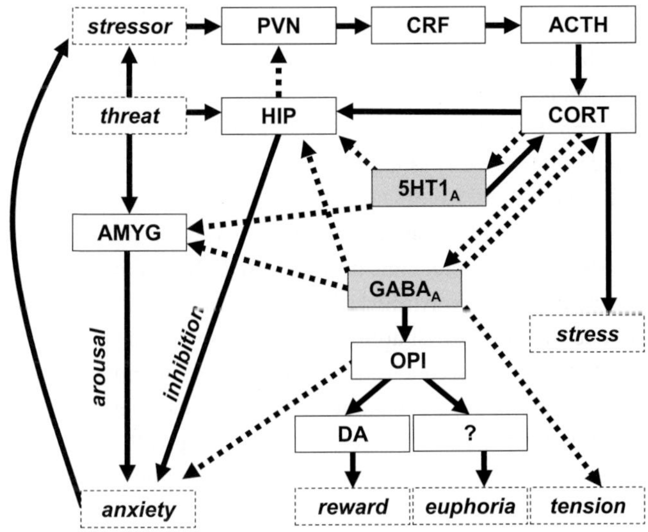

Fig. 13.9 Pathways for comorbidity beyond repulsion and conflict. A selection of sources of potential interaction between the GRS and GIS, primarily the amygdala and hippocampus, and other systems are shown. Solid lines represent net excitatory connections, and dashed lines represent net inhibitory connections. Of most immediate relevance to the long-term trait changes of Fig. 13.8 are the interactions with the stress system. Anxiety is a stressor, releasing corticosterone/cortisol (CORT) via activation of the paraventricular nucleus, release of corticotrophin releasing factor, and adrenocorticotropin hormone (ACTH). Negative feedback control of the release of CORT is achieved by its action on the hippocampus and its connection with the paraventricular nucleus. High levels of CORT can damage the hippocampus, reduce this feedback inhibition, and so result in progressive increases in CORT. Continuously high CORT can then result in depression as well as other problems. CORT will also reduce the effects of endogenous anxiolytic action mediated by 5-HT$_{1A}$ and GABA$_A$ (particular benzodiazepine site) receptors. At least in the short term, 5-HT$_{1A}$ activation releases CORT, but benzodiazepine activation inhibits it. (Both of these effects show tolerance.) The GABA$_A$ system is particularly important for comorbidity because it not only reduces anxiety (without tolerance) but also produces muscle relaxation, euphoria, and rewarding effects via endogenous opiate systems that cause the release of dopamine. These effects show tolerance and lead to addiction. Thus, use of anxiolytics can lead to substance use disorder, and via tolerance and withdrawal, substance use disorder can result in anxiety disorder (see text). Figure and adapted legend from McNaughton and Corr (2016) with permission.

to rebound anxiety upon withdrawal of the drugs. (Each of these classes of drug has its own binding site on the GABA$_A$ receptor system, through which all produce antianxiety actions as well as euphoria and muscle relaxation.) However, this antianxiety action, and the stressful nature of anxiety, gives it a capacity to generate SUD. SUD can often start with, and be substantially maintained by, self-medication particularly with alcohol. Once alcohol intake has started, the story is essentially the same as with recreational use leading to SUD. Here again we have the potential for a vicious cycle (as when anxiety and panic feed off each other), with anxiety and SUD reinforcing each other (for detailed reviews, see Stewart and Conrod, 2008). It should be emphasized that we are describing only one aspect of SUD, here, and that the causes of addiction go much deeper than a response to anxiety.

> An important point to note in relation to the self-medication story we have just presented is that SUD and the control of anxiety are linked through a complex web of endogenous interacting compounds (Fig. [13.9]). Serotonergic antianxiety drugs (such as buspirone or fluoxetine) impact on the neural structures that control anxiety (e.g. the hippocampus and amygdala) in much the same way as $GABA_A$ drugs, and without showing tolerance. Both classes of drug also (Fig. [13.9]) have their antianxiety action reduced by corticosterone/cortisol (CORT). However, 5-$HT1_A$ drugs differ from $GABA_A$ drugs in two important respects. The first (Fig. [13.9]) is that serotonergic drugs release CORT on initial use, while $GABA_A$ drugs inhibit it, with both classes of drug showing tolerance of their effects on CORT release. This partially explains the initial dysphoric effects of the serotonergics and the euphoric effects of the $GABA_A$ drugs. The second is that $GABA_A$ drugs, but not serotonergics, activate opiate systems that in turn activate dopamine systems producing rewarding and euphoriant actions that contribute to their abuse potential. We can argue, then, that the strong links between anxiety disorder and SUD relate to endogenous compounds that regulate not only anxiety but also reward systems.
>
> (McNaughton and Corr, 2016, pp. 1016–1062; our figure citation)

13.5.7 Cognition and panic

In this chapter so far, we have glibly talked about the relevant inputs to the PAG as if they were simple internal or external stimuli. But, of course, it is inherent in the idea of defensive distance that the stimulus must be interpreted as threatening for the reaction to be obtained. Rats and other animals, for example, can learn that that the 'innate predator', a human caregiver, is non-threatening. At this point, therefore, we must link our theory with ideas on the role of cognition in panic and panic disorder. This is especially so, since there is a tendency for people, mistakenly, to contrast biological and cognitive explanations of behaviour.

A succinct review of one cognitive theory of panic is provided by Clark and Ehlers (1993); (see also Clark, 1986; §14.2). This theory has many similarities with the analysis we have just provided. In particular, the main generator of the panic attack is presumed to be positive feedback between bodily sensations and perceived threat. In the theory 'it is assumed that the crucial event is a misinterpretation of certain bodily sensations' (*op. cit.*, p. 132). Such misinterpretation may result from an increased sensitivity of perception of some specific sensations such as heart rate (Näring and Van der Staak, 1995; but see Barsky et al., 1994). In favour of the theory is the fact that panic patients 'were significantly more likely to choose negative interpretations of the key bodily sensations ... but were no more likely to choose negative interpretations of the other ambiguous events' (Clark and Ehlers, 1993, p. 133); the fact that cognitive therapy can be effective with panic disorder (see Chapter 14); the fact that appropriate instructions before biological challenges reduce the probability of panic; and the fact that heart-beat discriminability predicts the maintenance of panic attacks (Ehlers and Breuer, 1996).

Differences between our analysis of panic and this cognitive theory occur at two points. First, the cognitive theory is intended to include only a subset of the phenomena we have included. Second, there are consequent terminological differences in the uses of words such as 'panic' and 'panic disorder'. We included in our analysis of panic disorder cases of, for example, 'benign heart pain', arguing that, in terms of the core biological component of panic, these cases are not essentially different from the 60% of the same heart pain population who received a subsequent diagnosis of panic disorder. These patients are excluded from the cognitive theory (and, of course, conventional diagnosis of panic disorder), but they are germane for the following reasons. 'Surveys suggest that 7–28% of the normal population will experience an occasional unexpected panic attack ... However, the cognitive theory assumes that an individual only goes on to develop the rarer condition of repeated panic attacks and panic disorder ... if he or she develops a tendency to interpret these perceived autonomic events in a catastrophic fashion' (Clark and Ehlers, 1993, p. 132). This 'tendency to interpret' is equivalent to the cognitive component of the conditioning we have postulated as occurring in a person with a neurotic introvert personality. However, if personality type were all there were to it, we would expect generalized anxiety disorder with occasional panic attacks to progress rapidly to full-blown panic disorder; and this does not appear generally to be the case. The cognitive theory can accommodate this by postulating a specific *additional* personality factor relating to the perception of somatic events. But the need for an additional explanatory factor when excluding some of the available data is not parsimonious.

13.5.8 Defensive quiescence

As we noted earlier, in the previous sections, we have been dealing with the dorsomedial PAG and treating it as the lowest component of the GRS (Fig. 6.2A). In contrast, there are now data (Silva and McNaughton, 2019) that led us to conclude that the external dorsolateral PAG and ventrolateral PAG are an equivalent lowest component of the GIS—and so should generate an anxious form of panic that produces defensive quiescence in rats (and likely humans too). This would require very high levels of balanced conflict as with very high levels of uncertainty as to the presence or absence of a predator. Importantly, whatever its symptomatology, it (but not classic panic) should be sensitive to anxiolytic drugs. It is likely, therefore, to be seen clinically as just a very high level of anxiety, not requiring a distinct classification.

13.6 Specific phobia

Let us now consider the individual disorders implied by our neurology, using our discussion of panic as a paradigm case for many of our arguments. We deal with them for convenience of exposition under the headings used by DSM-5-TR while noting divergence from it.

13.6.1 Specific phobia—background

Specific phobia[6] involves the active avoidance of a specific class of phobic object (e.g. spiders). Thus, in our theory, specific phobia is fear that will only generate anxiety when it also conflicts with a positive goal and so should be insensitive to anxiolytic drugs in the same way as the items in the Blanchards' fear/defence test battery (Chapters 2 and 4). This is indeed the case (Sartory et al., 1990) and the brain activity elicited by phobic objects is also insensitive to

[6] Consistent with DSM-5, we distinguish specific phobia from agoraphobia and social anxiety.

anxiolytic drugs (Fredrikson et al., 1995). However, specific phobic avoidance is *also not* sensitive to panicolytic anxiolytics (Sinclair and Nutt, 2007) suggesting that it is less a disorder of fear in general and more excessive input to fear systems from the circuits that detect the fear stimulus. It will therefore require deeper analysis than other, nominally more complex, conditions.

So, on psychological and pharmacological grounds, we must distinguish specific phobia from anxiety. This is true whether the specific fear constitutes a disorder or not—avoidance of spiders is adaptive in Australia; and the healthy population has a high sensitivity to snakes. That said, the presence of a phobic disorder should be capable, through normal conditioning processes, of giving rise to anticipatory anxiety. (The converse, however—anxiety, as in generalized anxiety disorder, leading on to specific phobia—theoretically should be rare.)

13.6.2 Specific phobia—theoretical context

First, let us look at phobia in the context of our theory. Following the Blanchards' analysis (Chapter 2), we would expect there to be both *innate* and conditioned fear stimuli to which an excessive neural reaction could produce a maladaptive response. Following LeDoux's analysis (Chapter 6), we would expect conditioned fear stimuli to have been created by strengthening of specific synapses in the amygdala, as a result of the conjunction of input to this region from lower and higher sensory processing areas with input from an appropriate unconditioned stimulus such as pain. This would apply to evolutionarily neutral sources of fear such as dental fear (Poulton and Menzies, 2002b); however, 'childhood fears deemed evolutionarily relevant may have different pathways and/or mechanisms underlying their emergence' (Poulton et al., 2023, p. 1).

A particularly simple explanation of the evolution and existence of innate fear stimuli (e.g. the cat for a rat, the snake for a human) would then be the selection of those members of a population in which conditioning to stimuli emanating from certain common sources of danger was particularly easy. A wide range of stimuli have access (via conditioning) to the fear mechanisms located in the amygdala. Provided random mutation (or the shuffling of multiple genes during sexual reproduction) continually maintains the variance in such a population despite a shift in its mean, the endpoint of such an evolutionary process will be animals demonstrating 'zero trial learning' (i.e. the production, as an unconditioned response, of what in previous generations was a conditioned response). The reverse process can also occur. A key technical feature of the Blanchards' experiments was the use of wild rats, for which the experimenter is an innate predatory stimulus, as compared to laboratory rats, which have largely lost this tendency as the result of selective breeding. We will discuss this in more detail in §13.6.7.

Given this view of conventional fears what would we expect of pathological phobias? First, there could be a super-sensitivity of the amygdala to fear conditioning (perhaps as the result of an overreactive reinforcement signal) or excessive output from the amygdala after fear conditioning has occurred. This should give us a patient who reacts with excessive fear to *both* conditioned *and* innate fear stimuli (and leaves open the possibility that humans do not have innate fear stimuli). §13.6.3 discusses the pure conditioning perspective. Second, the natural variation in the population (or possibly some special feature of ontogeny) would produce a greater than normal reaction to innate fear stimuli. Our 'conditioning' model of the evolution of the required connections has these (derived from the conditioned variant) being selective to specific fear stimuli. §13.6.4 discusses the non-randomness of phobic stimuli and 'prepared learning' and 'innate fear stimulus' explanations that follow on from this.

13.6.3 Specific phobia—the pure conditioning perspective

So, what is the aetiology of specific phobia as a disorder? Early theories of phobia, derived from a report (Watson and Rayner, 1920) of aversive classical conditioning of a 'stolid and unemotional' child, often referred to as 'Little Albert',[7] and the animal operant laboratory, emphasized conditioned fear as a model for phobias that have few and clearly delineated precipitating stimuli (Eysenck and Rachman, 1965; Gray, 1971). Consistent with this view, behaviour therapy was particularly successful in its treatment (e.g. Mathews, 1978), with exposure and cognitive-behavioural therapy now being the main treatments (Nutt, 2005).

> Some case reports of adult phobics confirm Watson's findings that phobias can be learned by association. The most interesting of these were described by Bagby in 1922. His first case was that of a young woman who had retained since childhood a severe fear of running water ... As a little girl of seven she had [become trapped alone] ... wedged between two rocks, with a waterfall noisily pouring over her head ... Although [this] and similar cases provide evidence that phobias can be acquired through the simple pairing of an alarming occurrence and a hitherto neutral situation, the sad fact [for conditioning theories] remains that such stories are rare. Few phobics can recall the precipitating incident for their fear. Furthermore, evidence from other sources raises problems that this theory, which claims that phobia is learned by association, cannot resolve ...
>
> War presents us with the conditions for a large-scale experiment when great numbers of civilians are exposed to bombing attacks. In such attacks loud noise is paired with a variety of hitherto neutral events. According to the theory of learning by association, this type of conditioning should generate a large number of phobias. Yet ... the vast majority of children, 96 percent, were unaffected ... This, then, is a failure of the conditioning theory of phobia on a gigantic scale.
>
> (Agras, 1985, pp. 45–47)

A second objection is to the learning mechanism invoked. The learning problem for clinical phobic patients, who have a chronic problem, should not be likelihood of association but failure to 'extinguish' the fear response. Discussion of extinction requires care. It might be thought (Eysenck, 1979) that phobic stimuli unaccompanied by their UCSs would undergo extinction. However, most well-learned responses are habitual and should persist unless conditions change (McNaughton, 1989b, pp. 124–128). In the specific case of avoidance learning, there are reports in the animal literature of an essential lack of extinction in the total absence of the reinforcer (Gray, 1987b).

[7] See Griggs (2014) for comments on problems with the study and distortions of reports of it in introductory psychology books.

On this view, the rapid extinction of *appetitively* motivated responses is an aberration. Appetitive extinction results, not because the response is no longer reinforced, but because '*omission* of an expected reward ... is a highly salient event which can actively suppress responding' (McNaughton, 1989b, p. 127, our emphasis; see also Appendix 7). However, strong resistance to extinction is not usually seen in classical, as opposed to instrumental, fear conditioning.

> Fears conditioned by association tend to be short-lived. Most conditioned reflexes will weaken and disappear after a few exposures to the fear-provoking event... [However,] avoidance of a feared situation blocks the normal process of unlearning the fear response... In the case of air raids, [mentioned earlier] which are unavoidable for a civilian, we would expect the fear response to be transient. *Only if the phobic situation is avoidable, as it usually is, would we expect the phobia to be long-lasting.*
>
> (Agras, 1985, p. 47)

Consistent with these arguments, the key therapeutic factor in the treatment of specific phobia is the total amount of time for which the patient is exposed to the phobic stimulus—the greater the exposure, the greater the therapeutic effect (Marks, 1973; Gelder et al., 1973; Teasdale, 1977) (Levis and Hare, 1977). (This issue is discussed in greater detail in the Chapter 14, §14.1.)

Note that, here, we are talking about specific object phobias where the stimuli are evolutionarily relevant objects and where common, regular, experience does not involve reinforcement via (e.g. pain). In contrast, as shown by the long-term prospective Dunedin Multidisciplinary Study 'Study members with greater caries experience at age 15 were almost five times more likely to report dental fear, but not other fears, at age 18. This finding suggests that... more extensive dental work with increased likelihood for aversive conditioning... was causally related to the onset of dental fear at age 18' (Poulton and Menzies, 2002b, p. 135). Here, no special explanation is required since we would expect similar, regular, painful experience to generate equivalent phobia with any situation.

13.6.1 Specific phobia—the prepared conditioning perspective

Eysenck (1979) objected to the simple conditioning theory because the stimuli that elicit phobias are not a random sample of stimuli: some (e.g. closed spaces, snakes, spiders) are greatly over-represented; others (e.g. cars, guns) that are associated with objectively stronger dangers, especially in the USA, are under-represented. Additionally, Gray (1979a) noted that the times of onset of phobias are not a random sample of ages; there is a predominance of onsets in early adult life (Marks, 1969).

Eysenck (1979), and others, saw Seligman's (1971) concept of 'preparedness' as providing an explanation. According to Seligman some stimuli are 'prepared' (by Darwinian evolution) to *enter into an association* with aversive UCSs. The evolutionary explanation for this would be a variant of the one we have provided in $13.6.2 for innate fear stimuli—but it differs in focusing on changes in the capacity for learning of a CR to a specific CS (reinforced by some negative event) rather than production of a UCR by a UCS.

In $11.3.1 of our 2nd edition we provide extensive discussion of experiments from Arne Öhman's laboratory using differential classical conditioning of autonomic responses (usually the skin conductance response) with an aversive UCS (usually a mild electric shock) and visual stimuli (presented as slides) as CSs. The experiments were conducted with healthy human subjects, most often undergraduates. The key innovation was the choice of CSs. These consisted of stimuli that are found as the objects of clinical simple phobias either commonly (e.g. snakes, spiders: 'fear-relevant stimuli') or rarely (e.g. flowers, mushrooms: 'fear-irrelevant stimuli').

Our general conclusions were that Öhman's results showed that the 'fear-relevant' stimuli come to elicit more persistent skin conductance responses as a result of association with an aversive UCS. This did not occur with fear-relevant but evolutionarily neutral CSs (rifles and revolvers; Öhman, 1979). So, 'fear-relevant' is really 'evolutionarily fear-relevant', fitting with Seligman's view of the stimuli (but not necessarily his view of the mechanism involved). However, the bulk of the evidence from a recent meta-analysis is that there is no increased resistance to extinction of fear *conditioning* with snake and spider pictures (Åhs et al., 2018). Even the contrary available positive evidence is weak; but may nonetheless have some theoretical importance (Del Giudice, 2021) particularly in the case of snakes (Kawai, 2019a, see also §13.6.4).

Importantly, Öhman's results did not usually fit with Seligman's 'preparedness': a greater readiness to become *conditioned fear stimuli* as the result of a Pavlovian conditioning process. 'Preparedness' does not explain the fact that the main skin conductance effects occur in the first half of the CS period. Nor does it explain the facts: that evolutionarily relevant stimuli have a special affinity for the skin conductance response relative to other responses; that they are susceptible to sensitization; that they are particularly easily differentiated into positive *and negative* (i.e. safety) fear stimuli; that their putative high associability may affect resistance to extinction, but does not speed up acquisition; and, critically, that they elicit strong skin conductance changes *in the absence of any conditioning*.

Further,

> just as people tend to develop phobias only to certain types of *objects*, they tend to respond to phobia conditioning only when certain types of *fear-evoking stimuli* are coupled with these objects. The observations from the mini-phobia experiments [such as Öhman's] provide the evidence here. Even with snakes and spiders, only stimuli such as electric shocks produce the mini-phobia. Loud noise does *not* produce a fear response to such animals. This result suggests that *only certain sensory pathways* are involved in the acquisition of this type of fear response. Could it be because snakes and spiders bite that tactile stimuli produce the fear?'
>
> Agras (1985, p. 49)

Öhman, with Mineka, then produced an 'Evolved Fear Module' theory that itself evolved somewhat between 2001–2003 (Öhman and Mineka, 2001; Mineka and Öhman, 2002; Öhman and Mineka, 2003; see also Öhman, 2009). The module has four key properties:

'[1] it is preferentially activated by stimuli related to survival threats in evolutionary history. Thus, fear-relevant stimuli lead to superior conditioning of aversive associations compared with fear-irrelevant stimuli.

[2] the module is automatically activated by fear-relevant stimuli, meaning that fear activation occurs before conscious cognitive analysis of the stimulus can occur.
[3] the fear module is relatively impenetrable to conscious cognitive control, and fear conditioning with fear-relevant stimuli can occur even with subliminal conditioned stimuli.
[4] the amygdala seems to be the central brain area dedicated to the fear module.
Finally, we propose that there are two levels of fear conditioning, with an emotional level that is relatively independent of the cognitive contingency level, each mediated by different brain areas [c.f. (LeDoux, 1994)].

(Mineka and Öhman, 2002, p. 927; reformatted)

Later added to this core (Öhman and Mineka, 2003, p.5, added emphasis) was a focus on snakes (and also, separately, human faces, Öhman, 2009, see also §13.8) as a particularly important case for humans:

> As reptiles, snakes may have signified deadly threats in the environment of early mammals.... Snakes remain special stimuli for humans. Intense snake fear is prevalent in both humans and other primates. Humans and monkeys learn snake fear more easily than fear of most other stimuli through direct or vicarious conditioning. Neither *the elicitation* nor the conditioning of snake fear in humans requires that snakes be consciously perceived; rather, both processes can occur with masked stimuli. Humans tend to perceive illusory correlations between snakes and aversive stimuli, and *their attention is automatically captured by snakes* in complex visual displays. Together, these and other findings delineate an evolved fear module in the brain. *This module is selectively and automatically activated by once-threatening stimuli*, is relatively encapsulated from cognition, and derives from specialized neural circuitry.

Throughout this theory development, but diminished towards the end, is an emphasis on the involvement of the Evolved Fear Module in conditioning. However, invoking evolution raises an immediate criticism of Seligman's (1971) view that also applies to a stimulus-specific-conditioning component of any later view. The criticism is that

> if we are biologically prepared to be afraid of certain objects that threaten our survival, why would we have to put ourselves in danger by experiencing the consequences of encounters with these objects? For example, if snakes are dangerous to our survival, it would be a great risk associated with meeting a snake and experience negative consequences of the encounter. If animals always had to learn which predators to avoid through encounters, they are likely to die.
>
> (Åhs et al., 2018, p. 431)

Indeed, according to one summary of Öhman's theory, he

> suggested that our brains are wired for fast, *pre-attentional visual detection* of salient stimuli such as snakes. Indeed, humans (even those without snake phobia) are able to detect pictures of snakes embedded in neutral backgrounds faster than objects that do not evoke fear.
>
> (Isbell, 2006, p. 10; see also Kawai, 2019a)

This secondary report sees no need to mention learning or extinction—after all changes in 'pre-attentional visual detection' or, more likely, attention (and arousal) proper will clearly have *indirect* but important consequences on learning.

13.6.5 Specific phobia—the innate fear stimulus perspective

It seems, then, that a small proportion of specific phobias can be established with brief intense experiences via conventional conditioning (§13.6.3) and that fear, e.g. of dentists can be generated by repeated pain experiences (Poulton and Menzies, 2002b). However, the over-representation of a relatively small set of evolutionarily relevant phobic objects in the bulk of specific phobias in the absence of any multi-trial conditioning history suggests that an evolutionary explanation is required for them. Possibly because it was being presented as an alternative to simple conditioning, the suggestion then (§13.6.4) was that evolution had *prepared stimuli for conditioning* (Seligman, 1971; Eysenck, 1979), potentially in the form of an Evolved Fear Module (Öhman and Mineka, 2001; Mineka and Öhman, 2002; Öhman and Mineka, 2003). But, is a conditioning assumption necessary if there can be innate fear stimuli? Is an Evolved Fear Module any more than a set of innate stimulus detectors?

The whole point of the concept of conditioning, as Pavlov noted at the outset of his research (Gray, 1979b), is to make sense of those cases in which there is *no* biologically prepared connection between the stimulus and the response it elicits. Once there is such a connection, it is hard to see what role conditioning need play. There is plenty of evidence for innate fears of a wide variety of stimuli in a diversity of species (Gray, 1987b), including fear of snakes in chimpanzees never before exposed to them (Hebb, 1946). One of the interesting features of such fears is that they are often subject to maturation; that is, they appear *without learning* at a given stage of ontogeny. This concept is well supported in the animal literature (Chapter 2 of Gray, 1987b) and fits the evidence that some phobias appear in human beings rather consistently at certain ages (Marks, 1969). To account for this age distribution, the preparedness hypothesis must have added to it the *ad hoc* and unlikely assumption that conditioning experiences involving the relevant stimuli cluster at the relevant ages.

So, the fear-relevant stimuli used by Öhman's group seem to us, quite simply, innate fear stimuli for humans (with snakes, in particular, shared by other primates, Öhman and Mineka, 2003; see also Kawai, 2019a). The emphasis is on the stimuli being innately 'conditioned' (in a phylogenetic sense, as for all innate stimuli of any type) while the connection to fear (or disgust, or appetite, etc.) simply depends on the motivational system into which they are plugged. This hypothesis makes immediate sense of several findings: the heightened response to fear-relevant stimuli *before* conditioning occurs; the sensitization by prior aversive stimulation; the greater response at CS onset; and the maturation and persistence of phobic avoidance. Similarly, with height phobia assessed *prospectively* 'falls resulting in serious injury between 5 and 9 years occurred with greater frequency in those without a fear at age 18 ... Most importantly, *no* individual who had a height phobia at age 18 had a history of a serious fall before the age of nine ... seriously damaging the relevance of associative learning models of height fear' (Poulton and Menzies, 2002b, p. 135).[8]

[8] For which see also evidence for the phylogenetic problems of hypophobia.

We must still account for the greater *discriminability* of innate fear stimuli in a Pavlovian conditioning paradigm, and for the minority of reports (Åhs et al., 2018; Del Giudice, 2021) of greater resistance to extinction of this *differential* conditioning. The key is that the skin conductance response was used, which has a special affinity for innate fear stimuli—heart rate does not show these effects (Fredrikson and Öhman, 1979). There is reason to see the skin conductance response as an orienting response. It is well known that this response participates in the orienting reflex (Sokolov, 1960). The orienting reflex can be conditioned, but it is not clear that this depends on the same processes as do other forms of Pavlovian conditioning; and, in any case, the preparedness theory is concerned with conditioned fear, not conditioned orienting. If so, according to our theory this effect of the innate fear stimuli (as opposed to any effects they have on avoidance) would be mediated by the GIS. This is consistent with the fact that the skin conductance response (unlike phobic avoidance in human beings or active avoidance in animals) is reduced after benzodiazepine or barbiturate administration (Marcy and Quermonne, 1974), as well as by septal lesions (Holdstock, 1969; Holdstock, 1970). Further, Fowles (1980) concluded that 'electrodermal activity increases when there is activation of the [GIS]', whereas heart rate does not change.

Innate fear stimuli then should have two effects; with the strength of effect in any species subject to the caveat that there is variation across primates in, e.g. their phylogenetic experience of snakes (see Öhman, 2009, p. 546). So, the innate strength of the fear stimulus in humans (as with a CS early in learning) could be insufficient to produce a reliable avoidance response absent other conditions such has high arousal. (The difference from chimpanzees could be due either to their progression or human regression relative to our common ancestor.)

First, innate fear stimuli would provide input (either quick and dirty or slow and sophisticated; Fig. 6.1) to the medial and central amygdala that elicits repulsion. This is like a conditioned stimulus except that the strength of the input is phylogenetically rather than ontogenetically driven. This is essentially the position taken by Öhman and Mineka (2001, p. 513); (following LeDoux, 1996; see also snake figure on p. 56 of LeDoux, 1994):

> Learning involves changes in the weights of excitatory connections according to a Hebbian learning rule. To interpret prepared connections in terms of this model, one would merely assume that some of the connections between units representing features of certain CS-UCS combinations for specific fear-relevant CSs and aversive UCSs rather than being given random weights in the beginning of simulation would start with positive weights, thus more rapidly gaining strength in the competition to control the next layer in the model.

Second, innate fear stimuli would act on the arousal/attention modules of the GIS (primarily the basolateral amygdala but also insula, Fig. 11.14B) to generate an orienting response, including the skin conductance component. If we adopt this hypothesis, we can account for one of the two remaining features of Öhman's results on which the preparedness theory stumbles: the ease with which innate fear stimuli are differentiated into CS+ and CS–. For this is predicted directly from the properties we have given to the GIS. One of the specific functions of this system is to increase level of arousal and spread of attention so as to enhance multidimensional analysis of the stimuli encountered in a threatening environment. Thus, in Öhman's experiments, the stimuli (snakes, spiders etc) are both the source and the target of this increased level of processing, and both the cause of increased discriminability and the means through which this discriminability is made evident.

The fact that this superior discrimination may be allied to greater resistance to extinction of the skin conductance response (as distinct from its speed of acquisition) can also be derived from this approach, if we bear in mind the evidence (Sutherland and Mackintosh, 1971; Mackintosh, 1974, pp. 438–439) that resistance to extinction increases as a positive function of the number of stimulus dimensions to which the subject attends during training. If it is activation of the GIS that causes an increase in multidimensional stimulus analysis, it follows that there should also be an increase in resistance to extinction of a differential CR. This strongly attentional view could fit with one possible answer to the 'intriguing question [of] why there were several reports of a fear relevancy effect on extinction in the 1970s but only two replications in later years ... we speculate that expectations may have played a role, as the participants in early studies were students in psychology and for the most part seem to have been aware of the study rationale' (Åhs et al., 2018, p. 434). That is, positive effects were obtained when attentional bias was higher and, speculatively, when participants were closer to the critical age for maturation of specific phobias.

13.6.6 Specific phobia—neurology

Let us now move from a top-down approach to a bottom-up one.

> In mammals, the amygdala, LC, SC, pulvinar, and the W/K visual pathway, particularly via its connection to the SC and pulvinar, are involved in *a danger detection system called the fear module that acts* ***pre-consciously*** *before action and perception occur*. Snakes were the first predators of crown-group placental mammals, and neurons in the visual systems of mammals appear to respond preferentially to cues that are characteristic of snakes. *Parts of the fear module have expanded in primates*, and in anthropoid primates, the fear module has dense connections with cortical areas that have also expanded. Primates have also expanded their visual systems beyond those of other mammals to include large areas of the neocortex, and cells in those areas also respond preferentially to the highly periodic patterns that are characteristic of snakes but are otherwise infrequent in nature. The connections of the fear module to the neocortex may allow more flexibility in responding to dangerous situations that require the animal's immediate attention.
>
> (Isbell, 2006, p. 12, emphasis added)

This approach fits generally with many of Ledoux's original (LeDoux, 1994) ideas but emphasizes evolutionarily appropriate stimuli and adds (Fig. 13.10; Isbell, 2006; for recent overview, see Kawai, 2019b) an extra, superfast, input (via superior colliculus and pulvinar) to the amygdala that can be viewed as dealing with orientation, prior to undirected escape (LGN), or avoidance (V1 ... V4). Critically, the arguments for a 'fear module' or 'snake detector' are based on expansion, in primates, of the visual system rather than the amygdala. We would see this expansion as involving distinct circuits that not only detect snakes but other visual objects such as spiders. Phobia related to the dark, or blood, or certain odours, would each have their own evolved circuits but in other brain areas. The visual expansion appears to have

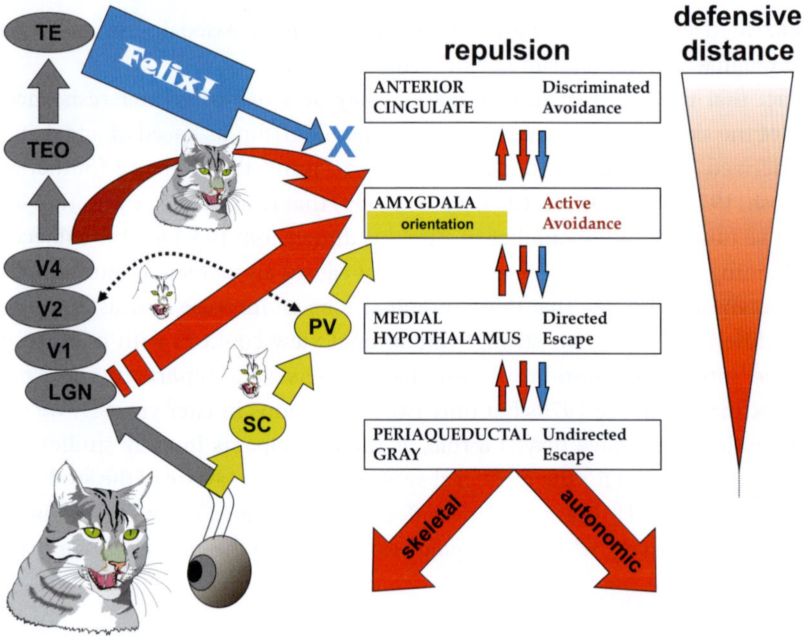

Fig. 13.10 Cats for rats / snakes for humans—fast pathways and specific innate fear stimuli. An adaptation of Fig. 6.1 including the circuits proposed by the Snake Detection Theory (based on Kawai, 2019b; see also Öhman, 2005). Dashes line represents a large number of reciprocal connections between the parallel systems. Contrary to 'fear module' approaches we see innate fear stimuli as simply 'pre-conditioned' stimuli with access to the fear system. Visual (especially for primates) stimuli can configure innate patterns that have privileged access to the amygdala. But note that the same would be true for appropriate auditory and, especially, olfactory stimuli processed by other pre-attentive systems. Also, this would be a simple genetic variant of the acquisition of fear responses by neutral stimuli via conditioning. Increased association strength could be achieved either ontogenetically or phylogenetically with the same ultimate consequence. *Abbreviations:* LGN = lateral geniculate nucleus; SC = superior colliculus; PV = pulvinar; TE/TEO = inferior temporal areas; V1, 2, 4 = visual cortex areas

involved both fast and slow pathways as well as attentive and object recognition circuits (note the indication in Fig. 13.10 of the extensive interconnections, e.g. [V2 ↔PV] between these systems).

> The koniocellular visual pathway, arising from the retina and connecting to the lateral geniculate nucleus, the superior colliculus, and the pulvinar, has expanded along with the parvocellular pathway, a visual pathway that is involved with color and object recognition. I suggest that *expansion of these pathways co-occurred*, with the koniocellular pathway being crucially involved (among other tasks) in pre-attentional visual detection of fearful stimuli, including snakes, and the parvocellular pathway being involved (among other tasks) in protecting the brain from increasingly greater metabolic demands to evolve the neural capacity to detect such stimuli quickly.
>
> (Isbell, 2006, p. 1)

Consistent with this, meta-analysis shows the expected increase in activity (as in fear conditioning paradigms) in the amygdala and insula in phobic subjects; with deactivation in right frontal and anterior cingulate cortex after exposure-based therapy (Ipser et al., 2013). Likewise, there is

> a double dissociation between the role of the amygdala in conditioning of the emotional response (SCR) and the role of the hippocampus in the development of CS-UCS contingency learning. Specifically, one patient with bilateral amygdala lesions did not acquire conditioned SCRs despite normal UCRs and normal acquisition of factual knowledge about the conditioning contingency. By contrast, another patient with bilateral hippocampal damage failed to learn the contingency at the cognitive level but did acquire differential conditioned SCRs. Thus, the amygdala circuit seems specifically dedicated to fear learning, whereas the hippocampus is important for conscious cognitive learning....
>
> We proposed that fear learning in humans occurs both at a basic associative level as evidenced by emotional responses (such as autonomic responses), mediated by the amygdala, and at a cognitive level of contingency learning, mediated by the hippocampus in at least its simple forms. When fear learning in human conditioning experiments involves fear-relevant stimuli that activate the fear module, the learning generally occurs at both levels simultaneously but independently. By contrast, when fear learning in human conditioning experiments involves fear-irrelevant stimuli, the learning would typically only engage at the cognitive level, without significant emotionality.
>
> (Mineka and Öhman, 2002, p. 934)

13.6.7 Specific phobia—individual variation

To sum up, evolutionarily relevant phobias do not seem to fit with a simple conditioning model (§13.6.3). The evolutionarily neutral dental fear appears to be conditioned; but not the more evolutionarily appropriate height phobia (Poulton and Menzies, 2002b). The preparedness hypothesis retained conditioning in a limited specialized form.

Here, we reject conditioning of any type for specific objects and see *evolutionarily appropriate* phobias as resulting from simple activation of innate fear *stimuli* via maturation, sensitization, dishabituation with non-specific stress and other '*different* learning processes' (Poulton et al., 2023, p. 1). With rats we need to see cats not only as visual stimuli like snakes for humans (albeit with stronger 'evolutionary conditioning') but also as olfactory stimuli (that need little processing for their functional signal). In this context, as others, humans can be treated as largely anosmic. Height, snake, and spider phobias are all visually driven in humans, consistent with phylogenetic, particularly primate, expansion of the pulvinar-related systems (§13.6.6). The specificity of specific phobia *must* be 'innate'.

So, with innate fear stimuli, why do some people become phobic and others not? The fast answer is that is how traits work. A normal distribution has extremes, each of which is nibbled away or expanded by selection. Absent the opposing maladaptations, there would be no trait (in the sense of individual variation).

Many people are reluctant to approach snakes or spiders or heights, or are nervous in the dark, but would not be classified as clinically phobic. Likewise, mean heritability of simple phobia is <50% (Torgersen, 1979; Van Houtem et al., 2013), so there is a strong environmental influence even on the emergence of phobic avoidance. Maturation in a given individual might involve more or less extreme ontogenetic factors. But we would also expect variation in genetic factors.

The modest heritable component is consistent with the evidence for evolved detectors of snakes (§13.6.5, §13.6.6), spiders etc. Following on from our 'conditioning' model of their evolution (§13.6.2), we see these as part of a 'fund of structural memory ... *phyletic memory*, or memory of the species. ... An unprovable but seemingly reasonable tenet ... is that the phyletic memory ... [has] developed in evolution by essentially the same mechanisms of association by co-occurrence and contiguity that contribute to the formation of individual memory in higher cortical systems, although the time scale of the two developments would be immensely different' (Fuster, 1995, p. 10; see also Mineka, 1992, on 'evolutionary memory').

This leads to three explanations of existing heritable variation. First, common phobic stimuli may be ones that are still becoming established in human populations subject to pressure from >150,000 human deaths per year due to snake venom (White, 2000). Second (and more likely given prosimian/platyrrhine/catarrhine differences, Isbell, 2006), common phobic stimuli were more powerful in our ancestors, and are undergoing regression ('phyletic forgetting' on analogy with Fuster's phyletic memory) due to increases in hominid defensive capacity (e.g. fire providing illumination at night). Third (and most likely) is that the presence of both progressive and regressive pressures has resulted in 'balancing selection' (Penke et al., 2007). All these explanations would give rise to genetic variation in the population; but the third would maintain it indefinitely—this is selection for standard deviation not mean. Particularly with the balancing case, the stimulus sensitivity can be regarded as trait variation (Penke et al., 2007, as per Chapter 12). Specific phobias reflect extreme values of personality factors.

13.6.8 Specific phobia—some conclusions

To conclude that specific object phobia often depends on the activation of innate fear stimuli is not to say that conditioning is never involved. In many cases phobic stimuli cannot be described as prepared/innate (Rachman and Seligman, 1976). Eysenck (1977), described a case in which a man developed a phobic reaction to a pattern of wall paper that had been on the walls of a bedroom in which he had been set upon by an irate husband. The stimulus source is irrelevant since the persistence of clinical phobic avoidance is what we would expect from the persistence of healthy active avoidance in general, absent *explicit countervailing* exposure-driven extinction (§13.6.3; Agras, 1985).

The more common, and cognitively complex, dental fear (Poulton and Menzies, 2002b) is also clearly not innate. Critically, it is not challenged with a period of exposure without pain but, instead, is frequently reinforced, most likely on a variable schedule that would have increased resistance to extinction. Again, persistence is understandable and it is, in any case, moot as to how far the fear is dysfunctional.

So, we would accept the proposal of at least 'three major pathways to the acquisition of fear ... [1] conditioning ... [2] vicarious acquisition ... [3] transmission of information and/or instruction' (Rachman, 1977, p. 383) as well as the arguments for 'adding a fourth, non-associative path to Rachman's' (Poulton and Menzies, 2002b, p. 127; see also Poulton and

Menzies, 2002a, for response to commentaries; Poulton et al., 2023, for update). All four pathways lead to patterns of strengthened connections that represent an engram capable of activating the fear system.

The role of exposure in extinction is most easily understood in terms of normal ritual sanitary precautions. Cleansing rituals (including mask wearing with COVID circulating) are clearly worth repeating in the *absence* of the punisher, disease. We attribute the continued absence of disease to the ritual (when we think about it at all). However, if such a ritual were regularly blocked and no disease followed, we would conclude that it was not needed.[9]

This type of explanation emphasizes cognitive factors more, and stimulus-response factors less, than in the original learning theory on which behaviour therapy was based. However, the original behaviourism was replaced by cognitive behaviourism (see, e.g. Dickinson, 1980)—although a cognitive orientation can be used even by those using classical behaviour therapy (Zinbarg, 1990). Thus, a major, and perhaps often the primary, effect of the various *behavioural* treatments of phobia is to alter the patient's *cognitions* in relation to the stimulus (whether conditioned or innately 'prepared'—they are just synaptic weights). Thus, the perception of the danger of the object can be reduced independently of the sensitivity of the fear system to dangers in general. Diagnostic systems should, therefore, categorically distinguish specific phobia from other forms of phobia and from anxiety.

13.7 Obsessions and compulsions

OCD shares with Panic Disorder that it has adaptive components (obsessions and compulsions) that can become maladaptive in individuals with a neurotic introvert personality (c.f., §13.5.4; making it sensitive to ketamine §13.2.2, §13.2.3; Martinotti et al., 2021). Its general aetiological relationship to anxiety is also like that of panic. We see OCD as primarily a fear disorder; but one that generates symptoms that, as they become more difficult to cope with under normal living conditions, can give rise to goal conflict and so anxiety.

Equally, it is clear that increases in anxiety can give rise to at least an increase in the frequency of obsessions and compulsions (c.f., Fig. 13.6). The repetitive checking of a toddler by a parent, for example, can seem obsessive to a non-parent; in this type of case, we attribute the increased checking to anxiety, rather than the other way round. As with panic and agoraphobia (§13.9), there is then the possibility that, in pathological cases, interactions of this kind could give rise to a vicious circle (c.f., Fig. 13.8); and also, that there may be different cases that are primarily anxious or primarily obsessional, respectively, both giving rise, however, to similar symptom patterns of mixed anxiety and obsession.

OCD is also, to some extent, like specific phobia in relation to its eliciting stimuli. But to most of us the symptoms of OCD are more mysterious than those of the specific phobias. If you say you are frightened of snakes, you are likely to be viewed as timid but rational. However, if you say you must wash your hands exactly 84 times and must do this every hour, you risk being viewed as irrational.

[9] That COVID spread among my mask-free highly educated academic colleagues (compared with the masked ones) provides me a vicarious counterfactual in New Zealand. So, don't try this experiment at home please! Just mask up. NMcN

Conditioning theories of the origin of this anxiety treat the compulsions as active avoidance behaviour (and so do we, but in a somewhat different fashion), maintained by a reduction in fear that follows them. As expected on the active avoidance model, environmental trigger stimuli (e.g. dirt in the case of hand washing) provoke the ritual in many cases, exposure to such stimuli without performance of the ritual increases subjective fear or anxiety, and performance of the ritual is followed by a decrease (Hodgson and Rachman, 1972; Röper and Rachman, 1976). The parallel with phobia, which we have also interpreted as a form of active avoidance behaviour or escape, extends to the resistance of compulsions to anxiolytic treatment and the fact that systematic exposure to 'anxiogenic thoughts' (equivalent, given the active avoidance model, to the phobic stimulus) tends to alleviate the compulsive rituals (e.g. Lovell et al., 1994).

However, obsessions call for a different type of explanation, as does the fact that (c.f. §13.6.4, §13.6.5) their rituals are not a random sample of those that could just happen to precede a reduction in anxiety; nor are obsessions a random sample of the ideas that could be threatening; and they are very similar in widely differing places. In New Delhi (Akhtar et al., 1975) as in England (Rachman, 1978), the commonest obsessions are with dirt, disease or contamination (50–60%), followed by orderliness or aggression (20–35%), and then by religion and sex (5–15%). Behavioural rituals, similarly, consist usually of cleaning, tidying up, and checking that various potential threats are absent (see also tables on p. 64 of Rapoport, 1989).

Many obsessions may, then, be responses to innate defensive stimuli (see also Jakes, 1996, especially p. xvii). What kind of stimuli might these be?

Dirt is one of the commonest obsessional preoccupations (Akhtar et al., 1975; Rachman, 1978) including in children and adolescents (Rapoport, 1989). It is likely that natural selection would reinforce the occurrence of grooming behaviour in response to dirt. Critically, in the case of organisms able to cause disease, grooming, and cleanliness, especially washing, *in the total absence of any perceptual evidence of contamination*, would also be adaptive. In at least some cases, therefore, it is likely that OCD involves the excessive activation of *normally adaptive* innate avoidance behaviour (and its accompanying cognitive complements). This excess is not surprising since, under normal ecological circumstances, there can be no external safety signal to terminate the behaviour (or the failure may be a failure of condensation and elimination within a planning sequence, Eilam, 2017). Thus, handwashing, checking that the door is locked, and so on, are usually done by patients tens or even hundreds of times. The disorder is in the failure to terminate the avoidance behaviour after a reasonable time not in the behaviour itself.

If obsessions and compulsions reflect innate avoidance tendencies, this does not link them directly with anxiety or even fear. As discussed in §13.6.3, normal avoidance behaviour can occur in the absence of any obvious fear as a simple habit. In some cases, therefore, especially early in the progression of the syndrome, we would expect ritual behaviour to occur in the absence of anxiety or fear (except that generated by the senseless intrusions and uncontrollable obsessions themselves). However, blocking of the ritual (as in blocking of a well-learned avoidance response) would be expected to result in fear. Furthermore, as occurrences of the ritual increase in frequency, its interaction with normal daily activity would have the consequence that it comes either to be blocked or to produce interference with normal activity, both of which could be equally disturbing. At this point we would expect the sufferer to seek clinical help.

Does this mean, then, that anxiety is simply a symptom of a more fundamental OCD? No more so than that anxiety is simply a symptom of Panic Disorder. One of the main functions of the GIS is to produce and control checking behaviour. High levels of anxiety would, then, be expected to produce (or increase) some obsessional ideation and compulsive ritual behaviour. Thus, there should often be positive feedback between obsessions and anxiety, analogous to the relationship between panic and anxiety. Pursuing the analogy further, there may be symptomatically similar patients who are primarily obsessional or primarily anxious, respectively; but it seems likely that in many cases OCD will be seen clinically in those who have a heightened sensitivity to both anxiety (via neuroticism) and obsession (c.f. Fig. 13.8—but substituting anterior cingulate for PAG).

Let us see how this analysis maps onto the available neurology. As concluded in Chapter 6, following Rapoport (1989), we can identify obsessions with increased activity in the anterior cingulate cortex (/caudal medial prefrontal and orbital frontal cortex, Graybiel and Rauch, 2000), and compulsions with excessive output from the basal ganglia, particularly caudate nucleus (Graybiel and Rauch, 2000) with decreased activity in the functionally inhibitory subthalamus (Welter et al., 2011). To some extent a system structured in this way can be viewed as autonomous in the normal production of a variety of innate motor programs. However, we have included the posterior cingulate in the SHS on the basis of its anatomical connections and its theta activity, and we attribute to this region at least part of the active risk assessment that can result from output from the hippocampal formation (see also §13.9). We would expect from this neurology, as previously suggested, that anxiety can be a source of obsessional checking. But *immediate* checking as such would remain located in the anterior cingulate, not in the SHS; while the latter, including the posterior cingulate, would generate future checking (i.e. risk assessment). This is consistent with the fact that anxiolytic drugs are not generally effective for the treatment of OCD *per se* (Appendix 1), although they would be expected to reduce any secondary anxiety consequent on this disorder (see next). Conversely the effectiveness of panicolytic drugs in OCD can be explained by an action on active avoidance with anterior cingulate reuptake systems (affected by clomipramine but not imipramine, Rapoport, 1989) somewhat different than those in areas controlling panic and depression that are sensitive to both clomipramine and imipramine.

For both functional and neurological reasons, then, we arrive at the following view of OCD. Obsessions and compulsions can arise from overactivity in the cingulate-basal ganglia circuitry. This is coupled with lost or reduced connectivity in fronto-striatal and fronto-parietal-limbic (including salience and default mode) networks. Often the overactivity will simply give rise to avoidance behaviour (or successful checking), will not produce major increases in anxiety, and will not lead to the seeking of clinical help. If rather less coherent components of the motor programs designed to cope with threatening stimuli are activated, this might be expected, as described by Rapoport (1989), to give rise to restricted and relatively anxiety-free cognitive variants of the motor tics characteristic of basal ganglia structural disease. Given current diagnostic categories, such conditions would still be classified as OCD. At the other end of the spectrum, where the frequency of fully fledged avoidance behaviour is very high, or the adequate stimuli elicit avoidance in problematic situations, or the avoidance response is in some other way blocked, then there will be conflict between this response and others. This conflict is likely to activate the GIS, with consequent anxiety. Such anxiety should be most likely (or will occur at a lower threshold) in those with a neurotic introvert personality. This is one scenario, given the normal progression of symptoms. However, the anterior cingulate is a direct target of the SHS. This suggests an alternative scenario: pathologically maintained anxiety (most likely generalized anxiety) could provide an unusually high level of input to the cingulate-basal ganglia circuitry (via the subicular input to posterior cingulate). This input could then trigger any latent obsessions and/or compulsions.

Finally, despite our focus on evolutionarily relevant scenarios and as with specific phobias, much the same arguments could apply to conditioned or instructed stimuli. The key steps would be a means of generating ritual avoidance behaviour to a threat or nominal threat where a safety signal would not be available.

13.8 Social anxiety

As detailed in Chapter 2, there can be both innate fear stimuli (e.g. a cat for a rat) and innate anxiety stimuli (e.g. the smell of the cat) with only the latter creating conflict and sensitive to anxiolytic drugs; and so, providing input to the GIS. Stimuli that arise in the course of social interaction are among the most important innate threats in many animal species (Gray, 1971); and social anxiety appears to result from conflicts generated by such stimuli (Marks, 1969). We can view sensitivity to social anxiety as a trait (du Rocher and Pickering, 2023); with 'Social Anxiety Disorder' having a quite arbitrary threshold separating an extreme portion of a continuous distribution that includes the normal population (Stein et al., 1994b).

In relation to the fear component of the conflict we can see the relevant stimuli as innate in the same way as snakes for simple phobia.

> Snakes are the prototypical stimulus in a predatory defense system promoting escape from predators, which prepares primates for efficient processing, attentional priority, and rapid fear acquisition to snakes and other stimuli related to predation. *The social submissiveness system plays a similar role* on the social arena by promoting yielding to dominant individuals without jeopardizing the protection of the group.... [There is] enhanced fear conditioning to snakes *and threatening faces* compared to neutral stimuli, as well as fast nonconscious processing of, and prioritized attention to, snakes and threatening faces. Human brain-imaging data show that these effects are mediated by an extensive fear-network centering on the amygdala.
>
> (Öhman, 2009, p. 543, added emphasis)

However, in social anxiety, it may not be detection of the individual stimuli that becomes disordered. Social anxiety

> is frequently multiphobic: fears of specific scrutiny situations (e.g. eating, writing, public speaking, appearing in public places, using public toilets) often co-existing together, and there may be a more pervasive anxiety about social interactions present ... A recent report indicates that two thirds of a large clinical sample suffer this generalised form of the disorder, in addition to fears of multiple specific situations ... While it seems likely that social [anxiety] can occur in a 'pure' form (e.g. public speaking anxiety), for many sufferers [social anxiety] and avoidant personality disorder are probably disorders on the same continuum ... In terms of other problems associated with social [anxiety], research

> has indicated that self-medication using alcohol, or other anxiolytics is frequent, and it is not unusual for this self-medication to escalate into significant substance abuse ... The presence of significant depressive symptoms is reported to be quite common, being found in half the patients in one study ... There are frequently clinically significant levels of generalized anxiety disorder.
>
> Mattick (1990, pp. 180–181)

Self-medication with alcohol and anxiolytics is consistent with the clinical effectiveness of benzodiazepines in SAD; but we should note that the SSRI, paroxetine, would be the likely first-line treatment, while the atypical antipsychotic, olanzepine (which affects dopamine 2 as well as $5HT_{1A}$ and $5HT_{2C}$ receptors), is highly effective (see Williams et al., 2020, for a meta-analysis of current drug treatments of SAD; also Table 4.1). There is reason to see both 5HT and dopamine as involved in SAD (Stein, 1998; Hjorth et al., 2021).

The lack of specificity of stimuli; the fact that, where specific stimuli are involved, we are dealing with anxiolytic-sensitive threat reactions; the fact that anxiolytics are used as self-medication; and the presence of depression as a, presumably long-term, consequence all fit with goal conflict as central to social anxiety. What, then, is its source?

The answer to this question lies in the theory's axioms: fear or phobia is a reaction to a set of stimuli that require exit from a dangerous situation; anxiety is a reaction to a set of stimuli that require entry into a dangerous situation, with resulting conflict. Specific phobias are correctly so named because the predominant required reaction is simple avoidance of a localized source of definite danger. The generally far from specific (Mattick, 1990) social anxieties are correctly so named because the predominant required reaction is entry into a diffuse source of a number of the most powerful rewards available to our species; but admixed with equivalent potential dangers. Here, 'eating, writing, public speaking, appearing in public places, using public toilets' etc. are clear and specific attractors—but approach to them opens one to potential diffuse dangers of unknown character that can appear without warning. This is not dissimilar to the case of OCD conflicting with everyday living—but involves complex social stimuli and (like novelty) a necessary admixture of diffuse attractive and diffuse (and uncertain) repulsive motivation. That is, unlike obsession, conflict is inherent to social anxiety and to its disorder.

One caveat should be entered here. There may be two types of trait social anxiety and so two types of social anxiety disorder—one more conflict-loaded and one more phobia-loaded. Both would engage the GIS but this need not be to the same extent.

> The social anxiety spectrum is considered to include two experientially distinct phenomena: social interaction anxiety (fearfulness and avoidance of situations where social interaction with other people is a requirement); and social observation/performance anxiety (fearfulness and avoidance of situations where observation or scrutiny from other people is likely). Elevated levels of trait social interaction anxiety tend to be more strongly related to the experience of low levels of positive affect, rather than to high levels of physiological arousal. By contrast, elevated levels of trait social phobia (social observation/performance anxiety[)] tend to be more strongly related to the experience of high levels of physiological arousal and symptoms similar to panic, rather than to low levels of positive affect.
>
> (du Rocher and Pickering, 2023, p. 2)

Anxiety, according to our theory, depends upon activity in the GIS. As shown in Fig. 13.2, we would see complex repulsion and complex attraction as processed by lateral and ventromedial orbital cortex, respectively. These are both reciprocally connected to rostromedial orbital cortex which we have strong reason to believe (§11.8.1) is one area that mediates anxiolytic action (in concert with the amygdala and hippocampus). In addition, we would see these orbital areas as optimizing goal selection policies (Fine and Hayden, 2022). All these areas also have direct links with the amygdala, which plays a central role in the perception of both facial (Adolphs et al., 1994; Calder et al., 1996; Morris et al., 1996a; Phillips et al., 1997; Rampino et al., 2019) and auditory (Phillips et al., 1998) expressions of fear. The anxiolytic, lorazepam, decreases activation induced by emotion face assessment in both the amygdala and insula (but not medial frontal cortex, Paulus et al., 2005).

It is notable that, as treatments of SAD, selective anxiolytics (other than pregabalin) are relatively weak (Table 4.1), as are noradrenaline reuptake inhibitors and tricylics. (Here the poor effect of clomipramine contrasts with its effect on OCD.) However, SSRIs, SNRIs, and monoamine oxidase inhibitors are more effective. Interestingly, 'SAD was associated with mainly increased expression and co-expression of the transporters for serotonin [SERT] and dopamine [DAT] in fear and reward-related brain regions' (Hjorth et al., 2021, p. 1) consistent with earlier suggestions that both 5HT and dopamine DA2 receptors are involved. DAT reduction in the putamen and SERT-DAT co-expression increase in the caudate both suggest disturbed attraction mechanisms (see du Rocher and Pickering, 2023, for comments on 'social anhedonia' in the context of both Reinforcement Sensitivity Theory and Attentional Control Theory). SERT reduction in the nucleus accumbens, SERT-DAT co-expression increase in the nucleus accumbens and amygdala, and DAT reduction in the amygdala are likely to have disturbed both attraction and repulsion. There were indications of higher DAT in the hippocampus.

> While our results on transporters are interesting in the light of pharmacologic and anatomical studies demonstrating functional reciprocity between serotonin and dopamine, the functionality of the altered SERT/DAT co-expression in SAD is not known. Transporter interactions may, however, impact the equilibrium between neural activations in fear and reward networks of the brain with resultant proneness for approach-avoidance conflicts at the behavioral level. Local coinciding increases of dopamine and SERT availability could thus play a causal or modulatory role in SAD.
>
> (Hjorth et al., 2021, p. 3975)

With this as background, we can perhaps attribute to the social anxieties the same innate or acquired strengthening of connections (in the orbital components of the GRS and perhaps GAS) as is postulated to occur in the amygdala in the case of specific phobias. However, in the case of the specific phobias, involvement of the GIS is limited to a modest orienting response (via the basolateral amygdala and insula, §13.6.5). In the case of the social anxieties, involvement of the GIS is much more extensive (including the orbital cortex as well as SHS and amygdala) because of the concurrent appetitive qualities of the aversive stimuli. This results in inhibition of the prepotent approach responses (i.e. inhibition of social involvement), as well as increased arousal and attention to negative stimuli (in this case negative social stimuli). The complex negative social consequences would be permanently anticipatory and, like obsessions, lack explicit safety signals.

Social anxiety can interact with panic in a manner that we will describe in detail for agoraphobia (§13.9), although the panic symptoms reported differ from those of agoraphobics (Page, 1994); and have the appearance more of consequences of high levels of social anxiety than causes. However, there may be cases where panic disorder is primary in social anxiety though not to the same extent as with agoraphobia. Most likely (as we will suggest for agoraphobia) is that social anxiety includes two or more quite different disorders. So, while social anxiety can be ameliorated by anxiolytic drugs, it may include a type that is particular sensitivity to selective serotonin reuptake inhibitors (Van Ameringen et al., 1994; Table 4.1). Thus, while excess anxiety appears to be characteristic of the disorder, the anxiety may in some cases be secondary to disturbance in some other part of the defence network; possibly panic disorder, but more likely an excess of social aversion mediated by the orbital cortex.

The theory presented here, then, suggests an important similarity between what used to be called 'social phobia' and agoraphobia: they are both anxieties rather than phobias; and both may depend on an excessive reaction to innate anxiety stimuli. As we will see, the theory also suggests an important difference between them. Agoranxiety/agoraphobia appears often to be an incidental consequence of the coincidence of a randomly occurring panic attack with the presence of otherwise affectively positive stimuli. Social anxiety, in contrast, involves social situations in which, as in the case of novel stimuli, both positive and negative affective value can be provided by one and the same object and in a particularly uncertain and anticipatory form.

13.9 Agoranxiety/Agoraphobia

Someone who is afraid of spiders/snakes etc. may curtail activities that bring them into contact with stimuli only secondarily associated with the negative stimuli. Similarly, one can generalize a fear of snakes to, e.g. a crocodile skin handbag. Such associations can spread through intricate stimulus and semantic generalization (Razran, 1971). But we should not assume that agoraphobia and social 'phobia' are simple *phobias* of complex stimuli. We have already made the case for social anxiety as a conflict in approaching people; here we make the case for 'agoranxiety' as a conflict in approaching the agora (the place people gather, or often anywhere outside your front door).

Agoraphobia commonly occurs together with panic attacks. Indeed, on one view, agoraphobia is *always* a means of avoiding, or avoiding the consequences of, panic attacks (e.g. Friend and Andrews, 1990; Joyce and Oakley-Browne, 1990). In contrast, Marks (1987) argued that panic is the result of extreme phobia produced by any of a variety of stimuli, and is more prominent in agoraphobia only because the fear stimuli are more difficult to avoid. In support of Marks' view, agoraphobia proper seems to precede panic in some cases (Lelliott et al., 1989). Moreover, as many as 1 in 20 of a mixed panic and/or agoraphobia sample can be diagnosed as agoraphobic without history of panic disorder, even after exclusion of phobias of specific stimuli such as crowds, tunnels etc. (Goisman et al., 1994). In §13.5.2, therefore, we agree with Marks, that high levels of anxiety can precipitate panic (as can a variety of other stimuli, such as a high partial pressure of carbon dioxide), and that agoraphobia can precipitate panic attacks in panic-prone individuals (Fig. 13.6). Agoraphobia, furthermore, is not the only such condition: generalized anxiety disorder, too, can on occasion predispose to panic disorder (e.g. Brawman-Mintzer et al., 1994). However, we accept also that, in many cases, panic *disorder* (i.e. the *inappropriate* occurrence of panic attacks) gives rise, through conditioning in individuals with a predisposing personality, to agoraphobia (§13.5.4; Fig. 13.7).

Taken together, these two views imply that agoraphobia as a clinical entity can, on occasion (c.f. Fig. 13.8), involve positive feedback between anxiety and panic in a vicious circle (independent of whether it is panic or anxiety that is causally primary)—but we view panic and anxiety as nonetheless distinct.

A particularly important way in which the conditioning process comes into play lies in the development of anxiety in relation to situations associated with the physiological consequences of fear itself. We say 'anxiety' here, because in most cases we are dealing with cases of conflict of potential appetitive activities (e.g. shopping) with potential, often unpredictable, negative events rather than simple repulsion from discrete, localizable, actual negative events. In many cases, this appears to be the way in which agoraphobia is generated.

For example, a person who experiences a panic attack in a particular environment may develop conditioned anxiety to, and avoidance of, that environment. The fact that the panic often cannot be attributed by the patient to a discrete, localizable external stimulus increases the chances of associational spread of the conditioned response, with the resultant development of a generalized agoraphobia.

Open spaces may act like this, as a diffuse set of poorly localized environmental stimuli; or, alternatively, they may themselves represent a source of uncertain threat able to act as an innate anxiety stimulus requiring risk assessment and behavioural inhibition. In either case, such spatially diffuse stimuli are particularly likely to activate the SHS (O'Keefe and Nadel, 1978) and, in particular, the posterior cingulate.

Crowded places similarly provide a complex set of diffuse and poorly localized social stimuli as a source of indefinite potential threat. The key point, given an analysis in terms of defensive direction, is that the specific phobias in general manifest as increased active avoidance of the specific phobic object while agoraphobia manifests as increased passive avoidance, *inhibiting entry into appetitive situations* because of a concurrent associated threat.

Given our theory, panic attacks in the classical sense would not be the only possible UCS at the origin of conditioned agoraphobia. Any other spontaneous, unpredictable aversive reaction could in principle produce the same conditioning. Agoraphobia without a history of panic disorder' seems in many cases to be the result of 'limited symptom' attacks that do not fulfil the criteria for full-blown panic, but may well provide a basis for conditioned avoidance (Goisman et al., 1995). Well established avoidance could then reduce the occurrence of the feared internal response through a general reduction in the level of arousal (§13.5.2).

So, agoraphobia coupled with panic attacks can arise either from a primary panic disorder, with resulting conditioning to the environment in which the panic occurs, or from a primary heightened anxiety that leads (via increased arousal) to the occurrence of panic attacks. This flexibility in the theory does not necessarily imply lack of testability. It should be possible, for example, to distinguish the types via carefully designed challenge tests. Manipulation of the partial pressure of CO_2, for example, could well determine whether an agoraphobic is particularly sensitive to panic attacks. Similarly, administration of cognitive tests could determine whether the patient is particularly sensitive to anxiety-provoking stimuli. These kinds of test are discussed further in §13.13.

13.10 Generalized anxiety disorder

> Generalized anxiety disorder was originally defined in DSM-III as a residual category. The hierarchical exclusion rules used in DSM-III obscured the independence of generalized anxiety disorder and were dropped in DSM-IIIR, thus allowing an independent diagnosis of generalized anxiety disorder in addition to other mental disorders and recognizing the importance and relative frequency of psychiatric comorbidity.
>
> (Brawman-Mintzer et al., 1993, p. 1216)

While there is very high comorbidity, it also seems clear that generalized anxiety can occur in isolation, with the same symptoms whether it is isolated or comorbid (Brawman-Mintzer et al., 1993; Brawman-Mintzer et al., 1994; Wittchen et al., 1994). Likewise, anxiety can precede depression, depression precede anxiety, or their onset can be concurrent (Poulton et al., 2023).

For our purposes, this is fortunate since, given the analysis so far, generalized anxiety disorder is, in essence, the only clearly identifiable primary anxiety disorder. That is, it is a case of maladaptive anxiety in which the primary pathology lies in the control of anxiety itself, as opposed to some mechanism (panic, phobia, innate stimulus detection) that then has consequential effects on the central control of anxiety.

13.10.1 Generalized anxiety, avoidance, and cognitive bias

Under normal circumstances, anxiety requires some eliciting source of conflict. According to our theory, the GIS will receive information about concurrently activated, conflicting, goals and this will result in inhibition of prepotent behaviour and, especially in cases involving aversive motivation, increases in arousal and aversion mediated by the amygdala. In all of the cases we have considered already, there has been an abnormality or oversensitivity of some area other than the GIS that has increased or replaced a normal aversive input and so engendered goal conflict and the resultant anxiety. By contrast, if there is GIS overactivity, we would expect maladaptive suppression of prepotent behaviour and the substitution of risk assessment, coupled with an increase in the relative weighting of affectively negative associations even in the absence of obvious external conflicting goals.

Increase in affectively negative cognitive bias is particularly important in this context. Approach-avoidance conflict could, in principle, be resolved by suppression of either approach or avoidance. However, it is fundamental to our theory (based as it is on the actions of the anti-anxiety drugs, and on the role of interference in hippocampal amnesia) that one part of the business of the hippocampus is to increase the power of negative at the expense of positive associations (i.e. risk aversion), and so to produce avoidance rather than approach via a positive input to the GRS (and potentially a negative one to the GAS; Fig. 5.1). In the pathological case this will result in the build-up of aversive memories.

Conversely, it is by decreasing activity in the GIS that anti-anxiety drugs decrease, but do not eliminate, avoidance. The putative overactivity of the GIS in patients with generalized anxiety disorder is consistent with the frequent inability of such patients to identify an explicit source of threat (in contrast, e.g. to the panic attacks that can often be identified in agoraphobia). Such overactivity is consistent also with the general picture of cognition in these patients.

> It has long been known that anxiety patients are pre-occupied with thoughts about threats, and that they have unrealistic beliefs about danger. There is also substantial evidence that correcting these distortions can decrease anxiety. Also, anxiety patients preferentially attend to and remember threatening cues. They interpret ambiguous words as threatening.
>
> (Nesse and Klaas, 1994, p. 465)

Why should overactivity in the GIS necessarily result in aversive output when we have argued that many of its normal operations involve the resolution of conflicts that are not particularly threatening? The answer is that frustration has the same effects as fear and even a conflict between two positive (but incompatible) goals involves the loss of whichever gain is not chosen—and so the situation elicits anticipatory frustration as a key element of the conflict. Indeed, given loss aversion, it could be thought that the essence of the choice is in avoiding the greater loss rather than obtaining the greater gain. Importantly, even the Stop Signal Task (where there is no extrinsic gain or loss) produces conflict-related 'theta' rhythm that is sensitive to anxiolytic drugs (§11.5.4).

In sum, generalized anxiety disorder reflects overactivity in one or more of the parts of the Central Nervous System (CNS) devoted to the resolution of conflict, repulsion, and risk assessment. At the present stage of development of the theory, it is most parsimonious to assume that this disorder is specific to overactivity of the GIS. Given the cognitive functions that we have ascribed to this system, this position is very close to the views of Andrew Mathews and of Michael Eysenck (see §13.2.5, §13.3.2). Importantly, the effect of the selective anxiolytic drugs will be to alter processing in the parallel Papez circuits (Fig. 9.9) that alter the motivational content of engrams. The drugs, then, will block the creation and maintenance of negative memories (but not the 'fear' memories themselves) and so allow their extinction. So, while the drugs have acute anxiolytic effects too, their *clinical* action on anxiety disorder proper (even with the benzodiazepines, §4.4) is delayed.

13.10.2 Generalized anxiety and goal-conflict-specific rhythmicity (GCSR)

For all the diagnostic categories we have considered so far, we have attempted to be clear (see particularly §13.5) that the labels refer to symptom packages that fractionate into cases where the brain area controlling the symptom is itself disordered, other cases where control of the symptom is normal but its input from some other brain area is disordered, and yet others where there can be interactions between disordered areas with, occasionally, vicious circles of positive feedback. Here we will argue that for generalized anxiety, as well, what we would see as the primary brain dysfunction cannot be equated with the current diagnostic label.

Our argument is based on the use of GCSR as an anxiety process biomarker (§11.5.4). Critically, the neurology of the response (Fig. 11.8, Fig. 11.10) makes it likely to be a measure of hippocampal output that is modulated by its RSA/'theta' input. Fig. 13.11 shows data from Shadli et al. (2021a) for a range of DSM diagnostic groups organized to have approximately equal numbers of participants in group (thus 'GAD' and 'GAD+MDD' are separated; SAD

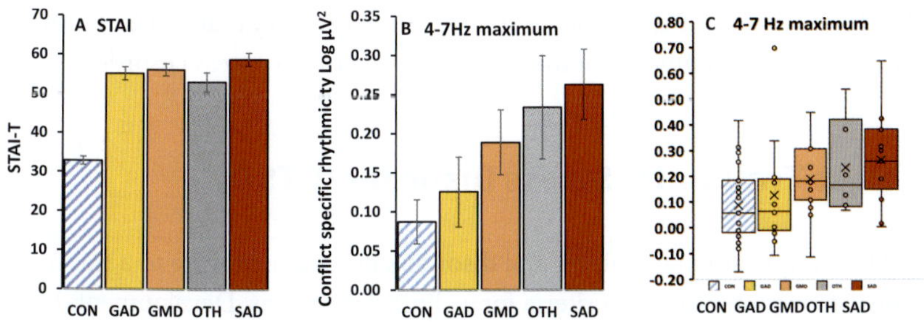

Fig. 13.11 Variation across DSM diagnostic groups in group averages of STAI and individual maximum GCSR in the range 4-7Hz. **A.** STAI-T (Spielberger et al., 1983) varied significantly with controls included ($F_{4,75} = 72.48$, $P < 0.0001$) but not between diagnoses with controls excluded (DSM, $F_{3,43} = 1.29$, NS). **B.** Average maximum 4-7Hz GCSR power varied significantly with controls included ($F_{4,75} = 3.53$, $P < 0.011$) but not between diagnoses with controls excluded ($F_{3,43} = 1.42$, NS). **C.** Distribution of maximum 4-7Hz GCSR scores across diagnostic groups. *Abbreviations:* CON = control; DSM = American Psychiatric Association's Diagnostic and Statistical Manual-IV; GAD = generalized anxiety disorder; GMD = generalized anxiety with major depression; OTH = other anxiety diagnoses (e.g., panic disorder); SAD = social anxiety disorder; STAI = Spielberger State Trait Anxiety Inventory; T = trait score on STAI. Figure and legend modified from Shadli et al. (2021a) with permission.

and comorbid SAD + GAD are combined; and a range of diagnoses are included in 'other'). STAI-T (Spielberger et al., 1983; see 12.1.1 for the view that STAI-T is general to neurotic disorders), showed no variation among the DSM diagnostic groups and a strong difference of all of them from control (Fig. 13.11A). GCSR is significantly elevated across DSM diagnoses compared to controls but its apparent variation among diagnoses was not significant with controls removed (Fig. 13.11B). It also varied across volunteer samples with the highest values in those with STAI-T above the clinical threshold (T>45) and becoming negligible at low values (T<33). Given our discussion of the disorders and their comorbidity so far, it is not surprising that GCSR (as a putative general anxiety process biomarker) has a broad distribution both within and between diagnostic groups (Fig.13.11C). It also appears to relate to some extent to comorbidity, with higher values in GAD cases with comorbid MDD (which is not sensitive to the anxiolytics that abolish GCSR) and the highest values in the SAD group (which contained five mixed diagnoses in a total of 13 cases).

Much further work, and more and better biomarkers (§12.14) will be needed to clarify the situation but at present it is reasonable to see hyper-reactive, RSA/'theta'-modulated, SHS output as generating a disorder that could sometimes be labelled GAD, but which clearly does not include all cases that would currently be diagnosed as such. Likewise, it is reasonable to expect the bulk of cases with such hyper-reactivity to present comorbid with other disorders, particularly SAD and depression. As noted already for GAD and depression, it seems that the occurrence of GAD can precede or follow or be concurrent with the occurrence of the disorder with which it is comorbid (Poulton et al., 2023)—with likely similar variations in dynamics to those shown in Figs. 13.6–13.8. When one asks either what causes these disorders to occur, or to develop in intensity, our earlier discussion provides some specific answers based on effects of internal dysfunction or personality extreme. But one important source that we must now consider is the effect of chronic or extreme-acute stress (Fig. 13.3). This can be usefully viewed through the lens of one final disorder category that, unlike all the others, is not primarily based on a simple symptom list—Post-Traumatic Stress Disorder.

13.11 Post-Traumatic Stress Disorder (PTSD)

> PTSD is unique among adult mental disorders because exposure to a traumatic event(s) is required to meet criteria for a clinical diagnosis. Developmental capacities and conditions of early childhood may increase both risk of trauma exposure and of PTSD. Rather than being solely a proximal response to trauma, the roots of PTSD involve predisposing developmental origins.... PTSD in adulthood rarely, if ever, develops in anything but the context of other disorders.... Both severe [childhood] maltreatment and prior history of mental disorders were found to independently predict adult PTSD. Note, the experience of mild trauma during childhood was not found to increase the risk of PTSD by the adult years, providing little evidence for the hypothesis of stress-sensitisation from moderate trauma.
>
> (Poulton et al., 2023, p. 3)[10]

A 'traumatic event' is described by ICD-11 (World Health Organization, 2023, 6B40; see also Payne et al., 2004, on 'What are stress and trauma?') as

> Exposure to an event or situation (either short- or long-lasting) of an extremely threatening or horrific nature. Such events include, but are not limited to, directly experiencing natural or human-made disasters, combat, serious accidents, torture, sexual violence, terrorism, assault or acute life-threatening illness (e.g. a heart attack); witnessing the threatened or actual injury or death of others in a sudden, unexpected, or violent manner; and learning about the sudden, unexpected or violent death of a loved one.

In some ways, this is like the unconditioned events that can condition evolutionarily neutral simple phobias (§13.6.4); and the symptoms of PTSD may subsequently be triggered or exacerbated by stimuli that are associated with, or in some way remind the patient of, that initial trauma. But these symptoms involve not only avoidance (which could be conditioned) but also re-experiencing (not just remembering) the event; they can occur without such an obvious environmental trigger (see the discussion of Adamec's experiments, next); and also, they can be more generalized:

> Persistent perceptions of heightened current threat, for example as indicated by hypervigilance or an enhanced startle reaction to stimuli such as unexpected noises. Hypervigilant persons constantly guard themselves against danger and feel themselves or others close to them to be under immediate threat either in specific situations or more generally. They may adopt new behaviours designed to ensure safety (e.g. not sitting with ones' back to the door, repeated checking in vehicles' rear-view mirrors).
>
> (World Health Organization, 2023, 6B40)

[10] §12.4 also discusses neuroticism and C&W BIS as PTSD risk factors.

Two features of PTSD are closer to panic disorder (PD) than to specific phobia. The first is the high level of arousal and autonomic disturbance seen. The second is that both PTSD and PD can manifest themselves during sleep, as nightmares or panic attacks, respectively. In the case of relaxation-induced panic, we accepted Graeff's (1994) hypothesis that this reflects the switching off during relaxation or sleep of descending inhibitory control from the GIS over the PAG. This could also be true of the mental activity (akin to flash backs) occurring during nightmares in PTSD. Note that, like PD (Dantendorfer et al., 1996) PTSD is associated with a decrease in hippocampal volume both in combat veterans (Bremner et al., 1995b; Gurvits et al., 1996) and survivors of childhood physical and sexual abuse (Bremner et al., 1997; Stein et al., 1997). This may require chronic trauma and not be linked to PTSD with acute trauma (Payne et al., 2004, p. 84), and so the damage may also explain the memory deficits in veterans (Bremner et al., 1995a) although perhaps not those with a history of childhood sexual abuse (Stein et al., 1997). Along with such *deficits* in memory, a key symptomatic feature of PTSD consists in *intrusive* memories (flashbacks), related to the traumatic incident.

Our discussion of the SHS damage seen in panic disorder (§13.5.5) indicated the two most likely aetiologies for this damage as perinatal anoxia or the neurotoxic effects of prolonged exposure to corticosteroids. In the case of PTSD, the latter is clearly the more likely (Payne et al., 2004). The hippocampus controls negative feedback of stress hormone release (McEwen et al., 1992) and its dysfunction may explain why patients with PTSD show abnormally high fluctuations in peripheral levels of cortisol (Southwick et al., 1994); with a potential vicious circle: an initial environmental insult, via prolonged activation of the SHS and stress-induced hormonal changes, can give rise to SHS damage, which then worsens the physiological and psychological consequences of further stress. The developmental contributions to later PTSD could involve less severe but nonetheless lasting changes in the stress system.

So far in this account we have concentrated on hippocampal *damage*, and the possible consequent *release* of other structures, particularly the amygdala, from hippocampal inhibitory control. In this context, a putative animal model of PTSD studied by Adamec (1998a); (Adamec, 1998b) is suggestive: just one or two systemic injections of an inverse benzodiazepine agonist, FG 7142 (*N*-methyl-β-carboline-3-carboxamide), with known anxiogenic properties in man, induced an increase in defensive behaviour that lasted more than 140 days; coupled with long-term potentiation of amygdala input to both the ventromedial hypothalamus and the PAG. Adamec advances a number of reasons to believe that the latter, electrophysiological, changes underlie the increased behavioural defensiveness caused by FG 7142. Predator stress has similar effects (that, as with PTSD, depend on the character of the traumatic event and show substantial individual differences).

> Predator stress has neurobiological and neuropharmacological features which recommend it as a model of aspects of PTSD. For example, there is evidence that predator stress induces lateralized lasting potentiation of right amygdala afferent and efferent neural transmission which likely mediates behavioral effects, paralleling right amygdala hyperexcitability in PTSD. In addition, propranolol given just after stress blocks lasting changes in affect in predator stressed rats, paralleling a similar effect of immediate post-trauma propranolol on PTSD symptom severity measured months later in humans.
>
> (Adamec et al., 2008, p. 1288)

These data suggest that a key process in PTSD is a 'lasting transformation in emotional disposition' (Pitman et al., 1993), that is, a general increase in the propensity to react with excessive defensive behaviour to all kinds of threat whether or not they closely resemble the original traumatic event. As noted in Chapter 12 this makes PTSD appear to involve a major change in a basic defensive trait.

While the PAG is likely to be involved in panic attacks, defensive analgesia, and a range of threat-related reactions, it does not look plausible as a location for producing all the symptoms of PTSD. In particular, flashbacks and nightmares are strongly perceptual in nature, suggesting a forebrain location. As we saw in Chapter 6, as well as its connections downstream to the hypothalamus and PAG, the amygdala has strong connections also with sensory systems. A reasonable hypothesis, therefore, places the perceptual phenomena of flashbacks and nightmares in these connections. Hippocampal inhibitory control (or, in PTSD, the loss of such control) could then influence the intensity of these perceptual phenomena either by way of the connections from the hippocampus to the amygdala itself, or by way of converging connections from the amygdala and the hippocampus to neocortical sensory processing areas. This hypothesis—that the amygdala plays a critical role in the laying down and retrieval of strongly emotional memories—was originally proposed by both LeDoux et al. (1989) and Pitman (1989).

Supplementing this 'amygdala boost' account for flashbacks is a memory-related account originally proposed by Nadel and Jacobs (1996), noting that high levels of stress-induced corticosteroids reduce hippocampal excitability while at the same time potentiating amygdala function. These changes could impair, at the time of initial exposure to trauma, the encoding (hippocampally mediated) and subsequent storage of information about context, while leaving intact encoding (via the amygdala) of associations between specific cues and the traumatic event. In consequence, 'when a person retrieves a traumatic event memory, the retrieved information is bereft of … context … [and] the memory takes on a quality of the here and now so strongly that the individual may literally *re-experience the event*' [Nadel & Jacobs, 1996, their emphasis]. Subsequent steroid-induced structural damage to the hippocampus might exacerbate the effects of these alterations in encoding processes by further weakening the capacity, at the time of retrieval, to analyse contextual differences between the past and current environments and use these to suppress retrieval.

> The stress that usually accompanies trauma) has identifiable effects on the hippocampus, impairing both the neuronal structure and the function of this brain region. As a direct consequence, stress (especially uncontrollable stressors) impairs various forms of memory. However, not all memories suffer this effect … [Hippocampal dysfunction means that some are] recorded in a fragmented manner, with the elements of the event not woven into a coherent remembered episode. At the same time, emotion works (via the amygdala) to promote memory for the … thematic content of an emotion event, but, again, without [coherence]'
>
> (Payne et al., 2004, p. 76, which see for detailed review)

Taking PTSD (and its apparent developmental origins, Poulton et al., 2023) as a guide, we can see anxiety-related disorders developing through an interaction of events (potentially including extensively repeated minor events, Dugan et al., 2023) with a tapestry of specific (anxiety, panic, obsession) and more general (neuroticism) traits that can give rise to recurring goal conflicts and so release of stress hormones with the potential for hippocampal damage and so dyscontrol of the pituitary–adrenal axis. This in turn can affect processing of approach-avoidance conflicts (Vogel and Schwabe, 2019). From this and our earlier diagnosis-specific perspective we can expect defensive disorders to present as a multidimensional spectrum of dysfunction (Fig. 13.1) that is not closely tied to the symptom patterns that result.

13.12 A typology of the anxiety-related disorders

This chapter has provided both ethological and neural (Fig. 13.2) reasons for distinguishing a variety of specific anxiety-related symptoms and syndromes. However, given the distinction between symptoms and syndromes, the use of our clinical typology is not quite so straightforward as the functional typology of defence (Fig. 13.5) on which it is based. We will start (§13.12.1) with our current theoretical typology of *primary* disorders. Note that this largely uses existing diagnostic labels but maps to only subsets of cases that would currently have this label (with others showing the equivalent symptoms for secondary reasons) and would expect the bulk of cases to have some comorbidity. We then discuss the implications of symptom/syndrome differences in the context of apparent and real comorbidity (§13.12.2). We will also discuss the implications of resistance to conventional treatment—which occurs with all the current diagnoses (§13.12.3). An important point is that our ultimate picture is of a multidimensional spectrum that largely overlaps the picture we have presented for personality (Chapter 12) and expects clinical presentations to involve multiple extreme personality factors (§13.2.3; Fig. 13.3).

13.12.1 The primary disorders

Panic Disorder (§13.5): an *excessive* reaction to proximity to an unavoidable major threat or to a stimulus, such as suffocation, which normally produces *undirected* escape responses. In spontaneous panic, and in many adaptive situations in the wild, freezing can occur rather than active escape attempts. The primary control centre for panic as a symptom and the primary location of dysfunction in 'pure' panic disorder (which would normally present in a cardiac not psychiatric clinic) and neurotic panic (with anxiety) is the PAG. The intensity of the syndrome may reflect loss of hippocampal inhibitory control of PAG.

Specific Phobic Disorder: an *excessive* production of a reaction normally generated by proximity to a specific avoidable major threat, or by a stimulus that predicts its presence, and which normally produces *directed* escape or active avoidance. The primary control centres (§13.6.6) for this are likely to lie in the medial hypothalamus and amygdala. The commonest cause of specific phobia, as a disorder, is likely to be a greater than average strength in the connections between detectors of evolutionarily relevant threat stimuli (e.g. snakes via the superior colliculus and pulvinar, Fig. 13.10) and their associated set of innate response production systems. Specific phobia can also result (although more rarely) from conditioned avoidance of evolutionarily neutral stimuli. The occurrence of the phobic avoidance response prevents its extinction; exposure to an innate or conditioned stimulus that has predicted, but is not in fact followed by, threat facilitates extinction.

Obsessive-Compulsive Disorder: at its most basic, involves excessive production of innate rituals generated both by specific environmental stimuli and, particularly, spontaneously. In the latter case the adaptive form of the behaviour fulfils the role of defence against threats that cannot be detected, such as disease organisms and, like Specific Phobic Disorder is likely to have an important innate component. It differs from simple phobia in the complexity of the eliciting stimuli and a usual lack of explicit safety signals that could terminate avoidance responding. We link the rituals to the various checking functions of the SHS, particularly the risk analysis output. However, the key control centres are the *anterior* cingulate cortex, caudal medial prefrontal cortex, and orbital frontal cortex (obsessions) and the basal ganglia (compulsions), and it is here, not the SHS, that any neuropathology would occur in 'pure' cases (lacking anxiety). As with Panic Disorder, pure cases would not normally present in the psychiatric clinic. Neurally induced spread of activity or conflict of the ritual with other goals and conditioning can result in the occurrence of, or increase in, anxiety (reflecting increased output from the SHS).

Social Anxiety Disorder: an excessive negative reaction to proximity to, or placement in, social interaction with conspecifics. This involves conflict between alternatives. It is likely to involve two types: social *interaction* anxiety (where conflict between positive and negative payoffs is primary); and social *observation/performance* anxiety (where conflict is derived from experience of panic-like symptoms). Such conflict may be between alternative goal objects or between alternative approach and avoidance tendencies (often driven by a fear of scrutiny) to a particular goal object. The primary control centres (i.e. the location of the mechanisms which detect and analyse social situations) appear to be the amygdala and orbital cortex. However, the primary site of pathology could be located either in these centres or in excessively strong connections from there to the SHS or result from increased reuptake of serotonin and dopamine—but is likely to involve all three. In all cases there is likely to be excessive activity in the SHS that constitutes part but not necessarily all of the functional problem.

Agoranxiety (overlapping some cases that would currently be diagnosed with agora-'phobia'): an excessive reaction most frequently resulting from the conditioning of anxiety by spontaneous panic, but which may also result from excessive responsiveness to a diffuse set of poorly localizable, innately aversive, spatial or social cues. This has similarities to social anxiety but with simpler stimuli. Here the primary site of excess activity of primary pathology (as with anxiety induced by approaching the dark) is likely to be in the posterior cingulate and its connections to the SHS and amygdala; but much of the distinctive behavioural pathology will be largely the result of conditioning and secondary to the panic attacks or other phobic stimuli that provided the reinforcement for that conditioning.

Nyctoanxiety (overlapping some cases that would currently be diagnosed with nycto-'phobia'). As for agoranxiety except linked to darkness (and its potential dangers including mythical monsters) rather than public places. It appears sensitive to benzodiazepines (https://www.choosingtherapy.com/nyctophobia/).

Generalized Anxiety Disorder is the one case where the pathology of anxiety itself is primary. This is anxiolytic-sensitive (and likely reflects overactivity in the GIS that is ameliorated most by the action of anxiolytics on ascending modulatory inputs). The delayed action of anxiolytic drugs (§4.4) and the role of iteration in memory formation and consolidation (§9.9.2) shows that the disorder is one of excess formation, or weighting, of aversive (e.g. fear) memories or an equivalent failure of emotional habituation. The mechanism is the one normally used by the GIS to amplify repulsion and arousal in the GRS when goal conflict is detected (Fig. 5.1) and so also increase the formation of aversive memory. Blockade of this hyperactive process by the drugs then allows the aversive component of the existing memories to be extinguished.

Anticipatory Panic Disorder: Based on Fig. 13.2, we postulate an *anxiolytic-sensitive* equivalent of panic based on high levels of (proximal) conflict and differing from conventional panic in the way that defensive quiescence differs from freezing. Such a disorder remains to be demonstrated—and would be confirmation of a prediction.

Post-Traumatic Stress Comorbidities is a loose class that reflects multiple primary disorders (including depression) that can be shown to have resulted from an extreme traumatic exposure or chronic high levels of stress. The symptoms that ensue can involve long-lasting conditioned responses but also include more general long-lasting increases in response to negative stimuli whether related to the original trauma or not. The comorbidities can involve intense activity (and re-activity) in all regions of the primary defence system, *viz* the PAG, hypothalamus, amygdala, and anterior cingulate; combined in some cases with loss of hippocampal inhibitory control, due to structural damage arising most probably from excessive and prolonged action of adrenocortical hormones within the hippocampus. Even given the traumatic circumstances that lead to this condition, differences in pre-trauma personality play a role (§12.4); conversely, the pervasive nature of the changes that ensue, including the structural damage sometimes affecting the hippocampus, represents in some degree a long-lasting change in personality. At present we see Post-Traumatic Stress Comorbidities as being a useful preliminary clinical category for triage, representing an important extreme area in the comorbidity spectrum but suspect it is not helpful to see it as a distinct primary disorder (i.e. dependent on the extreme of a single defining trait). Indeed, it is likely to be an extreme model for the generation of all of these disorders.

13.12.2 The symptom/syndrome and comorbidity problems

How is it that this inherently simple classification is not reflected in clear and discrete entities in the clinic? There are three reasons, one situational, one neurological, and one spectral.

In terms of situations, while the Blanchards' analysis allows one to categorize reactions in terms of defensive distance, it gives no guarantee that specific systems will be activated one by one. There is good evidence for blending of concurrent emotions (see Chapter 4 of McNaughton, 1989b); and, as noted earlier, when faced with a predator we must be prepared both to remain still and assess whether it has been detected (with a potential predator) and to flee (when it is proved to be an actual predator). Thus, both anxiety and fear will be present (fear here implying a high tendency to engage active avoidance). It is important to see the relevant behaviours as prepotently activated in parallel with action resulting from release of one from inhibition.

In terms of neurology, while we can equate individual symptoms with activity in individual areas, this gives no guarantee that the site producing the most evident *symptoms* is the critical dysfunctional site from a pathological point of view. (Note that high temperature appears adaptive with infection and, as a symptom, gives no indication as to specific causative pathology.) There are delayed links through the environment that are important for aetiology (e.g. the conditioning of agoraphobia by spontaneous panic); and there are neural links within the brain (so that, e.g. high levels of pathological anxiety can trigger otherwise adaptive panic). In some cases, inhibitory connections may blur the issue. In Graeff's view, the presence of moderate anxiety is generally inhibitory of panic, with resultant spontaneous panic attacks during sleep or relaxation. In this case, then, a secondary agoraphobia may partially suppress (via the serotonin system) the appearance of the panic attacks that were primarily responsible for the conditioning of anxiety in the first place.

We must, therefore, as does modern cognitive psychology, take a more iterative, network view of anxiety and its related phenomena. Under normal circumstances, in an anxiety-provoking situation, there will be some activation of each of the PAG, hypothalamus, amygdala, SHS, cingulate-basal ganglia loop, and prefrontal cortex including insula. The precise balance of activity between these areas will be determined by their interconnections and by the modulating influences of acetylcholine, noradrenaline, and serotonin, as well as a constellation of pituitary–adrenal hormones. Thus, in the majority of cases, a primary disturbance in any one area, whether of endogenous or environmental origin, will tend to spread to others (Fig. 13.12), giving rise to a mixture of symptoms. It follows that the primary disorder may not be obvious simply from the symptoms exhibited (even ignoring the effects of culturally specific display rules); and that, even if our typology of anxiety disorders were entirely correct, it would still not be easy to determine from symptoms the type applicable to a particular patient. We deal with this issue in the next section.

The final, spectral, reason for lack of current clinical clarity is one we have touched on both in considering panic and the disorders related to it (§13.5, especially Figs. 13.6–13.9) and in considering PTSD. In essence we expect disorders to be spectral in a way that goes beyond coincidental comorbidity of primary disorders. Chronic anxiety generates a stress response that can, in turn, contribute to disorder, most clearly in the case of PTSD. Acute traumatic stress or chronic stress thus acts against a baseline already determined by prior experience and which we would characterize as involving increased neuroticism, trait worry, or more

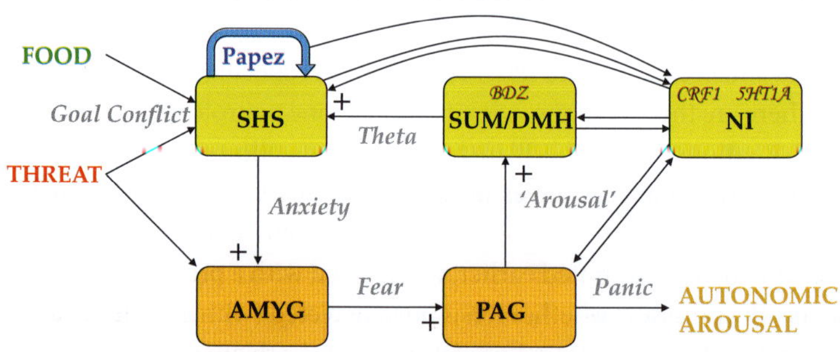

Fig. 13.12 One example of possible positive feedback loops involved in the control of anxiety shown with autonomic output only. Threat can activate both AMYG and SHS depending on whether conflict is present or not. There is a simple, potentially positive feedback loop, connecting them with the PAG and SUM/DMH. Additional short loops exist via NI and longer ones via the Papez circuits. Activity in the main loop can be controlled by BDZ receptors, CRF1 receptors, and 5HT1A receptors. *Abbreviations:* AMYG, amygdala; BDZ, benzodiazepine receptors; CRF1, corticotropin releasing factor 1 receptors; 5HT1A, serotonin 1A receptors; NI, nucleus incertus; PAG, periaqueductal gray; SHS, septo-hippocampal system; SUM/DMH, medial supramammillary and dorsomedial hypothalamic areas involved in the control of theta frequency.

specific changes in trait anxiety, trait panic, etc. Outputs such as panic can then condition further disorder or, themselves, be increased by a background elevation in arousal. Thus, not only will there be cases where a symptom is technically adaptive but driven by some other dysfunction but also cases where the control of the symptom itself can then be subject to progressive induced dysfunction.

13.12.3 Treatment resistance (TR) and typology

On this view, it is not surprising that there is substantial TR with all the neurotic disorders (§13.2.2). One simple explanation is that the expressed symptoms will often be secondary to the primary disorder, which may remain cryptic. However, we must note that, with drugs like SSRIs or treatments like Cognitive Behavioural Therapy (CBT) that have a broad spectrum of action, simple misdiagnosis is an unlikely explanation. Our alternative proposal is a double-hit hypothesis (§13.2.3) where not only is there a form of specific primary dysfunction in the form of high trait anxiety/panic/obsession/depression/etc. but also there is high neuroticism (taken to mean general threat sensitivity) and it is the combination of this with a high level of at least one primary trait that delivers disorder. On this view PTSD is likely to involve both extreme neuroticism (likely high initially and made extreme by trauma) but also several other extreme traits: panic, etc (also heightened by trauma) and so a high probability of TR.

For all the disorders, and especially their comorbidities, we would expect some cases to have a progressive course. Anxiety, in particular is likely to suffer positive feedback effects with chronic stress (particularly the positive feedback between dyscontrol of cortisol and hippocampal damage). Likewise, we have noted the likely role of the conditioning of anxiety (and its attendant arousal) in disorders such as agoranxiety. But most likely, with PTSD as a model, high background neuroticism or trait worry, coupled with 'semi-traumatic events' (Kehyayan et al., 2023) could lead to a progressive increase in neuroticism, where a sufficiently high level would generate a resultant specific-trait-linked disorder despite a normal level of that trait, rendering it insensitive to treatments other than ketamine and its relatives. We will discuss the nature of cases that are also resistant to ketamine in the next chapter.

13.13 Differential diagnosis

Our analysis of clinical anxiety has both optimistic and pessimistic consequences for diagnosis, and hence eventually for treatment. On the optimistic side, the separation of symptoms from syndromes, coupled with the conclusion that syndromes cannot be distinguished simply (or perhaps at all) in terms of symptoms, allows for a resolution of a number of controversies in the literature. Usually both sides are right: panic can be both the cause and the result of anxiety; anxiety can be both the source and the consequence of obsession. On the pessimistic side, we have largely explained away, or explained *post hoc*, rather than truly predictively explained the clinical situation (though many of our current suggestions are retained from the second edition). This is not to say, however, that the theory is compatible with *any* data that might be collected in future. An important conclusion from our analysis is that it should be possible to separate the different syndromes by using *theoretically based challenge tests* and ignoring the fact that different syndromes can present with much the same symptoms. Indeed, a key feature of the tests we propose is that they should seldom be directed towards the most obvious symptoms and (perhaps surprisingly to some) should be administered when state anxiety and hence symptoms are minimal (to avoid contagion).

The central idea behind our suggestions for differential diagnosis is that the specific nodes of the defence system should be selectively *challenged* to determine whether they are functioning normally, and that such challenges should be designed to produce *minimal* reactions from the rest of the defence system. Otherwise, given the recursive interactions characteristic of the defence system, simply making someone anxious (or fearful or panicky) will automatically spill over into activation of much of the system, so making it impossible to determine at which point excessive sensitivity resides. An important corollary of this iteration (and an idea gradually creeping into conventional diagnosis) is that there is likely, in any case, to be extensive genuine comorbidity. There is little reason to suppose that just one node of the overall defence system will be the only one hyper-sensitive in any one individual at any one time. Indeed, given what we saw in the section on PTSD, it is surprising that hyper-sensitivity is not usually more diffuse and widespread in syndromal terms (§13.12.2, §13.12.3).

Let us now briefly look at some possible challenge tests and ways in which they might contribute to a diagnostic scheme (and be used directly to test some aspects of the theory). What we need is a stimulus or paradigm maximally activating the region of interest with minimal activation of other parts of the defence system. With such a challenge we could then test patients for the extent to which the structure itself is overreactive, as opposed to being secondarily triggered by excessive activity elsewhere in the defence system. At present there are very few such tests and their use is not well developed—but they will provide a sketch of what is needed.

Starting at the bottom of the defence system, we have already discussed challenges of the PAG that can elicit panic (§13.5.1). CO_2 appears to be one candidate but its use has been 'impeded by the lack of standardization of the challenge methodology and by uncertainty concerning the optimal definition and assessment of laboratory panic' (Rassovsky and Kushner, 2003, p. 1); lactate infusion is an alternative, also linked to suffocation alarm, and both may tap into opioidergic disorder (Preter and Klein, 2008). (Technically CO_2 seems preferable except that they may tap different sensitivities.) CCK4 induces panic in controls and patients at different doses (Sandford et al., 2000) and orexin systems may also provide suitable targets (Johnson et al., 2010). Detailed work is need to see if some panic patients are characterized by physical reactions other than dyspnoea and to test how far patients with high levels of anxiety (with panic a potential secondary symptom) do not show such challenge sensitivity. The key point is that *threshold* measurements appear able to detect super-sensitivity in the PAG independent of other abnormalities in the defence system. There may also be relatively input-specific abnormalities of the PAG whose detection would require testing with, say, painful stimuli as well as asphyxia. Most important, is the notion of exclusion. A *lack* of positives on a range of such *primary* panic tests would suggest *secondary* panic. The idea that a panic symptom is adaptive and secondary to maladaptive anxiety, for example, is not common.

At the next level up, we have the hypothalamus and at least some aspects of amygdala function. If our current analysis is correct, no fundamentally new test is required here, as the disorders of major concern are the specific phobias, which are simply diagnosed with current methods comparing reactions to the specific phobic object versus other threatening objects. Recent improvements (that can also be used for exposure treatment) involve testing patients with moving images of the relevant objects using virtual reality (with some forms of delivery allowing brain imaging of treatment-induced changes, Alvarez-Perez et al., 2021).

Next are the aspects of amygdala function linked to the arousal component of anxiety. The most obvious relevant challenge would be 'fear'-potentiated startle, since this is not only sensitive to anxiolytic drugs (including when injected into the amygdala), but is also insensitive to hippocampal lesions. This challenge can have two different forms with more predictable and less predictable stimuli linked to stimulus-specific fear and anxiety relays respectively (Davis, 2006) and appears to involve circuits through the anterior insula, anterior cingulate, and PAG (Lindner et al., 2015).

Next is the SHS. What is required is a test sensitive to SHS damage and anti-anxiety drugs, but *not* to amygdala or PAG lesions (hypothalamic lesions would be likely to interrupt the theta frequency control system as well as escape and avoidance behaviour, and so their effects could not be used to rule out a proposed test). The most obvious tasks, here, are spatial navigation, delayed matching to sample and behaviour on a fixed interval schedule of reward. But all suffer, for clinical use, from the difficulty of finding a suitable source of positive motivation that can be applied in the clinic. This problem can be solved by using two-way avoidance. In the Joystick Operated Runway Task (Perkins et al., 2009; Perkins et al., 2013) both fear (flight intensity) and anxiety (risk assessment) can be assessed and 'demonstrates anxiolytic effects of lorazepam in dosages ≤1 mg in the absence of a drug effect on fear' (Marwood et al., 2022, p. 1). There is a potential risk with this task of changes in trait fear impacting on measures of anxiety and so both must be measured concurrently. There is also a risk of inducing panic. One potential alternative is GCSR (§11.5.4, §13.10.2); however, this currently lacks sensitivity and stability. What is needed is likely further development (12.14) of more complex virtual reality tasks that, like the Joystick Operated Runway Task, allow concurrent measurement of a range of traits, particularly via the use of trial-wise modelling (Fung et al., 2019; Qi et al., 2018).

As reviewed by Shephard et al. (2021), with the anterior cingulate and other circuits involved in OCD, there is now reason to see at least five circuits (fronto-limbic, sensorimotor, ventral cognitive, ventral affective, dorsal cognitive) as involved in generating a taxonomy of neurobiological variants. These circuits can be characterized in terms of more than one function (e.g. fronto-limbic including both dysregulated fear and intolerance of uncertainty). Importantly, these different functions are already associated with challenge tasks (Shephard et al., 2021, their Table 2); but where a 'battery' approach would need to be taken with, e.g. failure of 'response inhibition' not being specific to OCD. Further work is needed to identify any distinct OCD-specific challenge response; but, in the current context, a key exclusion is likely to be a high sensitivity to specific panic challenges.

We have only limited clues as to what might constitute useful diagnostic tests for other anxiety-related disorders. Tests of prefrontal hyperfunction could be based on the existing neuropsychological tests of prefrontal hypofunction.

13.14 Conclusion

There have been great strides in the last 20 years, particularly with imaging (e.g. Laumann et al., 2023). But much work still remains to be done before we have a complete neuropsychology of anxiety even for the rat, let alone of disorder in people. However, we believe that this book provides a skeleton of the former; and we have, in this chapter, attempted to provide at least some suggestions for the latter. Most hopefully, the bedrock of the theory of the present edition is essentially the same as the two previous editions, while its degree of contact with the clinical literature on both anxiety and amnesia is greater. The theory is certainly still not without flaws, probably multiple and major; but it already makes sense of a range of clinical issues—particularly TR. We expect a similar caveat if there is a 4th edition.

In the present chapter we have tried to pin-point loci in the brain at which the various symptoms and primary syndromes of anxiety and related states are mediated. This has led us to an appearance of a 'splitting' stance, emphasizing the different roles played in anxiety by different brain regions rather than what might unite them. However, we have also emphasized serial- and co-morbidity and, here and in Chapter 12, the idea that disorders are linked to extreme zones within a space of trait spectra. In the final major chapter, dealing with therapy, we will return to a firmly 'lumping' approach.

14
The treatment of anxiety and fear disorders

Chapter 13 unpacked our 2D hierarchical neurology into potential 'pure' primary anxiety disorders; but also emphasized that a primary disorder could produce secondary symptoms characteristic of another primary disorder. Further, our conclusion in Chapter 12 was that possession of a neurotic (trait anxious) personality increases reactivity to threat, and so creates a predisposition to the *whole range* of threat-related disorders (including anxiety but extending even to neurotic depression). This leads to a trait spectrum approach that anticipates comorbidity as well as serial morbidity. In this final chapter, we meld these two approaches via conclusions emerging from data on the treatment of defensive disorders. We will touch tangentially on the treatment of depression and its comorbidity with anxiety but with the caveat that proper analysis of stress and depression would take another book.

A key assumption that we make is that treatment failure will often result from a failure to identify the primary disorder trait involved. We will argue, particularly for GAD, that there will be cases, resistant to conventional treatment, where the primary problem is, instead, a major contribution to dysfunction from high levels of neuroticism. We finish on a positive note with a brief review of new psychedelic-based treatments that appear to target this neuroticism generally and, importantly, act immediately rather than requiring weeks for an effect.

The bulk of the chapter will review conventional therapies as if they are applied to *correctly diagnosed* cases of primary disorder. We will then consider combinations of therapies, comorbidity, and potential development of novel trait-oriented therapies.

14.1 Behaviour therapy/exposure

In Chapter 13 (§13.6) we discounted a role for classical conditioning in simple phobias except for a few rare cases (§13.6.5). This contrasts with the early successes of behaviour therapy in treating phobias as though they *were* conditioned reactions (e.g. Mathews, 1978) and theoretical accounts of these successes (e.g. Eysenck and Rachman, 1965). But, if not conditioning, what underlies the efficacy of behaviour therapy?

First applied to specific phobias (e.g. of snakes, spiders or heights), behaviour therapy then showed efficacy in much more complex and disabling conditions, including agoraphobia (Mathews et al., 1981; Marks and Marks, 1990) and post-traumatic stress disorder (Jaycox and Foa, 1998), for which the principal therapeutic ingredient was simple exposure; and obsessive-compulsive disorder, in which exposure was combined with 'response prevention', i.e. prevention of the compulsive rituals, leading to a surge of anxiety that was then able to extinguish (Baer and Minichiello, 1990). Critically, the most important variable appeared to

The Neuropsychology of Anxiety, Third Edition. Neil McNaughton and Jeffrey A. Gray, Oxford University Press.
 DOI: 10.1093/oso/9780198843313.003.0014

be total amount of exposure time to the phobic stimulus—the more the better (Marks, 1973; Gelder et al., 1973; Teasdale, 1977; Levis and Hare, 1977).

But, if one gets better by being exposed to the phobic stimulus, why did one get ill by being exposed to it in the first place? And why does one not get better in the natural course of exposure in the real world, without the help of a therapist? Our answer (§13.6) is that, in the bulk of cases (where conditioning is not involved), illness results from activation of an innate fear stimulus engram (§13.6.5); and the failure to get better is due to the phobic situation being avoidable, which prevents unlearning/habituation of the resultant response (§13.6.3).

There are currently a range of variations on the exposure theme: *in vivo*, desensitization, virtual reality (VR), and other treatments including Cognitive-Behavioural Therapy (CBT, see §14.2). The basic exposure/habituation principle is simple but delivery can face problems.

> Treatment gains are generally maintained for one year, but longer follow-up studies are needed to better understand and prevent relapse. Acutely, the treatments are not equally effective among the phobia subtypes. Most phobias respond robustly to *in vivo* exposure, but it is associated with *high dropout rates and low treatment acceptance*. Response to systematic desensitization is more moderate. A few studies suggest that virtual reality may be [as] effective [as *in vivo*] in flying and height phobia, but this needs to be substantiated by more controlled trials. Cognitive therapy is most helpful in claustrophobia, and blood-injury phobia is uniquely responsive to applied [muscle] tension. The limited data on medication have not been promising with the exception of adjunctive D-clycoserine. Despite the acute benefits of *in vivo* exposure, greater attention should be paid to improve treatment acceptance and retention, and *additional controlled studies of more acceptable treatments are needed*. . . . In contrast to flying phobia, the cost-effectiveness of virtual reality treatment for spider phobia is questionable given the ease of obtaining a spider for *in vivo* exposure.
>
> Choy et al. (2007, p. 266, p. 276; emphasis added)

An important point about our analysis of specific phobia as depending on very similar patterns of strengthened engram connections, independent of whether they are conditioned, vicarious, instructed, or innate, is that the best treatment involves experience of the phobic object. But, not only is *in vivo* exposure poorly tolerated, there are many cases where it is expensive (e.g. flying) or the phobic object difficult to control (e.g. sharks). Thus, while VR may not be cost-effective with spiders it will be in other cases. We also think it is important (albeit not yet properly tested) that the control of the object by VR allows for step-wise progression (e.g. of the number and motility of cockroaches) to reduce dropout.

Such VR has been shown to be effective with 'animal phobias with various types of animals such as spiders, sharks, and snakes . . . situational phobias such as driving phobia and flight phobia, natural phobias such as a height phobia, and blood-injection-injury phobia, which also includes dental phobias' (Albakri et al., 2022, p. 16). Consistent with our earlier analysis of simple phobia, agoranxiety, and social anxiety all depending on evolutionarily significant phobic stimuli, VR exposure is generally as effective as *in vivo* in all three (Wechsler et al., 2019). The same appears true (van Loenen et al., 2022) of VR-CBT compared to conventional exposure-based CBT (§14.2) for complex neurotic disorders.

In sum, at least with specific phobia, the original problem lies in the connections of an engram—and that engrams are a highly effective target of treatment. However, there may also be a contribution from neuroticism, especially in more treatment-resistant or avoidant cases, and we have previously predicted that specific phobia would be sensitive to ketamine (McNaughton and Glue, 2020, see also §14.4).

14.2 Cognitive-Behavioural Therapy (CBT)

14.2.1 From cognitive therapy to cognitive-behavioural therapy

Cognitive Therapy (CT; Beck, 1970; Beck, 1976; Ellis, 1962) started with the idea that psychological disorder was a result of maladaptive cognitive appraisal of events, which then affected behavioural and emotional responses. It aimed to teach patients how to monitor and alter these maladaptive cognitions, and so change their emotions and behaviour. Beck held that erroneous beliefs and dysfunctional information processing are not just a symptom of, e.g. depression, but play a central role in its initiation and maintenance. The 'cognitions' are 'stream-of consciousness or automatic thoughts that tend to be in an individual's awareness' (Beck et al., 1983, p. 2) and can be regarded as the surface manifestations of deeply held schemata. 'The cognitive model considers schematic change essential for significant and enduring symptom reduction' (Clark, 2014, p. 1). Beck's CT was supported by rigorous testing (Hawton et al., 1989; Gloaguen et al., 1998).

Cognitive distortions include (Beck, 1967; Beck, 1976): dichotomous thinking (the tendency to think in absolutist, all-or-nothing terms); over-generalization (unjustified extrapolation on the basis of a single instance); and arbitrary inference (jumping to conclusions when evidence is lacking or contradictory). They are automatic, involuntary, appear highly plausible to the thinker, and self-reinforcing. In depression, for example, negative cognitive shift influences perception, working memory, recall and long-term memory (Beck, 1987) that result in depressed mood and behaviour. This lower mood then increases the probability of further negative automatic thoughts, so creating a vicious circle that maintains the depression. Beck initially emphasized depression, but his cognitive model can be applied to psychopathology in general (Dobson and Block, 1988).

While behaviour therapy aimed (§14.1) to alter maladaptive behaviour directly, e.g. by exposing a patient to their phobic stimulus; CT attempted to alter behaviour by changing maladaptive patterns of thought. For some years the two approaches were seen as competing. However, clinical psychologists now use a combination of specific behavioural and cognitive techniques, selected depending upon the particular problem requiring resolution—with the Beck Institute for Cognitive Therapy now renamed the Beck Institute for Cognitive Behavior Therapy.[1] Indeed, one can see a key consequence of the exposure in behaviour therapy as altering beliefs about the specific phobic object, situation, or compulsive behaviour—matching our view that conditioning alters cognition in rats (§3.1; Dickinson, 1980). 'Both cognitive and experiential or behavioral interventions [can be] considered [cognitive restructuring] as long as the intention is cognitive or schematic change' (Clark, 2014, p. 2). Importantly for our understanding of it, CBT is a general model not a single treatment; and is applied across

[1] www.beckinstitute.org

a range of dimensions such as attention, cognition, cognitive re-appraisal, behaviour change, and emotion.

> Contemporary CBT is now an umbrella term for a set of empirically supported psychological interventions targeting specific processes. The overall goals of treatment are distress reduction and improvement in functioning, and ultimately, enhancement of well-being and quality of life. In order for these treatment outcomes to be achieved, the patient engages with the therapist in a particular style of therapeutic relationship, comprised of generic elements (e.g. alliance, expressed empathy, feedback, expressed positive regard) and CBT-specific elements (e.g. collaborative-empiricism, Socratic dialogue), and a particular session structure (e.g. agenda, homework, summary, feedback). Thus, contemporary CBT refers to a family of interventions that include both (a) in-session processes that are generic and specific, as well as (b) core treatment processes that target core dimensions in psychopathology.
>
> Kazantzis et al. (2018, p. 350)

Given the current mix of different types of technique, one can ask how far cognitive restructuring (CR) itself is important.

> There is initial evidence that CR promotes positive outcomes in individual psychotherapy. In the current review, therapist use of CR was positively related to intermediate (i.e. lower next-session depressive symptoms and greater cognitive change) and distal treatment outcomes (i.e. lower risk of relapse and lower attrition). The studies examining the therapeutic impact of CR within session have been limited to the treatment of depression. However, component analyses that have examined the additive effect of CR in relation to behavioral components have found CR to be at least as equally effective as behavioral components in the treatment of anxiety disorders and obsessive-compulsive disorder. In addition, evidence from component analyses suggests that CR may be more therapeutic than behavioral components in the treatment of social anxiety disorder and posttraumatic stress disorder. In a complementary body of work, mediation analyses have found cognitive change (i.e. the expected product of CR) to lead to symptom improvement across a variety of disorders.
>
> (Ezawa and Hollon, 2023, p. 9)

The treatments can also be seen as being tailored to the patient's specific condition. We already saw that, with simple phobia, exposure is to the specific phobic object—other objects, phobic for other people, would not be effective. Across the more complex neurotic disorders there will be differentiation of the target and appropriate treatment modality both between disorders (e.g. agoranxiety versus social anxiety versus generalized anxiety) and within (e.g. different sources of obsession in OCD). This variation makes it particularly useful that exposure via VR-CBT is as effective as conventional exposure-based CBT—allowing wide variation in the phobic stimuli used (van Loenen et al., 2022).

It is reasonable therefore to compare CBT, as a suite of treatment choices, with conventional pharmacotherapy, and its suite of drug choices. We think the symptom/syndrome problem in both cases may be a root cause of treatment resistance (defined as failure of several treatments including both conventional drug and psychological).

14.2.2 A closer look at panic, social anxiety, and PTSD . . .

It will be instructive to take a closer look at the way in which CBT has been applied to the highly proximal panic disorder, extremely distal social anxiety disorder, and more complex and general PTSD. In Chapter 13 we assigned these disorders largely different neural substrates. Yet CBT appears to work well and according to the same general principles in all three cases.

One explanation, of course, is that the CBT model is meant to be applied differently in different cases and its parts have different effects: panic being more sensitive to simple exposure and social anxiety to CR (Ezawa and Hollon, 2023); and PTSD having more complex targets (Ehlers and Wild, 2021). Chapter 12 suggests an alternative view: there are personality factors that operate on the defence system as a whole and which can, therefore, affect simultaneously all the different neural systems we were so careful to dissect from one another in Chapter 13. This has two perspectives; one we deal with here and one in the next section.

Our discussion of CBT in panic disorder and social anxiety is based on Clark's perspective (Clark, 1988; Clark and Wells, 1995; Clark, 1997; Clark, 2014) We start, like the cognitive approach to treatment, with a cognitive model of the presumed pathological processes thought to underlie each of these disorders.

The cognitive model of panic disorder states that:

> Individuals who experience recurrent panic attacks do so because they have a *relatively enduring tendency* to interpret certain bodily sensations in a catastrophic fashion. The sensations that are misinterpreted are mainly those involved in normal anxiety responses (e.g. palpitations, breathlessness, dizziness, paresthesias) but also include some other sensations. The catastrophic misinterpretation involves perceiving these sensations as much more dangerous than they really are and, in particular, interpreting the sensations as indicative of *immediately* impending physical or mental disaster—for example, perceiving a slight feeling of breathlessness as evidence of impending cessation of breathing and consequent death, perceiving palpitations as evidence of an impending heart attack, perceiving a pulsing sensation in the forehead as evidence of brain haemorrhage, or perceiving a shaky feeling as evidence of impending loss of control and insanity.
>
> Clark (1988, p. 149; early emphasis added)

This sequence of events is illustrated in Fig. 14.1.

> External stimuli (such as a department store for an [agoranxiety case]) and internal stimuli (body sensations, thoughts, images) can both provoke panic attacks. The sequence that culminates in an attack starts with the stimuli being interpreted as a sign of impending danger. This interpretation produces a state of apprehension, which is associated with a wide range of bodily sensations. If these anxiety-produced sensations are interpreted in a catastrophic fashion (impending insanity, death, loss of control etc.) a further increase in apprehension occurs, producing more bodily sensations, leading to a vicious circle which culminates in a panic attack.
>
> Clark (1997, pp. 124–125; c.f. Fig. 13.8)

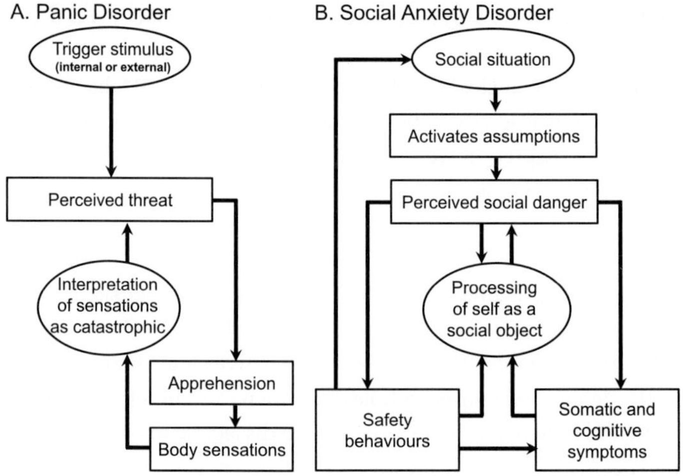

Fig. 14.1 **A.** The suggested vicious circle underlying a panic attack in panic disorder. Adapted from Clark (1986) with permission. **B.** The processes hypothesized to occur when a socially anxious person attempts to enter a feared situation. Redrawn from Clark and Wells (1995) with permission.

Further consequences of these tendencies to interpret bodily sensations in a potentially catastrophic fashion are that the subject becomes hypervigilant and repeatedly scans their inner sensations for signs of threat; and develops various patterns of 'safety' behaviour that avoid exposure to these threatening signs, but at the same time preclude any kind of disconfirmation of the erroneous beliefs that led to their being threatening in the first place. So, a patient afraid of suffering from heart disease will avoid exercise, precluding discovery of the fact that their heart rate may rise without the feared heart attack ensuing.

A central feature of this cognitive model of panic is, then, that attacks are due to an excessive weighting of adverse outcomes possibly associated with the stimuli that trigger the trains of thought illustrated in Clark's vignettes—but potentially more generally. This analysis of the way in which panic attacks arise was substantiated empirically (see Clark, 1996; Clark, 1997).

The cognitive model of social anxiety (Clark, 1997, Clark and Wells, 1995, see Fig. 14.1B) shares many features with the cognitive model of panic.

> Social [anxiety cases] are said to develop a series of assumptions about themselves and social situations. For example: 'Unless someone shows that they like me, they dislike me. Unless I am liked by everyone, I am worthless. If I show I am anxious people will think I am odd/will reject me.' These assumptions lead them to interpret normal social interactions in a negative way, viewing them as signs of danger. For example, if a social [anxiety case] is talking to someone at a party and the other person briefly looks out of the window the social [anxiety case] may think 'I'm being boring'. This interpretation triggers an 'anxiety programme' that can be usefully divided into three interlinked components.
>
> Clark (1997, pp. 126–127)

These three components are described by Clark (1997) as consisting of: 'the somatic and cognitive symptoms of anxiety that are reflexively triggered by the perception of danger' (e.g.

blushing, trembling, racing heart etc.); 'safety behaviours which patients engage in to try to reduce social threat and prevent feared outcomes from occurring' (e.g. trying not to attract attention, avoiding eye contact, censoring what one says, etc.); and a shift in attention, i.e. 'when social [anxiety cases] think they are in danger of negative evaluation by others, they shift their attention to detailed monitoring and observation of themselves'.

These are the same three components that operate in the cognitive model of panic (hypervigilance to bodily sensations in panic disorder being replaced, for example, by hypervigilance to aspects of one's own social performance in social anxiety, i.e. in each case to the relevant set of threat stimuli). In this way, a vicious circle is again set in motion, since *good* social performance is impeded by the very symptoms of anxiety, safety behaviours, and self-observation to which the social anxiety case is driven by fear of *poor* social performance. And, as before, we may see the whole process as depending upon the excessive weighting given to the potential adverse outcomes associated with specific stimuli, those stemming from social interaction taking, in social anxiety, the place of bodily sensations in panic disorder—except that social anxiety is linked to its own form of panic.

Our discussion of CBT in PTSD is based on the model (Fig. 14.2) provided by Ehlers and Clark (2000) and updated in Ehlers and Wild (2021).

> When trying to conceptualise PTSD from a cognitive perspective, one is immediately presented with a puzzle. PTSD is classified as an anxiety disorder. Within cognitive models, anxiety is a result of appraisals relating to impending threat. However, PTSD is a disorder in which the problem is a memory for an event that has already happened. We suggest that this apparent puzzle can be resolved by proposing that persistent PTSD occurs only *if individuals*

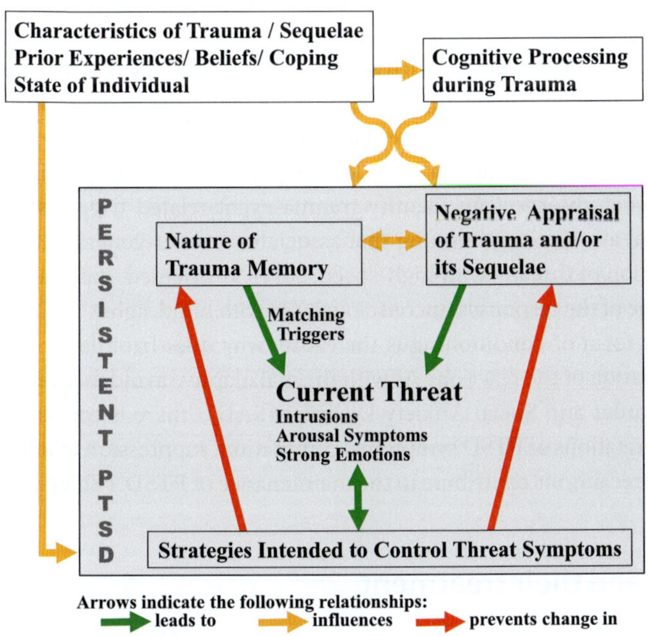

Fig. 14.2 A cognitive model of PTSD. For details see quote in text. Adapted from Ehlers and Clark (2000) with permission of the authors.

> *process the traumatic event and/or its sequelae in a way which produces a sense of a serious current threat.* The model proposes that two key processes lead to a sense of current threat.
> 1. individual differences in the appraisal of the trauma and/or its sequelae
> 2. individual differences in the nature of *the memory for the event and its link to other autobiographical memories.*
>
> Once activated, the perception of current threat is accompanied by intrusions and other reexperiencing symptoms, symptoms of arousal, anxiety and other emotional responses. The perceived threat also motivates a series of behavioural and cognitive responses that are intended to reduce perceived threat and distress in the short-term, but have the consequence of preventing cognitive change and therefore maintaining the disorder. Figure [14.3] summarises the key variables in the model.
>
> Ehlers and Clark (2000, p. 320; emphasis added; our figure reference)

The main recent elaboration of the 2000 'model is that we are now more precise about the nature of the problems with the autobiographical memory for the trauma and its relationship to reexperiencing. We use the term disjointedness of the worst moments in memory which then directly links to the rationale for the updating memories procedure in treatment' (Anke Ehlers, Personal Communication, 10 May 2023). This disjointedness of bad memories is related to intrusiveness and can go together with *better* memory recall of surrounding events. 'Memory disjointedness but not poor memory recall mediated the relationship between cognitive processing and intrusions. The findings suggest that different aspects of memory disorganization need to be distinguished to explain PTSD symptoms' (Sachschal et al., 2019, p. 1032).

Note here, that it is not the engram, as such, that is the focus here, but its recall or related associative effects. As emphasized by Ehlers (2015), unlike the single continuous sequence of normal episodic memory, trauma appears to result in distinct disjointed peri-event memories. The disorganization of the normal connectedness then provides an easy access point for perceptually biased simple-cue-driven re-experiencing linked to the worst events. But this re-experiencing is fragmented. Unlike intrusive memories in other disorders the memories are perceived as 'here and now', are usually of perceptions just prior to the trauma rather than of the trauma itself—and can include unexpected affect and physiological reactions, where an external observer can identify trauma-event-related trigger stimuli. All of this hints at classical aversive conditioning that associates an over-general set of simple stimuli to the anticipation of threat—with high-speed, survival-oriented, quick and dirty processes generating some of the responses unconsciously (as with blind sight).

But, if some form of conditioning is the cause, why does habituation or extinction not result in elimination of the reaction? As with the maladaptive avoidance reactions that maintain Panic Disorder and Social Anxiety Disorder (SAD), 'there is consistent evidence that negative interpretations of PTSD symptoms, rumination, suppression of intrusive memories, and excessive precautions contribute to the maintenance of PTSD' (Ehlers, 2015, p. 125).

14.2.3 . . . and their treatment

We have indicated earlier the general ways in which CBT re-educates the patient—altering maladaptive belief systems, with consequent desired change in both emotional and behavioural responses. Application of these general principles to panic disorder and social anxiety is reasonably straightforward.

For panic disorder, the key steps include: identifying the specific triggers for panic in the particular patient; the collation of evidence contradicting the patient's maladaptive beliefs about, e.g. the likelihood of having a heart attack; behavioural experiments, e.g. inducing feared bodily sensations in the clinic and demonstrating that no adverse consequences follow, or preventing safety behaviours to allow patients to disconfirm their expectations of adverse outcomes.

Mutatis mutandis, similar steps are involved in the treatment of social anxiety. For example, the patient may be asked to play a social role with and without the aid of their usual repertoire of safety behaviours while being videotaped, so that there is a record for later discussion with the therapist.

The original success rates reported with these therapies averaged, for panic disorder, 80% panic-free over a total of 97 patients across five studies (see Table 6.1 in Clark, 1997); and for social anxiety up to 65% (Heimberg et al., 1990; Clark, 1997). More recent meta-analysis with a range of generic measures of anxiety, using Hedge's g for effect size, found similar effect sizes in the range that 'only the effects of treatment for panic disorder as measured on the [Beck Anxiety Inventory] (13.33 points; 95% CI: 10.58–16.07[; g = 1.48]) were significantly (p = 0.001) larger than the effect sizes on GAD (6.06 points; 95% CI: 3.96–8.16[; g = 0.73]) and SAD (5.92 points; 95% CI: 4.64–7.20[; g =0.77]). The effects remained significant after adjusting for baseline severity and other major characteristics of the trials' (Cuijpers et al., 2016, p. 79). That is, all three conditions are significantly improved by CBT with a suggestion of a slightly greater effect with panic disorder but not as large a difference as with the early reports.

The cognitive component of CBT may be particularly important in some cases.

> Randomised controlled trials in the UK, Europe and Japan have established that individual cognitive therapy for social anxiety disorder (CT-SAD) based on the Clark and Wells model (1995) is an effective treatment that compares favourably with several other active interventions. In particular, CT-SAD has been shown to be superior to three versions of group [CBT], exposure therapy, interpersonal psychotherapy, psychodynamic therapy, paroxetine, fluoxetine, and medication based treatment as usual. . . . CT-SAD [may be] effective in patients who remain symptomatic following anti-depressant treatment.
>
> Clark et al. (2022, p. 1, which see for supporting citations)

In the case of panic disorder, internet- and mobile-based treatment appears to be as effective as face-to-face CBT and applied relaxation (Domhardt et al., 2020), while internet-based CT-SAD, 'when compared to conventional face-to-face therapy, . . . can more than double the amount of symptom change associated with each therapist hour' (Clark et al., 2022, p. 1).

With PTSD, as shown in Fig. 14.2 there are

> three factors (i.e. appraisals, memory characteristics, cognitive/behavioral strategies) that maintain a sense of current threat and PTSD symptoms according to Ehlers and Clark's (2000) model. . . . The model serves as the framework for an individualized formulation of the client's problems and treatment. The model suggests three treatment goals:

- Modify excessively negative appraisals (meanings) of the trauma and its sequelae.
- Reduce reexperiencing by elaboration of trauma memories and discrimination of triggers.
- Reduce behaviors and cognitive strategies that maintain the sense of current threat.

Ehlers and Wild (2021, p. 105)

The treatments then involve multiple procedures with what appears to need six common ingredients: psychoeducation (normalizing the patient's reactions), exposure (with *in vivo* being particularly effective), changing personal meanings, targeting multiple different emotions, emotion regulation, and memory change (via a coherent narrative). As with panic disorder and SAD, guided internet-based therapy was as effective as face-to-face and significantly cheaper (~60% less, Bisson et al., 2022); see also Thew et al. (2023, for likely effectiveness of early administration of a shortened version).

In the present context, the key feature of CBT is that it attempts (in the ways outlined above) to *reduce the excessive weighting* of potential adverse outcomes that gives rise to panic disorder and social anxiety in the first place; with PTSD involving more predictive stimuli. In this way, CBT attacks these disorders at the root and, despite some misconceptions, trauma-focussed CBT is applicable to a wide range of cases (Murray et al., 2022). The effects of CBT are also long-lasting, in contrast to much pharmacotherapy. But note that the general principle of weighting reduction involves targeting different parts of the brain (e.g. the snake detector, §13.6.6) for different cases.

14.2.4 CBT and the brain

Where in the brain might CBT act to prevent excessive weighting from being given to potential adverse outcomes? (This is a trick question.) The effectiveness of CBT is broad, from anxiolytic-insensitive panic (if simple, then, pure fear in our model, driven by the PAG) to generalized anxiety disorder (more or less pure anxiety driven by the GIS, particularly hippocampus) to social anxiety disorder. But the type of rational discourse that is central to CT can be mediated only via the neocortex (particularly the dorsolateral, ventrolateral, and medial prefrontal cortices, the anterior cingulate, the posterior cingulate/precuneus, and the insular cortices, Frewen et al., 2008) even in the case of panic disorder; whereas the BT component can clearly be either subcortical or (§3.1, §14.2.1) cortical. Further, we have already emphasized the smörgåsbord approach taken by CBT where, clearly, treatment of snake phobia will involve specific targeting of snake detecting neurons (e.g. in the pulvinar; see Section 3.17 in Kawai, 2019b). So, the quick answer to the question is 'CBT will act in different places depending on its varying procedures'.

Chapter 13 stressed the particular brain regions, activity in which results in specific symptoms (as adaptive reactions, consequences of dysfunction in other areas, or as a result of dysfunction of the area itself); for example, the PAG for symptoms of panic; the amygdala for arousal and attention changes due to affectively negative cues; and the septo-hippocampal system (SHS) for negative cognitive bias. But the neurology (Fig. 13.2) included strong iterative interactions that link the different structures making up the GAS, GRS, and GIS. When conflict is involved, the SHS occupies a nodal position within the multiple parallel ascending Papez circuits (McNaughton and Vann, 2022), while exercising both excitatory and inhibitory descending influences over the primary defence system.

The cortical circuits would be involved in GAD or SAD; where CBT would alter GAD- or SAD-specific neocortical inputs to the SHS (or wider GIS) as a result of verbally-coded re-descriptions of relevant stimuli. The SHS would then have reduced output to, for example, the amygdala—reducing risk aversion, arousal, and attention.

The descending excitatory influences lead to the wide-spread array of physiological and behavioural symptoms that can arise from even highly abstract sources of conflict in, e.g. OCD or GAD; the descending inhibitory influences are able to restrain panic behaviour (as analysed, e.g. in Graeff's work; see §13.4.1). So, CBT could recruit the descending route to achieve its beneficial effects on panic. If so, it would not reduce activity in the GIS but, rather, redirect and in some cases even enhance it. Altered frontal and parietal outputs to, in the case of snakes, the pulvinar would reduce the strength of the fear response (via direct input to the amygdala). This would tend to equalize repulsion versus attraction, potentially increasing conflict and so SHS activation, which would result in increased inhibitory control over lower centres mediating panic attacks. This predicts the interference by classical anxiolytics in Panic Disorder treatment with CBT (Sanderson and Wetzler, 1993) and simple exposure (§14.3).

14.2.5 CBT: Integrating personality and psychopathology

CBT is one area where the link between personality and psychopathology (Kotov et al., 2018; Krueger and Markon, 2014) seems obvious. CBT tries to change 'the way you think' (the thoughts themselves are simply evidence of fundamental change). CBT is not interested in current instances (except as evidence), it wants to reduce the frequency of a class of instances in the interminable future. It is not concerned with current fear but fearfulness. This may be where a classic 'treatment' model breaks down. Personality is, by definition, global and only slowly changing (absent trauma). Importantly, with neuroticism as a target of treatment for any particular neurotic disorder, one would expect a general long-lasting protection against the whole gamut of neurotic disorders (Andrews et al., 1990; Barlow et al., 2014). There are also potential practical advantages to such a high-order approach:

> The prevailing categorical approach in which patients are assigned diagnoses and treated with the associated CBT protocol(s) creates an enormous training burden for clinicians who must learn numerous discrete interventions in order to provide empirically supported care. Moreover, patients do not fit neatly within our nosological categories (i.e. subthreshold symptoms and diagnostic comorbidity), suggesting that our diagnosis-specific approach to treatment does not align with real-world clinical presentations. Thus, using CBT, or components thereof, to target a limited number of personality-informed dimensions (e.g. Neuroticism and Extraversion) has the potential to significantly streamline care....
>
> [However,] CBT clinicians and researchers may be hesitant to adopt such an approach because they simply do not know what it means to treat, for example, 'internalizing' or 'disinhibition'. Indeed, there are few CBT protocols aimed at altering personality features, though studies with nonclinical samples have demonstrated that setting and following through on behavior change goals is associated with personality change.
>
> (Sauer-Zavala et al., 2020, pp. 1–2)

This approach fits well with our 'double-hit' model (§13.2.3, Fig. 13.3), particularly, given the proposal that motivational and expectancy processes act as functional links between personality risk-factors such as neuroticism and resultant symptomatology (Sauer-Zavala et al., 2020). In our model neuroticism is both a risk factor for and a maintainer of neurotic disorder but (Fig. 13.3) must combine with both specific disorder-related traits and more or less specific events to generate disorder.

> This is consistent with the view that emotional disorders have their origin in
> three separate but interacting diatheses or vulnerabilities ... [1] a general biological (heritable) vulnerability common across disorders, [2] a general psychological vulnerability consisting of a heightened sense of unpredictability and uncontrollability and associated changes in brain function resulting from adverse early experiences, and [3] a more specific psychological vulnerability, also largely learned, accounting for why one particular emotional disorder may emerge instead of another. It seems increasingly evident that *the two generalized vulnerabilities identified in the triple vulnerability theory are implicated in the development and expression of neuroticism itself.* Indeed, we hypothesize that these two generalized vulnerabilities function as direct risk factors for the development of neuroticism, which in turn mediates risk for the development of anxiety and mood disorders. What is notable for our purposes is that *adverse experiences contribute strongly to changes in brain function and that later experiences may alter resulting temperamental expression and associated brain circuits.*
>
> (Barlow et al., 2014, pp. 348–349; emphasis added)

Importantly, neuroticism appears malleable using the 'unified protocol for transdiagnostic treatment of emotional disorders'; but there is need to further develop and assess 'interventions that target dimensions of temperament more directly' (Barlow et al., 2014, p. 357).

14.3 Conventional drug therapy and augmentation

14.3.1 Conventional drug therapy

The corner-stone of our theory is the *axiom* that selective anxiolytics (i.e. drugs that are not panicolytic, such as the barbiturates, benzodiazepines, buspirone, and pregabalin) reduce anxiety. This *defines* anxiety and differentiates it from fear. It also sees treatment resistance as a failure of diagnosis. The different therapeutic profiles of different classes of drug (§4.4, Table 4.1), or even specific drugs such as clomipramine versus imipramine, then guided us to the likely brain sites mediating different 'neurotic' symptoms and syndromes (Fig. 13.2).

Our theory, then, takes the clinical effects of the drugs as given rather than predicted; with one exception. Since the first linking of the effects of sodium amylobarbitone to impairment of control of hippocampal theta rhythm (Gray, 1970b; McNaughton and Sedgwick, 1978), all new types of selective anxiolytic drug (benzodiazepines, buspirone, pregabalin) have been found to also produce such impairment. Importantly, all new types of non-selective anxiolytics (e.g. SSRIs, ketamine) also impair theta rhythm (McNaughton et al., 2007; Munn and McNaughton, 2008; Engin et al., 2009).

As discussed in §4.4, like CBT, human clinical anxiolytic action (even with classical anxiolytics such as benzodiazepines) requires long-term administration of conventional drugs (Wheatley, 1990). In §13.4.3, we attributed this delayed action to the need to reverse long-term memory-related changes in responding (essentially anxious personality) resulting from chronic GIS hyperactivity (and supported by theta synchrony controlling iterative processing in the Papez circuits). Blockade of theta, then, blocks the formation and maintenance by goal conflict of aversive memories and allows them to habituate or extinguish. The immediate target of the drugs is, here, subcortical but the long-term therapeutic effects are on cortical engrams or schemata and so can be viewed as similar to the nominal primary targets of CBT.[2] Unlike CBT, however, cessation of drug treatment, particularly if abrupt, often results in relapse or (with benzodiazepines used as sleep medication) the perverse occurrence of anxiety disorder where there was none previously.

A roughly similar argument can be put for delayed effects on panic, obsession, and depression. While the anxiolytic action of panicolytic anti-depressants appears to be mediated by changes in theta, their other actions are not. For example, we have attributed OCD, at least in some cases, to low anterior cingulate serotonin. Our general picture, shown in Fig. 13.2, is that low serotonin (so low 'stability') shifts processing in the GRS, GIS and GAS towards reactive survival circuits and away from proactive planning circuits (§6.10). When chronic this would be expected to change engrams and schemata in a trait-like way that would then require extensive time for the effects to be reversed by treatment.

14.3.2 Conventional drug augmentation

With CBT and conventional anxiolytics both available it would seem obvious that combining them could be beneficial—especially if they have additive effects on the same ultimate cognitive target. So, for many years, benzodiazepines were combined with CBT to treat panic disorder with agoraphobia—but with little evidence of a beneficial drug effect and some for the opposite, particularly at follow-up (Hafner and Marks, 1976; Westra et al., 2002; see also Marks, 1976; Mathews, 1978; Wardle et al., 1994; see Marks et al., 1993, for high-dose alprazolam and exposure; see Sanderson and Wetzler, 1993, for similar conclusions on CBT). A negative effect fits with the fact that barbiturates and benzodiazepines sometimes block the effects on resistance to extinction of both partial reinforcement and partial punishment (Gray, 1977; Willner and Crowe, 1977; Feldon, 1977; Feldon et al., 1979; Feldon and Gray, 1981; Davis et al., 1981), viewed as habituation to frustration and fear, respectively.

Thus, there are probably two effects of classical anxiolytics used adjunctively. One, beneficial, is an acute relaxation that reduces the conflict of approach and increases the patient's exposure to the phobic object; the other, harmful, blocks the SHS-mediated habituation that results from this exposure. But the acute reduction in anxiety, particularly if the drug is used 'as needed' may be problematic in reducing the *exposure experience* that underlies the therapy (Westra et al., 2002). Interaction between these effects (and their likely schedule-dependence) may account for the mixed results obtained (Hussain, 1971; Johnston and Gath, 1973; Chambless et al., 1979; Westra et al., 2002). These results strongly caution, therefore, against long-term maintenance of patients on benzodiazepines (see Balon et al., 2020, for a

[2] Remember that simple exposure can be viewed as changing cognition.

recent contrary view) since, as noted earlier, this may reduce the chances of spontaneous development of tolerance to adversity.

'There is some evidence, albeit limited to certain drug classes, that the combination of medication and cognitive behavior therapy may be more effective than either strategy used alone' (Canton et al., 2012, p. 203; albeit marginally, see their Fig. 7). With panicolytic antidepressants (for which the mechanisms are unclear), in particular,

> despite some positive findings for combined treatment approaches in some groups of patients, many of the data do not support such an approach. However, combined treatment is often used in clinical practice. This is partly because of a need for better treatments than those offered by either pharmacotherapy or psychotherapy alone; each of these modalities is effective for only a subset of patients. There is also the consideration that even though trials of simultaneous pharmacotherapy and psychotherapy may not be more effective than either agent alone, it is possible that the sequenced use of pharmacotherapy and psychotherapy can optimize therapy by converting a partial response to a full response and by preventing recurrence of symptoms. Similarly, switching from one treatment to another after a good response to the first has also shown some benefit in some disorders.
>
> (Ganasen et al., 2010, p. 689)

For all the drugs, then, it appears that combination with CBT is generally non-additive and occasionally counterproductive. This is most likely due to the fact that the drugs are affecting subcortical mechanisms that, in one sense or another, *block* memory formation and so slowly reduce 'bad memories' while CBT operates via the neocortex to *generate* the formation of 'good memories' to replace the bad ones.

14.4 Novel psychedelic-based therapies and combinations

Specific memories (whether in strong flash-back or weak generalized association) will generate a specific defensive response or set of responses. Even generalized anxiety can be seen as a specific defensive response to a failure of specific memory (or of specific threat prediction). In terms of our current 'double-hit' model (§13.2.3, Fig. 13.3), the 'event strength' as an output of these specific memories will depend on both the activation of the engram as an input and its amplification as an output by the level of sensitivity of the matching trait system (GAD, SAD, panic, OCD, depression). Further, symptoms will also depend on the interaction of that specific event strength (driven by multiple, parallel, specific trait/aspect/facet, components) with the higher order trait of neuroticism. Note, here, that the generation of symptoms is multiplicative and that the aspects/facets are not contained within the superordinate trait. The relevant correlations involve intersection not complete overlap (hence they are usually weak—it's not just measurement error).

Our double-hit model depends on the fact that the many, specific, slow, weak effects of conventional treatment (whether this is psychological or pharmacological) show 'treatment resistance'. Medications often target only a subset of neurotic disorders (Muller et al., 2016; we have argued that CBT is more a set of treatments); and, as we have noted, they and CBT take months (Muller et al., 2016) to produce their full effects. Worse, 1/3rd of patients are resistant to *any conventional treatment* (Nemeroff, 2007; Muller et al., 2016), impacting public resources by doubling hospitalizations (Nemeroff, 2007) and suicide attempts; and requiring chronic care.

Change is afoot. As detailed in §4.2.2, a restricted range of low doses (Fig. 4.1) of ketamine (**K**) can *treat* 'treatment-resistant' major depressive disorder (MDD; Lai et al., 2014; George et al., 2017; Machado-Vieira et al., 2008), GAD, and SAD (Shadli et al., 2018b). **K** acts *within hours* (Zarate et al., 2013), to reduce symptoms including suicidal ideation and loss of life (DiazGranados et al., 2010). Importantly, **K** is also effective in other neurotic disorders: OCD (Rodriguez et al., 2013), and PTSD (Feder et al., 2014a; see Urban et al., 2023, on substance use disorder; see Burback et al., 2023, for an extensive review of PTSD and its treatment) including when this is comorbid with treatment-resistant depression (Veraart et al., 2023). Other promising psychedelics include psilocybin, lysergic acid diethylamide, mescaline (and other phenylalkylamines), and N,N-Dimethyltryptamine (Rucker et al., 2018; Timmermann et al., 2019; Nutt et al., 2020; Vollenweider and Preller, 2020; Vamvakopoulou et al., 2022), including actions on 'anxiety' as measured by the STAI and, typically, generated by life threatening illness (Dos Santos et al., 2016; Muttoni et al., 2019; Wolfson et al., 2020).

> However, concerns such as adverse side effects and potential misuse liability have limited [ketamine's] widespread use. Racemic ketamine has two enantiomers—(*S*)- and (*R*)-ketamine—that appear to have disparate underlying mechanisms.... Preclinical research suggests divergent mechanisms underlying (*S*)- and (*R*)-ketamine, with (*S*)-ketamine more directly affecting mechanistic target of rapamycin complex 1 (mTORC1) signaling and (*R*)-ketamine more directly affecting extracellular signal-related kinase (ERK) signaling. Clinical research suggests that (*R*)-ketamine has a milder side effect profile than (*S*)-ketamine and decreases depression rating scale scores, but recent randomized, controlled trials found that it had no significant antidepressant efficacy compared to placebo, suggesting that caution is warranted in interpreting its therapeutic potential. Future preclinical and clinical research is needed to maximize the efficacy of each enantiomer, either by optimizing dose, route of administration, or administration paradigm.
>
> (Johnston et al., 2023; see also §4.2.2)

For the standard racemic **K**, too, 'optimal dosing, modes of administration and the most effective forms of adjunctive psychotherapeutic support should be examined further' (Walsh et al., 2022, p. 1). The possibility of adjunctive use of **K** with psychotherapy is exciting and contrasts with conventional drugs. At least with substance use disorders, PTSD, and treatment-resistant depression, adding a range of psychotherapies to **K** treatment has tended to produce improved outcomes (Kew et al., 2023). One possible explanation both for this positive adjunctive effect, and its rapid therapeutic action is that **K** enhances engram re-organization; but this does not seem to match its action as an NMDA antagonist, nor its anxiolytic-like reduction of theta. As we shall see its actions appear complex but may well sum, instead, to a simple reduction in neuroticism, or some related general aspect of threat processing.

Particularly interesting, here, is Auvelity® (Axsome Therapeutics, 2022). This is a combination of dextromorphan (45 mg) and buproprion (105 mg) recently approved by the FDA for

Table 14.1 Comparison of overlapping aspects of the pharmacology of Auvelity® and ketamine

	Dextromorphan	Buproprion	D + B = Auvelity®	Ketamine	A = K
Dissociative?	√	×	√	√	√
Agonist	Sigma-1		Sigma-1	Sigma-2	Sigma↑
				5HT3A	
Antagonist		5HT3A			
	NMDA		NMDA	NMDA	NMDA↓
	SERT		SERT	Release 5HT	5HT↑
	NET-weak	NET	NET	Release NE	NE↑
		DAT-weak	DAT	Release DA	DA↑
	Nicotinic α3β4	Nicotinic α3β4	Nicotinic α3β4	Nicotinic α3β4	Nicotinic α3β4↓
	Nicotinic α4β2	Nicotinic α4β2	Nicotinic α4β2	Nicotinic α4β2	Nicotinic α4β2↓
	Nicotinic α7	Nicotinic α7	Nicotinic α7	Nicotinic α7	Nicotinic α7↓

Data as reviewed by Tully et al. (2022), Nguyen et al. (2016), Costa et al. (2019, p.293), Papakostas et al. (2008).
Abbreviations: A = K, functional actions shared by Auvelity and ketamine; D + B, predicted action from combination of individual dextromorphan and buproprion effects; DA, dopamine; DAT, DA transporter; NE, norepinephrine/noradrenaline; NET, NE transporter; NMDA, N-Methyl-d-aspartate glutamatergic receptor; SERT, serotonin transporter; 5HT, 5-hydroxy tryptamine/serotonin.

treatment of major depression.[3] Buproprion alone does not affect serotonin (it does interact with norepinephrine and dopamine transporters); but it not only produces similar anti-depressant effects to SSRIs but 'a comparable degree of improvement in anxiety symptoms' (Papakostas et al., 2008, p. 134). Its combination with dextromorphan (which, is like <u>K</u> in affecting serotonin, NMDA receptors, and Sigma receptors) is like the individual psychedelics in having a fast action and producing dissociation. As shown in Table 14.1, Auvelity® (based on the combined reported effects of its components) and <u>K</u> have a wide range of similar effects on NMDA, opiate, and nicotinic receptors and similar increases in the monoamines (albeit through different routes). One difference is their opposite interactions with 5HT3 receptors. They also have a range of non-matching actions.

This wide range of actions across multiple transmitter systems may seem surprising and does not offer a clean target for conventional drug development. However, given the role of stress in neuroticism and its disorders, it is less surprising. The monoamines tend to respond in a coordinated manner to stress (Hale and Lowry, 2015), 'blocking β2 or α7 nicotinic acetylcholine receptors (nAChRs) prevents, respectively, the development and the expression of social stress-induced neuroadaptations' (Morel et al., 2018, p. 1597; see Perkins et al., 2021, on α7 effects on human defensive behaviour and state anxiety), Sigma-1 opiate receptors appear to mediate the effects of stress on depression (Wang et al., 2022, Sigma-2 appear more metabolically oriented), and 'different types of environmental stress enhance glutamate

[3] Normally, dextromethorphan is metabolized very rapidly by CYP2D6 (half-life 2–4 hours, metabolized to dextrorphan which peaks at ~1.7 hours). Bupropion is one of the most potent CYP2D6 inhibitors available likely extending the half-life of dextromethorphan to ~25 hours, which could be a key to Auvelity®'s effects.

release/transmission in limbic/cortical areas and exert powerful structural effects, inducing dendritic remodeling, reduction of synapses and possibly volumetric reductions resembling those observed in depressed patients' (Sanacora et al., 2012), which implies a role for NMDA receptor antagonists. Auvelity® and K, then, seem to have a multi-system 'shotgun' approach to a stress-sensitive system, which at the moment we would see as generally coding for threat sensitivity via a trait such as neuroticism. A full picture of the system interactions involved would add to Fig. 13.9 explicit glutamate and nicotinic components; but, with so many reciprocal interactions both chemically and neurally (Fig. 11.15) a complex set of balanced changes across the systems involved would seem essential if some simple general function is to then emerge.

Our argument, then, would be to advance therapy not through some single wonder receptor but through balanced adjustments (seeking synergies and avoiding blocks) that may best be achieved through combinations of existing drugs, existing psychotherapies, and adjunctive use of each. We have already touched on the problems with the opposite interactions of benzodiazepines and buspirone with a stress response that generates anxiolytic antagonism. One simple step here would be to combine the two, summating their main anxiolytic effects, cancelling out their opposing effects on the stress system (and it's on them), and diluting the side effects they do not share. There is preliminary electrophysiological and behavioural evidence that this would be effective (Irvine, 2000). Auvelity® appears to take a similar approach—with the cost of development of combinations of older drugs being much less than that of completely new ones.

With both CBT and psychedelics there is an argument for targeting neuroticism in general. However, as with the more specific therapies, it may be that the combination of treatment modalities aimed at the same target is counterproductive. In which case, CBT targeting neuroticism might combine well with specific drug therapies, and specific CBT procedures with psychedelics, but not vice versa. As with application of the individual new treatments, more data are needed on the effects of combination. But, after years of drought, we can hope that the floodgate of novel (combination/broad target) treatments is about to open.

14.5 Prevention

We have used drugs as dissecting tools, while also staying open-minded about psychological therapies (in all cases, the target is the Conceptual Nervous System; and, in all cases, fundamental change must occur in the real Central Nervous System). In this chapter we have discussed both as 'treatments'. But, a trait-based approach—particularly one that emphasizes neuroticism—must look askance at both the concept of illness (with its categorical implications) and the concept of its mending (with its implications of reversal of categorical pathology).

If neuroticism is a trait, and the Big 5 a spectrum, we cannot identify a categorical boundary between pathology and wellness. Excessive/insufficient height and excessive/insufficient weight all carry their burdens in modern society (especially in combination)—but to be tall is not to be ill. This book has mostly been about specific state theory (are you currently anxious or fearful, if so where in your brain is most active?). But here we must stare traits in the face. By definition they are long-lasting and difficult to change (absent trauma). To achieve 'good' traits we must usually work for a long time. To prevent bad traits, we must start early. We must also note that a trait *per se* must be adaptive and both its extremes maladaptive to achieve balancing selection. Arguably, more has been done for public health via proper drainage than any medical marvels.

So, ideally, we would alter the trauma in early development that gives rise to the problems we are trying to solve at great cost for adults. Unfortunately, politicians (and much of the public) are averse to the necessary investment. An alternative is to accept that some damage will have been done but put in place early methods of reversing the long-term consequences—fixing what must euphemistically be labelled childhood 'difficulties' but in fact are the seeds, outside the child, of high neuroticism and other adverse factors.

> The current gold standard treatments for these childhood behavioral difficulties are behavior management and in more extreme cases, medication. While both are effective, they are not without their limitations. For example, medication compliance is often low, medications can have negative side effects, and not all children respond well to them. Behavioural interventions are often more palatable for parents than medication, but are generally more difficult to implement, can be quite costly, and are typically less effective than medications in the more severe cases. Given the high rates of behaviour problems in children, the fact that these are increasing, and that not all children are benefiting from our current treatments, we need to continue to diversify our offerings in order to increase the chances of successfully treating these problems early on, and hopefully changing the life course trajectory for these at-risk children.
>
> (Healey and Healey, 2019, p. 2)

Dione Healey[4] suggests that structured play, where parents are involved one-on-one with their children is 'an equally effective alternative way to manage difficult behavior in preschoolers [that] complements our current treatment options' (Healey and Healey, 2019, p. 1). Such methods could become absorbed into parenting rather than psychotherapy. From there to socio-therapy is not as big a step as currently.

[4] CoI: she is a member of my department, NMcN.

15
Coda

15.1 Coping with the data explosion

In the stock phrase, there was an 'explosion' of new data in the fields covered in this book in the 20 years after its first edition in 1982. At times we feared the theory would be exploded with the data. Certainly, the data exploded beyond the publishable confines of the second edition main text, generating 10 Appendices (republished here via URL and listed in pp. xxix–xxxi). Twenty more years later, the situation has morphed to the continuous controlled 'explosion' of a rocket launch. Ever more data were generated at an ever-increasing rate—powering our theory upwards, and generating 33 supporting published reviews (listed with their URLs on pp. xxix–xxxi). The advance of other theories to integrate all these data within a single theory is less obvious.

Our 'we have ignition' moment was the linking of anxiolytic action on decision conflict (Miller, 1944; Bailey and Miller, 1952) to the SHS. This linkage started our flight (1982) ever upward into multi-dimensional neuropsychological space, and remains a clear point of origin. The second edition (2000) appeared changed to some, but simply had an expanded view of the same terrain; and the view from this third edition (2023) is higher and wider again—with the GIS involving a hierarchical set of structures centred on the SHS. 'Toute Pensée émet un Coup de Dés'[1]; but the centre has held and—plus ça change, plus c'est la même chose—we see the hippocampus as more than ever 'an organ of hesitation and doubt'.[2]

But what if, in a defensive scenario, there is no hesitation or doubt?

In all three editions we have taken due account of three distinct classes of more direct reaction: (1) fight/flight/freeze mediated by the PAG (where it equates with panic, Graeff, 1994) and hypothalamus; (2) simple conditioned fear, mediated by the amygdala (LeDoux, 1996); and (3) cingulate and frontal cortex involvement in drug-resistant human defence, particularly obsession and compulsion (Rapoport, 1989). These brain areas support 'fear' that we distinguish categorically from 'anxiety' (Gray, 1987a). In the current edition we have renamed the fear system as a whole the Goal Repulsion System and restricted the label, Fight, Flight, Freeze System, to its original primordial components (see Flynn, 1967, p. 59, for original neural model; see Gray, 1971, p. 193-194, for application of the term 'fight/flight' system). The GRS, then, is also a hierarchically organized set of structures, not a single structure.

[1] 'All thoughts generate a roll of the dice' see front matter for non-linear layout, all editions. For some of the original graphics, see https://en.wikipedia.org/wiki/Un_coup_de_d%C3%A9s_jamais_n%27abolira_le_hasard_(Mallarm%C3%A9)

[2] Front matter editions 1 and 2, Chapter 1 header, this edition.

The Neuropsychology of Anxiety, Third Edition. Neil McNaughton and Jeffrey A. Gray, Oxford University Press.
 DOI: 10.1093/oso/9780198843313.003.0015

15.2 Conceptual expansion

There has also been functional fragmentation within the apparently unitary conceptual framework of the GIS. Conceptually, the GIS has always been held to output increases in: 1) goal inhibition; 2) arousal; and, 3) attention. But decision and arousal/attention have always involved opposite (subtraction/addition, respectively) operations (Gray and Smith, 1969) with consequences that we are only now neurologizing. Matching this mathematical split, while decision (via goal inhibition) is mediated most centrally by the SHS, increased arousal is mediated most centrally by the basolateral amygdala, bed nucleus of the stria terminalis, and insula (Fig. 11.15).

Our expanding view calls for ever-increasing clarity in our definition of terms and their relationship to conventional usage. Terminology is particularly a problem with 'reward' and 'punishment' (§12.7.1). Our remedy has been to avoid their use as far as possible; using gain/loss, attractor/repulsor, positive reinforcement/negative reinforcement, as appropriate. Unflagged variations in the meaning of 'punishment' in particular have caused major problems in the past, particularly with the translation of our neuropsychology into Reinforcement Sensitivity Theory (McNaughton and Corr, 2019b; Corr, 2008b).

Similar issues arise with 'fear' and 'anxiety' (McNaughton, 2018). We view fear as a set of panicolytic-sensitive adaptive reactions to repulsors that remove one from danger; and anxiety as a set of anxiolytic-sensitive adaptive reactions that allow one to approach danger cautiously (with conflicting attractors providing the reason for approach). DSM-5 'anxiety disorders' include both fear and anxiety (American Psychiatric Association, 2022)—providing a rich source of confusion. There is potentially less confusion with ICD-10's 'Neurotic, stress-related and somatoform disorders' (World Health Organization, 2010) but the boundaries of these go beyond the disorders we have discussed to depression; whereas, except for their exclusion of OCD, there is a good match with ICD-11's 'Anxiety or Fear-Related Disorders' (World Health Organization, 2023) and, with the exception of agoraphobia, with its use of the term phobia for what we would classify as fears. With such differing and ever-changing classifications one can only flag the necessity to not take the meaning of specific words as identical across different contexts.

15.3 Personality as a source of unity

Given our 2D hierarchical model of fear and anxiety (and their varied classifications) can we see *any* form of unity in the neural basis of anxiety or the 'anxiety-related disorders'? Perhaps the whole notion of 'anxiety-related disorders' is a spurious category of hopelessly disparate phenomena, nothing more than a heading in a textbook?

The data on predisposition to the comorbidity of the anxiety-related disorders, on the heritability of a related personality trait, and on the general sensitivity of anxiety-related disorders to cognitive-behavioural treatment (§14.2), monoamine reuptake inhibitors (Table 4.1), and ketamine (Table 4.1; §14.4), offer apparent antidotes to this counsel of despair—as does the concept of defensive distance. Strikingly, this unity binds both the states that we have considered as the core components of anxiety, whether normal or pathological (as e.g. in generalized anxiety disorder), and those we have seen as lying outside anxiety proper, such as panic disorder. What appears to be inherited is a set of enduring personality traits (measured as the degree of neuroticism) that predisposes to any of these neurotic conditions—so providing them a commonality.

It would be comforting if we could see in the neuropsychology of anxiety a matching common core that is genetically determined, neurologically and pharmacologically unified, and opposed by cognitive-behavioural therapy. However, we have preferred a more complex 'double-hit' model (§13.2.3, Fig. 13.3), where each hit has its own multifactorial control. The following somatic analogy may help to make this clearer.

An inherited low level of immune system function could predispose people to catch a variety of bacterial infections. These infections are extrinsic rather than intrinsic, are not the direct result of the inherited bias, and will differ markedly in their symptomatology, pathological characteristics, and required nursing. However, all might be treatable by the same or related antibiotics (for reasons that are independent of the nature of the inherited low level of immune function). This analogy shows how there can be a clear link between common predisposing factors and common treatments which relate to common properties of all the disease organisms, but which nonetheless allows the different diseases to be caused by different organisms and to involve different pathological pathways in different bodily organs. Pursuing the analogy further, such an inherited 'predisposition to infection' is not necessarily maladaptive (as we have argued anxiety also not to be), since it could result in a low level of autoimmune disease.

15.4 Cognitive bias . . .

Bearing this analogy in mind, then, what might be inherited as the predisposing factor of neuroticism; and what might be the common mode of action of Cognitive Behavioural Therapy (CBT) or selective serotonin reuptake inhibitors (SSRIs) in all the anxiety-related disorders? One possibility, touched upon in the previous chapter, is that neuroticism reflects principally a *cognitive* bias towards the identification or magnification of threat of all kinds. As emphasized in LeDoux's hierarchical system (see Fig. 6.1), threat is an input that is almost concurrent to all levels of the defensive system. Which of these responds most strongly depends upon defensive distance (as described in Chapter 2). But defensive distance is, itself, a cognitive construct and involves an interaction of the external size of the threat (a function of real distance and danger presented by the threat) with sensitivity to perception of threat as a personality trait (ranging, we think, from stable to neurotic).

The degree of bias towards the perception of threat (i.e. neuroticism) can then be seen as being influenced by polygenes, as discussed in the previous chapter, as well as by conditioning or trauma (as e.g. in the long-lasting changes observed in PTSD, §13.11). Ketamine and monoamine reuptake inhibitors would act directly or indirectly, respectively, to reduce such excessive perception of threat, so affecting both fear and anxiety. We have discussed arguments for developing a form of CBT that targets neuroticism rather than individual disorders (§14.2.4).

15.5 ... and specific sensitivities

With neuroticism as a risk and maintaining factor providing one 'hit', disorder still requires a second. With adaptive behaviour, the nature of the behaviour displayed and the specific emotion felt will depend in addition upon such factors as defensive direction (engaging fear or anxiety circuits), the presence of conflict, etc. as considered *in extenso* in this book. The strength of such behaviour, whether normal or requiring psychiatric treatment, will depend on the relevant trait sensitivity of the system controlling it. With high neuroticism and a high disorder-specific trait sensitivity (panic, goal conflict, etc.) we will have clinical disorder—but with complex symptom-syndrome mappings (§13.5).

If we are right, the main challenge for the future is to find means of identifying the underlying (often comorbid) system sensitivities and using this to guide our selection of components (within exposure therapy, or cognitive therapy) for psychological therapy and of drugs (and drug combinations) for pharmacological therapy. We expect optimal results to often require a combination of psychological and pharmacological therapy (concurrent and/or sequential).

On this view, the unity binding the anxiety-related disorders that is suggested by the data on personality, heritability, and those treatments that are generally effective can be reconciled with the diversity of underlying neural mechanisms that has occupied our attention for most of this book. That diversity remains (as does the selective and unified action of the anxiolytic drugs) – it has not been spirited away. Indeed, we would anticipate varying contributions from our general and specific 'hits', where conventional treatment resistance (with drugs and CBT acting on similar specific engrams and schemas, albeit via opposite fundamental actions) would result from a substantial input from neuroticism; while conventional treatment sensitivity (for a similar symptomatic presentation) would result from a relatively stronger input from disorder-specific trait sensitivities.

15.6 Envoi

That is as far as we can at present take the argument. The coming years will surely continue to be progressively more explosive as they have been since 1982. We wait with continued interest to see how far they will blow our theory apart or propel it upward in the next 20 years.

Another error is an impatience of doubt,
And haste to assert without due and mature suspension of doubt. . . .
If [you] will begin with certainties, [you] shall end in doubts;
but if [you] will be content to begin with doubts [you] shall end in certainties.

Francis Bacon. Advancement of Learning. I. V. 8

References

Abend, R. 2023. Understanding anxiety symptoms as aberrant defensive responding along the threat imminence continuum. *Neuroscience & Biobehavioral Reviews*, 105305. https://doi.org/10.1016/j.neubiorev.2023.105305

Abivardi, A., Khemka, S., & Bach, D. R. 2020. Hippocampal representation of threat features and behavior in a human approach–avoidance conflict anxiety task. *The Journal of Neuroscience*, 40, 6748–6758. https://doi.org/10.1523/jneurosci.2732-19.2020

Abler, B., Erk, S., Herwig, U., & Walter, H. 2007. Anticipation of aversive stimuli activates extended amygdala in unipolar depression. *Journal of Psychiatric Research*, 41, 511–522.

Aboitiz, F. 1995. Working memory networks and the origin of language areas in the human brain. *Medical Hypotheses*, 44, 504–506.

Abraham, W. C. 1988. Long-term potentiation as a possible associative memory mechanism in the brain. *New Zealand Journal of Psychology*, 17(2), 49–58.

Abraham, W. C. & Bear, M. F. 1996. Metaplasticity: the plasticity of synaptic plasticity. *Trends in Neuroscience*, 19, 126–130.

Ackil, J. E., Mellgren, R. L., Halgren, C. & Frommer, G. P. 1969. Effects of CS pre-exposures on avoidance learning in rats with hippocampal lesions. *Journal of Comparative and Physiological Psychology*, 69, 739–747.

Acuna, L. R., Back, F., Barp, C. G., Guilherme Tassoni Bortoloci, J., Assreuy, J. & Carobrez, A. P. 2023. Role of nitric oxide on defensive behavior and long-term aversive learning induced by chemical stimulation of the dorsolateral periaqueductal gray matter. *Neurobiology of Learning and Memory*, 200, 107735. https://doi.org/10.1016/j.nlm.2023.107735

Adamec, R. 1997. Transmitter systems involved in neural plasticity underlying increased anxiety and defense - implications for understanding anxiety following traumatic stress. *Neuroscience & Biobehavioral Reviews*, 21, 755–765.

Adamec, R., Holmes, A. & Blundell, J. 2008. Vulnerability to lasting anxiogenic effects of brief exposure to predator stimuli: sex, serotonin and other factors-Relevance to PTSD. *Neuroscience & Biobehavioral Reviews*, 32, 1287–1292.

Adamec, R. E. 1998a. Evidence that NMDA-dependent limbic neural plasticity in the right hemisphere mediates pharmacological stressor (FG-7142)- induced lasting increases in anxiety-like behavior - Study 1 - Role of NMDA receptors in efferent transmission from the cat amygdala. *Journal of Psychopharmacology*, 12, 122–128.

Adamec, R. E. 1998b. Evidence that NMDA-dependent limbic neural plasticity in the right hemisphere mediates pharmacological stressor (FG-7142)-induced lasting increases in anxiety-like behavior. Study 3- The effects on amygdala efferent physiology of block of NMDA receptors prior to injection of FG-7142 and its relationship to behavioral change. *Journal of Psychopharmacology*, 12, 227–238.

Adamec, R. E., Shallow, T. & Budgell, J. 1997. Blockade of CCKB but not CCKA receptors before and after the stress of predator exposure prevents lasting increases in anxiety-like behavior: implications for anxiety associated with posttraumatic stress disorder. *Behavioral Neuroscience*, 111, 435–449.

Adelman, H. M. & Maatsch, J. L. 1956. Learning and extinction based upon frustration, food reward, and exploratory tendency. *Journal of Experimental Psychology*, 52, 311–315.

Adolphs, R., Tranel, D., Damasio, H. & Damasio, A. 1994. Impaired recognition of emotion in facial expressions following bilateral damage to the human amygdala. *Nature*, 372, 669–672.

Aggleton, J. P. 1992. *The amygdala: neurobiological aspects of emotion, memory and mental dysfunction*, New York, Wiley-Liss.

Aggleton, J. P. 1993. The contribution of the amygdala to normal and abnormal emotional states. *Trends in Neuroscience*, 16, 328–333.

Aggleton, J. P., Hunt, P. R. & Shaw, C. 1990. The effects of mammillary body and combined amygdalar-fornix lesions on tests of delayed non-matching-to-sample in the rat. *Behavioural Brain Research*, 40, 145–157.

Aggleton, J. P., Yanakieva, S., Sengpiel, F. & Nelson, A. J. 2021. The separate and combined properties of the granular (area 29) and dysgranular (area 30) retrosplenial cortex. *Neurobiology of Learning and Memory*, 185, 107516. https://doi.org/https://doi.org/10.1016/j.nlm.2021.107516

Agras, W. S. 1985. *Panic: facing fears phobias and anxiety*, New York, W.H. Freeman.

Åhs, F., Rosen, J., Kastrati, G., Fredrikson, M., Agren, T. & Lundstrom, J. N. 2018. Biological preparedness and resistance to extinction of skin conductance responses conditioned to fear relevant animal pictures: a systematic review. *Neuroscience and Biobehavioural Reviews*, 95, 430–437. https://doi.org/10.1016/j.neubiorev.2018.10.017

Ait-Daoud, N., Hamby, A. S., Sharma, S. & Blevins, D. 2018. A review of alprazolam use, misuse, and withdrawal. *Journal of Addiction Medicine*, 12, 4–10. https://doi.org/10.1097/ADM.0000000000000350

Akhtar, S., Wig, N., Varma, O., Pershad, D. & Verma, S. 1975. A phenomenological analysis of symptoms in obsessive- compulsive neurosis. *British Journal of Psychiatry*, 127, 342–348.

Akimova, E., Lanzenberger, R. & Kasper, S. 2009. The serotonin-1A receptor in anxiety disorders. *Biological Psychiatry*, 66, 627–635. https://doi.org/https://doi.org/10.1016/j.biopsych.2009.03.012

Albakri, G., Bouaziz, R., Alharthi, W., Kammoun, S., Al-Sarem, M., Saeed, F. & Hadwan, M. 2022. Phobia exposure therapy using virtual and augmented reality: a systematic review. *Applied Sciences*, 12, e1672. https://doi.org/10.3390/app12031672

Albucher, R. C. & Liberzon, I. 2002. Psychopharmacological treatment in PTSD: a critical review. *Journal of Psychiatric Research*, 36, 355–367. https://doi.org/10.1016/S0022-3956(02)00058-4

Alemayehu, S., Bergey, G. K., Barry, E., Krumholz, A., Wolf, A., Fleming, C. P. & Frear, E. J., Jr. 1995. Panic attacks as ictal manifestations of parietal lobe seizures. *Epilepsia*, 36, 824–830.

Alger, B. E. & Teyler, T. J. 1976. Long-term and short-term plasticity in the CA1, CA3, and dentate regions of the rat hippocampal slice. *Brain Research*, 110, 463–480.

Alhaider, A. A., Ageel, A. M. & Ginawi, O. T. 1993. The quipazine- and YFMPP-increased conditioned avoidance response in rats: role of 5-HT1C/5-HT2 receptors. *Neuropharmacology*, 32, 1427–1432. https://doi.org/https://doi.org/10.1016/0028-3908(93)90040-A

Allegra, M., Posani, L., Gómez-Ocádiz, R. & Schmidt-Hieber, C. 2020. Differential relation between neuronal and behavioral discrimination during hippocampal memory encoding. *Neuron*, 108, 1103–1112.e6. https://doi.org/https://doi.org/10.1016/j.neuron.2020.09.032

Allman, J. M., Tetreault, N. A., Hakeem, A. Y., Manaye, K. F., Semendeferi, K., Erwin, J. M., Park, S., Goubert, V. & Hof, P. R. 2011. The von Economo neurons in the frontoinsular and anterior cingulate cortex. *Annals of the New York Academy of Sciences*, 1225, 59–71. https://doi.org/https://doi.org/10.1111/j.1749-6632.2011.06011.x

Alvarado, M. C. & Rudy, J. W. 1995a. Comparison of "configural" discrimination problems: implications for understanding the role of the hippocampal formation in learning and memory. *Psychobiology*, 23, 178–184.

Alvarado, M. C. & Rudy, J. W. 1995b. Rats with damage to the hippocampal-formation are impaired on the transverse-patterning problem but not on elemental discriminations. *Behavioral Neuroscience*, 109, 204–211.

Alvarez-Perez, Y., Rivero, F., Herrero, M., Vina, C., Fumero, A., Betancort, M. & Penate, W. 2021. Changes in brain activation through cognitive-behavioral therapy with exposure to virtual reality: a neuroimaging study of specific phobia. *Journal of Clinical Medicine*, 10. https://doi.org/10.3390/jcm10163505

Amaral, D. G., Price, J. L., Pitkänen, A. & Carmichael, S. T. 1992. Anatomical organization of the primate amygdaloid complex. *In:* Aggleton, J. P. (ed.) *The amygdala: neurobiological aspects of emotion, memory and mental dysfunction*. Wiley-Liss.

American Psychiatric Association 1987. *DSM-III: Diagnostic and statistical manual of mental disorders, 3rd edition—Revised*. Washington, DC, American Psychiatric Association.

American Psychiatric Association 1994. *DSM-IV: Diagnostic and statistical manual of mental disorders, 4th edition*. Washington, DC, American Psychiatric Association.

American Psychiatric Association 2013. *Diagnostic and statistical manual of mental disorders, fifth edition.* Arlington, VA, American Psychiatric Association.

American Psychiatric Association 2022. *Diagnostic and statistical manual of mental disorders fifth edition, text revision.* Washington, D.C., American Psychiatric Association.

Amsel, A. 1962. Frustrative nonreward in partial reinforcement and discrimination learning: some recent history and a theoretical extension. *Psychological Review*, 69, 306–328.

Amsel, A. 1972. Behavioural habituation, counterconditioning, and a general theory of persistence. *In:* Black, A. H. & Prokasy, W. F. (eds.) *Classical conditioning II: current research and theory* (pp. 409–426). New York: Appleton-Century-Crofts.

Amsel, A. 1992. *Frustration theory: an analysis of dispositional learning and memory.* Cambridge: Cambridge University Press.

Amsel, A. & Roussel, J. 1952. Motivational properties of frustration. I. Effect on a running response of the addition of frustration to the motivational complex. *Journal of Experimental Child Psychology*, 43, 363–368.

Andrade, T. G. C. S., Macedo, C. E. A., Zangrossi, H. & Graeff, F. G. 2004. Anxiolytic-like effects of median raphe nucleus lesion in the elevated T-maze. *Behavioural Brain Research*, 153, 55–60. https://doi.org/https://doi.org/10.1016/j.bbr.2003.10.036

Andrews, G., Stewart, G., Morris-Yates, A., Holt, P. & Henderson, S. 1990. Evidence for a general neurotic syndrome. *British Journal of Psychiatry*, 157, 6–12. https://doi.org/10.1192/bjp.157.1.6

Angulo-Garcia, D., Ferraris, M., Ghestem, A., Nallet-Khosrofian, L., Bernard, C. & Quilichini, P. P. 2020. Cell assemblies in the cortico-hippocampal-reuniens network during slow oscillations. *The Journal of Neuroscience*, 40, 8343–8354. https://doi.org/10.1523/jneurosci.0571-20.2020

Annese, J., Schenker-Ahmed, N. M., Bartsch, H., Maechler, P., Sheh, C., Thomas, N., Kayano, J., Ghatan, A., Bresler, N., Frosch, M. P., Klaming, R. & Corkin, S. 2014. Postmortem examination of patient H.M.'s brain based on histological sectioning and digital 3D reconstruction. *Nature Communications*, 5, A3122. https://doi.org/10.1038/ncomms4122

Anselme, P. 2008. Abnormal patterns of displacement activities: a review and reinterpretation. *Behavioural Processes*, 79, 48–58. https://doi.org/https://doi.org/10.1016/j.beproc.2008.05.001

Aoki, Y., Fujihara, S. & Kitamura, T. 1994. Panic attacks and panic disorder in a Japanese non-patient population: epidemiology and psychosocial correlates. *Journal of Affective Disorders*, 32, 51–59.

Arleo, A., Déjean, C., Allegraud, P., Khamassi, M., Zugaro, M. B. & Wiener, S. I. 2013. Optic flow stimuli update anterodorsal thalamus head direction neuronal activity in rats. *The Journal of Neuroscience*, 33, 16790–16795. https://doi.org/10.1523/jneurosci.2698-13.2013

Arnold, M. B. 1968. *The nature of emotion*. Harmondsworth: Penguin Books Ltd.

Aron, A. R. 2007. The neural basis of inhibition in cognitive control. *The Neuroscientist*, 13, 214–228.

Aron, A. R. 2011. From reactive to proactive and selective control: developing a richer model for stopping inappropriate responses. *Biological Psychiatry*, 69, e55–e68. https://doi.org/10.1016/j.biopsych.2010.07.024

Aron, A. R., Durston, S., Eagle, D. M., Logan, G. D., Stinear, C. M. & Stuphorn, V. 2007. Converging evidence for a fronto-basal-ganglia network for inhibitory control of action and cognition. *Journal of Neuroscience*, 27, 11860–11864. https://doi.org/10.1523/jneurosci.3644-07.2007

Aron, A. R., Fletcher, P. C., Bullmore, E. T., Sahakian, B. J. & Robbins, T. W. 2003. Stop-signal inhibition disrupted by damage to right inferior frontal gyrus in humans. *Nature Neuroscience*, 6, 115–116.

Aron, A. R., Robbins, T. W. & Poldrack, R. A. 2004. Inhibition and the right inferior frontal cortex. *Trends in Cognitive Sciences*, 8, 170–177.

Aron, A. R., Robbins, T. W. & Poldrack, R. A. 2014a. Inhibition and the right inferior frontal cortex: one decade on. *Trends in Cognitive Sciences*, 18, 177–85. https://doi.org/10.1016/j.tics.2013.12.003

Aron, A. R., Robbins, T. W. & Poldrack, R. A. 2014b. Right inferior frontal cortex: addressing the rebuttals. *Frontiers in Human Neuroscience*, 8. https://doi.org/10.3389/fnhum.2014.00905

Aronov, D., Nevers, R. & Tank, D. W. 2017. Mapping of a non-spatial dimension by the hippocampal–entorhinal circuit. *Nature*, 543, 719–722. https://doi.org/10.1038/nature21692

Ashton, H. 1994. Guidelines for the rational use of benzodiazepines: when and what to use. *Drugs*, 48, 25–40.

Ashton, M. C. & Lee, K. 2005. A defence of the lexical approach to the study of personality structure. *European Journal of Personality*, 19, 5–24. https://doi.org/10.1002/per.541

Asmundson, G. J. G. & Stein, M. B. 1994. Triggering the false suffocation alarm in panic disorder patients by using a voluntary breath-holding procedure. *American Journal of Psychiatry*, 151, 264–266.

Atmaca, M., Tezcan, E. T. & Kuloglu, M. 2003. An open clinical trial of reboxetine in the treatment of social phobia. *Journal of Clinical Psychopharmacology*, 23, 417–418.

Aupperle, R. L., Tankersley, D., Ravindran, L. N., Flagan, T., Stein, N. R., Stein, M. B. & Paulus, M. P. 2012. Pregabalin effects on neural response to emotional faces. *Frontiers in Human Neuroscience*, 6, Article 42. https://doi.org/10.3389/fnhum.2012.00042

Axsome Therapeutics 2022. Introducing Auvelity. *https://ml.globenewswire.com/media/8e8d153f-6231-4d74-be5c-6ce1b7b26c82/document/?v=08192022103000.*

Ayhan, F., Kulkarni, A., Berto, S., Sivaprakasam, K., Douglas, C., Lega, B. C. & Konopka, G. 2021. Resolving cellular and molecular diversity along the hippocampal anterior-to-posterior axis in humans. *Neuron*, 109, 2091–2105.e6. https://doi.org/https://doi.org/10.1016/j.neuron.2021.05.003

Bach, D. R. 2021. Cross-species anxiety tests in psychiatry: pitfalls and promises. *Molecular Psychiatry*, 27, 154–163. https://doi.org/10.1038/s41380-021-01299-4

Bach, D. R., Moutoussis, M., Bowler, A., Neuroscience in Psychiatry Network, c. & Dolan, R. J. 2020. Predictors of risky foraging behaviour in healthy young people. *Nature Human Behaviour*, 8, 832–843. https://doi.org/10.1038/s41562-020-0867-0

Baddeley, A. 1986. *Working memory*. Oxford, Clarendon Press.

Baddeley, A. 2011. Working memory: theories, models, and controversies. *Annual Review of Psychology*, 63, 1–29. https://doi.org/10.1146/annurev-psych-120710-100422

Baddeley, A. & Wilson, B. A. 1994. When implicit learning fails: amnesia and the problem of error elimination. *Neuropsychologia*, 32, 53–68.

Baddeley, H. 1981. Amnesia: a minimal model and an interpretation. *In:* Cermak, L. (ed.) *Human memory and amnesia*. Hillsdale, NJ: Erlbaum. https://www.taylorfrancis.com/chapters/edit/10.4324/9781315778105-15/amnesia-minimal-model-interpretation-alan-baddeley

Baenninger, R. 1967. Contrasting effects of fear and pain on mouse killing by rats. *Journal of Comparative and Physiological Psychology*, 63, 298–303.

Baer, L. & Minichiello, W. E. 1990. Behavioural treatment (BT) for obsessive-compulsive disorder. *In:* Noyes, R., Jr., Roth, M. & Burrows, D. (eds.) *Handbook of Anxiety, Vol 4: The Treatment of Anxiety*. Elsevier Science Publishers B.V.

Bailey, C. J. & Miller, N. E. 1952. The effect of sodium amytal on an approach-avoidance conflict in cats. *Journal of Comparative and Physiological Psychology*, 45, 205–208. https://doi.org/10.1037/h0055258

Bainbridge, T. F., Ludeke, S. G. & Smillie, L. D. 2022. Evaluating the Big Five as an organizing framework for commonly used psychological trait scales. *Journal of Personality and Social Psychology*, 122, 749–777. https://doi.org/10.1037/pspp0000395

Balaban, M. T. & Taussig, H. N. 1994. Salience of fear/threat in the affective modulation of the human startle blink. *Biological Psychology*, 38, 117–131.

Baldwin, D. S., Ajel, K., Masdrakis, V. G., Nowak, M. & Rafiq, R. 2013. Pregabalin for the treatment of generalized anxiety disorder: an update. *Neuropsychiatric Disorders and Treatment*, 9, 883–892.

Balleine, B. W. & Dickinson, A. 2000. The effect of lesions of the insular cortex on instrumental conditioning: evidence for a role in incentive memory. *Journal of Neuroscience*, 20, 8954–8964.

Balon, R., Starcevic, V., Silberman, E., Cosci, F., Dubovsky, S., Fava, G. A., Nardi, A. E., Rickels, K., Salzman, C., Shader, R. I. & Sonino, N. 2020. The rise and fall and rise of benzodiazepines: a return of the stigmatized and repressed. *Brazilian Journal of Psychiatry*, 42, 243–244. https://doi.org/10.1590/1516-4446-2019-0773

Bandelow, B., Michaelis, S. & Wedekind, D. 2017. Treatment of anxiety disorders. *Dialogues in Clinical Neuroscience*, 19, 93–107.

Bandler, R. & Carrive, P. 1988. Integrated defence reaction elicited by excitatory amino acid microinjection in the midbrain periaqueductal grey region of the unrestrained cat. *Brain Research*, 439, 95–106.

Bang, D., Kishida, K. T., Lohrenz, T., White, J. P., Laxton, A. W., Tatter, S. B., Fleming, S. M. & Montague, P. R. 2020. Sub-second dopamine and serotonin signaling in human striatum during perceptual decision-making. *Neuron*, 108, 999–1010.e6. https://doi.org/https://doi.org/10.1016/j.neuron.2020.09.015

Bannerman, D. M., Matthews, P., Deacon, R. M. J. & Rawlins, J. N. P. 2004a. Medial septal lesions mimic effects of both selective dorsal and ventral hippocampal lesions. *Behavioral Neuroscience*, 118, 1033–1041. https://doi.org/10.1037/0735-7044.118.5.1033

Bannerman, D. M., Rawlins, J. N. P., McHugh, S. B., Deacon, R. M. J., Yee, B. K., Bast, T., Zhang, W. N., Pothuizen, H. H. J. & Feldon, J. 2004b. Regional dissociation within the hippocampus - memory and anxiety. *Neuroscience & Biobehavioral Reviews*, 28, 273–283.

Bannerman, D. M., Sprengel, R., Sanderson, D. J., McHugh, S. B., Rawlins, J. N. P., Monyer, H. & Seeburg, P. H. 2014. Hippocampal synaptic plasticity, spatial memory and anxiety. *Nature Reviews Neuroscience*, 15, 181–192. https://doi.org/10.1038/nrn3677

Banov, M. D., Young, J. R., Dunn, T. & Szabo, S. T. 2019. Efficacy and safety of ketamine in the management of anxiety and anxiety spectrum disorders: a review of the literature. *CNS Spectrums*, 1–12. https://doi.org/10.1017/S1092852919001238

Banstola, A., Young, C. K., Parr-Brownlie, L. & McNaughton, N. 2022. Dynamic interaction between hippocampus, orbitofrontal cortex, and subthalamic nucleus during goal conflict in the stop signal task in rats. *Neuroscience Research*, 182, 65–75. https://doi.org/10.1016/j.neures.2022.06.006

Barbas, H. & Pandya, D. N. 1987. Architecture and frontal cortical connections of the premotor cortex (area 6) in the Rhesus monkey. *Journal of Comparative Neurology*, 256, 211–228.

Barbas, H. & Pandya, D. N. 1991. Patterns of connections of the prefrontal cortex in the rhesus monkey associated with cortical architecture. *In:* Levin, H. S., Eisenberg, H. M. & Benton, A. L. (eds.) *Frontal lobe function and dysfunction* (pp. 35–38). Oxford: Oxford University Press.

Barbier, M. & Risold, P.-Y. 2019. The claustrum is a target for projections from the supramammillary nucleus in the rat. *Neuroscience*, 409, 261–275. https://doi.org/https://doi.org/10.1016/j.neuroscience.2019.03.045

Bari, A., Mar, A. C., Theobald, D. E., Elands, S. A., Oganya, K. C. N. A., Eagle, D. M. & Robbins, T. W. 2011. Prefrontal and monoaminergic contributions to stop-signal task performance in rats. *The Journal of Neuroscience*, 31, 9254–9263. https://doi.org/10.1523/jneurosci.1543-11.2011

Bari, A., Xu, S., Pignatelli, M., Takeuchi, D., Feng, J., Li, Y. & Tonegawa, S. 2020. Differential attentional control mechanisms by two distinct noradrenergic coeruleo-frontal cortical pathways. *Proceedings of the National Academy of Sciences*, 202015635. https://doi.org/10.1073/pnas.2015635117

Barlow, D. H., Sauer-Zavala, S., Carl, J. R., Bullis, J. R. & Ellard, K. K. 2014. The nature, diagnosis, and treatment of neuroticism. *Clinical Psychological Science*, 2, 344–365. https://doi.org/10.1177/2167702613505532

Barnes, C. A., McNaughton, B. L., Mizumori, S. J. Y., Leonard, B. W. & Lin, L. H. 1990. Comparison of spatial and temporal characteristice of neuronal activity in sequentialstages of hippocampal processing. *Progress in Brain Research*, 83, 287–300.

Barnett, S. C., Parr-Brownlie, L. C., Perry, B. A. L., Young, C. K., Wicky, H. E., Hughes, S. M., McNaughton, N. & Dalrymple-Alford, J. C. 2021. Anterior thalamic nuclei neurons sustain memory. *Current Research in Neurobiology*, 2, e100022.

Barry, H. & Miller, N. E. 1965. Comparison of drug effects on approach, avoidance and escape motivation. *Journal of Comparative and Physiological Psychology*, 59, 18–24.

Barsky, A. J., Cleary, P. D., Sarnie, M. K. & Ruskin, J. N. 1994. Panic disorder, palpitations, and the awareness of cardiac activity. *Journal of Nervous and Mental Diseases*, 182, 63–71.

Bastin, J., Deman, P., David, O., Gueguen, M., Benis, D., Minotti, L., Hoffman, D., Combrisson, E., Kujala, J., Perrone-Bertolotti, M., Kahane, P., Lachaux, J.-P. & Jerbi, K. 2017. Direct recordings from human anterior insula reveal its leading role within the error-monitoring network. *Cerebral Cortex*, 27, 1545–1557. https://doi.org/10.1093/cercor/bhv352

Batalla, A., Homberg, J. R., Lipina, T. V., Sescousse, G., Luijten, M., Ivanova, S. A., Schellekens, A. F. A. & Loonen, A. J. M. 2017. The role of the habenula in the transition from reward to misery in substance use and mood disorders. *Neuroscience & Biobehavioral Reviews*, 80, 276–285. https://doi.org/10.1016/j.neubiorev.2017.03.019

Baxter, A. J., Vos, T., Scott, K. M., Ferrari, A. J. & Whiteford, H. A. 2014. The global burden of anxiety disorders in 2010. *Psychological Medicine*, 44, 2363–2374. https://doi.org/10.1017/S0033291713003243

Bechara, A., Tranel, D., Damasio, H., Adolphs, R., Rockland, C. & Damasio, A. R. 1995. Double dissociation of conditioning and declarative knowledge relative to the amygdala and hippocampus in humans. *Science*, 269, 1115–1118.

Beck, A. T. 1967. *Depression: clinical, experimental and theoretical aspects*, New York, Harper & Row.

Beck, A. T. 1970. Cognitive therapy: nature and relation to behaviour therapy. *Behavior Therapy*, 1, 184–200.

Beck, A. T. 1976. *Cognitive therapy and the emotional disorders*. New York: International Universities Press.

Beck, A. T. 1987. Cognitive models of depression. *Journal of Cognitive Psychotherapy: An International Quarterly*, 1, 5–37.

Beck, A. T., Epstein, N. & Harrison, R. 1983. Cognitions, attitudes, and personality dimensions in depression. *British Journal of Cognitive Psychology*, 1, 1–16.

Beck, C. H. M. & Fibiger, H. C. 1995. Conditioned fear-induced changes in behavior and in the expression of the immediate early gene c-fos: with and without diazepam pretreatment. *The Journal of Neuroscience*, 15, 709–720.

Beck, I., Smits, D. J. M., Claes, L., Vandereycken, W. & Bijttebier, P. 2009. Psychometric evaluation of the behavioral inhibition/behavioral activation system scales and the sensitivity to punishment and sensitivity to reward questionnaire in a sample of eating disordered patients. *Personality and Individual Differences*, 47, 407–412. https://doi.org/10.1016/j.paid.2009.04.007

Becker, A., Grecksch, G., Bernstein, H. G., Höllt, V. & Bogerts, B. 1999. Social behaviour in rats lesioned with ibotenic acid in the hippocampus: quantitative and qualitative analysis. *Psychopharmacology*, 144, 333–338.

Ben Shalom, D. 2009. The medial prefrontal cortex and integration in autism. *The Neuroscientist*, 15, 589–598.

Ben Shalom, D. 2022. The amygdala–insula–medial prefrontal cortex–lateral prefrontal cortex pathway and its disorders. *Frontiers in Neuroanatomy*, 16. https://doi.org/10.3389/fnana.2022.1028546

Ben Shalom, D. & Bonneh, Y. S. 2019. Editorial: the medial prefrontal cortex and Integration in ASD and typical cognition. *Frontiers in Human Neuroscience*, 13, A00074. https://doi.org/10.3389/fnhum.2019.00074

Bennett, A. T. D. 1996. Do animals have cognitive maps. *The Journal of Experimental Biology*, 199, 219–224.

Berger, T. W. & Alger, B. 1976. Neuronal substrates of classical conditioning in the hippocampus. *Science*, 192, 483–485.

Berger, T. W., Berry, S. D. & Thompson, R. F. 1986a. Role of the hippocampus in classical conditioning of aversive and appetitive behaviors. *In:* Isaacson, R. L. & Pribam, K. H. (eds.) *The Hippocampus* (vol. 4, pp. 203–239). Plenum Publishing, Corporation.

Berger, T. W., Rinaldi, P. C., Weisz, D. J. & Thompson, R. F. 1983. Single-unit analysis of different hippocampal cell types during classical conditioning of rabbit nictitating membrane response. *Journal of Neurophysiology*, 50, 1197–1219.

Berger, T. W. & Thompson, R. F. 1978a. Neuronal plasticity in the limbic system during classical conditioning of the rabbit nictitating membrane response. I. The hippocampus. *Brain Research*, 145, 323–346.

Berger, T. W. & Thompson, R. F. 1978b. Neuronal plasticity in the limbic system during classical conditioning of the rabbit nictitating membrane response. II: septum and mammillary bodies. *Brain Research*, 156, 293–314.

Berger, T. W., Weikart, C. L., Bassett, J. L. & Orr, W. B. 1986b. Lesions of the retrosplenial cortex produce deficits in reversal learning of the rabbit nictitating membrane response: implications for potential interactions between hippocampal and cerebellar brain systems. *Behavioral Neuroscience*, 100, 802–809.

Bermant, G. 1961a. *Regulation of sexual contact by female rats*. Boston, Harvard University.

Bermant, G. 1961b. Response latencies of female rats during sexual intercourse. *Science*, 133, 1771–1773.

Berners-Lee, A., Wu, X. & Foster, D. J. 2021. Prefrontal cortical neurons are selective for non-local hippocampal representations during replay and behavior. *The Journal of Neuroscience*, 41, 5894–5908. https://doi.org/10.1523/jneurosci.1158-20.2021

Berridge, K. C. 1996. Food reward: brain substrates of wanting and liking. *Neuroscience & Biobehavioral Reviews*, 20, 1–25.

Berridge, K. C. 2004. Motivation concepts in behavioral neuroscience. *Physiology and Behavior*, 81, 179–209.

Berry, A. S., White, R. L., Furman, D. J., Naskolnakorn, J. R., Shah, V. D., D'Esposito, M. & Jagust, W. J. 2019. Dopaminergic mechanisms underlying normal variation in trait anxiety. *The Journal of Neuroscience*, 39, 2735–2744. https://doi.org/10.1523/jneurosci.2382-18.2019

Besharat, M. A., Atari, M. & Mirjalili, R. S. 2019. Transdiagnostic processes in generalized anxiety disorder and obsessive-compulsive disorder: worry, cognitive avoidance, intolerance of uncertainty, and metacognitive beliefs. *Practice in Clinical Psychology*, 7, 281–290. https://doi.org/10.32598/jpcp.7.4.281

Bevandić, J., Genzel, L. & Ólafsdóttir, H. F. 2021. Shining a light on hippocampal remapping. *Neuron*, 109, 913–915. https://doi.org/https://doi.org/10.1016/j.neuron.2021.02.020

Bhasin, G. & Nair, I. R. 2022. Dynamic hippocampal CA2 responses to contextual spatial novelty. *Frontiers in Systems Neuroscience*, 16, A923911. https://doi.org/10.3389/fnsys.2022.923911

Bienvenu, O. J., Hettema, J. M., Neale, M. C., Prescott, C. A. & Kendler, K. S. 2007. Low extraversion and high neuroticism as indices of genetic and environmental risk for social phobia, agoraphobia, and animal phobia. *American Journal of Psychiatry*, 1714–1721.

Bignami, G. 1965. Selection for high rates and low rates of avoidance conditioning in the rat. *Animal Behaviour*, 13, 221–227.

Bisson, J. I., Ariti, C., Cullen, K., Kitchiner, N., Lewis, C., Roberts, N. P., Simon, N., Smallman, K., Addison, K., Bell, V., Brookes-Howell, L., Cosgrove, S., Ehlers, A., Fitzsimmons, D., Foscarini-Craggs, P., Harris, S. R. S., Kelson, M., Lovell, K., McKenna, M., McNamara, R., Nollett, C., Pickles, T. & Williams-Thomas, R. 2022. Guided, internet based, cognitive behavioural therapy for post-traumatic stress disorder: pragmatic, multicentre, randomised controlled non-inferiority trial (RAPID). *BMJ*, 377, e069405. https://doi.org/10.1136/bmj-2021-069405

Blackman, D. E. 1983. On cognitive theories of animal learning: extrapolation from humans to animals. *In:* Davey, G. C. L. (ed.) *Animal models of human behaviour* (pp. 37–50). New York: John Wiley.

Blair, H. T. & Sharp, P. E. 1995. Anticipatory head direction signals in anterior thalamus: evidence for a thalamocortical circuit that integrates angular head motion to compute head direction. *The Journal of Neuroscience*, 15, 6260–6270.

Blanchard, D. C. 2017. Translating dynamic defense patterns from rodents to people. *Neuroscience & Biobehavioral Reviews*, 76, 22–28. https://doi.org/10.1016/j.neubiorev.2016.11.001

Blanchard, D. C. 2018. Risk assessment: at the interface of cognition and emotion. *Current Opinion in Behavioral Sciences*, 24, 69–74. https://doi.org/10.1016/j.cobeha.2018.03.006

Blanchard, D. C. 2023. Are cognitive aspects of defense a core feature of anxiety and depression? *Neuroscience & Biobehavioral Reviews*, 144, 104947. https://doi.org/https://doi.org/10.1016/j.neubiorev.2022.104947

Blanchard, D. C. & Blanchard, R. J. 1988. Ethoexperimental approaches to the biology of emotion. *In:* Rosenzweig, M. K. & Porter, L. W. (eds.) *Annual review of psychology* (pp. 43–68). Palo Alto.

Blanchard, D. C. & Blanchard, R. J. 1990a. Effects of ethanol, benzodiazepines and serotonin compounds on ethopharmacological models of anxiety. *In:* McNaughton, N. & Andrews, G. (eds.) *Anxiety*. Dunedin: University of Otago Press, p. 188–200.

Blanchard, D. C., Hynd, A. L., Minke, K. A., Minemoto, T. & Blanchard, R. J. 2001. Human defensive behaviors to threat scenarios show parallels to fear- and anxiety-related defense patterns of non-human mammals. *Neuroscience & Biobehavioral Reviews*, 25, 761–770. https://doi.org/10.1016/S0149-7634(01)00056-2

Blanchard, D. C. & Meyza, K. 2017. Risk assessment and serotonin: animal models and human psychopathologies. *Behavioural Brain Research*, 357–358, 9–17. https://doi.org/10.1016/j.bbr.2017.07.008

Blanchard, D. C., Williams, G., Lee, E. M. C. & Blanchard, R. J. 1981. Taming of wild *Rattus* norvegicus by lesions of the mesencephalic central gray. *Physiological Psychology*, 9, 157–163.

Blanchard, R. J. & Blanchard, D. C. 1972. Effects of hippocampal lesions on the rat's reaction to a cat. *Journal of Comparative and Physiological Psychology*, 78, 77–82.

Blanchard, R. J. & Blanchard, D. C. 1989. Antipredator defensive behaviors in a visible burrow system. *Journal of Comparative Psychology*, 103, 70–82.

Blanchard, R. J. & Blanchard, D. C. 1990b. Anti-predator defense as models of animal fear and anxiety. *In:* Brain, P. F., Parmigiani, S., Blanchard, R. J. & Mainardi, D. (eds.) *Fear and Defence* (pp. 89–108). Chur: Harwood Academic Publishers.

Blanchard, R. J. & Blanchard, D. C. 1990c. An ethoexperimental analysis of defense, fear and anxiety. *In:* McNaughton, N. & Andrews, G. (eds.) *Anxiety* (pp. 124–133). Dunedin: Otago University Press.

Blanchard, R. J. & Blanchard, D. C. 1994. Environmental targets and sensorimotor systems in aggression and defence. *In:* Cooper, S. J. & Hendrie, C. A. (eds.) *Ethology and Psychopharmacology* (pp. 133–157). John Wiley & Sons Ltd.

Blanchard, R. J. & Blanchard, D. C. 1996. Defensive quiescence to social stress: relationship to other "immobile" defenses. *Society for Neuroscience Abstracts*, 22, 1138–1138.

Blanchard, R. J., Flannelly, K. J. & Blanchard, D. C. 1986. Defensive behaviors of laboratory and wild Rattus norvegicus. *Journal of Comparative Psychology*, 100, 101–107.

Blanchard, R. J., Flores, T., Magee, L., Weiss, S. & Blanchard, D. C. 1996. Pregrouping aggression and defense scores influences alcohol consumption for dominant and subordinate rats in visible burrow systems. *Aggressive Behaviour*, 18, 459–467.

Blanchard, R. J., Griebel, G., Guardiola-Lemaître, B., Brush, M. M., Lee, J. & Blanchard, D. C. 1997a. An ethopharmacological analysis of selective activation of 5-HT1A receptors: the mouse 5-HT1A syndrome. *Pharmacology, Biochemistry and Behavior*, 57, 897–908.

Blanchard, R. J., Griebel, G., Henrie, J. A. & Blanchard, D. C. 1997b. Differentiation of anxiolytic and panicolytic drugs by effects on rat and mouse defense test batteries. *Neuroscience & Biobehavioral Reviews*, 21, 783–789. https://doi.org/10.1016/S0149-7634(96)00062-0

Blanchard, R. J., Parmigiani, S., Bjornson, C., Masuda, C., Weiss, S. M. & Blanchard, D. C. 1995. Antipredator behaviour of Swiss-Webster mice in a visible burrow system. *Aggressive Behaviour*, 21, 123–136.

Blanchard, R. J., Yudko, E. B., Rodgers, R. J. & Blanchard, D. C. 1993. Defense system psychopharmacology: an ethological approach to the pharmacology of fear and anxiety. *Behavioural Brain Research*, 58, 155–165.

Bland, B. H., Colom, L. V., Konopacki, J. & Roth, S. H. 1988. Intracellular records of carbachol-induced theta rhythm in hippocampal slices. *Brain Research*, 447, 364–368.

Blaxton, T. A., Zeffiro, T. A., Gabrieli, J. D. E., Bookheimer, S. Y., Carrillo, M. C., Theodore, W. H. & Disterhoft, J. F. 1996. Functional mapping of human learning: a positron emission tomography activation study of eyeblink conditioning. *The Journal of Neuroscience*, 16, 4032–4040.

Bliss, T. V. P. & Lomo, T. 1973. Long-lasting potentiation of synaptic transmission in the dentate area of the anaethsetised rabbit following stimulation of the perforant path. *Journal of Physiology*, 232, 331–356.

Blizard, D. A. 1981. The Maudsley Reactive and Nonreactive strains: a North American perspective. *Behavior Genetics*, 11, 469–489. https://doi.org/10.1007/BF01070004

Blizard, D. A., Adams, N. & Boomsma, D. I. 2023. The genetics of neuroticism: insights from the Maudsley rat model and human studies *Personality Neuroscience*, 6, e6.

Blizard, D. A. & Liang, B. 1979. Plasma catecholamines under basal and stressful conditions in rat strains selectively bred for differences in response to stress. *In:* Usdin, E., Kopin, I. J. & Bachas, J. (eds.) *Catecholamines: basic and clinical frontiers* (pp. 1795–1797). New York: Pergamon.

Boccara, C. N., Nardin, M., Stella, F., O'Neill, J. & Csicsvari, J. 2019. The entorhinal cognitive map is attracted to goals. *Science*, 363, 1443–1447. https://doi.org/10.1126/science.aav4837

Boccardi, M., Frisoni, G. B., Hare, R. D., Cavedo, E., Najt, P., Pievani, M., Rasser, P. E., Laakso, M. P., Aronen, H. J., Repo-Tiihonen, E., Vaurio, O., Thompson, P. M. & Tiihonen, J. 2011. Cortex and amygdala morphology in psychopathy. *Psychiatry Research: Neuroimaging*, 193, 85–92. https://doi.org/https://doi.org/10.1016/j.pscychresns.2010.12.013

Boden, P. R. & Woodruff, G. N. 1994. Benzodiazepine/cholecystokinin interactions at functional CCK receptors in rat brain. *British Journal of Pharmacology*, 112, 429–434.

Boehner, P. (ed.) 1957. *Ockham: philosophical writings*. Edinburgh: Nelson.

Bogdan, R., Baranger, D. A. A. & Agrawal, A. 2018. Polygenic risk scores in clinical psychology: bridging genomic risk to individual differences. *Annual Review of Clinical Psychology*, 14, 119–157. https://doi.org/10.1146/annurev-clinpsy-050817-084847

Bokma, W. A., Wetzer, G., Gehrels, J. B., Penninx, B., Batelaan, N. M. & van Balkom, A. 2019. Aligning the many definitions of treatment resistance in anxiety disorders: a systematic review. *Depression and Anxiety*, 36, 801–812. https://doi.org/10.1002/da.22895

Bonnici, H. M., Chadwick, M. J., Lutti, A., Hassabis, D., Weiskopf, N. & Maguire, E. A. 2012. Detecting representations of recent and remote autobiographical memories in vmpfc and hippocampus. *The Journal of Neuroscience*, 32, 16982–16991. https://doi.org/10.1523/jneurosci.2475-12.2012

Borkovec, T. D., Robinson, E., Pruzinsky, T. & DePree, J. A. 1983. Preliminary exploration of worry: some characteristics and processes. *Behaviour Research and Therapy*, 21, 9–16.

Bottini, G., Corcoran, R., Sterzi, R., Paulesu, E., Schenone, P., Scarpa, P., Frackowiak, R. S. J., & Frith, C. D. 1994. The role of the right hemisphere in the interpretation of figurative aspects of language. A positron emission tomography activation study. *Brain*, 117, 1241–1253.

Botvinick, M. 2007. Conflict monitoring and decision making: reconciling two perspectives on anterior cingulate function. *Cognitive Affective & Behavioral Neuroscience*, 7, 356–366.

Botvinick, M., Nystrom, L. E., Fissell, K., Carter, C. S. & Cohen, J. D. 1999. Conflict monitoring versus selection-for-action in anterior cingulate cortex. *Nature*, 402, 179–181.

Botvinick, M. M., Cohen, J. D. & Carter, C. S. 2004. Conflict monitoring and anterior cingulate cortex: an update. *Trends in Cognitive Science*, 8, 539–46. https://doi.org/10.1016/j.tics.2004.10.003

Bouton, M. E., Broomer, M. C., Rey, C. N. & Thrailkill, E. A. 2020. Unexpected food outcomes can return a habit to goal-directed action. *Neurobiology of Learning and Memory*, 169, 107163. https://doi.org/https://doi.org/10.1016/j.nlm.2020.107163

Bowyer, C., Brush, C. J., Threadgill, H., Harmon-Jones, E., Treadway, M., Patrick, C. J. & Hajcak, G. 2021. The effort-doors task: examining the temporal dynamics of effort-based reward processing using ERPs. *Neuroimage*, 228, 117656. https://doi.org/10.1016/j.neuroimage.2020.117656

Bradfield, L. A., Leung, B. K., Boldt, S., Liang, S. & Balleine, B. W. 2020. Goal-directed actions transiently depend on dorsal hippocampus. *Nature Neuroscience*, 23, 1194–1197. https://doi.org/10.1038/s41593-020-0693-8

Braestrup, C. & Nielsen, M. 1980. Benzodiazepine receptors. *Arzneimittelforschung*, 30, 852–857.

Braestrup, C. & Squires, R. F. 1977. Specific benzodiazepine receptors in rat brain characterized by high-affinity [3H]-diazepam binding. *Proceedings of the National Academy of Sciences of the United States of America*, 74, 3805–3809.

Brain, P. F. 2017. Bob Blanchard: a neurobiological legacy and appreciation. *Neuroscience & Biobehavioral Reviews*, 76, Part A, 2–3. https://doi.org/10.1016/j.neubiorev.2017.01.001

Brawman-Mintzer, O., Lydiard, R. B., Crawford, M. M., Emmanuel, N., Payeur, R., Johnson, M., Knapp, R. G. & Ballenger, J. C. 1994. Somatic symptoms in generalized anxiety disorder with and without comorbid psychiatric disorders. *American Journal of Psychiatry*, 151, 930–932.

Brawman-Mintzer, O., Lydiard, R. B., Emmanuel, N., Payeur, R., Johnson, M., Roberts, J., Jarrell, M. P. & Ballenger, J. C. 1993. Psychiatric comorbidity in patients with generalized anxiety disorder. *American Journal of Psychiatry*, 150, 1216–1218.

Breese, C. R., Hampson, R. E. & Deadwyler, S. A. 1989. Hippocampal place cells: stereotypy and plasticity. *Journal of Neuroscience*, 9, 1097–1111.

Bremner, J. D., Krystal, J. H., Southwick, S. M. & Charney, D. S. 1995a. Functional neuroanatomical correlates of the effects of stress on memory. *Journal of Traumatic Stress*, 8, 527–???

Bremner, J. D., Randall, P., Scott, T. M., Bronen, R. A., Seibyl, J. P., Southwick, S. M., Delaney, R. C., McCarthy, G., Charney, D. S. & Innis, R. B. 1995b. MRI-based measurement of hippocampal volume in patients with combat-related posttraumatic stress disorder. *American Journal of Psychiatry*, 152, 973–981.

Bremner, J. D., Randall, P., Vermetten, E., Staib, L., Bronen, R. A., Mazure, C., Capeli, S., McCarthy, G., Innes, R. B. & Charney, D. S. 1997. Magnetic resonance imaging-based measurement of hippocampal volume in post-traumatic stress disorder related to childhood physical and sexual abuse—a preliminary report. *Biological Psychiatry*, 41, 23–32.

Broadbent, D. E. 1971. *Decision and stress*. London, Academic Press.

Broadhurst, P. L. 1957. Emotionality and the Yerkes-Dodson law. *Journal of Experimental Psychology*, 54, 345–351. https://doi.org/10.1037/h0049114

Broadhurst, P. L. 1960. Applications of biometrical genetics to the inheritance of behaviour. *In:* Eysenck, H. J. (ed.) *Experiments in personality, Vol 1 Psychogenetics and psychopharmacology* (pp. 1–102). London: Routledge Kegan Paul.

Broadhurst, P. L. 1975. The Maudsley reactive and nonreactive strains of rats: a survey. *Behavior Genetics*, 5, 299–319.

Brodt, S. & Born, J. 2021. Ripples for recall: the hippocampus constructing the context? *Neuron*, 109, 2646–2648. https://doi.org/https://doi.org/10.1016/j.neuron.2021.08.010

Brodt, S., Inostroza, M., Niethard, N. & Born, J. 2023. Sleep—A brain-state serving systems memory consolidation. *Neuron*, 111, 1050–1075. https://doi.org/10.1016/j.neuron.2023.03.005

Broekkamp, C. L. E., Berendsen, H. H. G., Jenck, F. & Van Delft, A. M. L. 1989. Animal models for anxiety and response to serotonergic drugs. *Psychopathology*, 22(suppl), 2–12.

Bromberg-Martin, E. S., Matsumoto, M. & Hikosaka, O. 2010. Dopamine in motivational control: rewarding, aversive, and alerting. *Neuron*, 68, 815–834.

Brooks, V. B. 1979. Motor programs revisited. *In:* Talbott, R. E. & Humphrey, D. R. (eds.) *Posture and movement* (pp. 13–49). New York: Raven Press.

Brown, J., Lewis, V., Brown, M., Horn, G. & Bowes, J. B. 1982. A comparison between transient amnesias induced by two drugs (diazepam or lorazepam) and amnesia of organic origin. *Neuropsychologia*, 20, 55–70.

Brown, J. S. 1961. *The motivation of behavior*. New York, McGraw Hill.

Brown, J. W. 1985. Frontal lobe syndromes. *In:* Frederiks, J. A. M. (ed.) *Handbook of clinical neurology: clinical neuropsychology*. Elsevier Science Publishers.

Brown, L. Y., Alexander, G. M., Cushman, J. & Dudek, S. M. 2020. Hippocampal CA2 organizes CA1 slow and fast gamma oscillations during novel social and object interaction. *eNeuro*, ENEURO.0084-20.2020. https://doi.org/10.1523/eneuro.0084-20.2020

Brown, M. F. 1992. Does a cognitive map guide choices in the radial-arm maze? *Journal of Experimental Psychology: Animal Behaviour Processes*, 18, 56–66.

Brown, M. W. 1982. Effect of context on the response of single units recorded from the hippocampal region of behaviourally trained monkeys. *In:* Marsan, C. A. & Matthies, H. (eds.) *Neuronal plasticity and memory formation* (pp. 557–573). New York: Raven Press.

Browne, T. R. & Perry, J. K. 1973. Benzodiazepines in the treatment of epilepsy. *Epilepsia*, 14, 277–310.

Brunec, I. K. 2016. Unified and separable hippocampal representations of time and space. *Journal of Neuroscience*, 36, 12293–12295. https://doi.org/10.1523/jneurosci.2860-16.2016

Brunec, I. K., Robin, J., Olsen, R. K., Moscovitch, M. & Barense, M. D. 2020. Integration and differentiation of hippocampal memory traces. *Neuroscience & Biobehavioral Reviews*, 118, 196–208. https://doi.org/https://doi.org/10.1016/j.neubiorev.2020.07.024

Brunzell, D. H. & Kim, J. J. 2001. Fear conditioning to tone, but not to context, is attenuated by lesions of the insular cortex and posterior extension of the intralaminar complex in rats. *Behavioral Neuroscience*, 115, 365–375.

Brush, F. R., Baron, S., Froehlich, J. C., Ison, J. R., Pelligrino, L. J., Phillips, D. S., Sakellaris, P. C. & Williams, V. N. 1985. Genetic differences in avoidance learning by rattus norvegicus: escape/avoidance responding, sensitivity to electric shock, discrimination learning, and open-field behavior. *Journal of Comparative Psychology*, 99, 60–73.

Bryant, K. G. & Barker, J. M. 2020. Arbitration of approach-avoidance conflict by ventral hippocampus. *Frontiers in Neuroscience*, 14, A615337. https://doi.org/10.3389/fnins.2020.615337

Buhusi, C. V., Gray, J. A. & Schmajuk, N. A. 1998. Perplexing effects of hippocampal lesions on latent inhibition: a neural network solution. *Behavioral Neuroscience*, 112, 316–351.

Bunsey, M. & Eichenbaum, H. 1996. Conservation of hippocampal memory function in rats and humans. *Nature*, 379, 255–257.

Burback, L., Bremault-Phillips, S., Nijdam, M. J., McFarlane, A. & Vermetten, E. 2023. Treatment of posttraumatic stress disorder: a state-of-the-art review. *Current Neuropharmacology*, online. https://doi.org/10.2174/1570159X21666230428091433

Burgess, N. 2014. The 2014 Nobel Prize in Physiology or Medicine: a spatial model for cognitive neuroscience. *Neuron*, 84, 1120–5. https://doi.org/10.1016/j.neuron.2014.12.009

Burke, S. N., Maurer, A. P., Nematollahi, S., Uprety, A. R., Wallace, J. L. & Barnes, C. A. 2011. The influence of objects on place field expression and size in distal hippocampal CA1. *Hippocampus*, 21, 783–801. https://doi.org/10.1002/hipo.20929

Butters, N. & Cermak, L. S. 1975. Some analyses of amnesic syndromes in braindamaged patients. *In:* Isaacson, R. L. & Pribram, K. H. (eds.) *The hippocampus, Vol. 2 Neurophysiology and behaviour* (pp. 377–409). New York: Plenum Press.

Butters, N., Delis, D. C. & Lucas, J. A. 1995. Clinical assessment of memory disorders in amnesia and dementia. *Annual Review of Psychology*, 46, 493–523.

Buzsáki, G. 2005. Theta rhythm of navigation: link between path integration and landmark navigation, episodic and semantic memory. *Hippocampus*, 15, 827–840.

Buzsáki, G. 2006. *Rhythms of the brain*. Oxford, Oxford University Press.

Buzsáki, G. & Haas, H. L. 1988. Hippocampal sharp waves: a physiological correlate of LTP. *In:* Buzsáki, G. & Haas, H. L. (eds.) *Synaptic plasticity in the hippocampus*. Heidelberg: Springer-Verlag.

Buzsáki, G. & Vöröslakos, M. 2023. Brain rhythms have come of age. *Neuron*, 111, 922–926. https://doi.org/10.1016/j.neuron.2023.03.018

Cahill, L., McGaugh, J. L. & Weinberger, N. M. 2001. The neurobiology of learning and memory: some reminders to remember. *Trends in Neurosciences*, 24, 578–581.

Cahusac, P. M. B. & Miyashita, Y. 1988. Hippocampal activity related to the processing of single sensory-motor associations. *Neuroscience Letters*, 90, 265–272.

Cahusac, P. M. B., Miyashita, Y. & Rolls, E. T. 1989. Responses of hippocampal formation neurons in the monkey related to delayed spatial response and object-place memory tasks. *Behavioural Brain Research*, 33, 229–240.

Cai, W., Ryali, S., Chen, T., Li, C.-S. R. & Menon, V. 2014. Dissociable roles of right inferior frontal cortex and anterior insula in inhibitory control: evidence from intrinsic and task-related functional parcellation, connectivity, and response profile analyses across multiple datasets. *The Journal of Neuroscience*, 34, 14652–14667. https://doi.org/10.1523/jneurosci.3048-14.2014

Calder, A. J., Young, A. W., Rowland, D., Perrett, D. I., Hodges, J. R. & Etcoff, N. L. 1996. Facial emotion recognition after bilateral amygdala damage: differentially severe impairment of fear. *Cognitive Neuropsychology*, 13, 699–740.

Calhoon, G. G. & Tye, K. M. 2015. Resolving the neural circuits of anxiety. *Nature Neuroscience*, 18, 1394–1404. https://doi.org/10.1038/nn.4101

Çalışkan, G. & Stork, O. 2018. Hippocampal network oscillations as mediators of behavioural metaplasticity: insights from emotional learning. *Neurobiology of Learning and Memory*, 154, 37–53. https://doi.org/10.1016/j.nlm.2018.02.022

Cameron, O. G., Huang, G. C., Nichols, T., Koeppe, R. A., Minoshima, S., Rose, D. & Frey, K. A. 2007. Reduced γ-aminobutyric acidA–benzodiazepine binding sites in insular cortex of individuals with panic disorder. *Archives of General Psychiatry*, 64, 793–800. https://doi.org/10.1001/archpsyc.64.7.793

Canteras, N. S. 2002. The medial hypothalamic defensive system: hodological organizationa and functional implications. *Pharmacology, Biochemistry and Behavior*, 71, 481–491.

Canteras, N. S. & Graeff, F. G. 2014. Executive and modulatory neural circuits of defensive reactions: implications for panic disorder. *Neuroscience & Biobehavioral Reviews*. https://doi.org/10.1016/j.neubiorev.2014.03.020

Canton, J., Scott, K. M. & Glue, P. 2012. Optimal treatment of social phobia: systematic review and meta-analysis. *Neuropsychiatric Disease and Treatment*, 8, 203–15. https://doi.org/10.2147/NDT.S23317

Carcone, D. & Ruocco, A. C. 2017. Six years of research on the National Institute of Mental Health's Research Domain Criteria (RDoC) initiative: a systematic review. *Frontiers in Cellular Neuroscience*, 11, A046. https://doi.org/10.3389/fncel.2017.00046

Carli, M. & Samanin, R. 1992. 8-Hydroxy-2-(di-n-propylamino) tetralin impairs spatial learning in a water maze: role of postsynaptic 5-HT1A receptors. *British Journal of Pharmacology*, 105, 720–726.

Carlson, J. M., Greenberg, T., Rubin, D. & Mujica-Parodi, L. R. 2011. Feeling anxious: anticipatory amygdalo-insular response predicts the feeling of anxious anticipation. *Social Cognitive and Affective Neuroscience*, 6, 74–81. https://doi.org/10.1093/scan/nsq017

Carlton, C. N., Sullivan-Toole, H., Ghane, M. & Richey, J. A. 2020. Reward circuitry and motivational deficits in social anxiety disorder: what can be learned from mouse models? *Frontiers in Neuroscience*, 14. https://doi.org/10.3389/fnins.2020.00154

Carthy, E. & Ellender, T. 2021. Histamine, neuroinflammation and neurodevelopment: a review. *Frontiers in Neuroscience*, 15, A608214. https://doi.org/10.3389/fnins.2021.680214

Carver, C. S., Johnson, S. L. & Joormann, J. 2008. Serotonergic function, two-mode models of self-regulation, and vulnerability to depression: what depression has in common with impulsive aggression. *Psychological Bulletin*, 134, 912–943. https://doi.org/10.1037/a0013740

Carver, C. S. & White, T. L. 1994. Behavioral inhibition, behavioral activation, and affective responses to impending reward and punishment: the BIS/BAS scales. *Journal of Personality and Social Psychology*, 67, 319–333.

Caspi, A., Houts, R. M., Belsky, D. W., Goldman-Mellor, S. J., Harrington, H., Israel, S., Meier, M. H., Ramrakha, S., Shalev, I., Poulton, R. & Moffitt, T. E. 2014. The p factor: one general psychopathology factor in the structure of psychiatric disorders? *Clinical Psychological Science*, 2, 119–137. https://doi.org/10.1177/2167702613497473

Cassaday, H. J., Muir, C., Stevenson, C. W., Bonardi, C., Hock, R. & Waite, L. 2023. From safety to frustration: the neural substrates of inhibitory learning in aversive and appetitive conditioning procedures. *Neurobiology of Learning and Memory*, 202, 107757. https://doi.org/10.1016/j.nlm.2023.107757

Castegnetti, G., Tzovara, A., Khemka, S., Melinscak, F., Barnes, G. R., Dolan, R. J. & Bach, D. R. 2020. Representation of probabilistic outcomes during risky decision-making. *Nature Communications*, 11, e2419. https://doi.org/10.1038/s41467-020-16202-y

Cattell, R. B. 1965. *The scientific analysis of personality*. Harmondsworth, Pelican.

Cauda, F., D'Agata, F., Sacco, K., Duca, S., Geminiani, G. & Vercelli, A. 2011. Functional connectivity of the insula in the resting brain. *NeuroImage*, 55, 8–23. https://doi.org/10.1016/j.neuroimage.2010.11.049

Cavada, C., Compañy, T., Tejedor, J., Cruz-Rizzolo, R. J. & Reinoso-Suárez, F. 2000. The anatomical connections of the macaque monkey orbitofrontal cortex. A review. *Cerebral Cortex*, 10, 220–242.

Cermak, L. S. & Butters, N. 1972. The role of interference and encoding in the short-term memory deficits of Korsakoff patients. *Neuropsychologia*, 10, 89–95.

Cermak, L. S., Butters, N. & Gerrein, J. 1973. The extent of the verbal encoding ability of Korsakoff patients. *Neuropsychologia*, 11, 85–94.

Cermak, L. S., Butters, N. & McReines, J. 1974. Some analyses of the verbal encoding deficit of alcoholic Korsakoff patients. *Brain and Language*, 2, 141–150.

Chambers, C. D., Garavan, H. & Bellgrove, M. A. 2009. Insights into the neural basis of response inhibition from cognitive and clinical neuroscience. *Neuroscience and Biobehavioral Reviews*, 33, 631–646.

Chambless, D. L., Foa, E. B., Groves, G. A. & Goldstein, A. J. 1979. Flooding with Brevital in the treatment of agoraphobia: counter- effective? *Behaviour Research and Therapy*, 17, 243–252.

Chang, L. J., Yarkoni, T., Khaw, M. W. & Sanfey, A. G. 2013. Decoding the role of the insula in human cognition: functional parcellation and large-scale reverse inference. *Cerebral Cortex*, 23, 739–749. https://doi.org/10.1093/cercor/bhs065

Chang, W., Lv, Z., Pang, X., Nie, L. & Zheng, J. 2022. The local neural markers of MRI in patients with temporal lobe epilepsy presenting ictal panic: a resting resting-state postictal fMRI study. *Epilepsy & Behavior*, 129, 108490. https://doi.org/https://doi.org/10.1016/j.yebeh.2021.108490

Chao, L. L. & Knight, R. T. 1995. Human prefrontal lesions increase distractibility to irrelevant sensory inputs. *Neuroreport*, 6, 1605–1610.

Chee, S.-S. A., Menard, J. L. & Dringenberg, H. C. 2014. Behavioral anxiolysis without reduction of hippocampal theta frequency after histamine application in the lateral septum of rats. *Hippocampus*, 24, 615–627. https://doi.org/10.1002/hipo.22244

Chen, L., Ke, Y., Ma, H., Gao, L., Zhou, Y., Huaqiang, Z., Liu, H., Zhang, F. & Zhou, W. 2021. Fluoxetine and ketamine reverse the depressive but not anxiety behavior induced by lesion of cholinergic neurons in the horizontal limb of the diagonal band of broca in male rat. *Frontiers in Behavioral Neuroscience*, 15, A602708. https://doi.org/10.3389/fnbeh.2021.602708

Chen, S., He, L., Huang, A. J. Y., Boehringer, R., Robert, V., Wintzer, M. E., Polygalov, D., Weitemier, A. Z., Tao, Y., Gu, M., Middleton, S. J., Namiki, K., Hama, H., Therreau, L., Chevaleyre, V., Hioki, H., Miyawaki, A., Piskorowski, R. A. & McHugh, T. J. 2020. A hypothalamic novelty signal modulates hippocampal memory. *Nature*, 586, 270–274. https://doi.org/10.1038/s41586-020-2771-1

Chen, Y.-L., Sherwood, S. N. & Freeman, A. J. 2023. Multidimensional item response theory of the BIS/BAS scales: evidence for a bifactor model structure. *Journal of Psychopathology and Behavioral Assessment*, online. https://doi.org/10.1007/s10862-023-10064-6

Chen, Y. C., Thaler, D., Nixon, P. D., Stern, C. E. & Passingham, R. E. 1995. The functions of the medial premotor cortex. II. The timing and selection of learned movements. *Experimental Brain Research*, 102, 461–473.

Cheng, D. T., Disterhoft, J. F., Power, J. M., Ellis, D. A. & Desmond, J. E. 2008. Neural substrates underlying human delay and trace eyeblink conditioning. *PNAS*, 195, 8108–8113.

Chi, C. C. 1965. The effect of amobarbital sodium on conditioned fear as measured by the potentiated startle response in rats. *Psychopharmacologia*, 7, 115–122.

Chiba, A. A., Kesner, R. P. & Reynolds, A. M. 1994. Memory for spatial location as a function of temporal lag in rats: role of hippocampus and medial prefrontal cortex. *Behavioral and Neural Biology*, 61, 123–131.

Cho, J. R., Chen, X., Kahan, A., Robinson, J. E., Wagenaar, D. A. & Gradinaru, V. 2021. Dorsal raphe dopamine neurons signal motivational salience dependent on internal state, expectation, and behavioral context. *The Journal of Neuroscience*, 41, 2645–2655. https://doi.org/10.1523/jneurosci.2690-20.2021

Chockanathan, U. & Padmanabhan, K. 2021. Divergence in population coding for space between dorsal and ventral CA1. *eNeuro*, ENEURO.0211-21.2021. https://doi.org/10.1523/eneuro.0211-21.2021

Choi, J. S., Lindquist, D. H. & Brown, T. H. 2001. Amygdala lesions block conditioned enhancement of the early component of the rat eyeblink reflex. *Behavioral Neuroscience*, 115, 764–775.

Choi, W. Y. Y., Balsam, P. D. r. D. & Horvitz, J. C. C. 2005. Extended habit training reduces dopamine mediation of appetitive response expression. *Journal of Neuroscience*, 25, 6729–6733.

Cholvin, T., Hainmueller, T. & Bartos, M. 2021. The hippocampus converts dynamic entorhinal inputs into stable spatial maps. *Neuron*, 109, 3135–3148.e7. https://doi.org/https://doi.org/10.1016/j.neuron.2021.09.019

Choy, Y., Fyer, A. J. & Lipsitz, J. D. 2007. Treatment of specific phobia in adults. *Clinical Psychology Review*, 27, 266–286. https://doi.org/10.1016/j.cpr.2006.10.002

Cieciuch, J. & Strus, W. 2017. Two-factor model of personality. *In:* Zeigler-Hill, V. & Shackelford, T. K. (eds.) *Encyclopedia of personality and individual differences* (pp. 1–17). Springer International Publishing AG.

Clare, L., Wright, J. J. & Bourke, P. D. 2002. Spatial eigenmodes and synchronous oscillation: coincidence detection in simulated cerebral cortex. *Journal of Mathematical Biology*, 45, 57–78.

Clark, B. J., Rice, J. P., Akers, K. G., Candelaria-Cook, F. T., Taube, J. S. & Hamilton, D. A. 2013. Lesions of the dorsal tegmental nuclei disrupt control of navigation by distal landmarks in cued, directional, and place variants of the Morris water task. *Behavioral Neuroscience*, 127, 566–581. https://doi.org/https://doi.org/10.1037/a0033087

Clark, D. A. 2014. Cognitive restructuring. *In:* Dozois, D. (ed.) *The Wiley handbook of cognitive behavioral therapy*. online: John Wiley & Sons.

Clark, D. M. 1986. A cognitive approach to panic. *Behaviour Research and Therapy*, 24, 461–470.

Clark, D. M. 1988. A cognitive model of panic. *In:* Rachman, S. & Maser, J. (eds.) *Panic: psychological perspectives*. Hillsdale: Erlbaum.

Clark, D. M. 1996. Panic disorder: from theory to therapy. *In:* Salkovskis, P. M. (ed.) *Frontiers of cognitive therapy* (pp. 318–344). Guildford Publications.

Clark, D. M. 1997. Panic disorder and social phobia. *In:* Clark, D. M. & Fairburn, C. G. (eds.) *Science and practice of cognitive behaviour therapy* (pp. 121–153). Oxford, Oxford University Press.

Clark, D. M. & Ehlers, A. 1993. An overview of the cognitive theory and treatment of panic disorder. *Applied & Preventative Psychology*, 2, 131–139.

Clark, D. M. & Wells, A. 1995. A cognitive model of social phobia. *In:* Heimberg, R. G., Liebowitz, M. R., Hope, D. A. & Schneier, F. R. (eds.) *Social phobia: diagnosis, assessment & treatment* (pp. 69–93). New York: Guildford.

Clark, D. M., Wild, J., Warnock-Parkes, E., Stott, R., Grey, N., Thew, G. & Ehlers, A. 2022. More than doubling the clinical benefit of each hour of therapist time: a randomised controlled trial of internet cognitive therapy for social anxiety disorder. *Psychological Medicine*, online, 1–11. https://doi.org/10.1017/S0033291722002008

Clewett, D., Dunsmoor, J., Bachman, S. L., Phelps, E. A. & Davachi, L. 2022. Survival of the salient: aversive learning rescues otherwise forgettable memories via neural reactivation and post-encoding hippocampal connectivity. *Neurobiology of Learning and Memory*, 187, 107572. https://doi.org/https://doi.org/10.1016/j.nlm.2021.107572

Cloninger, C. R., Svrakic, D. M. & Przybecky, T. R. 1993. A psychobiological model of temperament and character. *Archives of General Psychiatry*, 50, 975–990. https://doi.org/10.1001/archpsyc.1993.01820240059008

Cohen, A. O. & Meyer, H. C. 2020. Ventral hippocampus projections to prelimbic cortex support contextual fear memory. *The Journal of Neuroscience*, 40, 8410–8412. https://doi.org/10.1523/jneurosci.1285-20.2020

Cohen, N. J. & Eichenbaum, H. 1993. *Memory, amnesia, and the hippocampal memory system.* Cambridge, MA: The MIT Press.

Cole, B. J. & Hillmann, M. 1994. Effects of benzodiazepine receptor ligands on the performance of an operant delayed matching to position task in rats: opposite effects of FG 7142 and lorazepam. *Psychopharmacology (Berl)*, 115, 350–357.

Cole, B. J., Jones, G. H. & Turner, J. D. 1994. 5-HT1A receptor agonists improve the performance of normal and scopolamine-impaired rats in an operant delayed matching to position task. *Psychopharmacology (Berl)*, 116, 135–142.

Cole, J. C. & Rodgers, R. J. 1993. An ethological analysis of the effects of chlordiazepoxide and bretazenil (Ro 16-6028) in the murine elevated plus- maze. *Behavioural Pharmacology*, 4, 573–580.

Colgin, L. L. 2013. Mechanisms and functions of theta rhythms. *Annual Review of Neuroscience*, 36, 295–312.

Colgin, L. L. 2020. Five decades of hippocampal place cells and EEG rhythms in behaving rats. *The Journal of Neuroscience*, 40, 54–60. https://doi.org/10.1523/jneurosci.0741-19.2019

Colombo, M., Eickhoff, A. E. & Gross, C. G. 1993. The effects of inferior temporal and dorsolateral frontal lesions on serial-order behavior and visual imagery in monkeys. *Cognitive Brain Research*, 1, 211–217.

Combe, C. L. & Gasparini, S. 2021. Ih from synapses to networks: HCN channel functions and modulation in neurons. *Progress in Biophysics and Molecular Biology*, 166, 119–132. https://doi.org/https://doi.org/10.1016/j.pbiomolbio.2021.06.002

Commissaris, R. L., Verbanac, J. S., Markovska, V. L., Altman, H. J. & Hill, T. J. 1996. Anxiety-like and depression-like behavior in Maudsley reactive (MR) and non-reactive (MNRA) rats. *Progress in Neuropsychopharmacology and Biological Psychiatry*, 20, 491–501.

Conejo, N. M., González-Pardo, H., Gonzalez-Lima, F. & Arias, J. L. 2010. Spatial learning of the water maze: progression of brain circuits mapped with cytochrome oxidase histochemistry. *Neurobiology of Learning and Memory*, 93, 362–371.

Coop, C. F. & McNaughton, N. 1991. Buspirone affects hippocampal rhythmical slow activity through serotonin1A rather than dopamine D2 receptors. *Neuroscience*, 40, 169–174.

Coop, C. F., McNaughton, N. & Lambie, I. 1991. Effects of GABAA and GABAB receptor agonists on reticular-elicited hippocampal rhythmical slow activity. *European Journal of Pharmacology*, 192, 103–108.

Coop, C. F., McNaughton, N. & Scott, D. J. 1992. Pindolol antagonizes the effects on hippocampal rhythmical slow activity of clonidine, baclofen and 8-OH-DPAT, but not chlordiazepoxide and sodium amylobarbitone. *Neuroscience*, 46, 83–90.

Coop, C. F., McNaughton, N., Warnock, K. & Laverty, R. 1990. Effects of ethanol and Ro 15-4513 in an electrophysiological model of anxiolytic action. *Neuroscience*, 35, 669–674.

Cooper, A. J., Duke, E., Pickering, A. D. & Smillie, L. D. 2014. Individual differences in reward prediction error: contrasting relations between feedback-related negativity and trait measures of reward sensitivity, impulsivity and extraversion. *Frontiers in Human Neuroscience*, 8, 248. https://doi.org/10.3389/fnhum.2014.00248

Coray, R. & Quednow, B. B. 2022. The role of serotonin in declarative memory: a systematic review of animal and human research. *Neuroscience & Biobehavioral Reviews*, 139, 104729. https://doi.org/https://doi.org/10.1016/j.neubiorev.2022.104729

Corkin, S. 1968. Acquisition of motor skill after bilateral medial temporal-lobe excision. *Neuropsychologia*, 6, 255–265.

Corr, P. J. 2008a. Reinforcement sensitivity theory (RST): introduction. *In:* Corr, P. J. (ed.) *The Reinforcement Sensitivity Theory of Personality*. Cambridge. Cambridge University Press.

Corr, P. J. (ed.) 2008b. The *reinforcement sensitivity theory of personality*. Cambridge: Cambridge University Press.

Corr, P. J. 2013. Approach and avoidance behavior: multiple systems and their interactions. *Emotion Review*, 5, 286–291.

Corr, P. J. & Cooper, A. J. 2016. The reinforcement sensitivity theory of personality questionnaire (RST-PQ): development and validation. *Psychological assessment*, 28, 1427–1440.

Corr, P. J. & McNaughton, N. 2008. Reinforcement sensitivity theory and personality. *In:* Corr, P. J. (ed.) *The reinforcement sensitivity theory of personality*. Cambridge: Cambridge University Press.

Corr, P. J. & McNaughton, N. 2012. Neuroscience and approach/avoidance personality traits: a two stage (valuation-motivation) approach. *Neuroscience & Biobehavioral Reviews*, 36, 2339–2354. https://doi.org/10.1016/j.neubiorev.2012.09.013

Corr, P. J. & McNaughton, N. 2016. Neural mechanisms of low trait anxiety and risk for externalizing behaviour. *In:* Beauchaine, T. P. & Hinshaw, S. P. (eds.) *The Oxford Handbook of Externalizing Spectrum Disorders* (pp. 220–238). Oxford Handbooks Online: Oxford University Press. https://doi.org/10.1093/oxfordhb/9780199324675.013.1.

Corr, P. J. & Mobbs, D. 2023. Editorial: an emerging field with bright prospects. *Personality Neuroscience*, 6, e1, 1–7.

Costa de Melo, N., Sánchez-Ortiz, B. L., dos Santos Sampaio, T. I., Matias Pereira, A. C., Pinheiro da Silva Neto, F. L., Ribeiro da Silva, H., Alves Soares Cruz, R., Keita, H., Soares Pereira, A. M. & Tavares Carvalho, J. C. 2019. Anxiolytic and antidepressant effects of the hydroethanolic extract from the leaves of Aloysia polystachya (Griseb.) Moldenke: a study on zebrafish (*Danio rerio*). *Pharmaceuticals*, 12. https://doi.org/10.3390/ph12030106

Costa, P. T., Jr. & McCrae, R. R. 1995. Domains and facets: hierarchical personality assessment using the revised NEO personality inventory. *Journal of Personality Assessment*, 64, 21–50. https://doi.org/10.1207/s15327752jpa6401_2

Costa, P. T. & McCrae, R. R. 1985. *The NEO personality inventory manual*. Odessa FL, Psychological Assessment Resources.

Costa, R., Oliveira, N. G. & Dinis-Oliveira, R. J. 2019. Pharmacokinetic and pharmacodynamic of bupropion: integrative overview of relevant clinical and forensic aspects. *Drug Metabolism Reviews*, 51, 293–313. https://doi.org/10.1080/03602532.2019.1620763

Cowley, D. S., Roy-Byrne, P. P., Radant, A., Ritchie, J. C., Greenblatt, D. J., Nemeroff, C. B. & Hommer, D. W. 1995. Benzodiazepine sensitivity in panic disorder: effects of chronic alprazolam treatment. *Neuropsychopharmacology*, 12, 147–157.

Craig, A. D. 2002. How do you feel? Interoception: the sense of the physiological condition of the body. *Nature Reviews Neuroscience*, 3, 655–666.

Craig, A. D. 2009. How do you feel — now? The anterior insula and human awareness. *Nature Reviews Neuroscience*, 10, 59–70. https://doi.org/10.1038/nrn2555

Crawley, J. N. & Corwin, R. L. 1994. Biological actions of cholecystokinin. *Peptides*, 15, 731–755.

Crespi, F. 2019. On the role of cholecystokinin (CCK) in fear and anxiety: a review and research proposal. *Journal of Human Psychology*, 1, 1–10. https://doi.org/10.14302/issn.2644-1101.jhp-19-2766

Crestani, F., Lorez, M., Baer, K., Essrich, C., Benke, D., Laurent, J. P., Belzung, C., Fritschy, J. M., Lüscher, B. & Mohler, H. 1999. Decreased GABAA-receptor clustering results in enhanced anxiety and a bias for threat cues. *Nature Neuroscience*, 2, 833–839.

Cristina, O. 2018. Brain-heart interaction in perseverative cognition. *Psychophysiology*, 55, e13082. https://doi.org/doi:10.1111/psyp.13082

Criswell, H. E., Knapp, D. J., Overstreet, D. H. & Breese, G. R. 1994. Effects of ethanol, chlordiazepoxide, and MK-801 on performance in the elevated-plus maze and on locomotor activity. *Alcohol Clinical Experimental Research*, 18, 596–601.

Cruz, A. P. M., Castro-Gomes, V. & Landeira-Fernandez, J. 2023. An animal model of trait anxiety: Carioca High Freezing rats as a model of generalized anxiety disorder. *Personality Neuroscience*, in press.

Cryan, J. F. & Sweeney, F. F. 2011. The age of anxiety: role of animal models of anxiolytic action in drug discovery. *British Journal of Pharmacology*, 164, 1129–1161. https://doi.org/10.1111/bph.2011.164.issue-4

Cui, R.-s., Ruan, H., Liu, L.-y. & Li, X.-w. 2020a. Involvement of noradrenergic and serotonergic systems in risk-based decisions between options of equivalent expected value in rats. *Neurobiology of Learning and Memory*, 175, 107310. https://doi.org/https://doi.org/10.1016/j.nlm.2020.107310

Cui, W., Aida, T., Ito, H., Kobayashi, K., Wada, Y., Kato, S., Nakano, T., Zhu, M., Isa, K., Kobayashi, K., Isa, T., Tanaka, K. & Aizawa, H. 2020b. Dopaminergic signaling in the nucleus accumbens modulates stress-coping strategies during inescapable stress. *The Journal of Neuroscience*, 40, 7241–7254. https://doi.org/10.1523/jneurosci.0444-20.2020

Cuijpers, P., Gentili, C., Banos, R. M., Garcia-Campayo, J., Botella, C. & Cristea, I. A. 2016. Relative effects of cognitive and behavioral therapies on generalized anxiety disorder, social anxiety disorder and panic disorder: a meta-analysis. *Journal of Anxiety Disorders*, 43, 79–89. https://doi.org/10.1016/j.janxdis.2016.09.003

Cullinan, W. E., Herman, J. P. & Watson, S. J. 1993. Ventral subicular interaction with the hypothalamic paraventricular nucleus: evidence for a relay in the bed nucleus of the stria terminalis. *Journal of Comparative Neurology*, 332, 1–20. https://doi.org/https://doi.org/10.1002/cne.903320102

Curran, H. V. 1991. Benzodiazepines, memory and mood: a review. *Psychopharmacology*, 105, 1–8.

Cutler, N. R., Sramek, J. J., Keppel Hesselink, J. M., Krol, A., Roeschen, J., Rickels, K. & Schweizer, E. 1993. A double-blind, placebo-controlled study comparing the efficacy and safety of ipsapirone versus lorazepam in patients with generalized anxiety disorder: a prospective multicenter trial. *Journal of Clinical Psychopharmacology*, 13, 429–437.

da Silva, G. N., Seiffert, N. & Tovote, P. 2023. Cerebellar contribution to the regulation of defensive states. *Frontiers in Systems Neuroscience*, 17, A1160083. https://doi.org/10.3389/fnsys.2023.1160083

Dalgleish, T. & Power, M. 1999. *Handbook of cognition and emotion*. Chichester: Wiley and Sons.

Dalrymple-Alford, J. C., Harland, B., Loukavenko, E. A., Perry, B., Mercer, S., Collings, D. A., Ulrich, K., Abraham, W. C., McNaughton, N. & Wolff, M. 2015. Anterior thalamic nuclei lesions and recovery of function: relevance to cognitive thalamus. *Neuroscience & Biobehavioural Reviews*, 54, 154 – 60.

Danion, J. M., Weingartner, H., File, S. E., Jaffard, R., Sunderland, T., Tulving, E. & Warburton, D. M. 1993. Pharmacology of human memory and cognition: illustrations from the effects of benzodiazepines and cholinergic drugs. *Journal of Psychopharmacology*, 7, 371–377.

Dantendorfer, K., Amering, M., Baischer, W., Berger, P., Steinberger, K., Windhaber, J. & Katschnig, H. 1995a. Is there a pathophysical and therapeutic link between panic disorder and epilepsy. *Acta Psychiatrica Scandanavica*, 91, 430–432.

Dantendorfer, K., Prayer, D., Kramer, J., Amering, M., Baischer, W., Berger, P., Schoder, M., Steinberger, K., Windhaber, J., Imhof, H. & Katschnig, H. 1996. High frequency of EEG and MRI brain abnormalities in panic disorder. *Psychiatry Research: Neuroimaging Section*, 68, 41–53.

Dantendorfer, K., Windhaber, J. & Maierhofer, D. 1995b. Jackson seizure and panic disorder relieved by carbamazepine. *European Journal of Psychiatry*, 10, 370–371.

Daum, I. & Ackermann, H. 1994. Dissociation of declarative and nondeclarative memory after bilateral thalamic lesions: a case report. *International Journal of Neuroscience*, 75, 153–165.

Daum, I., Channon, S., Polkey, C. E. & Gray, J. A. 1991. Classical conditioning after temporal lobe lesions in man: impairment in conditional discrimination. *Behavioral Neuroscience*, 105, 396–408.

Davidson, T. L. & Jarrard, L. E. 1992. Support for configural association theory: now you see it, now you don't. *Hippocampus*, 2, 90–91.

Davidson, T. L. & Jarrard, L. E. 1993. A role for hippocampus in the utilization of hunger signals. *Behavioral and Neural Biology*, 59, 167–171.

Davidson, T. L., McKernan, M. G. & Jarrard, L. E. 1993. Hippocampal lesions do not impair negative patterning: a challenge to configural association theory. *Behavioral Neuroscience*, 107(2), 227–234.

Davies, M. F., Onaivi, E. S., Chen, S. W., Maguire, P. A., Tsai, N. F. & Loew, G. H. 1994. Evidence for central benzodiazepine receptor heterogeneity from behavior tests. *Pharmacology, Biochemistry and Behavior*, 49, 47–56.

Davis, K. L. & Panksepp, J. 2018. The emotional foundations of personality: a neurobiological and evolutionary approach. New York (dowloaded from https://play.google.com/books): W. W. Norton & Co.

Davis, M. 1992a. The role of the amygdala in conditioned fear. *In:* Aggleton, J. P. (ed.) *The amygdala: neurobiological aspects of emotion, memory, and mental function* (pp. 255–305). Wiley-Liss Inc.

Davis, M. 1992b. The role of the amygdala in fear-potentiated startle: implications for animal models of anxiety. *Trends in Pharmacological Science*, 13(1), 35–41.

Davis, M. 1992c. The role of the amygdala in fear and anxiety. *Annual Review of Neuroscience*, 15, 353–375.

Davis, M. 2002. Role of NMDA receptors and MAP kinase in the amygdala in extinction of fear: clinical implications for exposure therapy. *European Journal of Neuroscience*, 16, 395–398.

Davis, M. 2006. Neural systems involved in fear and anxiety measured with fear-potentiated startle. *American Psychologist*, 61, 741–756.

Davis, M., Falls, W. A., Campeau, S. & Kim, M. 1993. Fear-potentiated startle: a neural and pharmacological analysis. *Behavioural Brain Research*, 58, 175–198.

Davis, M., Rainnie, D. & Cassell, M. 1994. Neurotransmission in the rat amygdala related to fear and anxiety. *Trends in Neuroscience*, 17, 208–214.

Davis, N. M., Brookes, S., Gray, J. A. & Rawlins, J. N. P. 1981. Chlordiazepoxide and resistance to punishment. *Quarterly Journal of Experimental Psychology*, 33b, 227–239.

Davitz, J. R. 1969. *The language of emotion*. New York: Academic Press.

Dawson, G. R., Crawford, S. P., Collinson, N., Iversen, S. D. & Tricklebank, M. D. 1995. Evidence that the anxiolytic-like effects of chlordiazepoxide on the elevated plus maze are confounded by increases in locomotor activity. *Psychopharmacology (Berl)*, 118, 316–323.

Dawson, G. R. & Tricklebank, M. D. 1995. Use of the elevated plus maze in the search for novel anxiolytic agents. *Trends in Pharmacological Science*, 16, 33–36.

de Abreu, M. S., Genario, R., Giacomini, A. C. V. V., Demin, K. A., Lakstygal, A. M., Amstislavskaya, T. G., Fontana, B. D., Parker, M. O. & Kalueff, A. V. 2020. Zebrafish as a model of neurodevelopmental disorders. *Neuroscience*, 445, 3–11. https://doi.org/https://doi.org/10.1016/j.neuroscience.2019.08.034

De Gregorio, D., Aguilar-Valles, A., Preller, K. H., Heifets, B. D., Hibicke, M., Mitchell, J. & Gobbi, G. 2021. Hallucinogens in mental health: preclinical and clinical studies on LSD, psilocybin, MDMA, and ketamine. *The Journal of Neuroscience*, 41, 891–900. https://doi.org/10.1523/jneurosci.1659-20.2020

de Paiva, J. P. Q., Bueno, A. P. A., Dos Santos Corrêa, M., Oliveira, M. G. M., Ferreira, T. L. & Fornari, R. V. 2021. The posterior insular cortex is necessary for the consolidation of tone fear conditioning. *Neurobiology of Learning and Memory*, 179, 107402. https://doi.org/https://doi.org/10.1016/j.nlm.2021.107402

De Silva, A., Salem, V., Matthews, P. M. & Dhillo, W. S. 2012. The use of functional MRI to study appetite control in the CNS. *Experimental Diabetes Research*, 2012, A764017. https://doi.org/10.1155/2012/764017

De Souza Silva, M. A. & Tomaz, C. 1995. Amnesia after diazepam infusion into basolateral but not central amygdala of Rattus norvegicus. *Neuropsychobiology*, 32, 31–36.

Deacon, R. M. J., Bannerman, D. M. & Rawlins, J. N. P. 2002. Anxiolytic effects of cytotoxic hippocampal lesions in rats. *Behavioral Neuroscience*, 116, 494–497. https://doi.org/10.1037/0735-7044.116.3.494

Deacon, R. M. J. & Rawlins, J. N. P. 1995. Serial position effects and duration of memory for nonspatial stimuli in rats. *Journal of Experimental Psychology: Animal Behaviour*, 21, 285–292.

Deakin, J. F. W. 1993. A review of clinical efficacy of 5-HT1A agonists in anxiety and depression. *Journal of Psychopharmacology*, 7, 283–289.

Deakin, J. F. W. & Graeff, F. G. 1991. 5-HT and mechanisms of defence. *Journal of Psychopharmacology*, 5, 305–315.

Del Giudice, M. 2021. Ahs et al.'s (2018) Systematic review on biological preparedness and resistance to extinction: a commentary and reanalysis. *Neuroscience & Biobehavioural Reviews*, 120, 13–15. https://doi.org/10.1016/j.neubiorev.2020.11.009

Dellemijn, P. L. I. & Fields, H. L. 1994. Do benzodiazepines have a role in chronic pain management? *Pain*, 57, 137–152.

den Boer, J. A. & Westenberg, H. G. 1988. Effect of a serotonin and noradrenaline uptake inhibitor in panic disorder: a double-blind comparative study with fluvoxamine and maprotiline. *International Clinical Psychopharmacology*, 3, 59–74. https://doi.org/10.1097/00004850-198801000-00005

Deng, J., Zhou, H., Lin, J.-K., Shen, Z.-X., Chen, W.-Z., Wang, L.-H., Li, Q., Mu, D., Wei, Y.-C., Xu, X.-H. & Sun, Y.-G. 2020. The parabrachial nucleus directly channels spinal nociceptive signals to the intralaminar thalamic nuclei, but not the amygdala. *Neuron*, 107, 909–923.e6. https://doi.org/https://doi.org/10.1016/j.neuron.2020.06.017

Depue, R. A. & Collins, P. F. 1999. Neurobiology of the structure of personality: dopamine, facilitation of incentive motivation and extraversion. *Behavioral and Brain Sciences*, 22, 491–569. https://doi.org/https://www.cambridge.org/core/journals/behavioral-and-brain-sciences/article/neurobiology-of-the-structure-of-personality-dopamine-facilitation-of-incentive-motivation-and-extraversion/E8AC4097F3DBB5EE4A7EFE822482D8E4

Descarries, L., Watkins, K. C. & Lapierre, Y. 1977. Noradrenergic axon terminals in the cerebral cortex of rat: III. Topometric ultrastructural analysis. *Brain Research*, 133, 197–222.

Devenport, L., Stidhan, J. & Hale, R. 1989. Ethanol and spatial localisation. *Behavioral Neuroscience*, 103, 1259–1266.

DeYoung, C. G. 2006. Higher-order factors of the Big Five in a multi-informant sample. *Journal of Personality and Social Psychology*, 91, 1138–51. https://doi.org/10.1037/0022-3514.91.6.1138

DeYoung, C. G. 2010. Personality neuroscience and the biology of traits. *Social and Personality Psychology Compass*, 4, 1165–1180. https://doi.org/10.1111/j.1751-9004.2010.00327.x

DeYoung, C. G. 2013. The neuromodulator of exploration: a unifying theory of the role of dopamine in personality. *Frontiers in Human Neuroscience*, 7, A762. https://doi.org/10.3389/fnhum.2013.00762

DeYoung, C. G. 2015. Cybernetic Big Five Theory. *Journal of Research in Personality*, 56, 33–58. https://doi.org/10.1016/j.jrp.2014.07.004

DeYoung, C. G., Beaty, R. E., Genc, E., Latzman, R. D., Passamonti, L., Servaas, M. N., Shackman, A. J., Smillie, L. D., Spreng, R. N., Viding, E. & Wacker, J. 2022. Personality neuroscience: an emerging field with bright prospects. *Personality Science*, 3, e7269. https://doi.org/10.5964/ps.7269

DeYoung, C. G. & Krueger, R. F. 2018. A cybernetic theory of psychopathology. *Psychological Inquiry*, 29, 117–138. https://doi.org/10.1080/1047840X.2018.1513680

DeYoung, C. G., Peterson, J. B. & Higgins, D. M. 2002. Higher-order factors of the Big Five predict conformity: are there neuroses of health? *Personality and Individual Differences*, 33, 533–552.

Diamond, A. 1995. Evidence of robust recognition memory early in life even when assessed by reaching behaviour. *Journal of Experimental Child Psychology*, 59, 419–456.

Díaz, A. & Pickering, A. D. 1993. The relationship between Gray's and Eysenck's personality spaces. *Personality and Individual Differences*, 15, 297–305.

DiazGranados, N., Ibrahim, L. A., Brutsche, N. E., Ameli, R., Henter, I. D., Luckenbaugh, D. A., Machado-Vieira, R. & Zarate, C. A., Jr. 2010. Rapid resolution of suicidal ideation after a single infusion of an N-methyl-D-aspartate antagonist in patients with treatment-resistant major depressive disorder. *Journal of Clinical Psychiatry*, 71, 1605–1611. https://doi.org/10.4088/JCP.09m05327blu

Dickinson, A. 1974. Response suppression and facilitation by aversive stimuli following septal lesions in rats: a review and model. *Physiological Psychology*, 2, 444–456.

Dickinson, A. 1980. *Contemporary animal learning theory*. Cambridge, Cambridge University Press.

Dickson, C. R., Holmes, G. L. & Barry, J. M. 2022. Dynamic θ frequency coordination within and between the prefrontal cortex-hippocampus circuit during learning of a spatial avoidance task. *eNeuro*, 9, ENEURO.0414-21.2022. https://doi.org/10.1523/eneuro.0414-21.2022

Dickson, C. T., Magistretti, J., Shalinsky, M. H., Fransén, E., Hasselmo, M. E. & Alonso, A. 2000. Properties and role of I*h* in the pacing of subthreshold oscillations in entorhinal cortex layer II neurons. *Journal of Neurophysiology*, 83, 2562–2579. https://doi.org/10.1152/jn.2000.83.5.2562

Do, Q. & Hasselmo, M. E. 2021. Neural circuits and symbolic processing. *Neurobiology of Learning and Memory*, 186, 107552. https://doi.org/https://doi.org/10.1016/j.nlm.2021.107552

Doble, A. & Martin, I. L. 1992. Multiple benzodiazepine receptors: no reason for anxiety. *Trends in Pharmacological Science*, 13, 76–81.

Dobson, K. S. & Block, L. 1988. Historical and philosophical bases of the cognitive-behavioural therapies. *In:* Dobson, K. S. (ed.) *Handbook of Cognitive-Behavioural Therapies* (pp. 3–38). New York: The Guildford Press.

Domhardt, M., Letsch, J., Kybelka, J., Koenigbauer, J., Doebler, P. & Baumeister, H. 2020. Are internet- and mobile-based interventions effective in adults with diagnosed panic disorder and/or agoraphobia? A systematic review and meta-analysis. *Journal of Affective Disorders*, 276, 169–182. https://doi.org/10.1016/j.jad.2020.06.059

Domino, E. F. 2010. Taming the ketamine tiger. 1965. *Anesthesiology*, 113, 678–84. https://doi.org/10.1097/ALN.0b013e3181ed09a2

Dong, C., Madar, A. D. & Sheffield, M. E. J. 2021. Distinct place cell dynamics in CA1 and CA3 encode experience in new environments. *Nature Communications*, 12, e2977. https://doi.org/10.1038/s41467-021-23260-3

Dong, M.-X., Chen, G.-H. & Hu, L. 2020. Dopaminergic system alteration in anxiety and compulsive disorders: a systematic review of neuroimaging studies. *Frontiers in Neuroscience*, 14, A608520. https://doi.org/10.3389/fnins.2020.608520

Donovick, P. J., Burright, R. G. & Fink, E. A. 1979. Discrimination behavior of rats with septal lesions in a cue addition-deletion paradigm. *Physiology and Behavior*, 22, 125–131.

Dorfman, A., Weiss, O., Hagbi, Z., Levi, A. & Eilam, D. 2021. Social spatial cognition. *Neuroscience & Biobehavioral Reviews*, 121, 277–290. https://doi.org/https://doi.org/10.1016/j.neubiorev.2020.12.023

Dos Santos, R. G., Osorio, F. L., Crippa, J. A., Riba, J., Zuardi, A. W. & Hallak, J. E. 2016. Antidepressive, anxiolytic, and antiaddictive effects of ayahuasca, psilocybin and lysergic acid diethylamide (LSD): a systematic review of clinical trials published in the last 25 years. *Therapeutic Advances in Psychopharmacology*, 6, 193–213. https://doi.org/10.1177/2045125316638008

Douglas, R. J. 1967. The hippocampus and behavior. *Psychological Bulletin*, 67, 416–442.

Doyère, V., Dębiec, J., Monfils, M.-H., Schafe, G. E. & LeDoux, J. E. 2007. Synapse-specific reconsolidation of distinct fear memories in the lateral amygdala. *Nature Neuroscience*, 1–3.

Drewe, E. A. 1975a. An experimental investigation of Luria's theory on the effects of frontal lobe lesions in man. *Neuropsychologia*, 13, 421–429.

Drewe, E. A. 1975b. Go-no go learning after frontal lobe lesions in humans. *Cortex*, 11, 8–16.

Drewett, R. F., Gray, J. A., James, D. T. D., McNaughton, N., Valero, I. & Dudderidge, H. J. 1977. Sex and strain differences in septal driving of the hippocampal theta rhythm as a function of frequency: effects of gonadectomy and gonadal hormones. *Neuroscience*, 2, 1033–1041.

Du Rocher, A. R. & Pickering, A. D. 2023. Social interaction anxiety, social phobia, and cognitive control: controlled reactions to facial affect during an emotional face flanker task. *Current Psychology*, online. https://doi.org/10.1007/s12144-023-04624-y

Duann, J.-R., Ide, J. S., Luo, X. & Li, C.-S. R. 2009. Functional connectivity delineates distinct roles of the inferior frontal cortex and presupplementary motor area in stop signal inhibition. *The Journal of Neuroscience*, 29, 10171–10179.

Dudai, Y., Karni, A. & Born, J. 2015. The consolidation and transformation of memory. *Neuron*, 88, 20–32. https://doi.org/https://doi.org/10.1016/j.neuron.2015.09.004

Dugan, K. A., Vogt, R. L., Zheng, A., Gillath, O., Deboeck, P. R., Fraley, R. C. & Briley, D. A. 2023. Life events sometimes alter the trajectory of personality development: effect sizes for 25 life events estimated using a large, frequently assessed sample. *Journal of Personality*, online, e12837. https://doi.org/10.1111/jopy.12837

Dugatkin, L. A. 2018. The silver fox domestication experiment. *Evolution: Education and Outreach*, 11, e16. https://doi.org/10.1186/s12052-018-0090-x

Duvelle, É., Grieves, R. M., Hok, V., Poucet, B., Arleo, A., Jeffery, K. J. & Save, E. 2019. Insensitivity of place cells to the value of spatial goals in a two-choice flexible navigation task. *The Journal of Neuroscience*, 39, 2522–2541. https://doi.org/10.1523/jneurosci.1578-18.2018

Eagle, D. M. & Baunez, C. 2010. Is there an inhibitory-response-control system in the rat? Evidence from anatomical and pharmacological studies of behavioral inhibition. *Neuroscience & Biobehavioral Reviews*, 34, 50–72.

Eagle, D. M., Lehmann, O., Theobald, D. E. H., Pena, Y., Zakaria, R., Ghosh, R., Dalley, J. W. & Robbins, T. W. 2009. Serotonin depletion impairs waiting but not stop-signal reaction time in rats: implications for theories of the role of 5-HT in behavioral inhibition. *Neuropsychopharmacology*, 34, 1311–1321. https://doi.org/10.1038/npp.2008.202

Eagle, D. M. & Robbins, T. W. 2003. Inhibitory control in rats performing a stop-signal reaction-time task: effects of lesions of the medial striatum and *d*-amphetamine. *Behavioral Neuroscience*, 117, 1302–1317.

Ehlers, A. 2015. Intrusive reexperiencing in posttraumatic stress disorder: memory processes and their implications for therapy. *In:* Watson, L. A. & Berntsen, D. (eds.) *Clinical perspectives on autobiographical memory* (pp. 109–132). Cambridge: Cambridge University Press.

Ehlers, A. & Breuer, P. 1996. How good are patients with panic disorder at perceiving their heartbeats. *Biological Psychology*, 42, 165–182.

Ehlers, A. & Clark, D. M. 2000. A cognitive model of posttraumatic stress disorder. *Behaviour Research and Therapy*, 38, 319–345.

Ehlers, A. & Wild, J. 2021. Cognitive behavior therapies for posttraumatic stress disorder. *Handbook of cognitive behavioral therapy: applications (Vol. 2).*

Eibl-Eibesfeldt, I. & Sutterlin, C. 1990. Fear, defense and aggression in animals and man: some ethological perspectives. *In:* Brain, P. F., Parmigian, S., Blanchard, R., Mainardi, R. & Harwood, D. (eds.) *Fear and defense* (pp. 381–408). Chur: Academic Publishers.

Eichenbaum, H. 1996. Is the rodent hippocampus just for 'place'? *Current Opinion in Neurobiology*, 6, 187–195.

Eichenbaum, H., Kuperstein, M., Fagan, A. & Nagode, J. 1987. Cue-sampling and goal-approach correlates of hippocampal unit activity in rats performing an odor-discrimination task. *The Journal of Neuroscience*, 7(3), 716–732.

Eichenbaum, H., Otto, T. & Cohen, N. J. 1994. Two functional components of the hippocampal memory system. *Behavioral and Brain Sciences*, 17, 449–518.

Eichenbaum, H., Otto, T. & Cohen, N. J. 1996. The hippocampal system: dissociating its functional components and recombining them in the service of declarative memory. *Behavioral and Brain Sciences*, 19, 772–776.

Eichenbaum, H., Shedlack, K. J. & Eckmann, K. W. 1980. Thalamocortical mechanisms in odor-guided behavior. I. Effects of lesions of the mediodorsal thalamic nucleus and frontal cortex on olfactory discrimination in the rat. *Brain Behaviour and Evolution*, 17, 255–275.

Eichenbaum, H., Steward, C. & Morris, R. G. M. 1990. Hippocampal representation in place learning. *The Journal of Neuroscience*, 10(11), 3531–3542.

Eilam, D. 2017. From an animal model to human patients: an example of a translational study on obsessive compulsive disorder (OCD). *Neuroscience & Biobehavioral Reviews*, 76, Part A, 67–76. https://doi.org/10.1016/j.neubiorev.2016.12.034

Ekman, P. 1982. *Emotion in the human face*. Cambridge, Cambridge University Press.

Ekman, P. & Friesen, W. V. 1986. A new pan-cultural facial expression of emotion. *Motivation and Emotion*, 10, 159–168.

Ekstrom, A. D., Caplan, J. B., Ho, E., Shattuck, K., Fried, I. & Kahana, M. J. 2005. Human hippocampal theta activity during virtual navigation. *Hippocampus*, 15, 881–889.

Elliott, K. & Whelan, J. 1978. *Functions of the septo-hippocampal system. CIBA Foundation Symposium 58 (New Series)*. Amsterdam: Elsevier.

Elliott, R., Zahn, R., Deakin, J. F. & Anderson, I. M. 2011. Affective cognition and its disruption in mood disorders. *Neuropsychopharmacology*, 36, 153–182.

Ellis, A. 1962. *Reason and emotion in psychotherapy*. Secaucus, NJ: Citadel Press.

Engin, E. & Treit, D. 2008. The effects of intra-cerebral drug infusions on animals' unconditioned fear reactions: a systematic review. *Progress in Neuro-Psychopharmacology and Biological Psychiatry*, 32, 1399–1419.

Engin, E., Treit, D. & Dickson, C. T. 2009. Anxiolytic- and antidepressant-like properties of ketamine in behavioral and neurophysiological animal models. *Neuroscience*, 161, 359–369.

Ennis, M., Xu, S. j. & Rizvi, T. A. 1997. Discrete subregions of the rat midbrain periaqueductal gray project to nucleus ambiguus and the periambigual region. *Neuroscience*, 80, 829–845. https://doi.org/https://doi.org/10.1016/S0306-4522(97)00051-1

Esbenshade, T. A., Fox, G. B. & Cowart, M. D. 2006. Histamine H3 receptor antagonists: preclinical promise for treating obesity and cognitive disorders. *Molecular Interventions*, 6, 77–88, 59.

Espinoza Oyarce, D. A., Burns, R., Butterworth, P. & Cherbuin, N. 2021. Bridging classical and revised Reinforcement Sensitivity Theory research: a longitudinal analysis of a large population study. *Frontiers in Psychology*, 12, A737117. https://doi.org/10.3389/fpsyg.2021.737117

Espinoza Oyarce, D. A., Burns, R. A., Butterworth, P. & Cherbuin, N. 2023. A new measure of the Revised Reinforcement Sensitivity Theory. *Social Psychology*, 53, 327–340. https://doi.org/10.1027/1864-9335/a000502

Espinoza Oyarce, D. A., Burns, R. A., Shaw, M. D., Butterworth, P. & Cherbuin, N. 2021–2022. Brain and behaviour: how the reinforcement sensitivity theory links neuroscience and behavioural output. *Poster presented at the Society for Mental Health Research (SMHR) Conference*. Hotel Grand Chancellor, Hobart, TAS.

Esteban Masferrer, M., Silva, B. A., Nomoto, K., Lima, S. Q. & Gross, C. T. 2020. Differential encoding of predator fear in the ventromedial hypothalamus and periaqueductal grey. *The Journal of Neuroscience*, 40, 9283–9292. https://doi.org/10.1523/jneurosci.0761-18.2020

Esteves, I. M., Chang, H., Neumann, A. R., Sun, J., Mohajerani, M. H. & McNaughton, B. L. 2021. Spatial information encoding across multiple neocortical regions depends on an intact hippocampus. *The Journal of Neuroscience*, 41, 307–319. https://doi.org/10.1523/jneurosci.1788-20.2020

Estrada, V. B., Matsubara, N. K., Gomes, M. V., Corrêa, F. M. A. & Pelosi, G. G. 2016. Noradrenaline microinjected into the dorsal periaqueductal gray matter causes anxiolytic-like effects in rats tested in the elevated T-maze. *Life Sciences*, 152, 94–98. https://doi.org/https://doi.org/10.1016/j.lfs.2016.03.011

Evrard, H. C. 2019. The organization of the primate insular cortex. *Frontiers in Neuroanatomy*, 13, 43. https://doi.org/10.3389/fnana.2019.00043

Evrard, H. C. 2022. Interoceptive integration in the primate insular cortex. *In:* Nguyen, D., Isnard, J. & Kahane, P. (eds.) *Insular epilepsies* (Chapter 6, pp. 52–66). Cambridge: Cambridge University Press.

Eysenck, H. J. 1957. *The dynamics of anxiety and hysteria*. New York, Preger.

Eysenck, H. J. 1960. Classification and the problem of diagnosis. *In:* Eysenck, H. J. (ed.) *Handbook of abnormal psychology* (pp. 1–31). London: Pitman.

Eysenck, H. J. 1977. *You and neurosis*. London, Temple Smith.

Eysenck, H. J. 1979. The conditioning model of neurosis. *Behavioral and Brain Sciences*, 2, 155–166.

Eysenck, H. J. & Eysenck, H. J. 1967. *Handbook of abnormal psychology: the biological basis of personality*. Springfield, Ill., Thomas.

Eysenck, H. J. & Eysenck, S. B. G. 1964. *Eysenck personality inventory*. London: University of London Press.

Eysenck, H. J. & Eysenck, S. B. G. 1969. *The structure and measurement of personality*. London: Routledge and Kegan Paul.

Eysenck, H. J. & Eysenck, S. B. G. 1976. *Psychoticism as a dimension of personality*. London: Hodder and Stoughton.

Eysenck, H. J. & Rachman, S. 1965. *The causes and cures of neurosis*. San Diego: Knapp.

Eysenck, M. W. 1992a. *Anxiety: the cognitive perspective*, Lawrence Erlbaum Associates.

Eysenck, M. W. 1992b. The nature of anxiety. *In:* Gale, A. & Eysenck, M. W. (eds.) *Handbook of individual differences; biological perspectives* (pp. 157–178). John Wiley and Sons.

Eysenck, M. W. & Calvo, M. G. 1992. Anxiety and performance; the processing efficiency theory. *Cognition and Emotion*, 6, 409–434.

Eysenck, M. W. & Derakshan, N. 2011. New perspectives in attentional control theory. *Personality and Individual Differences*, 50, 955–960.

Eysenck, M. W., Derakshan, N., Santos, R. & Calvo, M. G. 2007. Anxiety and cognitive performance: attentional control theory. *Emotion*, 7, 336–353.

Eysenck, M. W., Moser, J. S., Derakshan, N., Hepsomali, P. & Allen, P. 2022. A neurocognitive account of attentional control theory: how does trait anxiety affect the brain's attentional networks? *Cognition and Emotion*, 37, 220–237. https://doi.org/10.1080/02699931.2022.2159936

Eysenck, S. B., Barrett, P. & Eysenck, H. J. 1984. *Eysenck personality questionnaire-revised*, Pergamon Press.

Ezawa, I. D. & Hollon, S. D. 2023. Cognitive restructuring and psychotherapy outcome: a meta-analytic review. *Psychotherapy, 60, 396-406.* https://doi.org/10.1037/pst0000474

Facklam, M., Schoch, P. & Haefely, W. E. 1992. Relationship between benzodiazepine receptor occupancy and potentiation of aminobutyric acid-stimulated chloride flux in vitro of four ligands of differing intrinsic efficacies. *Journal of Pharmacology and Experimental Therapeutics*, 261, 1106–1112.

Fanselow, M. S. 1991. The midbrain periaqueductal gray as a coordinator of action in response to fear and anxiety. *In:* Depaulis, A. & Bandler, R. (eds.) *The midbrain periaqueductal gray matter* (pp. 151–173). New York: Plenum Press.

Farkas, E., Jansen, A. S. P. & Loewy, A. D. 1997. Periaqueductal gray matter projection to vagal preganglionic neurons and the nucleus tractus solitarius. *Brain Research*, 764, 257–261. https://doi.org/https://doi.org/10.1016/S0006-8993(97)00592-1

Fattahi, M., Sharif, F., Geiller, T. & Royer, S. 2018. Differential representation of landmark and self-motion information along the ca1 radial axis: self-motion generated place fields shift toward landmarks during septal inactivation. *The Journal of Neuroscience*, 38, 6766–6778. https://doi.org/10.1523/jneurosci.3211-17.2018

Feder, A., Parides, M. K., Murrough, J. W., Perez, A. M., Morgan, J. E., Saxena, S., Kirkwood, K., Aan Het Rot, M., Lapidus, K. A., Wan, L. B., Iosifescu, D. & Charney, D. S. 2014a. Efficacy of intravenous ketamine for treatment of chronic posttraumatic stress disorder: a randomized clinical trial. *JAMA Psychiatry*, 71, 681–8. https://doi.org/10.1001/jamapsychiatry.2014.62

Feder, A., Parides, M. K., Murrough, J. W., Perez, A. M., Morgan, J. E., Saxena, S., Kirkwood, K., aan het Rot, M., Lapidus, K. A. B., Wan, L.-B., Iosifescu, D. & Charney, D. S. 2014b. Efficacy of intravenous ketamine for treatment of chronic posttraumatic stress disorder. *JAMA Psychiatry*, 71. https://doi.org/10.1001/jamapsychiatry.2014.62

Feder, R. & Ranck, J. B., Jr. 1973. Studies on single neurons in dorsal hippocampal formation and septum in unrestrained rats. II. Hippocampal slow waves and theta cell firing during bar pressing and other behaviours. *Experimental Neurology*, 41, 532–555.

Feighner, J. P. 1987. Buspirone in the long-term treatment of generalized anxiety disorder. *The Journal of Clinical Psychiatry*, 48(12), 3–6.

Feinstein, J. S., Buzza, C., Hurlemann, R., Follmer, R. L., Dahdaleh, N. S., Coryell, W. H., Welsh, M. J., Tranel, D. & Wemmie, J. A. 2013. Fear and panic in humans with bilateral amygdala damage. *Nature Neuroscience*, 16, 270–273. https://doi.org/http://www.nature.com/neuro/journal/vaop/ncurrent/abs/nn.3323.html#supplementary information

Feinstein, J. S., Stein, M. B. & Paulus, M. P. 2006. Anterior insula reactivity during certain decisions is associated with neuroticism. *Social Cognitive and Affective Neuroscience*, 1, 136–142.

Feldon, J. 1977. *The effects of anti-anxiety drugs and selective lesions of the septo-hippocampal system on behavioural responses to non-reward and punishment*, Unpublished D.Phil. thesis, University of Oxford.

Feldon, J. & Gray, J. A. 1981. The partial reinforcement extinction effect after treatment with chlordiazepoxide. *Psychopharmacology*, 73, 269–275.

Feldon, J., Guillamon, A., Gray, J. A., De Wit, H. & McNaughton, N. 1979. Sodium amylobarbitone and responses to nonreward. *Quarterly Journal of Experimental Psychology*, 31, 19–50.

Fellous, J.-M. & Sejnowski, T. J. 2000. Cholinergic induction of oscillations in the hippocampal slice in the slow (0.5–2 Hz), theta (5–12 Hz), and gamma (35–70 Hz) bands. *Hippocampus*, 10, 187–197. https://doi.org/https://doi.org/10.1002/(SICI)1098-1063(2000)10:2<187::AID-HIPO8>3.0.CO;2-M

Feltner, D. E., Liu-Dumaw, M., Schweizer, E. & Bielski, R. 2011. Efficacy of pregabalin in generalized social anxiety disorder: results of a double-blind, placebo-controlled, fixed-dose study. *International Clinical Psychopharmacology*, 26, 213–20. https://doi.org/10.1097/YIC.0b013e32834519bd

Ferber, S., Shoval, G., Zalsman, G., Mikulincer, M. & Weller, A. 2021. Between action and emotional survival during the COVID-19 era: sensorimotor pathways as control systems of transdiagnostic anxiety-related intolerance to uncertainty. *Frontiers in Psychiatry*, 12, 680403. https://doi.org/10.3389/fpsyt.2021.680403

Fernandez-Teruel, A. & McNaughton, N. 2023. Post-encounter freezing during approach-avoidance conflict: the role of the hippocampus. *Nature Reviews Neuroscience*, 24, 451-452. https://doi.org/10.1038/s41583-023-00703-y

Fernández-Teruel, A. & Tobeña, A. 2020. Revisiting the role of anxiety in the initial acquisition of two-way active avoidance: pharmacological, behavioural and neuroanatomical convergence. *Neuroscience & Biobehavioral Reviews*, 118, 739–758. https://doi.org/https://doi.org/10.1016/j.neubiorev.2020.08.014

Ferraris, M., Cassel, J.-C., Pereira de Vasconcelos, A., Stephan, A. & Quilichini, P. P. 2021. The nucleus reuniens, a thalamic relay for cortico-hippocampal interaction in recent and remote memory consolidation. *Neuroscience & Biobehavioral Reviews*, 125, 339–354. https://doi.org/https://doi.org/10.1016/j.neubiorev.2021.02.025

Ferraris, M., Ghestem, A., Vicente, A. F., Nallet-Khosrofian, L., Bernard, C. & Quilichini, P. P. 2018. The nucleus reuniens controls long-range hippocampo–prefrontal gamma synchronization during slow oscillations. *The Journal of Neuroscience*, 38, 3026–3038. https://doi.org/10.1523/jneurosci.3058-17.2018

Ferreira, A., Picazo, O., Uriarte, N., Pereira, M. & Fernández-Guasti, A. 2000. Inhibitory effect of buspirone and diazepam, but not of 8-OH-DPAT, on maternal behavior and aggression. *Pharmacology Biochemistry and Behavior*, 66, 389–396. https://doi.org/https://doi.org/10.1016/S0091-3057(00)00211-2

Fiebig, F., Herman, P. & Lansner, A. 2020. An indexing theory for working memory based on fast Hebbian plasticity. *eNeuro*, ENEURO.0374-19.2020. https://doi.org/10.1523/eneuro.0374-19.2020

Field, M. J., Oles, R. J. & Singh, L. 2001. Pregabalin may represent a novel class of anxiolytic agents with a broad spectrum of activity. *British Journal of Pharmacology*, 132, 1–4.

File, S. E. 1992. Behavioural detection of anxiolytic action. *In:* Elliott, J. M., Heal, D. J. & Marsden, C. A. (eds.) *Experimental approaches to anxiety and depression* (pp. 25–44). London: John Wiley & Sons Ltd.

File, S. E. & Cooper, S. J. 1985. Benzodiazepines and behavior. *Neuroscience & Biobehavioral Reviews*, 9, 1–3.

Fine, J. M. & Hayden, B. Y. 2022. The whole prefrontal cortex is premotor cortex. *Philosophical Transactions of the Royal Society B: Biological Sciences*, 377, 20200524. https://doi.org/doi:10.1098/rstb.2020.0524

Fiorillo, C. D. 2013. Two dimensions of value: dopamine neurons represent reward but not aversiveness. *Science*, 341, 546–549. https://doi.org/10.1126/science.1238699

Flesch, T., Juechems, K., Dumbalska, T., Saxe, A. & Summerfield, C. 2022. Orthogonal representations for robust context-dependent task performance in brains and neural networks. *Neuron*, 110, 1258–1270.e11. https://doi.org/https://doi.org/10.1016/j.neuron.2022.01.005

Floden, D. & Stuss, D. T. 2006. Inhibitory control is slowed in patients with right superior medial frontal damage. *Journal of Cognitive Neuroscience*, 18, 1843–1849.

Floderus-Myhred, B., Pedersen, N. & Rasmuson, I. 1980. Assessment of heritability for personality, based on a short-form of the Eysenck Personality Inventory: a study of 12,898 twin pairs. *Behavior Genetics*, 10, 153–162.

Flynn, J. P. 1967. The neural basis of aggression in cats. *In:* Glass, D. C. (ed.) *Neurophysiology and Emotion* (pp. 40–60). New York: Rockefeller University Press.

Flynn, J. P. 1969. Neural aspects of attack behaviour in cats. *Annals of the New York Academy of Sciences*, 159, 1008–1012.

Formica, S., González-García, C., Senoussi, M., Marinazzo, D. & Brass, M. 2022. Theta-phase connectivity between medial prefrontal and posterior areas underlies novel instructions implementation. *eNeuro*, ENEURO.0225-22.2022. https://doi.org/10.1523/eneuro.0225-22.2022

Foster, T. C., Castro, C. A. & McNaughton, B. L. 1989. Spatial selectivity of rat hippocampal neurons: dependence on preparedness for movement. *Science*, 244, 1580–1582.

Fowles, D. C. 1980. The three arousal model: implications of Gray's two-factor learning theory for heart rate, electrodermal activity and psychopathy. *Psychophysiology*, 17, 87–104.

Franchina, V., Klackl, J. & Jonas, E. 2023. The reinforcement sensitivity theory affects questionnaire (RST-AQ). A validation study of a new scale targeting affects related to anxiety, approach motivation and fear. *Current Psychology*. https://doi.org/10.1007/s12144-023-04623-z

Franck, J. E., Pokorny, J., Kunkel, D. D. & Schwartzkroin, P. A. 1995. Physiologic and morphologic characteristics of granule cell circuitry in human epileptic hippocampus. *Epilepsia*, 36, 543–558.

Frankland, P. W. & Yeomans, J. S. 1995. Fear-potentiated startle and electrically evoked startle mediated by synapses in rostrolateral midbrain. *Behavioral Neuroscience*, 109, 669–680.

Franklin, J. A. 1990. Behavioural treatment for panic disorder. *In:* McNaughton, N. & Andrews, G. (eds.) *Anxiety* (pp. 84–91). Dunedin: University of Otago.

Fredes, F. & Shigemoto, R. 2021. The role of hippocampal mossy cells in novelty detection. *Neurobiology of Learning and Memory*, 183, 107486. https://doi.org/https://doi.org/10.1016/j.nlm.2021.107486

Fredrikson, M. & Öhman, A. 1979. Cardiovascular and electrodermal responses conditioned to fear-relevant stimuli. *Psychophysiology*, 16, 1–7.

Fredrikson, M., Wik, G., Annas, P., Ericson, K. & Stone-Elander, S. 1995. Functional neuroanatomy of visually elicited simple phobic fear: additional data and theoretical analysis. *Psychophysiology*, 32, 43–48.

Freed, D. M., Corkin, S. & Cohen, N. J. 1987. Forgetting in H.M.: a second look. *Neuropsychologia*, 25, 461–471.

Frewen, P. A., Dozois, D. J. A. & Lanius, R. A. 2008. Neuroimaging studies of psychological interventions for mood and anxiety disorders: empirical and methodological review. *Clinical Psychology Review*, 28, 228–246.

Friedman, N. P. & Robbins, T. W. 2022. The role of prefrontal cortex in cognitive control and executive function. *Neuropsychopharmacology*, 47, 72–89. https://doi.org/10.1038/s41386-021-01132-0

Friend, P. & Andrews, G. 1990. Agoraphobia without panic attacks. *In:* McNaughton, N. & Andrews, G. (eds.) *Anxiety* (pp. 67–73). Dunedin: University of Otago Press.

Frisby, J. P. 1979. Seeing. Oxford, Oxford University Press.

Frost, B. E., Cafalchio, M., Martin, S. K., Islam, M. N., Aggleton, J. P. & O'Mara, S. M. 2020. Spatial coding in the subiculum requires anterior thalamic inputs. *BioRxiv*, e928762. https://doi.org/10.1101/2020.01.31.928762

Frost, B. E., Martin, S. K., Cafalchio, M., Islam, M. N., Aggleton, J. P. & O'Mara, S. M. 2021. Anterior thalamic inputs are required for subiculum spatial coding, with associated consequences for hippocampal spatial memory. *The Journal of Neuroscience*, 41, 6511–6525. https://doi.org/10.1523/jneurosci.2868-20.2021

Frost, R. & McNaughton, N. 2017. The neural basis of delay discounting: a review and preliminary model. *Neuroscience & Biobehavioral Reviews*, 79, 48–65. https://doi.org/10.1016/j.neubiorev.2017.04.022

Funahashi, S., Inoue, M. & Kubota, K. 1993. Delay-related activity in the primate prefrontal cortex during sequential reaching tasks with delay. *Neuroscience Research*, 18, 171–175.

Funahashi, S. & Kubota, K. 1994. Working memory and prefrontal cortex. *Neuroscience Research*, 21, 1–11.

Fung, B. J., Qi, S., Hassabis, D., Daw, N. & Mobbs, D. 2019. Slow escape decisions are swayed by trait anxiety. *Nature Human Behaviour*, 3, 702–708. https://doi.org/10.1038/s41562-019-0595-5

Furey, M. L., Khanna, A., Hoffman, E. M. & Drevets, W. C. 2010. Scopolamine produces larger antidepressant and antianxiety effects in women than in men. *Neuropsychopharmacology*, 35, 2479–2488. https://doi.org/10.1038/npp.2010.131

Fuster, J. M. 1990. Behavioral electrophysiology of the prefrontal cortex of the primate. *In:* Uylings, H. B. M., Van Eden, C. G., De Bruin, J. P. C., Corner, M. A. & Feenstra, M. G. P. (eds.) *Progress in brain research* (pp. 313–324). Elsevier Science publishers B. V. (Biomed division).

Fuster, J. M. 1995. *Memory in the cerebral cortex*. Cambridge, MIT Press.

Fuster, J. M. 2015. Overview of prefrontal functions: E Pluribus Unum – coordinating new sequences of purposeful action. *In:* Fuster, J. M. (ed.) *The prefrontal cortex (fifth edition)* (Chapter 8, pp. 275–425). San Diego: Academic Press.

Fuster, J. M. 2022. Cognitive networks (cognits) process and maintain working memory. *Frontiers in Neural Circuits*, 15, 790691. https://doi.org/10.3389/fncir.2021.790691

Fuxe, K., Agnati, L. F., Bolme, P., Hokfelt, T., Lidbrink, P., Ljungdahl, A., Perez de la Mora, M. & Ogren, S. O. 1975. The possible involvement of GABA mechanisms in the action of benzodiazepines on central catecholamine neurons. *Advances in Biochemistry and Pharmacology*, 14, 45–61.

Gaffan, D. 1972. Loss of recognition memory in rats with lesions of the fornix. *Neuropsychologia*, 10, 327–341.

Gaffan, D. 1974. Recognition impaired and association intact in the memory of monkeys after transection of the fornix. *Journal of Comparative and Physiological Psychology*, 86, 1100–1109.

Gaffan, D. 1977a. Monkey's recognition memory for complex pictures and the effect of fornix transection. *Quarterly Journal of Experimental Psychology.*, 29, 505–514

Gaffan, D. 1977b. Monkeys' recognition memory for complex pictures and the effect of fornix transection. *Quarterly Journal of Experimental Psychology*, 29, 505–514.

Gaffan, D. 1977c. Recognition memory after short retention intervals in fornix- transected monkeys. *Quarterly Journal of Experimental Psychology.*, 29, 577–588.

Gaffan, D. 1977d. Recognition memory after short retention intervals in fornix-transected monkeys. *Quarterly Journal of Experimental Psychology*, 29, 577–588.

Gaffan, D. 1994. Scene-specific memory for objects: a model of episodic memory impairment in monkeys with fornix transection. *Cognitive Neuroscience*, 6, 305–320.

Galaj, E. & Ranaldi, R. 2021. Neurobiology of reward-related learning. *Neuroscience & Biobehavioral Reviews*, 124, 224–234. https://doi.org/https://doi.org/10.1016/j.neubiorev.2021.02.007

Gallay, D. S., Gallay, M. N., Jeanmonod, D., Rouiller, E. M. & Morel, A. 2011. The insula of Reil revisited: multiarchitectonic organization in macaque monkeys. *Cerebral Cortex*, 22, 175–190. https://doi.org/10.1093/cercor/bhr104

Ganasen, K. A., Ipser, J. C. & Stein, D. J. 2010. Augmentation of cognitive behavioral therapy with pharmacotherapy. *Psychiatric Clinics of North America*, 33, 687–99. https://doi.org/10.1016/j.psc.2010.04.008

Gandal, M. J., Haney, J. R., Parikshak, N. N., Leppa, V., Ramaswami, G., Hartl, C., Schork, A. J., Appadurai, V., Buil, A., Werge, T. M., Liu, C., White, K. P., Horvath, S. & Geschwind, D. H. 2018. Shared molecular neuropathology across major psychiatric disorders parallels polygenic overlap. *Science*, 359, 693–697. https://doi.org/10.1126/science.aad6469

Garakani, A., Murrough, J. W., Freire, R. C., Thom, R. P., Larkin, K., Buono, F. D. & Iosifescu, D. V. 2020. Pharmacotherapy of anxiety disorders: current and emerging treatment options. *Frontiers in Psychiatry*, 11, Article 595584. https://doi.org/10.3389/fpsyt.2020.595584

Gastaut, H. & Lammers, H. J. 1961. *Anatomie du Rhinencéphale*. Paris, Masson et Cie.

Gaykema, R. P. A. 1992. *The basal forebrain cholinergic system: organization of connections and long-term effects of lesions in the rat*. PhD Thesis, University of Groningen.

Gehrlach, D. A., Weiand, C., Gaitanos, T. N., Cho, E., Klein, A. S., Hennrich, A. A., Conzelmann, K. K. & Gogolla, N. 2020. A whole-brain connectivity map of mouse insular cortex. *eLife*, 9. https://doi.org/10.7554/eLife.55585

Gelder, M. G., Bancroft, J. H. J., Gath, D. H., Johnston, D. W., Mathews, A. M. & Shaw, P. M. 1973. Specific and non-specific factors in behaviour therapy. *British Journal of Psychiatry*, 123, 445–462.

Gemzik, Z. M., Donahue, M. M. & Griffin, A. L. 2021. Optogenetic suppression of the medial septum impairs working memory maintenance. *Learning & Memory*, 28, 361–370. https://doi.org/10.1101/lm.053348.120

Gener, T., Perez-Mendez, L. & Sanchez-Vives, M. V. 2013. Tactile modulation of hippocampal place fields. *Hippocampus*, 23, 1453–1462. https://doi.org/10.1002/hipo.22198

Genetics of Personality Consortium 2015. Meta-analysis of genome-wide association studies for neuroticism, and the polygenic association with major depressive disorder. *JAMA Psychiatry*, 72, 642–650. https://doi.org/10.1001/jamapsychiatry.2015.0554

George, D., Galvez, V., Martin, D., Kumar, D., Leyden, J., Hadzi-Pavlovic, D., Harper, S., Brodaty, H., Glue, P., Taylor, R., Mitchell, P. B. & Loo, C. K. 2017. Pilot randomized controlled trial of titrated subcutaneous ketamine in older patients with treatment-resistant depression. *American Journal of Geriatric Psychiatry*, 25, P1199–P1209. https://doi.org/10.1016/j.jagp.2017.06.007

George, F. & Johnson, L. 1985. *Purposive behaviour and teleological explanations*. New York, Gordon and Breach.

Geuze, E., van Berckel, B. N. M., Lammertsma, A. A., Boellaard, R., de Kloet, C. S., Vermetten, E. & Westenberg, H. G. M. 2007. Reduced GABAA benzodiazepine receptor binding in veterans with post-traumatic stress disorder. *Molecular Psychiatry*, 13, 74–83.

Ghaem, O., Mellet, E., Crivello, F., Tzourio, N., Mazoyer, B., Berthoz, A. & Denis, M. 1997. Mental navigation along memorized routes activates the hippocampus, precuneus, and insula. *Neuroreport*, 8, 739–744.

Gidyk, D. C., McDonald, R. J. & Sutherland, R. J. 2021. Intact behavioral expression of contextual fear, context discrimination, and object discrimination memories acquired in the absence of the hippocampus. *The Journal of Neuroscience*, 41, 2437–2446. https://doi.org/10.1523/jneurosci.0546-20.2020

Gilboa, A. & Moscovitch, M. 2021. No consolidation without representation: correspondence between neural and psychological representations in recent and remote memory. *Neuron*, 109, 2239–2255. https://doi.org/https://doi.org/10.1016/j.neuron.2021.04.025

Giovanniello, J., Yu, K., Furlan, A., Nachtrab, G. T., Sharma, R., Chen, X. & Li, B. 2020. A central amygdala-globus pallidus circuit conveys unconditioned stimulus-related information and controls fear learning. *The Journal of Neuroscience*, 40, 9043–9054. https://doi.org/10.1523/jneurosci.2090-20.2020

Gisquet-Verrier, P. & Schenk, F. 1994. Selective hippocampal lesions in rats do not affect retrieval processes promoted by prior cuing with the conditioned stimulus or the context. *Psychobiology*, 22, 289–303.

Givens, B. 1996a. Behavioral correlates of single units in the medial septal area: the effect of ethanol. *Neuroscience*, 71, 417–427.

Givens, B. 1996b. Stimulus-evoked resetting of the dentate theta rhythm: relation to working memory. *Neuroreport*, 8, 159–163.

Glaser, T. 1994. Ipsapirone, a potent and selective 5-HT1A receptor ligand with anxiolytic and antidepressant properties. *Correlates in Pharmacostructures*, 13(5), 430–439.

Glassman, R. B., Garvey, K. J., Elkins, K. M., Kasal, K. L. & Couillard, N. L. 1994. Spatial working memory score of humans in a large radial maze, similar to published score of rats, implies capacity close to the magical number 7 ± 2. *Brain Research Bulletin*, 34, 151–159.

Glimcher, P. W., Camerer, C. F., Fehr, E. & Poldrack, R. A. 2009. *Neuroeconomics: decision making and the brain*. Amsterdam, Elsevier.

Glimcher, P. W. & Rustichini, A. 2004. Neuroeconomics: the consilience of brain and decision. *Science*, 306, 447–452.

Gloaguen, V., Cottraux, J., Cucherat, M. & Blackburn, I. M. 1998. A meta-analysis of the effects of cognitive therapy in depressed patients. *Journal of Affective Disorders*, 49, 59–72.

Glue, P., Gulati, A., Le Nedelec, M. & Duffull, S. 2011. Dose- and exposure-response to ketamine in depression. *Biological Psychiatry*, 70, [illegible] 10. https://doi.org/10.1016/j.biopsych.2010.11.031

Glue, P., Medlicott, N. J., Harland, S., Neehoff, S., Anderson-Fahey, B., Le Nedelec, M., Gray, A. & McNaughton, N. 2017. Ketamine's dose-related effects on anxiety symptoms in patients with treatment refractory anxiety disorders. *Journal of Psychopharmacology*, 31, 1302–1305. https://doi.org/10.1177/0269881117705089

Glue, P., Medlicott, N. J., Surman, P., Lam, F., Hung, N. & Hung, C. T. 2020. Ascending-dose study of controlled-release ketamine tablets in healthy volunteers: pharmacokinetics, pharmacodynamics, safety, and tolerability. *The Journal of Clinical Pharmacology*, n/a, in press. https://doi.org/10.1002/jcph.1573

Glue, P., Neehoff, S., Sabadel, A., Broughton, L., Le Nedelec, M., Shadli, S., McNaughton, N. & Medlicott, N. J. 2019. Effects of ketamine in patients with treatment-refractory generalized anxiety and social anxiety disorders: exploratory double-blind psychoactive-controlled replication study. *Journal of Psychopharmacology*, online 269881119874457. https://doi.org/10.1177/0269881119874457

Glue, P., Neehoff, S. M., Medlicott, N. J., Gray, A., Kibby, G. & McNaughton, N. 2018. Safety and efficacy of maintenance ketamine treatment in patients with treatment-refractory generalised anxiety and social anxiety disorders. *Journal of Psychopharmacology*, 32, 663–667. https://doi.org/10.1177/0269881118762073

Glykys, J. & Mody, I. 2007. Activation of GABAA receptors: views from outside the synaptic cleft. *Neuron*, 56, 763–770.

Goeders, N. E., Ritz, M. C. & Kuhar, M. J. 1988. Buspirone enhances benzodiazepine receptor binding in vivo. *Neuropharmacology*, 27, 275–280.

Goel, V. & Grafman, J. 1995. Are the frontal lobes implicated in 'planning' functions? Interpreting data from the Tower of Hanoi. *Neuropsychologia*, 33, 623–642.

Goisman, R. M., Warshaw, M. G., Peterson, L. G., Rogers, M. P., Cuneo, P., Hunt, M. F., Tomlin-Albanese, J. M., Kazim, A., Gollan, J. K., Epstein-Kaye, T., Reich, J. H. & Keller, M. B. 1994. Panic, agoraphobia, and panic disorder with agoraphobia: data from a multicenter anxiety disorders study. *Journal of Nervous and Mental Diseases*, 182, 72–79.

Goisman, R. M., Warshaw, M. G., Steketee, G. S., Fierman, E. J., Rogers, M. P., Goldenberg, I., Weinshenker, N. J., Vasile, R. G. & Keller, M. B. 1995. DSM-IV and the disappearance of agoraphobia without a history of panic disorder: new data on a controversial diagnosis. *American Journal of Psychiatry*, 152, 1438–1443.

Goldberg, H. L. 1990. Modern treatment modalities in anxiety. *In:* McNaughton, N. & Andrews, G. (eds.) *Anxiety* (pp. 102–107). Dunedin: Otago University press.

Goldberg, H. L. & Finnerty, R. J. 1979. Comparative efficacy of buspirone and diazepam in the treatment of anxiety. *American Journal of Psychiatry*, 136, 1184–1187.

Goldman-Rakic, P. S. 1992. Working memory and the mind. *Scientific American*, 267, 73–79.

Goldman-Rakic, P. S. & Porrino, L. J. 1985. The primate mediodorsal (MD) nucleus and its projection to the frontal lobe. *The Journal of Comparative Neurology*, 242, 535–560.

González-Pardo, H., Conejo, N. M., Lana, G. & Arias, J. L. 2012. Different brain networks underlying the acquisition and expression of contextual fear conditioning: a metabolic mapping study. *Neuroscience*, 202, 234–242. https://doi.org/10.1016/j.neuroscience.2011.11.064

Goode, T. D., Tanaka, K. Z., Sahay, A. & McHugh, T. J. 2020. An integrated index: engrams, place cells, and hippocampal memory. *Neuron*, 107, 805–820. https://doi.org/https://doi.org/10.1016/j.neuron.2020.07.011

Gordon, E. M., Chauvin, R. J., Van, A. N., Rajesh, A., Nielsen, A., Newbold, D. J., Lynch, C. J., Seider, N. A., Krimmel, S. R., Scheidter, K. M., Monk, J., Miller, R. L., Metoki, A., Montez, D. F., Zheng, A., Elbau, I., Madison, T., Nishino, T., Myers, M. J., Kaplan, S., Badke D'Andrea, C., Demeter, D. V., Feigelis, M., Ramirez, J. S. B., Xu, T., Barch, D. M., Smyser, C. D., Rogers, C. E., Zimmermann, J., Botteron, K. N., Pruett, J. R., Willie, J. T., Brunner, P., Shimony, J. S., Kay, B. P., Marek, S., Norris, S. A., Gratton, C., Sylvester, C. M., Power, J. D., Liston, C., Greene, D. J., Roland, J. L., Petersen, S. E., Raichle, M. E., Laumann, T. O., Fair, D. A. & Dosenbach, N. U. F. 2023. A somato-cognitive action network alternates with effector regions in motor cortex. *Nature*, 617, 351–359. https://doi.org/10.1038/s41586-023-05964-2

Gorenstein, E. E. & Newman, J. P. 1969. Disinhibitory psychopathology: a new perspective and a model for research. *Psychological Review*, 87, 301–315.

Gorman, J. M., Kent, J. M., Sullivan, G. M. & Coplan, J. D. 2000. Neuroanatomical hypothesis of panic disorder, revised. *American Journal of Psychiatry*, 157, 493–505.

Gorman, J. M., Liebowitz, M. R., Fyer, A. J. & Stein, J. 1989. A neuroanatomical hypothesis for panic disorder. *American Journal of Psychiatry*, 146, 148–161.

Gothard, K. M., Skaggs, W. E., Moore, K. M. & McNaughton, B. L. 1996. Binding of hippocampal CA1 neural activity to multiple reference frames in a landmark-based navigation task. *The Journal of Neuroscience*, 16, 823–835.

Goyal, A., Miller, J., Qasim, S. E., Watrous, A. J., Zhang, H., Stein, J. M., Inman, C. S., Gross, R. E., Willie, J. T., Lega, B., Lin, J.-J., Sharan, A., Wu, C., Sperling, M. R., Sheth, S. A., McKhann, G. M., Smith, E. H., Schevon, C. & Jacobs, J. 2020. Functionally distinct high and low theta oscillations in the human hippocampus. *Nature Communications*, 11, e02469. https://doi.org/10.1038/s41467-020-15670-6

Graeff, F. G. 1991. Neurotransmitters in the dorsal periaqueductal grey and animal models of panic anxiety. *In:* Briley, M. & File, S. E. (eds.) *New concepts in anxiety* (pp. 288–312). MacMillan Press.

Graeff, F. G. 1994. Neuroanatomy and neurotransmitter regulation of defensive behaviors and related emotions in mammals. *Brazilian Journal of Medical and Biological Research*, 27, 811–829.

Graeff, F. G. & Del-Ben, C. M. 2008. Neurobiology of panic disorder: from animal models to brain neuroimaging. *Neuroscience & Biobehavioral Reviews*, 32, 1326–1335.

Graeff, F. G., Netto, C. F. & Zangrossi, H., Jr. 1998. The elevated T-maze as an experimental model of anxiety. *Neuroscience & Biobehavioral Reviews*, 23, 237–246.

Graeff, F. G., Viana, M. B. & Tomaz, C. 1993. The elevated T maze, a new experimental model of anxiety and memory: effect of diazepam. *Brazilian Journal of Medical and Biological Research*, 26, 67–70.

Graeff, F. G. & Zangrossi, H., Jr. 2002. Animal models of anxiety disorders. *In:* D'Haenen, H., Den Boer, J. & Willner, P. (eds.) *Biological psychiatry* (pp. 879–893). John Wiley & Sons Ltd.

Grafman, J. 1995. Similarities and distinctions among current models of prefrontal cortical functions. *Annals of the New York Academy of Sciences*, 769, 337–368.

Granon, S., Vidal, C., Thinus-Blanc, C., Changeux, J. P. & Poucet, B. 1994. Working memory, response selection, and effortful processing in rats with medial prefrontal lesions. *Behavioral Neuroscience*, 108, 883–891.

Gravielle, M. C. 2018. Regulation of GABAA receptors by prolonged exposure to endogenous and exogenous ligands. *Neurochemistry International*, 118, 96–104. https://doi.org/https://doi.org/10.1016/j.neuint.2018.05.015

Gray, J. A. 1964. Strength of the nervous system as a dimension of personality in man. *In:* Gray, J. A. (ed.) *Pavlov's typology* (pp. 289–366). Oxford: Pergamon.

Gray, J. A. 1967. Disappointment and drugs in the rat. *Advancement of Science*, 23, 595–605.

Gray, J. A. 1969. Sodium amobarbital and effects of frustrative nonreward. *Journal of Comparative and Physiological Psychology*, 69, 55–64.

Gray, J. A. 1970a. The psychophysiological basis of introversion-extraversion. *Behaviour Research and Therapy*, 8, 249–266. https://doi.org/10.1016/0005-7967(70)90069-0

Gray, J. A. 1970b. Sodium amobarbital, the hippocampal theta rhythm and the partial reinforcement extinction effect. *Psychological Review*, 77, 465–480.

Gray, J. A. 1971. *The psychology of fear and stress*. London: Weidenfeld and Nicolson.

Gray, J. A. 1972. The structure of the emotions and the limbic system. *In:* Porter, R. & Knight, J. (eds.) *Physiology, emotion and psychosomatic illness, Ciba Foundation Symposium 8 (New Series)* (pp. 87–130). Amsterdam: Associated Scientific Publishers.

Gray, J. A. 1975. *Elements of a two-process theory of learning*. London, Academic Press.

Gray, J. A. 1976. The behavioural inhibition system: a possible substrate for anxiety. *In:* Feldman, M. P. & Broadhurst, A. M. (eds.) *Theoretical and experimental bases of behaviour modification* (pp. 3–41). London: Wiley.

Gray, J. A. 1977. Drug effects on fear and frustration: possible limbic site of action of minor tranquilizers. *In:* Iversen, L. L., Iversen, S. D. & Snyder, S. H. (eds.) *Handbook of psychopharmacology. Vol 8: drugs, neurotransmitters and behaviour* (pp. 433–529). New York: Plenum Press.

Gray, J. A. 1979a. Is there any need for conditioning in Eysenck's conditioning model of neurosis? *Behavioral and Brain Sciences*, 2, 169–171.

Gray, J. A. 1979b. *Pavlov*. London: Fontana.

Gray, J. A. 1981. A critique of Eysenck's theory of personality. *In:* Eysenck, H. J. (ed.) *A model for personality* (pp. 246–276). New York: Springer.

Gray, J. A. 1982. *The neuropsychology of anxiety: an enquiry in to the functions of the septo-hippocampal system*. Oxford: Oxford University Press.

Gray, J. A. 1987a. Interactions between drugs and behaviour therapy. *In:* Eysenck, H. J. & Martin, I. (eds.) *Theoretical foundations of behaviour therapy* (pp. 433–447). New York: Plenum Press.

Gray, J. A. 1987b. *The psychology of fear and stress*. London, Cambridge University Press.

Gray, J. A. 1995. The contents of consciousness: a neuropsychological conjecture. *Behavioral and Brain Sciences*, 18, 659–722.

Gray, J. A. 2004. *Consciousness: creeping up on the hard problem*, Oxford University Press.

Gray, J. A., Buhusi, C. V. & Schmajuk, N. A. 1997. The transition from automatic to controlled processing. *Neural Networks*, 10, 1257–1268.

Gray, J. A., Feldon, J., Rawlins, J. N. P., Hemsley, D. R. & Smith, A. D. 1991. The neuropsychology of schizophrenia. *Behavioral and Brain Sciences*, 14, 1–20.

Gray, J. A. & McNaughton, N. 1983. Comparison between the behavioural effect of septal and hippocampal lesions: a review. *Neuroscience & Biobehavioral Reviews*, 7, 119–188. https://doi.org/10.1016/0149-7634(83)90014-3

Gray, J. A. & McNaughton, N. 2000. *The neuropsychology of anxiety: an enquiry into the functions of the septo-hippocampal system (2 ed.)*. Oxford: Oxford University Press.

Gray, J. A., McNaughton, N., James, D. T. D. & Kelly, P. H. 1975. Effect of minor tranquillisers on hippocampal theta rhythm mimicked by depletion of forebrain noradrenaline. *Nature*, 258, 424–425.

Gray, J. A. & Smith, P. T. 1969. An arousal-decision model for partial reinforcement and discrimination learning. *In:* Gilbert, R. & Sutherland, N. S. (eds.) *Animal discrimination learning* (pp. 243–272). London: Academic Press.

Graybiel, A. M. & Rauch, S. L. 2000. Toward a neurobiology of Obsessive-Compulsive Disorder. *Neuron*, 28, 343–347.

Graziano, M. S. A. 2023. Fundamental principles of cortical organization reflected in a new study. *Neuron*, 111, 1524–1525. https://doi.org/10.1016/j.neuron.2023.04.024

Green, J. T. & Arenos, J. D. 2007. Hippocampal and cerebellar single-unit activity during delay and trace eyeblink conditioning in the rat. *Neurobiology of Learning and Memory*, 87, 269–284.

Grella, S. L., Neil, J. M., Edison, H. T., Strong, V. D., Odintsova, I. V., Walling, S. G., Martin, G. M., Marrone, D. F. & Harley, C. W. 2019. Locus Coeruleus Phasic, But Not Tonic, Activation Initiates Global Remapping in a Familiar Environment. *The Journal of Neuroscience*, 39, 445–455. https://doi.org/10.1523/jneurosci.1956-18.2018

Griebel, G. 1995. 5-hydroxytryptamine-interacting drugs in animal models of anxiety disorders: more than 30 years of research. *Pharmacology and Therapeutics*, 65, 319–395.

Griffin, A. L. 2021. The nucleus reuniens orchestrates prefrontal-hippocampal synchrony during spatial working memory. *Neuroscience & Biobehavioral Reviews*, 128, 415–420. https://doi.org/https://doi.org/10.1016/j.neubiorev.2021.05.033

Griffith, J. W., Zinbarg, R. E., Craske, M. G., Mineka, S., Rose, R. D., Waters, A. M. & Sutton, J. M. 2010. Neuroticism as a common dimension in the internalizing disorders. *Psychological Medicine*, 40, 1125–1136. https://doi.org/10.1017/S0033291709991449

Griggs, R. A. 2014. The continuing saga of Little Albert in introductory psychology textbooks. *Teaching of Psychology*, 41, 309–317. https://doi.org/10.1177/0098628314549702

Grillner, S. 2018. The enigmatic "indirect pathway" of the basal ganglia: a new role. *Neuron*, 99, 1105–1107. https://doi.org/10.1016/j.neuron.2018.08.040

Grillner, S. & Robertson, B. 2016. The basal ganglia over 500 million years. *Current Biology*, 26, R1088–R1100. https://doi.org/https://doi.org/10.1016/j.cub.2016.06.041

Grillner, S. & Thompson, W. S. 2021. Basal ganglia reign through downstream control of motor centers in midbrain and brain stem while updating cortex with efference copy information. *Neuron*, 109, 1587–1589. https://doi.org/https://doi.org/10.1016/j.neuron.2021.04.015

Grillon, C., Ameli, R., Foot, M. & Davis, M. 1993. Fear-potentiated startle: relationship to the level of state/trait anxiety in healthy subjects. *Biological Psychiatry*, 33, 566–574.

Grillon, C. & Ernst, M. 2020. A way forward for anxiolytic drug development: testing candidate anxiolytics with anxiety-potentiated startle in healthy humans. *Neuroscience & Biobehavioral Reviews*, 119, 348–354. https://doi.org/https://doi.org/10.1016/j.neubiorev.2020.09.024

Grogans, S. E., Bliss-Moreau, E., Buss, K. A., Clark, L. A., Fox, A. S., Keltner, D., Cowen, A. S., Kim, J. J., Kragel, P. A., MacLeod, C., Mobbs, D., Naragon-Gainey, K., Fullana, M. A. & Shackman, A. J. 2023. The nature and neurobiology of fear and anxiety: state of the science and opportunities for accelerating discovery. *Neuroscience and Biobehavioral Reviews*, 151, 105237. https://doi.org/10.1016/j.neubiorev.2023.105237

Gross, C. G. 1994. How inferior temporal cortex became a visual area. *Cerebral Cortex*, 5, 455–469.

Grossberg, S. 2021. A neural model of intrinsic and extrinsic hippocampal theta rhythms: anatomy, neurophysiology, and function. *Frontiers in Systems Neuroscience*, 15, A665052. https://doi.org/10.3389/fnsys.2021.665052

Guidotti, A., Toffano, G. & Costa, E. 1978. An endogenous protein modulates the affinity of GABA and benzodiazepine receptors in rat brain. *Nature*, 275, 553–555.

Gurvits, T. V., Shenton, M. E., Hokama, H., Ohta, H., Lasko, N. B., Gilbertson, M. W., Orr, S. P., Kikinis, R., Jolesz, F. A., McCarley, R. W. & Pitman, R. K. 1996. Magnetic resonance imaging study of hippocampal volume in chronic, combat-related posttraumatic stress disorder. *Biological Psychiatry*, 40, 1091–1099.

Gutiérrez, H., Hernández-Echeagaray, E., Ramírez-Amaya, V. & Bermúdez-Rattoni, F. 1999. Blockade of N-methyl-D-aspartate receptors in the insular cortex disrupts taste aversion and spatial memory formation. *Neuroscience*, 89, 751–758.

Haber, S. N. & Calzavara, R. 2009. The cortico-basal ganglia integrative network: the role of the thalamus. *Brain Research Bulletin*, 78, 69–74.

Hackmann, A., Surawy, C. & Clark, D. M. 1998. Seeing yourself through others' eyes: a study of spontaneously occurring images in social phobia. *Behavioural and Cognitive Psychotherapy*, 26, 3–12.

Haefely, W. 1990a. Benzodiazepine receptor and ligands: structural and functional differences. *In:* Hindmarch, I., Beaumont, G., Brandon, S. & Leonard, B. E. (eds.) *Benzodiazepines: current concepts* (pp. 165–187, pp. 1–18). John Wiley and Sons Ltd.

Haefely, W. 1990b. The GABAa-benzodiazepine receptor: biology and pharmacology. *In:* Burrows, G. D., Roth, M. & Noyes, R. (eds.) *Handbook of anxiety: the neurobiology of anxiety* (pp. 165–187). Elsevier Science Publishers B.V.

Haefely, W. 1991. Comparative pharmacology of benzodiazepine receptor ligands with differing intrinsic efficacy. *In:* Barnard, E. A. & Costa, E. (eds.) *Transmitter amino acid receptors: structures, transduction and models for drug development* (pp. 91–111). New York: Thieme Medical Publishers.

Haefely, W. 1992. The role of GABA in anxiolytic/antidepressant drug action. *In:* Elliott, J. M., Heal, D. J. & Marsden, C. A. (eds.) *Experimental approaches to anxiety and depression* (pp. 151–168). John Wiley and Sons Ltd.

Haefely, W., Facklam, M., Schoch, P., Martin, J. R., Bonetti, E. P., Moreau, J. L., Jenck, F. & Richards, J. G. 1992. Partial agonists of benzodiazepine receptors for the treatment of epilepsy, sleep, and anxiety disorders. *In:* Biggio, G., Concas, A. & Costa, E. (eds.) *GABAergic synaptic transmission* (pp. 379–394). New York: Raven Press.

Haefely, W., Martin, J. R. & Schoch, P. 1990. Novel anxiolytics that act as partial agonists at benzodiazepine receptors. *Trends in Pharmacological Science*, 11, 452–456.

Haefely, W. E. 1990c. The GABAa-benzodiazepine receptor complex and anxiety. *In:* Sartorius, N., Andreoli, V., Cassano, G., Eisenberg, L., Kielholz, P., Pancheri, P. & Racagni, G. (eds.) *Anxiety: psychobiological and clinical perspectives* (pp. 23–36). New York: Hemisphere Publishing Corporation.

Haegelen, C., Rouaud, T., Darnault, P. & Morandi, X. 2009. The subthalamic nucleus is a key-structure of limbic basal ganglia functions. *Medical Hypotheses*, 72, 421–426.

Hafner, J. & Marks, I. 1976. Exposure in vivo of agoraphobics: contributions of diazepam, group exposure, and anxiety evocation. *Psychological Medicine*, 6, 71–88.

Hale, M. W. & Lowry, C. A. 2015. Brain Monoaminergic Systems in Stress Neuroendocrinology. *In:* Russell, J. A. & Shipston, M. J. (eds.) *Neuroendocrinology of Stress* (pp. 19–41). www.wiley.com/go/russell/stress: John Wiley & Sons, Ltd.

Hall, C. S. 1951. The genetics of behavior. *In:* Stevens, S. S. (ed.) *Handbook of experimental psychology* (pp. 304–329). New York: Wiley.

Hall, G., Purves, D. & Bonardi, C. 1996. Contextual control of conditioned responding in rats with dorsal hippocampal lesions. *Behavioral Neuroscience*, 110, 933–945.

Hall, P. J., Chong, W., McNaughton, N. & Corr, P. J. 2011. A economic perspective on the reinforcement sensitivity theory of personality. *Personality and Individual Differences*, 51, 242–247.

Haller, J. 2018. The role of central and medial amygdala in normal and abnormal aggression: a review of classical approaches. *Neuroscience & Biobehavioral Reviews*, 85, 34–43. https://doi.org/https://doi.org/10.1016/j.neubiorev.2017.09.017

Hamid, A. A., Frank, M. J. & Moore, C. I. 2021. Wave-like dopamine dynamics as a mechanism for spatiotemporal credit assignment. *Cell*, 184, 2733–2749 e16. https://doi.org/10.1016/j.cell.2021.03.046

Hampson, R. E., Byrd, D. R., Konstantopoulos, J. K., Bunn, T. & Deadwyler, S. A. 1996. Hippocampal place fields: relationship between degree of field overlap and cross-correlations within ensembles of hippocampal neurons. *Hippocampus*, 6, 281–293.

Handley, S. L. 1995. 5-hydroxytryptamine pathways in anxiety and its treatment. *Pharmacology and Therapeutics*, 66, 103–148.

Handley, S. L., McBlane, J. W., Critchley, M. A. E. & Njung'e, K. 1993. Multiple serotonin mechanisms in animal models of anxiety: environmental, emotional and cognitive factors. *Behavioural Brain Research*, 58, 203–210.

Hanganu-Opatz, I. L., Klausberger, T., Sigurdsson, T., Nieder, A., Jacob, S. N., Bartos, M., Sauer, J.-F., Durstewitz, D., Leibold, C. & Diester, I. 2023. Resolving the prefrontal mechanisms of adaptive cognitive behaviors: a cross-species perspective. *Neuron*, 111, 1020–1036. https://doi.org/10.1016/j.neuron.2023.03.017

Hannesson, D. K. & Skelton, R. W. 1998. Recovery of spatial performance in the Morris water maze following bilateral transection of the fimbria/fornix in rats. *Behavioural Brain Research*, 90, 35–56.

Harland, B., Contreras, M., Souder, M. & Fellous, J.-M. 2021. Dorsal CA1 hippocampal place cells form a multi-scale representation of megaspace. *Current Biology*. https://doi.org/10.1016/j.cub.2021.03.003

Harper, C. A., Satchell, L. P., Fido, D. & Latzman, R. D. 2021. Functional fear predicts public health compliance in the COVID-19 pandemic. *International Journal of Mental Health and Addiction*, 19, 1875–1888. https://doi.org/10.1007/s11469-020-00281-5

Harris, J. A. & Westbrook, R. F. 1995. Effects of benzodiazepine microinjection into the amygdala or periaqueductal gray on the expression of conditioned fear and hypoalgesia in rats. *Behavioral Neuroscience*, 109, 295–304.

Harro, J., Vasar, E. & Bradwejn, J. 1993. CCK in animal and human research on anxiety. *Trends in Pharmacological Science*, 14, 244–249.

Harvey, R. E., Robinson, H. L., Liu, C., Oliva, A. & Fernandez-Ruiz, A. 2023. Hippocampo-cortical circuits for selective memory encoding, routing, and replay. *Neuron*. https://doi.org/10.1016/j.neuron.2023.04.015

Haslam, N., McGrath, M. J., Viechtbauer, W. & Kuppens, P. 2020. Dimensions over categories: a meta-analysis of taxometric research. *Psychological Medicine*, 50, 1418–1432. https://doi.org/10.1017/s003329172000183x

Hasler, G. 2012. Can the neuroeconomics revolution revolutionize psychiatry? *Neuroscience & Biobehavioral Reviews*, 36, 64–78. https://doi.org/10.1016/j.neubiorev.2011.04.011

Hasselmo, M. E. 2006. The role of acetylcholine in learning and memory. *Current Opinion in Neurobiology*, 16, 710–5.

Hasselmo, M. E. & Bower, J. M. 1993. Acetylcholine and memory. *Trends in Neuroscience*, 16, 218–222.

Hauser, W., Petzke, F. & Sommer, C. 2010. Comparative efficacy and harms of duloxetine, milnacipran, and pregabalin in fibromyalgia syndrome. *The Journal of Pain*, 11, 505–21. https://doi.org/10.1016/j.jpain.2010.01.002

Hawton, K., Salkovskis, P. M., Kirk, J. & Clark, D. M. 1989. *Cognitive behaviour therapy for psychiatric problems*. Oxford: Oxford University Press.

Hayne, H. 1998. Age-related changes in deferred imitation: the development of declarative memory. A paper presented at the annual meeting of the International Society for Developmental Biology, Orleans, France, July 1998.

Hayne, H., MacDonald, S. & Barr, R. 1997. Developmental changes in the specificity of memory over the second year of life. *Infant Behavior and Development*, 20, 233–245.

He, H., Boehringer, R., Huang, A. J. Y., Overton, E. T. N., Polygalov, D., Okanoya, K. & McHugh, T. J. 2021. CA2 inhibition reduces the precision of hippocampal assembly reactivation. *Neuron*, 109, 3674–3687.e7. https://doi.org/https://doi.org/10.1016/j.neuron.2021.08.034

Healey, D. & Healey, M. 2019. Randomized Controlled Trial comparing the effectiveness of structured-play (ENGAGE) and behavior management (TRIPLE P) in reducing problem behaviors in preschoolers. *Scientific Reports*, 9, A3497. https://doi.org/10.1038/s41598-019-40234-0

Hebb, D. O. 1946. On the nature of fear. *Psychological Review*, 53, 259–276.

Hebb, D. O. 1949. *The organization of behavior: a neuropsychological theory*. New York, Wiley-Interscience.

Hebb, D. O. 1955. Drives and the C.N.S. (conceptual nervous system). *Psychological Review*, 62, 243–254.

Heimberg, R. G., Dodge, C. S., Hope, D. A., Kennedy, C. R. & Zollo, L. J. 1990. Cognitive behavioural group treatment for social phobia: comparison with a credible placebo control. *Cognitive Therapy and Research*, 17, 235–248.

Hellewell, J. S. E., Guimaraes, F. S., Wang, M. & Deakin, J. F. W. 1999. Comparison of buspirone with diazepam and fluvoxamine on aversive classical conditioning in humans. *Journal of Psychopharmacology*, 13, 122–127.

Henke, P. G. 1977. Dissociation of the frustration effect and the partial reinforcement extinction effect after limbic lesions in rats. *Journal of Comparative and Physiological Psychology*, 91, 1032–1038.

Hensman, R., Guimaraes, F. S., Wang, M. & Deakin, J. F. W. 1991. Effects of ritanserin on aversive classical conditioning in humans. *Psychopharmacology*, 104, 220–224.

Hernandes, P. M., Batistela, M. F., Vilela-Costa, H. H., Sant'Ana, A. B., Kumpel, V. D., Tirapelle, M. C., Bom, A. d. O. P., de Andrade, T. G. C. S. & Zangrossi, H. 2021. Role of 5-HT1A receptors in the ventral hippocampus in the regulation of anxiety- and panic-related defensive behaviors in rats. *Behavioural Brain Research*, 408, 113296. https://doi.org/https://doi.org/10.1016/j.bbr.2021.113296

Herremans, A. H. J., Hijzen, T. H., Olivier, B. & Slangen, J. L. 1995. Relation between stimulus discriminability and response bias in a delayed conditional discrimination task in the rat. *Journal of Neuroscience Methods*, 63, 29–35.

Herrup, K. 2010. Reimagining Alzheimer's disease—an age-based hypothesis. *Journal of Neuroscience.*, 30, 16755–16762. https://doi.org/10.1523/jneurosci.4521-10.2010

Hertel, P. T. & Mathews, A. 2011. Cognitive bias modification: past perspectives, current findings, and future applications. *Perspectives in Psychological Science*, 6, 521–536.

Herz, R. S. & Cupchik, G. C. 1995. The emotional distinctiveness of odor-evoked memories. *Chemical Senses*, 20, 517–528.

Heym, N., Ferguson, E. & Lawrence, C. 2008. An evaluation of the relationship between Gray's revised RST and Eysenck's PEN: distinguishing BIS and FFFS in Carver and White's BIS/BAS scales. *Personality and Individual Differences*, 45, 709–715. https://doi.org/10.1016/j.paid.2008.07.013

Heymann, G., Jo, Y. S., Reichard, K. L., McFarland, N., Chavkin, C., Palmiter, R. D., Soden, M. E. & Zweifel, L. S. 2020. Synergy of distinct dopamine projection populations in behavioral reinforcement. *Neuron*, 105, 909–920.e5. https://doi.org/https://doi.org/10.1016/j.neuron.2019.11.024

Hill, A. J. 1978. First occurrence of hippocampal spatial firing in a new environment. *Experimental Neurology*, 62, 282–297.

Hill, A. J. & Best, P. J. 1981. Effects of deafness and blindness on the spatial correlates of hippocampal unit activity in the rat. *Experimental Neurology*, 74, 204–217.

Hinde, R. A. 1998. *Animal behaviour*. New York: McGraw-Hill.

Hinton, G. E., Plaut, D. C. & Shallice, T. 1993. Simulating brain damage. *Scientific American*, 269 (October), 58–66.

Hirsh, R. 1974. The hippocampus and contextual retrieval of information from memory: a theory. *Behavioural Biology*, 12, 421–434.

Hitchcock, J. M. & Davis, M. 1991. Efferent pathway of the amygdala involved in conditioned fear as measured with the fear-potentiated startle paradigm. *Behavioral Neuroscience*, 105(6), 826–842.

Hjorth, O. R., Frick, A., Gingnell, M., Hoppe, J. M., Faria, V., Hultberg, S., Alaie, I., Månsson, K. N. T., Wahlstedt, K., Jonasson, M., Lubberink, M., Antoni, G., Fredrikson, M. & Furmark, T. 2021. Expression and co-expression of serotonin and dopamine transporters in social anxiety disorder: a multitracer positron emission tomography study. *Molecular Psychiatry*, 26, 3970–3979. https://doi.org/10.1038/s41380-019-0618-7

Hodges, H. & Green, S. 1986. Effects of chlordiazepoxide on cued radial maze performance in rats. *Psychopharmacology (Berl)*, 88, 460–466.

Hodges, H., Green, S. & Glenn, B. 1987. Evidence that the amygdala is involved in benzodiazepine and serotonergic effects on punished responding but not on discrimination. *Psychopharmacology (Berl)*, 92, 491–504.

Hodgson, R. & Rachman, S. 1972. The effects of contamination and washing in obsessional patients. *Behaviour Research and Therapy*, 10, 111–117.

Hoehn-Saric, R., Merchant, A. F., Keyser, M. C. & Smith, V. K. 1981. Effects of clonidine on anxiety disorders. *Archives of General Psychiatry*, 38, 1278–1286.

Hofer, M. A. 1972. Physiological and behavioural processes in early maternal deprivation. *In:* Porter, R. & Knight, J. (eds.) *Physiology, emotion and psychosomatic illness. CIBA symposium No. 8 (new series).* Elsevier.

Holdstock, T. L. 1969. Autonomic reactivity following septal and amygdaloid lesions in white rats. *Physiology and Behavior*, 4, 603–607.

Holdstock, T. L. 1970. Plasticity of autonomic functions in rats with septal lesions. *Neuropsychologia*, 8, 147–160.

Holley, L. A., Turchi, J., Apple, C. & Sarter, M. 1995. Dissociation between the attentional effects of infusions of a benzodiazepine receptor agonist and an inverse agonist into the basal forebrain. *Psychopharmacology (Berl)*, 120, 99–108.

Hollup, S. A., Molden, S., Donnett, J. G., Moser, M. B. & Moser, E. I. 2001. Accumulation of hippocampal place fields at the goal location in an annular watermaze task. *Journal of Neuroscience*, 21, 1635–1644.

Holmes, A. J., Lee, P. H., Hollinshead, M. O., Bakst, L., Roffman, J. L., Smoller, J. W. & Buckner, R. L. 2012. Individual differences in amygdala-medial prefrontal anatomy link negative affect, impaired social functioning, and polygenic depression risk. *The Journal of Neuroscience*, 32, 18087–18100. https://doi.org/10.1523/JNEUROSCI.2531-12.2012

Holt, P. 1990. Panic disorder: some historical trends. *In:* McNaughton, N. & Andrews, G. (eds.) *Anxiety* (pp. 54–65). Dunedin: University of Otago Press.

Homskaya, E. D. 1964. Verbal regulation of the vegetative components of the orienting reflex in focal brain lesions. *Cortex*, 1, 63–76.

Hones, V. I. & Mizumori, S. J. Y. 2022. Response flexibility: the role of the lateral habenula. *Frontiers in Behavioral Neuroscience*, 16, A852235. https://doi.org/10.3389/fnbeh.2022.852235

Horii, N., Nomoto, K., Endo, N., Yamanaka, A., Kikusui, T. & Nishi, M. 2020. Hypothalamic perifornical urocortin-3 neurons modulate defensive responses to a potential threat stimulus. *iScience*, 24, 101908. https://doi.org/10.1016/j.isci.2020.101908

Hormigo, S., Shanmugasundaram, B., Zhou, J. & Castro-Alamancos, M. A. 2021. A signaled locomotor avoidance action is fully represented in the neural activity of the midbrain tegmentum. *The Journal of Neuroscience*, 41, 4262–4275. https://doi.org/10.1523/jneurosci.0027-21.2021

Hormigo, S., Vega-Flores, G. & Castro-Alamancos, M. A. 2016. Basal Ganglia Output Controls Active Avoidance Behavior. *The Journal of Neuroscience*, 36, 10274–10284. https://doi.org/10.1523/jneurosci.1842-16.2016

Hosie, A. M., Wilkins, M. E., da Silva, H. M. & Smart, T. G. 2006. Endogenous neurosteroids regulate GABAA receptors through two discrete transmembrane sites. *Nature*, 444, 486–9.

Houser, C. R., Peng, Z., Wei, X., Huang, C. S. & Mody, I. 2021. Mossy cells in the dorsal and ventral dentate gyrus differ in their patterns of axonal projections. *The Journal of Neuroscience*, 41, 991–1004. https://doi.org/10.1523/jneurosci.2455-20.2020

Humphries, M. D. & Prescott, T. J. 2010. The ventral basal ganglia, a selection mechanism at the crossroads of space, strategy, and reward. *Progress in Neurobiology*, 90, 385–417. https://doi.org/10.1016/j.pneurobio.2009.11.003

Hunsaker, M. R. & Kesner, R. P. 2018. Unfolding the cognitive map: the role of hippocampal and extra-hippocampal substrates based on a systems analysis of spatial processing. *Neurobiology of Learning and Memory*, 147, 90–119. https://doi.org/https://doi.org/10.1016/j.nlm.2017.11.012

Hunt, P. S., Richardson, R. & Campbell, B. A. 1994. Delayed development of fear-potentiated startle in rats. *Behavioral Neuroscience*, 108, 69–80.

Huo, H., Zhang, R., Seger, C. A., Feng, T. & Chen, Q. 2020. The effect of trait anxiety on risk-taking: functional coupling between right hippocampus and left insula. *Psychophysiology*, 57, e13629. https://doi.org/10.1111/psyp.13629

Hur, J., Smith, J. F., DeYoung, K. A., Anderson, A. S., Kuang, J., Kim, H. C., Tillman, R. M., Kuhn, M., Fox, A. S. & Shackman, A. J. 2020. Anxiety and the neurobiology of temporally uncertain threat anticipation. *The Journal of Neuroscience*, in press, JN-RM-0704-20. https://doi.org/10.1523/jneurosci.0704-20.2020

Huron, C., Servais, C. & Danion, J. M. 2001. Lorazepam and diazepam impair true, but not false, recognition in healthy volunteers. *Psychopharmacology*, 155, 204–209.

Hussain, M. Z. 1971. Desensitization and flooding (implosion) in treatment of phobias. *American Journal of Psychiatry*, 127, 1509–1514.

Iacono, R. P. & Nashold, B. S. 1982. Mental and behavioral effects of brain stem and hypothalamic stimulation in man. *Human Neurobiology*, 1, 273–279.

Iacovides, A., Fountoulakis, K. N., Fotiou, F., Fokas, K., Nimatoudis, I. & Kaprinis, G. 2002. Relation of pesonality disorders to subtypes of major depression according both to DSM-IV and ICD-10. *Canadian Journal of Psychiatry*, 47, 196–197.

Illescas-Huerta, E., Ramirez-Lugo, L., Sierra, R. O., Quillfeldt, J. A. & Sotres-Bayon, F. 2021. Conflict test battery for studying the act of facing threats in pursuit of rewards. *Frontiers in Neuroscience*, 15, A645769. https://doi.org/10.3389/fnins.2021.645769

Inostroza, M. & Born, J. 2013. Sleep for preserving and transforming episodic memory. *Annual Review of Neuroscience*, 36, 79–102. https://doi.org/doi:10.1146/annurev-neuro-062012–170429

Insel, T. 2013. *Transforming Diagnosis* [Online]. NIMH Director's Blog: National Institutes of Mental Health. Available: http://www.nimh.nih.gov/about/director/2013/transforming-diagnosis.shtml [Accessed April 29 2013].

Insel, T., Cuthbert, B., Garvey, M. G., Heinssen, R., Pine, D. S., Quinn, K., Sanislow, C. & Wang, P. 2010. Research Domain Criteria (RDoC): toward a new classification framework for research on mental disorders. *American Journal of Psychiatry*, 167, 748–751.

Ipser, J. C., Singh, L. & Stein, D. J. 2013. Meta-analysis of functional brain imaging in specific phobia. *Psychiatry Clin Neurosci*, 67, 311–22. https://doi.org/10.1111/pcn.12055

Irvine, G. I. 2000. *Combining novel and classical anxiolytic drugs: implications for treatment*. MSc, University of Otago.

Isbell, L. A. 2006. Snakes as agents of evolutionary change in primate brains. *Journal of Human Evolution*, 51, 1–35. https://doi.org/10.1016/j.jhevol.2005.12.012

Ison, J. R., Glass, D. H. & Bohmer, H. M. 1966. Effects of sodium amytal on the approach to stimulus change. *Proceedings of the American Psychological Association*, 2, 5–6.

Ivkovich, D. & Stanton, M. E. 2001. Effects of early hippocampal lesions on trace, delay, and long-delay eyeblink conditioning in developing rats. *Neurobiology of Learning and Memory*, 76, 426–46. https://doi.org/10.1006/nlme.2001.4027

Jackson, C. J. 2009. Jackson-5 scales of revised reinforcement sensitivity theory (r-RST) and their application to dysfunctional real world outcomes. *Journal of Research in Personality*, 43, 556–569. https://doi.org/https://doi.org/10.1016/j.jrp.2009.02.007

Jacobs, J. 2014. Hippocampal theta oscillations are slower in humans than in rodents: implications for models of spatial navigation and memory. *Philosophical Transactions of the Royal Society B: Biological Sciences*, 369, 20130304. https://doi.org/doi:10.1098/rstb.2013.0304

Jacobs, J., Korolev, I. O., Caplan, J. B., Ekstrom, A. D., Litt, B., Baltuch, G., Fried, I., Schulze-Bonhage, A., Madsen, J. R. & Kahana, M. J. 2010. Right-lateralized brain oscillations in human spatial navigation. *Journal of Cognitive Neuroscience*, 22, 824–836.

Jacobson, S., Butters, N. & Tovsky, N. J. 1978. Afferent and efferent subcortical projections of behaviorally defined sectors of prefrontal granular cortex. *Brain Research*, 159, 279–296.

Jacobson, S. & Trojanowski, J. Q. 1977. Prefrontal granular cortex of the rhesus monkey. I. Intrahemispheric cortical afferents. *Brain Research*, 132, 209–233. https://doi.org/https://doi.org/10.1016/0006-8993(77)90417-6

Jakes, I. 1996. *Theoretical approaches to obsessive-compulsive disorder*. Cambridge, Cambridge University Press.

James, D. T. D., McNaughton, N., Rawlins, J. N. P., Feldon, J. & Gray, J. A. 1977. Septal driving of hippocampal theta rhythm as a function of frequency in the free-moving male rat. *Neuroscience*, 2, 1007–1017.

James, W. 1884. What is an emotion? *Mind (reprinted in Arnold, 1968, The nature of emotion)*, 9, 188–205.

Janacsek, K., Evans, T. M., Kiss, M., Shah, L., Blumenfeld, H. & Ullman, M. T. 2022. Subcortical cognition: the fruit below the rind. *Annual Review of Neuroscience*, 45, 361–386. https://doi.org/10.1146/annurev-neuro-110920-013544

Jang, K. L., Livesley, W. J. & Vernon, P. A. 1996. Heritability of the big five personality dimensions and their facets: a twin study. *Journal of Personality*, 64, 577–91. https://doi.org/10.1111/j.1467-6494.1996.tb00522.x

Jann, M. 1988. Buspirone: an update on a unique anxiolytic agent. *Pharmacotherapy*, 8(2), 100–116.

Jansen, D. M. & Frijda, N. H. 1994. Modulation of the acoustic startle response by film-induced fear and sexual arousal. *Psychophysiology*, 31, 565–571.

Jardim, M. C. & Guimaraes, F. S. 2001. GABAergic and glutamatergic modulation of exploratory behavior in the dorsomedial hypothalamus. *Pharmacology, Biochemistry and Behavior*, 69, 579–584.

Jardim, M. C., Nogueira, R. L., Graeff, F. G. & Nunes-de-Souza, R. L. 1999. Evaluation of the elevated T-maze as an animal model of anxiety in the mouse. *Brain Research Bulletin*, 48, 407–411.

Jarrard, L. E. 1975. Role of interference in retention by rats with hippocampal lesions. *Journal of Comparative and Physiological Psychology*, 89, 400–408.

Jarrard, L. E. 1978. Selective hippocampal lesions: differential effects on performance by rats of spatial task with preoperative versus postoperative training. *Journal of Comparative and Physiological Psychology*, 92, 1119–1127.

Jarrard, L. E. 1983. Selective hippocampal lesions and behavior: effects of kainic acid lesions on performance of place and cue tasks. *Behavioral Neuroscience*, 97, 873–889.

Jarrard, L. E. 1991. On the neural basis of the spatial mapping system: hippocampus versus hippocampal formation. *Hippocampus*, 2, 236–239.

Jarrard, L. E., Feldon, J., Rawlins, J. N. P., Sinden, J. D. & Gray, J. A. 1986. The effects of intrahippocampal ibotenate on resistance to extinction after continuous or pertial reinforcement. *Experimental Brain Research*, 61, 519–530.

Jaycox, L. H. & Foa, E. B. 1998. Post-traumatic stress disorder. *In:* Bellack, A. S. & Hersen, M. (eds.) *Comprehensive clinical psychology* (pp. 499–517). Oxford: Elsevier Science.

Jean-Richard-dit-Bressel, P., Killcross, S. & McNally, G. P. 2018. Behavioral and neurobiological mechanisms of punishment: implications for psychiatric disorders. *Neuropsychopharmacology*, 43, 1639–1650. https://doi.org/10.1038/s41386-018-0047-3

Jean-Richard-dit-Bressel, P. & McNally, G. P. 2015. The role of the basolateral amygdala in punishment. *Learning & Memory*, 22, 128–37. https://doi.org/10.1101/lm.035907.114

Jean-Richard-dit-Bressel, P., Tran, J., Didachos, A. & McNally, G. P. 2021. Instrumental aversion coding in the basolateral amygdala and its reversion by a benzodiazepine. *bioRxiv*, 2021.07.08.451726. https://doi.org/10.1101/2021.07.08.451726

Jezek, K., Henriksen, E. J., Treves, A., Moser, E. I. & Moser, M.-B. 2011. Theta-paced flickering between place-cell maps in the hippocampus. *Nature*, 478, 246–249. https://doi.org/http://www.nature.com/nature/journal/v478/n7368/abs/nature10439.html#supplementary-information10.1038/nature10439

Jhou, T. C., Fields, H. L., Baxter, M. G., Saper, C. B. & Holland, P. C. 2009. The rostromedial tegmental nucleus (RMTg), a GABAergic afferent to midbrain dopamine neurons, encodes aversive stimuli and inhibits motor responses. *Neuron*, 61, 786–800. https://doi.org/10.1016/j.neuron.2009.02.001

Jiang, F. & Khanna, S. 2004. Reticular stimulation evokes suppression of CA1 synaptic responses and generation of theta through separate mechanisms. *European Journal of Neuroscience*, 19, 295–308.

Jobst, B. C. & Cascino, G. D. 2015. Resective epilepsy surgery for drug-resistant focal epilepsy: a review. *JAMA*, 313, 285–293. https://doi.org/10.1001/jama.2014.17426

Joensen, B. H., Bush, D., Vivekananda, U., Horner, A. J., Bisby, J. A., Diehl, B., Miserocchi, A., McEvoy, A. W., Walker, M. C. & Burgess, N. 2023. Hippocampal theta activity during encoding promotes subsequent associative memory in humans. *Cerebral Cortex*. https://doi.org/10.1093/cercor/bhad162

Johansen-Berg, H., Behrens, T. E., Robson, M. D., Drobnjak, I., Rushworth, M. F., Brady, J. M., Smith, S. M., Higham, D. J. & Matthews, P. M. 2004. Changes in connectivity profiles define functionally distinct regions in human medial frontal cortex. *Proceedings of the National Academy of Sciences U S A*, 101, 13335–40. https://doi.org/10.1073/pnas.0403743101

John, Y. J., Zikopoulos, B., García-Cabezas, M. Á. & Barbas, H. 2022. The cortical spectrum: a robust structural continuum in primate cerebral cortex revealed by histological staining and magnetic resonance imaging. *Frontiers in Neuroanatomy*, 16, A897237. https://doi.org/10.3389/fnana.2022.897237

Johnsen, S. H. W. & Rytter, H. M. 2021. Dissociating spatial strategies in animal research: critical methodological review with focus on egocentric navigation and the hippocampus. *Neuroscience & Biobehavioral Reviews*, 126, 57–78. https://doi.org/https://doi.org/10.1016/j.neubiorev.2021.03.022

Johnson, D. M. G., Illig, K. R., Behan, M. & Haberly, L. B. 2000. New features of connectivity in piriform cortex visualized by intracellular injection of pyramidal cells suggest that "primary" olfactory cortex functions like "association" cortex in other sensory systems. *Journal of Neuroscience*, 20, 6974–6982.

Johnson, P. L., Truitt, W., Fitz, S. D., Minick, P. E., Dietrich, A., Sanghani, S., Traskman-Bendz, L., Goddard, A. W., Brundin, L. & Shekhar, A. 2010. A key role for orexin in panic anxiety. *Nature Medicine*, 16, 111–115. https://doi.org/10.1038/nm.2075

Johnson, S. L., Turner, R. J. & Iwata, N. 2003. BIS/BAS levels and psychiatric disorder: an epidemiological study. *Journal of Psychopathology and Behavioral Assessment*, 25, 25–36.

Johnson, T. N., Rosvold, H. E. & Mishkin, M. 1968. Projections from behaviorally-defined sectors of the prefrontal cortex to the basal ganglia, septum and diencephalon of the monkey. *Experimental Neurology*, 21, 20–34.

Johnston, A. L. & File, S. E. 1988. Effects of ligands for specific 5-HT receptor subtypes in two animal tests of anxiety. *In:* Lader, M. (ed.) *Buspirone: a new introduction to the treatment of anxiety. Royal Society of Medicine Services International Congress and Symposium Series No. 133* (pp. 31–37). Royal Society of Medicine Services Ltd.

Johnston, D. & Gath, D. 1973. Arousal levels and attribution effects in diazepam-assisted flooding. *British Journal of Psychiatry*, 123, 463–466.

Johnston, J. N., Henter, I. D. & Zarate, C. A., Jr. 2023. The antidepressant actions of ketamine and its enantiomers. *Pharmacology and Therapeutics*, in press, 108431. https://doi.org/10.1016/j.pharmthera.2023.108431

Joshi, A., Salib, M., Viney, T. J., Dupret, D. & Somogyi, P. 2017. Behavior-dependent activity and synaptic organization of septo-hippocampal GABAergic neurons selectively targeting the hippocampal CA3 area. *Neuron*, 96, 1342–1357 e5. https://doi.org/10.1016/j.neuron.2017.10.033

Joyce, P. R. & Oakley-Browne, M. A. 1990. The epidemiology of panic and agoraphobia. *In:* McNaughton, N. & Andrews, G. (eds.) *Anxiety* (pp. 32–38). Dunedin: University of Otago Press.

Jung, M. W. & McNaughton, B. L. 1993. Spatial selectivity of unit activity in the hippocampal granular layer. *Hippocampus*, 3, 165–182.

Jung, M. W., Wiener, S. I. & McNaughton, B. L. 1994. Comparison of spatial firing characteristics of units in dorsal and ventral hippocampus of the rat. *The Journal of Neuroscience*, 14, 7347–7356.

Kaada, B. R., Rasmussen, E. W. & Kveim, O. 1962. Impaired acquisition of passive avoidance behavior by subcallosal, septal, hypothalamic, and insular lesions in rats. *Journal of Comparative and Physiological Psychology*, 55, 661–670.

Kahneman, D. 2011. *Thinking, fast and slow*. London, UK: Penguin Books.

Kahneman, D. & Tversky, A. 1979. Prospect theory: an analysis of decision under risk. *Econometrica*, 47, 263–291.

Kamin, L. J. 1968. 'Attention-like' processes in classical conditioning. *In:* Jones, M. R. (ed.) Miami symposium on the prediction of behaviour: aversive stimulation (pp. 9–31). Miami: University of Miami Press.

Kamin, L. J., Brimer, C. J. & Black, A. H. 1963. Conditioned suppression as a monitor of the fear of the CS in the course of avoidance training. *Journal of Comparative and Physiological Psychology*, 56, 497–501.

Kandel, E. R. & Hawkins, R. D. 1992. The biological basis of learning and individuality. *Scientific American*, 267, 79–86.

Kane, S. P. 2020. *Buspirone Hydrochloride, ClinCalc DrugStats Database, Version 20.1* [Online]. Available at: https://clincalc.com/DrugStats/Drugs/BuspironeHydrochloride [Accessed 7 September 2020].

Kant, G. J., Wylie, R. M., Vasilakis, A. A. & Ghosh, S. 1996. Effects of triazolam and diazepam on learning and memory as assessed using a water maze. *Pharmacology, Biochemistry and Behavior*, 53, 317–322.

Kapczinski, F., Curran, H. V., Gray, J. & Lader, M. 1994. Flumazenil has an anxiolytic effect in simulated stress. *Psychopharmacology (Berl)*, 114, 187–189.

Katherine Shear, M. D., Robert Jin, M. A., Ayelet Meron Ruscio, P. D., Ellen E. Walters, M. S. & Ronald C. Kessler, P. D. 2006. Prevalence and correlates of estimated DSM-IV child and adult separation anxiety disorder in the national comorbidity survey replication. *American Journal of Psychiatry*, 163, 1074–1083. https://doi.org/10.1176/ajp.2006.163.6.1074

Katz, R. J., Landau, P. S., Lott, M., Bystritsky, A., Diamond, B., Hoehn-Saric, R., Rosenthal, M. & Weise, C. 1993. Serotonergic (5-HT2) mediation of anxiety-therapeutic effects of serazepine in generalized anxiety disorder. *Biological Psychiatry*, 34, 41–44.

Kaviani, H., Gray, J. A., Checkley, S. A., Kumari, V. & Wilson, G. D. 1999. Modulation of the human acoustic startle reflex by emotionally-toned film-clips. *International Journal of Psychophysiology*, 32, 47–54.

Kawai, N. 2019a. Are snakes special in human fear learning and cognition? The preparedness theory of phobia and the fear module theory. *In:* Kawai, N. (ed.) *The fear of snakes* (Chapter 2, pp. 19–31). Singapore: Springer Nature Singapore Pte Ltd.

Kawai, N. 2019b. The underlying neuronal circuits of fear learning and the Snake Detection Theory (SDT). *In:* Kawai, N. (ed.) *The fear of snakes* (Chapter 3, pp. 33–58). Singapore: Springer Nature Singapore Pte Ltd.

Kazantzis, N., Luong, H. K., Usatoff, A. S., Impala, T., Yew, R. Y. & Hofmann, S. G. 2018. The processes of cognitive behavioral therapy: a review of meta-analyses. *Cognitive Therapy and Research*, 42, 349–357. https://doi.org/10.1007/s10608-018-9920-y

Kazmierska-Grebowska, P., Jankowski, M. M. & MacIver, M. B. 2023. Missing puzzle pieces in dementia research: HCN channels and theta oscillations. *Aging and Disease*, online. https://doi.org/10.14336/AD.2023.0607

Keck, P. E., Jr., McElroy, S. L., Tugrul, K. C., Bennett, J. A. & Smith, J. M. R. 1993. Antiepileptic drugs for the treatment of panic disorder. *Neuropsychobiology*, 27, 150–153.

Kehyayan, A., Wright, P., Marks, J., Matura, J. M., Axmacher, N., Herpertz, S. & Kessler, H. 2023. The influence of the behavioural inhibition system on the development of PTSD-like symptoms after presentation of a traumatic film in healthy subjects. *European Journal of Psychotraumatology*, 14, 2172258. https://doi.org/10.1080/20008066.2023.2172258

Kelly, D., Walter, C. J. S., Mitchell-Heggs, N. & Sargant, W. 1972. Modified leucotomy assessed clinically, physiologically and psychologically at six weeks and eighteen months. *British Journal of Psychiatry*, 120, 19–29.

Kendler, K. S., Neale, M. C., Kessler, R. C., Heath, A. C. & Eaves, L. J. 1992a. Generalized anxiety disorder in women: a population-based twin study. *Archives of General Psychiatry*, 49, 267–272.

Kendler, K. S., Neale, M. C., Kessler, R. C., Heath, A. C. & Eaves, L. J. 1992b. The genetic epidemiology of phobias in women: the interrelationship of agoraphobia, social phobia, situational phobia and simple phobia. *Archives of General Psychiatry*, 49, 273–281.

Kendler, K. S., Neale, M. C., Kessler, R. C., Heath, A. C. & Eaves, L. J. 1992c. Major depression and generalized anxiety disorder. Same genes, (partly) different environments? *Archives of General Psychiatry*, 49, 716–722.

Kensinger, E. A., Ullman, M. T. & Corkin, S. 2001. Bilateral medial temporal lobe damage does not affect lexical or grammatical processing: evidence from amnesic patient HM. *Hippocampus*, 11, 347–360.

Kesner, A. J., Calva, C. B. & Ikemoto, S. 2022. Seeking motivation and reward: roles of dopamine, hippocampus and supramammillo-septal pathway. *Progress in Neurobiology*, 102252. https://doi.org/https://doi.org/10.1016/j.pneurobio.2022.102252

Kesner, R. P. 1993. Paired associate learning in the rat: role of hippocampus, medial prefrontal cortex, and parietal cortex. *Psychobiology*, 21, 183–192.

Kesner, R. P. 1996. Parallels between animals and humans in terms of the neural foundations of memory: implication for Alzheimer's disease. *In:* Altman, H. J. & Altman, B. N. (eds.) *Alzheimer's and Parkinson's diseases* (pp. 209–220). New York: Plenum Press.

Kesner, R. P., Chiba, A. A. & Jackson-Smith, P. 1994a. Rats do show primacy and recency effects in memory for lists of spatial locations: a reply to Gaffan. *Animal Learning and Behaviour*, 22, 214–218.

Kesner, R. P. & DeSpain, M. J. 1988. Correspondence between rats and humans in the utilization of retrospective and prospective codes. *Animal Learning and Behaviour*, 16, 299–302.

Kesner, R. P. & Holbrook, T. 1987. Dissociation of item and order spatial memory in rats following medial prefrontal cortex lesions. *Neuropsychologia*, 25, 653–664.

Kesner, R. P., Hopkins, R. O. & Fineman, B. 1994b. Item and order dissociation in humans with prefrontal cortex damage. *Neuropsychologia*, 32, 881–891.

Kesner, R. P. & Novak, J. M. 1982. Serial position curve in rats: role of the dorsal hippocampus. *Science*, 218, 173–175.

Kessler, J., Irle, E. & Markowitsch, H. J. 1986. Korsakoff and alcoholic subjects are severely impaired in animal tasks of associative memory. *Neuropsychologia*, 24, 671–680.

Kessler, R. C. 2007. The global burden of anxiety and mood disorders: putting the European Study of the Epidemiology of Mental Disorders (ESEMeD) findings into perspective. *Journal of Clinical Psychiatry*, 68[suppl2], 10–19.

Kessler, R. C., Chiu, W. T., Demler, O., Merikangas, K. R. & Walters, E. E. 2005. Prevalence, severity, and comorbidity of 12-month DSM-IV disorders in the National Comorbidity Survey Replication. *Archives of General Psychiatry*, 62, 617–27. https://doi.org/10.1001/archpsyc.62.6.617

Kessler, R. C., Petukhova, M., Sampson, N. A., Zaslavsky, A. M. & Wittchen, H. U. 2012. Twelve-month and lifetime prevalence and lifetime morbid risk of anxiety and mood disorders in the United States. *International Journal of Methods in Psychiatric Research*, 21, 169–84. https://doi.org/10.1002/mpr.1359

Kew, B. M., Porter, R. J., Douglas, K. M., Glue, P., Mentzel, C. L. & Beaglehole, B. 2023. Ketamine and psychotherapy for the treatment of psychiatric disorders: systematic review. *BJPsych Open*, 9, e79. https://doi.org/10.1192/bjo.2023.53

Kim, A. J. & Anderson, B. A. 2020. Arousal-biased competition explains reduced distraction by reward cues under threat. *eNeuro*, ENEURO.0099-20.2020. https://doi.org/10.1523/eneuro.0099-20.2020

Kim, S. D., Rivers, S., Bevins, R. A. & Ayres, J. J. B. 1996. Conditioned stimulus determinants of conditioned response form in Pavlovian fear conditioning. *Journal of Experimental Psychology: Animal Behaviour*, 22, 87–104.

Kimble, D. P. 1969. Possible inhibitory functions of the hippocampus. *Neuropsychologia*, 7, 235–244.

Kimble, D. P. 1975. Choice behavior in rats with hippocampal lesions. *In:* Isaacson, R. L. & Pribam, K. H. (eds.) *The hippocampus, Vol. 2. Neurophysiology and behavior* (pp. 309–326). New York: Plenum Press.

Kinsbourne, M. & Wood, F. 1975. Short-term memory processes and the amnesic syndrome. *In:* Deutsch, D. & Deutsch, J. A. (eds.) *Short-term memory* (pp. 258–291). New York: Academic Press.

Király, B. & Hangya, B. 2020. Cartographers of the cognitive map: locus coeruleus is part of the guild. *Neuron*, 105, 951–953. https://doi.org/https://doi.org/10.1016/j.neuron.2020.02.020

Kirk, I. J. & McNaughton, N. 1991. Supramammillary cell firing and hippocampal rhythmical slow activity. *Neuroreport*, 2, 723–725.

Kirk, I. J. & McNaughton, N. 1993. Mapping the differential effects of procaine on frequency and amplitude of reticularly elicited hippocampal rhythmical slow activity. *Hippocampus*, 3, 517–526.

Kirk, I. J., Oddie, S. D., Konopacki, J. & Bland, B. H. 1996. Evidence for differential control of posterior hypothalamic, supramammillary, and medial mammillary theta-related cellular discharge by ascending and descending pathways. *The Journal of Neuroscience*, 16, 5547–5554.

Kirk, R. C., White, K. G. & McNaughton, N. 1988a. Low dose scopolamine affects discriminability but not rate of forgetting in delayed conditional discrimination. *Psychopharmacology*, 96, 541–546. https://doi.org/10.1007/BF02180037

Kirk, R. C., White, K. G. & McNaughton, N. 1988b. Low dose scopolamine affects discriminability but not rate of forgetting in delayed conditional discrimination. *Psychopharmacology*, 96, 541–546.

Kita, T., Nishijo, H., Eifuku, S., Terasawa, K. & Ono, T. 1995. Place and contingency differential responses of monkey septal neurons during conditional place-object discrimination. *The Journal of Neuroscience*, 15, 1683–1703.

Kjelstrup, K. G., Tuvnes, F. A., Steffenach, H.-A., Murison, R., Moser, E. I. & Moser, M.-B. 2002. Reduced fear expression after lesions of the ventral hippocampus. *Proceedings of the National Academy of Sciences*, 99, 10825–10830. https://doi.org/10.1073/pnas.152112399

Klein-Flügge, M. C., Bongioanni, A. & Rushworth, M. F. S. 2022. Medial and orbital frontal cortex in decision-making and flexible behavior. *Neuron*, 110, 2743–2770. https://doi.org/https://doi.org/10.1016/j.neuron.2022.05.022

Klein, D. F. 1993. The treatment of atypical depression. *European Journal of Psychiatry*, 8, 251–255.

Klein, D. F. 1995. Recognising panic disorder. *European Journal of Psychiatry*, 10 Suppl. 2, 61S–63S.

Knierim, J. J., Kudrimoti, H. S. & McNaughton, B. L. 1995. Place cells, head direction cells, and the learning of landmark stability. *The Journal of Neuroscience*, 15, 1648–1659.

Knowlton, B. J., Lavond, D. G. & Thompson, R. F. 1988. The effect of lesions of cerebellar cortex on retention of the classically conditioned eyeblink response when stimulation of the lateral reticular nucleus is used as the conditioned stimulus. *Behavioral and Neural Biology*, 49, 293–301.

Kocsis, B. & Kaminski, M. 2006. Dynamic changes in the direction of the theta rhythmic drive between supramammillary nucleus and the septo-hippocampal system. *Hippocampus*, 16, 531–540.

Kocsis, B. & Li, S. 2004. In vivo contribution of h-channels in the septal pacemaker to theta rhythm generation. *European Journal of Neuroscience*, 20, 2149–2158.

Kocsis, B., Martínez-Bellver, S., Fiáth, R., Domonkos, A., Sviatkó, K., Schlingloff, D., Barthó, P., Freund, T. F., Ulbert, I., Káli, S., Varga, V. & Hangya, B. 2022. Huygens synchronization of medial septal pacemaker neurons generates hippocampal theta oscillation. *Cell Reports*, 40, 111149. https://doi.org/10.1016/j.celrep.2022.111149

Koenigsberg, H. W., Pollak, C. P., Fine, J. & Kakuma, T. 1994. Cardiac and respiratory activity in panic disorder: effects of sleep and sleep lactate infusions. *American Journal of Psychiatry*, 151, 1148–1152.

Koh, M. T., Wheeler, D. S. & Gallagher, M. 2009. Hippocampal lesions interfere with long-trace taste aversion conditioning. *Physiology & Behavior*, 98, 103–107. https://doi.org/https://doi.org/10.1016/j.physbeh.2009.04.017

Kolb, B. 1984. Functions of the frontal cortex of the rat: a comparative review. *Brain Research Reviews*, 8, 65–98.

Kolb, B. 2010. Do all mammals have a prefrontal cortex? *Evolution of Nervous Systems*, 3, 443–450.

Kolb, B., Buhrmann, K., McDonald, R. & Sutherland, R. J. 1994. Dissociation of the medial prefrontal, posterior parietal, and posterior temporal cortex for spatial navigation and recognition memory in the rat. *Cerebral Cortex*, 6, 664–680.

Komisaruk, B. R. 1970. Synchrony between limbic system theta activity and rhythmical behaviours in rats. *Journal of Comparative and Physiological Psychology*, 70, 482–492.

Koolschijn, R. S., Emir, U. E., Pantelides, A. C., Nili, H., Behrens, T. E. J. & Barron, H. C. 2019. The hippocampus and neocortical inhibitory engrams protect against memory interference. *Neuron*, 101, 528–541.e6. https://doi.org/https://doi.org/10.1016/j.neuron.2018.11.042

Kopchia, K. L., Altman, H. J. & Commissaris, R. L. 1992. Effects of lesions of the central nucleus of the amygdala on anxiety-like behaviors in the rat. *Pharmacology, Biochemistry and Behavior*, 43, 453–461.

Korn, C. W. & Bach, D. R. 2019. Minimizing threat via heuristic and optimal policies recruits hippocampus and medial prefrontal cortex. *Nature Human Behaviour*, 3, 733–745. https://doi.org/10.1038/s41562-019-0603-9

Korotkova, T., Ponomarenko, A., Monaghan, C. K., Poulter, S. L., Cacucci, F., Wills, T., Hasselmo, M. E. & Lever, C. 2018. Reconciling the different faces of hippocampal theta: the role of theta oscillations in cognitive, emotional and innate behaviors. *Neuroscience & Biobehavioral Reviews*, 85, 65–80. https://doi.org/10.1016/j.neubiorev.2017.09.004

Koster, R., Chadwick, M. J., Chen, Y., Berron, D., Banino, A., Duzel, E., Hassabis, D. & Kumaran, D. 2018. Big-loop recurrence within the hippocampal system supports integration of information across episodes. *Neuron*, 99, 1342–1354 e6. https://doi.org/10.1016/j.neuron.2018.08.009

Kotov, R., Gamez, W., Schmidt, F. & Watson, D. 2010. Linking 'big' personality traits to anxiety, depressive, and substance use disorders: a meta-analysis. *Psychological Bulletin*, 136, 768–821. https://doi.org/10.1037/a0020327

Kotov, R., Jonas, K. G., Carpenter, W. T., Dretsch, M. N., Eaton, N. R., Forbes, M. K., Forbush, K. T., Hobbs, K., Reininghaus, U., Slade, T., South, S. C., Sunderland, M., Waszczuk, M. A., Widiger, T. A., Wright, Aidan G. C., Zald, D. H., Krueger, R. F., Watson, D. & Workgroup, H. U. 2020. Validity and utility of Hierarchical Taxonomy of Psychopathology (HiTOP): I. Psychosis superspectrum. *World Psychiatry*, 19, 151–172. https://doi.org/https://doi.org/10.1002/wps.20730

Kotov, R., Krueger, R. F. & Watson, D. 2018. A paradigm shift in psychiatric classification: the Hierarchical Taxonomy Of Psychopathology (HiTOP). *World Psychiatry*, 17 (February), 24–25. https://doi.org/10.1002/wps.20478

Kotov, R., Krueger, R. F., Watson, D., Achenbach, T. M., Althoff, R. R., Bagby, R. M., Brown, T. A., Carpenter, W. T., Caspi, A., Clark, L. A., Eaton, N. R., Forbes, M. K., Forbush, K. T., Goldberg, D., Hasin, D., Hyman, S. E., Ivanova, M. Y., Lynam, D. R., Markon, K., Miller, J. D., Moffitt, T. E., Morey, L. C., Mullins-Sweatt, S. N., Ormel, J., Patrick, C. J., Regier, D. A., Rescorla, L., Ruggero, C. J., Samuel, D. B., Sellbom, M., Simms, L. J., Skodol, A. E., Slade, T., South, S. C., Tackett, J. L., Waldman, I. D., Waszczuk, M. A., Widiger, T. A., Wright, A. G. & Zimmerman, M. 2017. The Hierarchical Taxonomy of Psychopathology (HiTOP): a dimensional alternative to traditional nosologies. *Journal of Abnormal Psychology*, 126, 454–477. https://doi.org/10.1037/abn0000258

Kotov, R., Krueger, R. F., Watson, D., Cicero, D. C., Conway, C. C., DeYoung, C. G., Eaton, N. R., Forbes, M. K., Hallquist, M. N., Latzman, R. D., Mullins-Sweatt, S. N., Ruggero, C. J., Simms, L. J., Waldman, I. D., Waszczuk, M. A. & Wright, A. G. C. 2021. The Hierarchical Taxonomy of Psychopathology (HiTOP): a quantitative nosology based on consensus of evidence. *Annual Review of Clinical Psychology*, 17, 83–108. https://doi.org/10.1146/annurev-clinpsy-081219-093304

Kovács, K. A. 2020. Episodic memories: how do the hippocampus and the entorhinal ring attractors cooperate to create them? *Frontiers in Systems Neuroscience*, 14, A559186. https://doi.org/10.3389/fnsys.2020.559186

Kowalczyk, T., Staszelis, A., Kaźmierska-Grębowska, P., Tokarski, K. & Caban, B. 2021. The role of the posterior hypothalamus in the modulation and production of rhythmic theta oscillations. *Neuroscience*, 470, 100–115. https://doi.org/https://doi.org/10.1016/j.neuroscience.2021.07.001

Krebs, J. R., Stephens, D. W. & Sutherland, W. J. 1983. Perspectives in optimal foraging. *In:* Clark, G. A. & Brush, A. H. (eds.) *Perspectives in ornithology* (pp. 165–221). Cambridge: Cambridge University Press.

Kropff, E., Carmichael, J. E., Moser, E. I. & Moser, M.-B. 2021. Frequency of theta rhythm is controlled by acceleration, but not speed, in running rats. *Neuron*, 109, 1029–1039.e8. https://doi.org/https://doi.org/10.1016/j.neuron.2021.01.017

Krout, K. E., Jansen, A. S. P. & Loewy, A. D. 1998. Periaqueductal gray matter projection to the parabrachial nucleus in rat. *Journal of Comparative Neurology*, 401, 437–454. https://doi.org/https://doi.org/10.1002/(SICI)1096-9861(19981130)401:4<437::AID-CNE2>3.0.CO;2-5

Krueger, J. N., Wilmot, J. H., Teratani-Ota, Y., Puhger, K. R., Nemes, S. E., Crestani, A. P., Lafreniere, M. M. & Wiltgen, B. J. 2020. Amnesia for context fear is caused by widespread disruption of hippocampal activity. *Neurobiology of Learning and Memory*, 175, 107295. https://doi.org/https://doi.org/10.1016/j.nlm.2020.107295

Krueger, R. F., Hobbs, K. A., Conway, C. C., Dick, D. M., Dretsch, M. N., Eaton, N. R., Forbes, M. K., Forbush, K. T., Keyes, K. M., Latzman, R. D., Michelini, G., Patrick, C. J., Sellbom, M., Slade, T., South, S. C., Sunderland, M., Tackett, J., Waldman, I., Waszczuk, M. A., Wright, A. G. C., Zald, D. H., Watson, D., Kotov, R. & HiTOP Utility Workgroup 2021. Validity and utility of Hierarchical Taxonomy of Psychopathology (HiTOP): II. Externalizing superspectrum. *World Psychiatry*, 20, 171–193.

Krueger, R. F. & Markon, K. E. 2014. The role of the DSM-5 personality trait model in moving toward a quantitative and empirically based approach to classifying personality and psychopathology. *Annual Review of Clinical Psychology*, 10, 477–501. https://doi.org/10.1146/annurev-clinpsy-032813-153732

Krupić, D., Corr, P. J., Ručević, S., Križanić, V. & Gračanin, A. 2016. Five reinforcement sensitivity theory (RST) of personality questionnaires: comparison, validity and generalization. *Personality and Individual Differences*, 97, 19–24. https://doi.org/https://doi.org/10.1016/j.paid.2016.03.012

Krystal, J. H., Abdallah, C. G., Sanacora, G., Charney, D. S. & Duman, R. S. 2019. Ketamine: a paradigm shift for depression research and treatment. *Neuron*, 101, 774–778. https://doi.org/10.1016/j.neuron.2019.02.005

Krzywkowski, P., Penna, B. & Gross, C. T. 2020. Dynamic encoding of social threat and spatial context in the hypothalamus. *eLife*, 9, e57148. https://doi.org/10.7554/eLife.57148

Kubie, J. L., Levy, E. R. J. & Fenton, A. A. 2020. Is hippocampal remapping the physiological basis for context? *Hippocampus*, 30, 851–864. https://doi.org/https://doi.org/10.1002/hipo.23160

Kubie, J. L. & Ranck, J. B., Jr. 1983. Sensory-behavioural correlates in individual hippocampus neurons in three situations: space and context. *In:* Seifert, W. (ed.) *Neurobiology of the hippocampus* (pp. 433–448). London: Academic Press.

Kunz, L., Brandt, A., Reinacher, P. C., Staresina, B. P., Reifenstein, E. T., Weidemann, C. T., Herweg, N. A., Patel, A., Tsitsiklis, M., Kempter, R., Kahana, M. J., Schulze-Bonhage, A. & Jacobs, J. 2021. A neural code for egocentric spatial maps in the human medial temporal lobe. *Neuron*, 109, 2781–2796.e10. https://doi.org/https://doi.org/10.1016/j.neuron.2021.06.019

Kurth, F., Zilles, K., Fox, P. T., Laird, A. R. & Eickhoff, S. B. 2010. A link between the systems: functional differentiation and integration within the human insula revealed by meta-analysis. *Brain Structure and Function*, 214, 519–34. https://doi.org/10.1007/s00429-010-0255-z

La-Vu, M. Q., Sethi, E., Maesta-Pereira, S., Schuette, P. J., Tobias, B. C., Reis, F., Wang, W., Torossian, A., Bishop, A., Leonard, S. J., Lin, L., Cahill, C. M. & Adhikari, A. 2022. Sparse genetically defined neurons refine the canonical role of periaqueductal gray columnar organization. *eLife*, 11. https://doi.org/10.7554/eLife.77115

LaChance, P. A., Dumont, J. R., Ozel, P., Marcroft, J. L. & Taube, J. S. 2020. Commutative properties of head direction cells during locomotion in 3D: are all routes equal? *The Journal of Neuroscience*, 40, 3035–3051. https://doi.org/10.1523/jneurosci.2789-19.2020

Lader, M. H. 1967. Palmar skin conductance measures in anxiety and phobic states. *Journal of Psychosomatic Research*, 11, 271–281.

Lader, M. H. 1975. *The psychophysiology of mental illness*. London, Routledge & Kegan Paul.

Lader, M. H. 1990. Introduction: use and abuse. *In: In the anxiolytic jungle: where next?* (ed. D. Wheatley), pp. 3–7. Chichester: Wiley.

Lader, M. H. & Mathews, A. 1970. Physiological changes during spontaneous panic attacks. *Journal of Psychosomatic Research*, 14, 377–382.

Lader, M. & Tyrer, P. 1975. Vegetative system and emotion. *In:* Levi, L. (ed.) *Emotions: their parameters and measurement*. New York: Raven Press.

Lader, M. H. & Wing, L. 1966. *Physiological measures, sedative drugs, and morbid anxiety. Maudsley Monographs, Vol. 18*. London: Oxford University Press.

Lages, Y. V. & McNaughton, N. 2022. Non-human contributions to personality neuroscience – from fish through primates. An introduction to the special issue. *Personality Neuroscience*, 5, e11. https://doi.org/10.1017/pen.2022.4

Lai, C. H. 2019. Fear network model in panic disorder: the past and the future. *Psychiatry Investigations*, 16, 16–26. https://doi.org/10.30773/pi.2018.05.04.2

Lai, R., Katalinic, N., Glue, P., Somogyi, A. A., Mitchell, P. B., Leyden, J., Harper, S., & Loo, C. K. 2014. Pilot dose-response trial of i.v. ketamine in treatment-resistant depression. *World Journal of Biological Psychiatry*, 15, 579–84. https://doi.org/10.3109/15622975.2014.922697

Lamprecht, R., Dracheva, S., Assoun, S. & LeDoux, J. E. 2009. Fear conditioning induces distinct patterns of gene expression in lateral amygdala. *Genes, Brain and Behavior*, 8, 735–743.

LaRocco, J., Le, M. D. & Paeng, D. G. 2020. A systemic review of available low-cost eeg headsets used for drowsiness detection. *Frontiers in Neuroinformatics*, 14, 553352. https://doi.org/10.3389/fninf.2020.553352

Lathe, R. 2001. Hormones and the hippocampus. *Journal of Endocrinology*, 169, 205–231. https://doi.org/10.1677/joe.0.1690205

Latuske, P., Kornienko, O., Kohler, L. & Allen, K. 2018. Hippocampal remapping and its entorhinal origin. *Frontiers in Behavioral Neuroscience*, 11, A0253. https://doi.org/10.3389/fnbeh.2017.00253

Laumann, T. O., Zorumski, C. F. & Dosenbach, N. U. F. 2023. Precision neuroimaging for localization-related psychiatry. *JAMA Psychiatry*, online. https://doi.org/10.1001/jamapsychiatry.2023.1576

Laurent, G., Fournier, J., Hemberger, M., Muller, C., Naumann, R., Ondracek, J. M., Pammer, L., Reiter, S., Shein-Idelson, M., Tosches, M. A. & Yamawaki, T. 2016. Cortical Evolution: introduction to the reptilian cortex. *In:* Buzsaki, G. & Christen, Y. (eds.) *Micro-, meso- and macro-dynamics of the brain* (pp. 23–33). Cham (CH).

Layfield, D., Sidell, N., Blankenberger, K. & Newman, E. L. 2023. Hippocampal inactivation during rearing on hind legs impairs spatial memory. *Scientific Reports*, 13, 6136. https://doi.org/10.1038/s41598-023-33209-9

Leake, J., Zinn, R., Corbit, L. H., Fanselow, M. S. & Vissel, B. 2021. Engram size varies with learning and reflects memory content and precision. *The Journal of Neuroscience*, 41, 4120–4130. https://doi.org/10.1523/jneurosci.2786-20.2021

Leal, G. C., Bandeira, I. D., Correia-Melo, F. S., Telles, M., Mello, R. P., Vieira, F., Lima, C. S., Jesus-Nunes, A. P., Guerreiro-Costa, L. N. F., Marback, R. F., Caliman-Fontes, A. T., Marques, B. L. S., Bezerra, M. L. O., Dias-Neto, A. L., Silva, S. S., Sampaio, A. S., Sanacora, G., Turecki, G., Loo, C., Lacerda, A. L. T. & Quarantini, L. C. 2021. Intravenous arketamine for treatment-resistant depression: open-label pilot study. *European Archives of Psychiatry and Clinical Neuroscience*, 271, 577–582. https://doi.org/10.1007/s00406-020-01110-5

Leaton, R. N. & Borszcz, G. S. 1985. Potentiated startle: its relation to freezing and shock intensity in rats. *Journal of Experimental Psychology: Animal Behaviour Processes*, 11, 421–428.

LeDoux, J. & Daw, N. D. 2018. Surviving threats: neural circuit and computational implications of a new taxonomy of defensive behaviour. *Nature Reviews Neuroscience*. https://doi.org/10.1038/nrn.2018.22

LeDoux, J. E. 1992. Emotion and the amygdala. *In:* Aggleton, J. P. (ed.) *The amygdala: neurobiological aspects of emotion, memory and mental dysfunction* (pp. 339–351). New York, Wiley-Liss.

LeDoux, J. E. 1994. Emotion, memory and the brain. *Scientific American*, 270, June, 50–59.

LeDoux, J. E. 1995. Emotion: clues from the brain. *Annual Review of Psychology*, 46, 209–235.

LeDoux, J. E. 1996. *The emotional brain*. New York: Simon and Schuster.

LeDoux, J. E. 2000. Emotion circuits in the brain. *Annual Review of Neuroscience*, 23, 155–184.

LeDoux, J. E. 2002. *Synaptic self*. Harmondsworth: Viking Penguin.

LeDoux, J. E. 2012. Rethinking the Emotional Brain. *Neuron*, 73, 653–676. https://doi.org/10.1016/j.neuron.2012.02.004

LeDoux, J. E. 2014. Coming to terms with fear. *Proceedings of the National Academy of Sciences*, 111, 2871–8. https://doi.org/10.1073/pnas.1400335111

LeDoux, J. E. 2015. *Anxious: the modern mind in the age of anxiety*. London: Oneworld Publications.

LeDoux, J. E. 2021. As soon as there was life, there was danger: the deep history of survival behaviours and the shallower history of consciousness. *Philosophical Transactions of the Royal Society B: Biological Sciences*, 377, 20210292. https://doi.org/doi:10.1098/rstb.2021.0292

LeDoux, J. E., Romanski, L. & Xagoraris, A. 1989. Indelibility of subcortical emotional memories. *Journal of Cognitive Neuroscience*, 1, 238–243.

Lee, M. G., Chrobak, J. J., Sik, A., Wiley, R. G. & Buzsáki, G. 1994. Hippocampal theta activity following selective lesion of the septal cholinergic system. *Neuroscience*, 62, 1033–1047.

Lee, S.-C., Amir, A., Haufler, D. & Pare, D. 2017. Differential recruitment of competing valence-related amygdala networks during anxiety. *Neuron*, 96, 81–88.e5. https://doi.org/10.1016/j.neuron.2017.09.002

Lee, S. L. T., Timmerman, B., Pflomm, R., Roy, N., Kumar, M. & Markus, E. J. 2023. Sequential order spatial memory in male rats: characteristics and impact of medial prefrontal cortex and hippocampus disruption. *Neurobiology of Learning and Memory*, 200, 107739. https://doi.org/10.1016/j.nlm.2023.107739

Lehr, A. B., Kumar, A., Tetzlaff, C., Hafting, T., Fyhn, M. & Stöber, T. M. 2021. CA2 beyond social memory: evidence for a fundamental role in hippocampal information processing. *Neuroscience & Biobehavioral Reviews*, 126, 398–412. https://doi.org/https://doi.org/10.1016/j.neubiorev.2021.03.020

Leichnetz, G. P. & Astruc, J. 1976. The efferent projections of the medial prefrontal cortex in the squirrel monkey (Saimiri sciureus). *Brain Research*, 109, 455–472.

Lelliott, P., Marks, I., McNamee, G. & Tobeña, A. 1989. Onset of panic disorder with agoraphobia. *Archives of General Psychiatry*, 46, 1000–1004.

Lenneberg, E. H. 1967. *Biological foundations of language*. New York: Wiley.

León, L. A., Castro-Gomes, V., Zárate-Guerrero, S., Corredor, K., Mello Cruz, A. P., Brandão, M. L., Cardenas, F. P., & Landeira-Fernandez, J. 2017. Behavioral effects of systemic, infralimbic and prelimbic injections of a serotonin 5-HT2a antagonist in carioca high- and low-conditioned freezing rats. *Frontiers in Behavioral Neuroscience*, 11, A117. https://doi.org/10.3389/fnbeh.2017.00117

Leonard, K. & Abramovitch, A. 2019. Cognitive functions in young adults with generalized anxiety disorder. *European Psychiatry*, 56, 1–7. https://doi.org/10.1016/j.eurpsy.2018.10.008

Lerner, I., Lupkin, S. M., Tsai, A., Khawaja, A. & Gluck, M. A. 2021. Sleep to remember, sleep to forget: rapid eye movement sleep can have inverse effects on recall and generalization of fear memories. *Neurobiology of Learning and Memory*, 180, 107413. https://doi.org/https://doi.org/10.1016/j.nlm.2021.107413

Leue, A., Reuter, M., Corr, P. J. & Ettinger, U. 2022. Construct validity of questionnaires for the original and revised reinforcement sensitivity theory. *Frontiers in Psychology*, 13, A1026894. https://doi.org/10.3389/fpsyg.2022.1026894

Levinson, A. R., Speed, B. C., Infantolino, Z. P. & Hajcak, G. 2017. Reliability of the electrocortical response to gains and losses in the doors task. *Psychophysiology*, in press. https://doi.org/10.1111/psyp.12813

Levis, D. J. & Hare, N. P. 1977. A review of the theoretical rationale and empirical support for the extinction approach of implosive (flooding) therapy. *In:* Hersen, M., Eisler, R. M. & Moller, P. M. (eds.) *Progressive behavior modification, Vol. 4* (pp. 299–376). New York: Academic Press.

Li, M., Kinney, J. L., Jiang, Y. Q., Lee, D. K., Wu, Q., Lee, D., Xiong, W. C. & Sun, Q. 2023. Hypothalamic supramammillary nucleus selectively excites hippocampal CA3 interneurons to suppress CA3 pyramidal neuron activity. *Journal of Neuroscience*, 43, 4612–4624. https://doi.org/10.1523/JNEUROSCI.1910-22.2023

Li, R. C. C.-s., Huang, C. n., Constable, R. T. d. & Sinha, R. j. 2006. Imaging response inhibition in a stop-signal task: neural correlates independent of signal monitoring and post-response processing. *Journal of Neuroscience*, 26, 186–192.

Li, S. & Kirouac, G. J. 2012. Sources of inputs to the anterior and posterior aspects of the paraventricular nucleus of the thalamus. *Brain Structure and Function*, 217, 257–273. https://doi.org/10.1007/s00429-011-0360-7

Li, X. B., Inoue, T., Hashimoto, S. & Koyama, T. 2001. Effect of chronic administration of flesinoxan and fluvoxamine on freezing behavior induced by conditioned fear. *European Journal of Pharmacology*, 425, 43–50.

Lian, Y. & Burkitt, A. N. 2021. Learning an efficient hippocampal place map from entorhinal inputs using non-negative sparse coding. *eNeuro*, 8, ENEURO.0557-20.2021. https://doi.org/10.1523/eneuro.0557-20.2021

Lickley, R. A. & Sebastian, C. L. 2018. The neural basis of reactive aggression and its development in adolescence. *Psychology, Crime & Law*, 24, 313–333. https://doi.org/10.1080/1068316x.2017.1420187

Liebman, J. M., Mayer, D. J. & Liebeskind, J. C. 1970. Mesencephalic central gray lesions and fear-motivated behavior in rats. *Brain Research*, 23, 353–370.

Lin, J., Li, L., Pan, N., Liu, X., Zhang, X., Suo, X., Kemp, G. J., Wang, S. & Gong, Q. 2023. Neural correlates of neuroticism: a coordinate-based meta-analysis of resting-state functional brain imaging studies. *Neuroscience & Biobehavioural Reviews*, 146, 105055. https://doi.org/10.1016/j.neubiorev.2023.105055

Linden, D. J. 1999. The return of the spike: postsynaptic action potentials and the induction of LTP and LTD. *Neuron*, 22, 661–666.

Lindner, K., Neubert, J., Pfannmoller, J., Lotze, M., Hamm, A. O. & Wendt, J. 2015. Fear-potentiated startle processing in humans: parallel fMRI and orbicularis EMG assessment during cue conditioning and extinction. *International Journal of Psychophysiology*, 98, 535–45. https://doi.org/10.1016/j.ijpsycho.2015.02.025

Lindquist, D. H. 2020. Emotion in motion: a three-stage model of aversive classical conditioning. *Neuroscience & Biobehavioral Reviews*, 115, 363–377. https://doi.org/https://doi.org/10.1016/j.neubiorev.2020.04.025

Lindsay, G. W., Rigotti, M., Warden, M. R., Miller, E. K. & Fusi, S. 2017. Hebbian Learning in a Random Network Captures Selectivity Properties of the Prefrontal Cortex. *The Journal of Neuroscience*, 37, 11021–11036. https://doi.org/10.1523/jneurosci.1222-17.2017

Lindsley, O. R. 1990. Precision teaching: by teachers for children. *Teaching Exceptional Children*, 22, 10–15.

Lingawi, N. W., Laurent, V., Westbrook, R. F. & Holmes, N. M. 2021. Acquisition and extinction of second-order context conditioned fear: role of the amygdala. *Neurobiology of Learning and Memory*, 183, 107485. https://doi.org/https://doi.org/10.1016/j.nlm.2021.107485

Lippold, J. V., Ettinger, U., Hurlemann, R., Corr, P. J., Reuter, M. & Perkins, A. M. 2020. Differentiating anxiety from fear: an experimental-pharmacological approach. *Personality Neuroscience*, 3, e6. https://doi.org/10.1017/pen.2020.1

Liu, J., Lin, L. & Wang, D. V. 2021. Representation of fear of heights by basolateral amygdala neurons. *The Journal of Neuroscience*, 41, 1080–1091. https://doi.org/10.1523/jneurosci.0483-20.2020

Liu, Z., Le, Q., Lv, Y., Chen, X., Cui, J., Zhou, Y., Cheng, D., Ma, C., Su, X., Xiao, L., Yang, R., Zhang, J., Ma, L. & Liu, X. 2022. A distinct D1-MSN subpopulation down-regulates dopamine to promote negative emotional state. *Cell Research*, 32, 139-156 https://doi.org/10.1038/s41422-021-00588-5

Livermore, J. J. A., Klaassen, F. H., Bramson, B., Hulsman, A. M., Meijer, S. W., Held, L., Klumpers, F., de Voogd, L. D. & Roelofs, K. 2021. Approach-avoidance decisions under threat: the role of autonomic psychophysiological states. *Frontiers in Neuroscience*, 15, A621517. https://doi.org/10.3389/fnins.2021.621517

Logan, C. G. & Grafton, S. T. 1995. Functional anatomy of human eyeblink conditioning determined with regional cerebral glucose metabolism and positron-emission tomography. *Proceedings of the National Academy of Sciences of the United States of America*, 92, 7500–7504.

Lomi, E., Mathiasen, M. L., Yin Cheng, H., Zhang, N., Aggleton, J. P., Mitchell, A. S. & Jeffery, K. J. 2021. Evidence for two distinct thalamocortical circuits in retrosplenial cortex. *Neurobiology of Learning and Memory*, 185, 107525. https://doi.org/https://doi.org/10.1016/j.nlm.2021.107525

Lommen, M. J. J., Engelhard, I. M., van de Schoot, R. & van den Hout, M. A. 2014. Anger: cause or consequence of posttraumatic stress? A prospective study of Dutch soldiers. *Journal of Traumatic Stress*, 27, 200–207. https://doi.org/https://doi.org/10.1002/jts.21904

Loo, C. K., Gálvez, V., O'Keefe, E., Mitchell, P. B., Hadzi-Pavlovic, D., Leyden, J., Harper, S., Somogyi, A. A., Lai, R., Weickert, C. S. & Glue, P. 2016. Placebo-controlled pilot trial testing dose titration and intravenous, intramuscular and subcutaneous routes for ketamine in depression. *Acta Psychiatrica Scandinavica*, 134, 48–56. https://doi.org/10.1111/acps.12572

Loonen, A. J. & Ivanova, S. A. 2018a. The evolutionary old forebrain as site of action to develop new psychotropic drugs. *Journal of Psychopharmacology*, 32, 1277–1285. https://doi.org/10.1177/0269881118798617

Loonen, A. J. M. & Ivanova, S. A. 2015. Circuits regulating pleasure and happiness: the evolution of reward-seeking and misery-fleeing behavioral mechanisms in vertebrates. *Frontiers in Neuroscience*, 9, A304. https://doi.org/10.3389/fnins.2015.00394

Loonen, A. J. M. & Ivanova, S. A. 2016. Circuits regulating pleasure and happiness: the evolution of the amygdalar-hippocampal-habenular connectivity in vertebrates. *Frontiers in Neuroscience*, 10, A539. https://doi.org/10.3389/fnins.2016.00539

Loonen, A. J. M. & Ivanova, S. A. 2018b. Circuits regulating pleasure and happiness: evolution and role in mental disorders. *Acta Neuropsychiatrica*, 30, 29–42. https://doi.org/10.1017/neu.2017.8

Loonen, A. J. M. & Ivanova, S. A. 2019. Evolution of circuits regulating pleasure and happiness with the habenula in control. *CNS Spectrums*, 24, 233–238. https://doi.org/10.1017/S1092852917000748

Loonen, A. J. M. & Ivanova, S. A. 2022. Circuits regulating pleasure and happiness - focus on potential biomarkers for circuitry including the habenuloid complex. *Acta Neuropsychiatrica*, 34, 229–239, 1–11. https://doi.org/10.1017/neu.2022.15

Lopes-dos-Santos, V., van de Ven, G. M., Morley, A., Trouche, S., Campo-Urriza, N, & Dupret, D. 2018. Parsing hippocampal theta oscillations by nested spectral components during spatial exploration and memory-guided behavior. *Neuron*, 100, 940–952.e7. https://doi.org/10.1016/j.neuron.2018.09.031

Lovell, K., Marks, I. M., Noshirvani, H. & O'Sullivan, G. 1994. Should treatment distinguish anxiogenic from anxiolytic obsessive-compulsive ruminations? Results of a pilot controlled study and of a clinical audit. *Psychotherapy and Psychosomatics*, 61, 150–155.

Low, I. I. C., Williams, A. H., Campbell, M. G., Linderman, S. W. & Giocomo, L. M. 2021. Dynamic and reversible remapping of network representations in an unchanging environment. *Neuron*, 109, 2967–2980.e11. https://doi.org/https://doi.org/10.1016/j.neuron.2021.07.005

Ludwig, V. U., Nüsser, C., Goschke, T., Wittfoth-Schardt, D., Wiers, C. E., Erk, S., Schott, B. H. & Walter, H. 2015. Delay discounting without decision-making: medial prefrontal cortex and amygdala activations reflect immediacy processing and correlate with impulsivity and anxious-depressive traits. *Frontiers in Behavioral Neuroscience*, 9, A280. https://doi.org/10.3389/fnbeh.2015.00280

Luyten, L., Vansteenwegen, D., van Kuyck, K., Gabriëls, L. & Nuttin, B. 2011. Contextual conditioning in rats as an animal model for generalized anxiety disorder. *Cognitive, Affective, & Behavioral Neuroscience*, 11, 228–244. https://doi.org/10.3758/s13415-011-0021-6

Lynch, M. A., Lindsay, J. & Ounsted, C. 1975. Tranquilizers causing aggression. *British Medical Journal*, No. 5952, 260–260.

Maack, D. J. & Ebesutani, C. 2018. A re-examination of the BIS/BAS scales: evidence for BIS and BAS as unidimensional scales. *International Journal of Methods in Psychiatric Research*, in press, e1612. https://doi.org/doi:10.1002/mpr.1612

Maas, J. W. 1963. Neurochemical differences between two strains of mice. *Nature*, 197, 255–257.

Machado-Vieira, R., Salvadore, G., Luckenbaugh, D. A., Manji, K. H. & Zarate, C. A. 2008. Rapid onset of antidepressant action: a new paradigm in the research and treatment of major depression. *Journal of Clinical Psychiatry* 69, 946–958.

MacKay, D. G. 1987. *The organization of perception and action: a theory for language and other cognitive skills*. New York, Springer-Verlag.

Mackintosh, N. J. 1973. Stimulus selection: learning to ignore stimuli that predict no change in reinforcement. *In:* Hinde, R. A. & Stevenson-Hinde, J. T. (eds.) *Constraints on learning* (pp. 75–96). London: Academic Press.

Mackintosh, N. J. 1974. *The psychology of animal learning*. New York, Academic Press.

Mackintosh, N. J. 1978. Cognitive or associative theories of conditioning: implications of an analysis of blocking. *In:* Hulse, S. H., Fowler, H. & Honig, W. K. (eds.) *Cognitive processes in animal behavior* (pp. 155–175). Hillsdale, NJ: Erlbaum.

Macphail, E. M. 1996. Cognitive function in mammals: the evolutionary perspective. *Cognitive Brain Research*, 3, 279–290.

Macrides, F., Davis, B. J., Youngs, W. M., Nadi, N. S. & Margolis, F. L. 1981. Cholinergic and catecholaminergic afferents to the olfactory bulb in the hamster: a neuroanatomical, biochemical, and histochemical investigation. *The Journal of Comparative Neurology*, 203, 495–514.

Magee, J. C. 1998. Dendritic hyperpolarization-activated currents modify the integrative properties of hippocampal CA1 pyramidal neurons. *The Journal of Neuroscience*, 18, 7613–7624. https://doi.org/10.1523/jneurosci.18-19-07613.1998

Mahut, H. 1971. Spatial and object reversal learning in monkeys with partial temporal lobe ablations. *Neuropsychologia*, 9, 409–424.

Maierhofer, D., Anderer, P. & Dantendorfer, K. Impaired conditional discrimination in panic disorder patients. 21st Conference of Collegium Internationale Neuropsychopharmacologicum, Glasgow, 12th - 16th July. 1998 1998.

Mair, W. G. P., Warrington, E. K. & Weiskrantz, L. 1979. Memory disorder in Korsakoff's psychosis: a neuropathological and neuropsychological investigation of two cases. *Brain*, 102, 749–783.

Mao, D., Kandler, S., McNaughton, B. L. & Bonin, V. 2017. Sparse orthogonal population representation of spatial context in the retrosplenial cortex. *Nature Communications*, 8, A243. https://doi.org/10.1038/s41467-017-00180-9

Marcy, R. & Quermonne, M. A. 1974. An improved method for studying the psychogalvanic reaction in mice and its inhibition by psycholeptic drugs: comparison with the effects of other pharmacological agents. *Psychopharmacologia*, 34, 335–349.

Markon, K. E., Krueger, R. F. & Watson, D. 2005. Delineating the structure of normal and abnormal personality: an integrative hierarchical approach. *Journal of Personality and Social Psychology*, 88, 139–157.

Markou, A. & Cryan, J. F. 2012. Stress, anxiety and depression: toward new treatment strategies. *Neuropharmacology*, 62, 1–2. https://doi.org/10.1016/j.neuropharm.2011.09.023

Markowitsch, H. J. 1982. Thalamic mediodorsal nucleus and memory: a critical evaluation of studies in animals and man. *Neuroscience & Biobehavioral Reviews*, 6, 351–380.

Markowitsch, H. J., von Cramon, Y. D. & Schuri, U. 1993. Mnestic performance profile of a bilateral diencephalic infarct patient with preserved intelligence and severe amnesic disturbances. *Journal of Clinical and Experimental Neuropsychology*, 15, 627–652.

Marks, I. & Marks, M. 1990. Exposure treatment of agoraphobia/panic. *In:* Noyes, R., Jr., Roth, M. & Burrows, G. D. (eds.) *Handbook of anxiety, Vol 4: the treatment of anxiety* (pp. 293–310). Elsevier Science Publishers B.V.

Marks, I. M. 1969. *Fears and phobias*. London, Heinemann.

Marks, I. M. 1973. Reduction of fear: towards a unifying theory. *Canadian Psychiatry Association Journal*, 18, 9–12.

Marks, I. M. 1976. `Psychopharmacology': the use of drugs combined with psychological treatment. *In:* Spitzer, R. L. E. K. (ed.) *Evaluation of psychological therapies* (pp. 108–126). Baltimore: Johns Hopkins University Press.

Marks, I. M. 1987. Behavioural aspects of panic disorder. *American Journal of Psychiatry*, 144, 1160–1165.

Marks, I. M. 1988. The syndromes of anxious avoidance: classification of phobic and obsessive-compulsive phenomena. *In:* Noyes, R., Jr., Roth, M. & Burrows, G. D. (eds.) *Handbook of anxiety, Vol 2: classification, etiological factors and associated disturbances* (pp. 109–146). Elsevier Science Publishers B.V.

Marks, I. M., Birley, J. L. T. & Gelder, M. G. 1966. Modified Leucotomy in severe agoraphobia: a controlled serial inquiry. *British Journal of Psychiatry*, 112, 757–769.

Marks, I. M. & Nesse, R. M. 1994. Fear and fitness: an evolutionary analysis of anxiety disorders. *Ethology and Sociobiology*, 15, 247–261.

Marks, I. M., Swinson, R. P., Basoglu, M., Kuch, K., Noshirvani, H., O'Sullivan, G., Lelliott, P. T., Kirby, M., McNamee, G., Sengun, S. & Wickwire, K. 1993. Alprazolam and exposure alone and combined in panic disorder with agoraphobia. *British Journal of Psychiatry*, 162, 776–787.

Marks, J. 1990. The current role of benzodiazepines in anxiety. *In:* McNaughton, N. & Andrews, G. (eds.) *Anxiety* (pp. 109–113). Dunedin: University of Otago Press.

Markus, E. J., Barnes, C. A., McNaughton, B. L., Gladden, V. L. & Skaggs, W. E. 1994. Spatial information content and reliability of hippocampal CA1 neurons: effects of visual input. *Hippocampus*, 4, 410–421.

Markus, E. J., Qin, Y. L., Leonard, B., Skaggs, W. E., McNaughton, B. L. & Barnes, C. A. 1995. Interactions between location and task affect the spatial and directional firing of hippocampal neurons. *The Journal of Neuroscience*, 15, 7079–7094.

Maron, E. & Nutt, D. 2017. Biological markers of generalized anxiety disorder. *Dialogues in Clinical Neuroscience*, 19, 147–157.

Marr, D. & Poggio, T. 1976. Cooperative computation of stereo disparity. *Science*, 194, 283–287. https://doi.org/10.2307/1742217

Martinotti, G., Chiappini, S., Pettorruso, M., Mosca, A., Miuli, A., Di Carlo, F., D'Andrea, G., Collevecchio, R., Di Muzio, I., Sensi, S. L. & Di Giannantonio, M. 2021. Therapeutic potentials of ketamine and esketamine in obsessive–compulsive disorder (OCD), substance use disorders (SUD) and eating disorders (ED): a review of the current literature. *Brain Sciences*, 11, e856.

Martins, D., Rademacher, L., Gabay, A. S., Taylor, R., Richey, J. A., Smith, D. V., Goerlich, K. S., Nawijn, L., Cremers, H. R., Wilson, R., Bhattacharyya, S. & Paloyelis, Y. 2021. Mapping social reward and punishment processing in the human brain: a voxel-based meta-analysis of neuroimaging findings using the social incentive delay task. *Neuroscience & Biobehavioral Reviews*, 122, 1–17. https://doi.org/https://doi.org/10.1016/j.neubiorev.2020.12.034

Marwood, L., Wise, T., Kerr-Gaffney, J., Strawbridge, R., Williams, S. C. R., Cleare, A. J. & Perkins, A. 2022. Brain activity during pursuit and goal-conflict threat avoidance in major depressive disorder. *Personality Neuroscience*, 5, e9. https://doi.org/10.1017/pen.2022.1

Masserman, J. H. & Yum, K. S. 1946. An analysis of the influence of alcohol on experimental neuroses in cats. *Psychosomatic Medicine*, 8, 36–52.

Masuoka, T., Mikami, A., Yasuda, M., Shinomiya, K. & Kamei, C. 2007. Effects of histamine H(1) receptor antagonists on hippocampal theta rhythm during spatial memory performance in rats. *European Journal of Pharmacology*, 576, 77–82.

Matheson, G. K., Raess, B. U. & Tunnicliff, G. 1996. Effects of repeated doses of azapirones on rat brain 5-HT1A receptors and plasma corticosterone levels. *General Pharmacology*, 27, 355–361.

Mathews, A. 1978. Fear-reduction research and clinical phobias. *Psychological Bulletin*, 85, 390–404.

Mathews, A. 1993. Biases in processing emotional information. *The Psychologist*, 6, 493–499.

Mathews, A. & MacLeod, C. 1994. Cognitive approaches to emotion and emotional disorders. *Annual Review of Psychology*, 45, 25–50.

Mathews, A. & MacLeod, C. 2005. Cognitive vulnerability to emotional disorders. *Annual Review of Clinical Psychology*, 1, 167–95. https://doi.org/10.1146/annurev.clinpsy.1.102803.143916

Mathews, A., Yiend, J. & Lawrence, A. D. 2004. Individual differences in the modulation of fear-related brain activation by attentional control. *Journal of Cognitive Neuroscience*, 16, 1683–1694. https://doi.org/10.1162/0898929042947810

Mathews, A. M., Gelder, M. G. & Johnston, D. W. 1981. *Agoraphobia: nature and treatment*. New York: Guildford Press.

Mathiasen, M. L., Aggleton, J. P. & Witter, M. P. 2023. Projections of the insular cortex to orbitofrontal and medial prefrontal cortex: a tracing study in the rat. *Frontiers in Neuroanatomy*, 17, A1131167. https://doi.org/10.3389/fnana.2023.1131167

Mathuru, A. S. & Jesuthasan, S. 2013. The medial habenula as a regulator of anxiety in adult zebrafish. *Frontiers in Neural Circuits*, 7, Article 99. https://doi.org/10.3389/fncir.2013.00099

Matsumoto, M. & Hikosaka, O. 2009. Two types of dopamine neuron distinctly convey positive and negative motivational signals. *Nature*, 459, 837–41. https://doi.org/10.1038/nature08028

Matthews, G. & Gilliland, K. 1999. The personality theories of H. J. Eysenck and J. A Gray: a comparative review. *Personality and Individual Differences*, 26, 583–626.

Mattick, R. P. 1990. Social phobia: an overview of psychological concepts and treatments. *In:* McNaughton, N. & Andrews, G. (eds.) *Anxiety* (pp. 179–185). Dunedin: University of Otago Press.

Matveychuk, D., Thomas, R. K., Swainson, J., Khullar, A., MacKay, M.-A., Baker, G. B. & Dursun, S. M. 2020. Ketamine as an antidepressant: overview of its mechanisms of action and potential predictive biomarkers. *Therapeutic Advances in Psychopharmacology*, 10, 2045125320916657. https://doi.org/10.1177/2045125320916657

Mayes, A., Meudell, P. & Neary, D. 1980. Do amnesics adopt inefficient encoding strategies with faces and random shapes? *Neuropsychologia*, 18, 527–540. https://doi.org/https://doi.org/10.1016/0028-3932(80)90154-2

Mayes, A. R., Hunkin, N. M., Isaac, C. & Muhlert, N. 2019. Are there distinct forms of accelerated forgetting and, if so, why? *Cortex*, 110, 115–126. https://doi.org/https://doi.org/10.1016/j.cortex.2018.04.005

McCleary, R. A. 1966. Response-modulating functions of the limbic system: initation and suppression. *In:* Stellar, E. & Spargue, J. M. (eds.) *Progress in physiological psychology, Vol. 1* (pp. 209–272). New York: Academic Press.

McCrae, R. R. & Costa, P. T. J. 2008. The five-factor theory of personality. *In:* John, O. P., Robins, R. W. & Pervin, L. A. (eds.) *Handbook of personality: theory and research* (pp. 159–181). New York: Guilford Press.

McDonald, A. J., Mascagni, F. & Guo, L. 1996. Projections of the medial and lateral prefrontal cortices to the amygdala: a phaseolus vulgaris leucoagglutinin study in the rat. *Neuroscience*, 71, 55–75.

McEchron, M. D. & Disterhoft, J. F. 1997. Sequence of single neuron changes in CA1 hippocampus of rabbits during acquisition of trace eyeblink conditioned responses. *Journal of Neurophysiology*, 78, 1030–1044.

McEwen, B. S. & Akil, H. 2020. Revisiting the stress concept: implications for affective disorders. *The Journal of Neuroscience*, 40, 12–21. https://doi.org/10.1523/jneurosci.0733-19.2019

McEwen, B. S., Gould, E. A. & Sakai, R. R. 1992. The vulnerability of the hippocampus to protective and destructive effects of glucocorticoids in relation to stress. *British Journal of Psychiatry*, 154, 221–228.

McFarlane, A. C. 1989. The aetiology of post-traumatic morbidity: predisposing, precipitating and perpetuating factors. *British Journal of Psychiatry*, 154, 221–228. https://doi.org/10.1192/bjp.154.2.221

McGaughy, J., Kaiser, T. & Sarter, M. 1996. Behavioral vigilance following infusions of 192 IgG-saporin into the basal forebrain: selectivity of behavioral impairment and relation to cortical AChE-positive fiber density. *Behavioral Neuroscience*, 110, 247–265.

McGaughy, J. & Sarter, M. 1995. Behavioral vigilance in rats: task validation and effects of age, amphetamine, and benzodiazepine receptor ligands. *Psychopharmacology (Berl)*, 117, 340–357.

McGonigle, B., McFarland, D. J. & Collier, P. 1967. Rapid extinction following drug-inhibited incidental learning. *Nature*, 214, 531–532.

McKenzie, S., Huszár, R., English, D. F., Kim, K., Christensen, F., Yoon, E. & Buzsáki, G. 2021. Preexisting hippocampal network dynamics constrain optogenetically induced place fields. *Neuron*, 109, 1040–1054.e7. https://doi.org/https://doi.org/10.1016/j.neuron.2021.01.011

McLaughlin, I., Dani, J. A. & De Biasi, M. 2017. The medial habenula and interpeduncular nucleus circuitry is critical in addiction, anxiety, and mood regulation. *Journal of Neurochemistry*, 142, 130–143. https://doi.org/https://doi.org/10.1111/jnc.14008

McLaughlin, K. A., Borkovec, T. D. & Sibrava, N. J. 2007. The effects of worry and rumination on affect states and cognitive activity. *Behavior Therapy*, 38, 23–38. https://doi.org/https://doi.org/10.1016/j.beth.2006.03.003

McNally, G. P. 2021. Motivational competition and the paraventricular thalamus. *Neuroscience & Biobehavioral Reviews*, 125, 193–207. https://doi.org/https://doi.org/10.1016/j.neubiorev.2021.02.021

McNally, G. P., Johansen, J. P. & Blair, H. T. 2011. Placing prediction into the fear circuit. *Trends in Neurosciences*, 34, 283–292. https://doi.org/https://doi.org/10.1016/j.tins.2011.03.005

McNally, R. J. 2016. The legacy of Seligman's *Phobias and Preparedness* (1971). *Behavior Therapy*, 47, 585–594.

McNamara, R. K. & Skelton, R. W. 1991. Diazepam impairs acquisition but not performance in the Morris water maze. *Pharmacology, Biochemistry and Behavior*, 38, 651–658.

McNamara, R. K. & Skelton, R. W. 1992. Like diazepam, CL 218,872, a selective ligand for the benzodiazepine Omega-1 receptor subtype, impairs place learning in the Morris water maze. *Psychopharmacology (Berl)*, 107, 347–351.

McNamara, R. K. & Skelton, R. W. 1993. Effects of intracranial infusions of chlordiazepoxide on spatial learning in the Morris water maze. I. Neuroanatomical specificity. *Behavioural Brain Research*, 59, 175–191.

McNaughton, B. L., Barnes, C. A., Gerrard, J. L., Gothard, K., Jung, M. W., Knierim, J. J., Kudrimoti, H., Qin, Y., Skaggs, W. E., Suster, M. & Weaver, K. L. 1996a. Deciphering the hippocampal polyglot: the hippocampus as a path integration system. *The Journal of Experimental Biology*, 199, 173–185.

McNaughton, B. L., Barnes, C. A. & O'Keefe, J. 1983. The contributions of position, direction, and velocity to single unit activity in the hippocampus of freely-moving rats. *Experimental Brain Research*, 52, 41–49.

McNaughton, B. L., Battaglia, F. P., Jensen, O., Moser, E. I. & Moser, M. B. 2006a. Path integration and the neural basis of the 'cognitive map'. *Nature Reviews Neuroscience*, 7, 663–678.

McNaughton, B. L., Chen, L. L. & Markus, E. J. 1991. "Dead reckoning," landmark learning, and the sense of direction: a neurophysiological and computational hypothesis. *Journal of Cognitive Neuroscience*, 3, 190–202.

McNaughton, B. L., Leonard, B. & Chen, L. 1989. Cortical-hippocampal interactions and cognitive mapping: a hypothesis based on reintegration of the parietal and inferotemporal pathways for visual processing. *Psychobiology*, 17, 236–246.

McNaughton, N. 1985a. Chlordiazepoxide and successive discrimination: different effects on acquisition and performance. *Pharmacology, Biochemistry and Behavior*, 23, 487–494.

McNaughton, N. 1985b. The effects of systemic and intraseptal injections of sodium amylobarbitone on rearing and ambulation in rats. *Australian Journal of Psychology*, 37, 15–27.

McNaughton, N. 1985c. Is the hippocampus a store, intermediate or otherwise? *Behavioral and Brain Sciences*, 8, 508–509.

McNaughton, N. 1989a. Anxiety: one label for many processes. *New Zealand Journal of Psychology*, 18, 51–59.

McNaughton, N. 1989b. *Biology and emotion*. Cambridge: Cambridge University Press.

McNaughton, N. 1993. Stress and behavioural inhibition. *In:* Stanford, S. C. & Salmon, P. (eds.) *Stress: an integrated approach* (pp. 191–206). Academic Press.

McNaughton, N. 1994. The hippocampus: relational processor or anti-processor? *Behavioral and Brain Sciences*, 17, 487–488.

McNaughton, N. 1997. Cognitive dysfunction resulting from hippocampal hyperactivity - A possible cause of anxiety disorder. *Pharmacology, Biochemistry and Behavior*, 56, 603–611.

McNaughton, N. 2002. Aminergic transmitter systems. *In:* D'Haenen, H., Den Boer, J. A., Westenberg, H. & Willner, P. (eds.) *Textbook of biological psychiatry* (pp. 895–914). Chichester: John Wiley & Sons.

McNaughton, N. 2005. *Fears and anxieties: a map of your dark side*. Dunedin: University of Otago.

McNaughton, N. 2008a. The neurobiology of anxiety: potential for comorbidity of anxiety and substance use disorders. *In:* Stewart, S. H. & Conrod, P. J. (eds.) *Anxiety and substance use disorders: the vicious cycle of comorbidity* (pp. 19–33). New York: Springer Science+Business Media.

McNaughton, N. 2008b. Unscrambling the personality 0melette. *European Journal of Personality*, 22, 403–405.

McNaughton, N. 2011. Fear, anxiety and their disorders: past, present and future neural theories. *Psychology & Neuroscience*, 4, 173–181. https://doi.org/10.3922/j.psns.2011.2.002

McNaughton, N. 2018. What do you mean 'anxiety'? Developing the first anxiety syndrome biomarker. *Journal of the Royal Society of New Zealand*, 48, 177–190. https://doi.org/10.1080/03036758.2017.1358184

McNaughton, N. 2019. Brain maps of fear and anxiety. *Nature Human Behaviour*, 3, 662–663. https://doi.org/10.1038/s41562-019-0621-7

McNaughton, N. 2020. Personality neuroscience and psychopathology: should we start with biology and look for neural-level factors? *Personality Neuroscience*, 3, e4. https://doi.org/10.1017/pen.2020.5

McNaughton, N. 2022. Neuropsychological theory as a basis for clinical translation of animal models of neuropsychiatric disorder. *Frontiers in Behavioral Neuroscience*, 16. https://doi.org/10.3389/fnbeh.2022.877633

McNaughton, N., Azmitia, E. C., Williams, J. H., Buchan, A. & Gray, J. A. 1980a. Septal elicitation of hippocampal theta rhythm after localized deafferentation of serotoninergic fibres. *Brain Research*, 200, 259–269.

McNaughton, N. & Bannerman, D. 2024. The homogenous hippocampus: How hippocampal cells process goals. OSF, preprint. https://doi.org/10.31219/osf.io/a458n

McNaughton, N. & Coop, C. F. 1991. Neurochemically dissimilar anxiolytic drugs have common effects on hippocampal rhythmic slow activity. *Neuropharmacology*, 30, 855–863.

McNaughton, N. & Corr, P. J. 2004. A two-dimensional neuropsychology of defense: fear/anxiety and defensive distance. *Neuroscience & Biobehavioral Reviews*, 28, 285–305. https://doi.org/10.1016/j.neubiorev.2004.03.005

McNaughton, N. & Corr, P. J. 2008. Animal cognition and human personality. *In:* Corr, P. J. (ed.) *The reinforcement theory of personality* (pp. 95–119). Cambridge: Cambridge University Press. http://www.philipcorr.net/uploads/downloads/41.pdf.

McNaughton, N. & Corr, P. J. 2009. Central theories of motivation and emotion. *In:* Berntson, G. G. & Cacioppo, J. T. (eds.) *Handbook of neuroscience for the behavioural sciences. Vol. 2* (Chapter 36, pp. 710–730). Hoboken, New Jersey: John Wiley & Sons Inc. https://doi.org/10.1002/9780470478509.neubb00203.

McNaughton, N. & Corr, P. J. 2014. Approach, avoidance, and their conflict: the problem of anchoring. *Frontiers in Systems Neuroscience*, 8, A0124. https://doi.org/10.3389/fnsys.2014.00124

McNaughton, N. & Corr, P. J. 2016. Mechanisms of comorbidity, continuity, and discontinuity in anxiety-related disorders. *Development and Psychopathology*, 28, 1053–1069. https://doi.org/10.1017/S0954579416000699

McNaughton, N. & Corr, P. J. 2018. Survival circuits and risk assessment. *Current Opinion in Behavioral Sciences*, 24, 14–20. https://doi.org/10.1016/j.cobeha.2018.01.018

McNaughton, N. & Corr, P. J. 2019a. Hierarchical levels of control: the state-trait distinction. *Psychological Inquiry*, 30, 158–164. https://doi.org/10.1080/1047840x.2019.1646058

McNaughton, N. & Corr, P. J. 2019b. Sensitivity to punishment and reward: revisiting Gray (1970). *In:* Corr, P. J. (ed.) *Personality and individual differences: revisiting the classic studies* (Chapter 7, pp. 115–136). Los Angeles: Sage.

McNaughton, N. & Corr, P. J. 2022. The non-human perspective on the neurobiology of temperament, personality, and psychopathology: what's next? *Current Opinion in Behavioral Sciences*, 43, 255–262. https://doi.org/10.1016/j.cobeha.2021.11.005

McNaughton, N., Davis, N. M., Brookes, S., Rawlins, J. N. P., Feldon, J. & Gray, J. A. 1980b. Minor tranquillisers and hippocampal connections- some behavioural dissociations. *In:* Sinz, R. & Rosenzweig, M. R. (eds.) *Psychophysiology* (pp. 183–189). Amsterdam: Elsevier Biomedical Press.

McNaughton, N., DeYoung, C. G. & Corr, P. J. 2016. Approach/avoidance. *In:* Absher, J. R. & Cloutier, J. (eds.) *Neuroimaging personality, social cognition and character* (Chapter 2, pp. 25–49). San Diego: Elsevier.

McNaughton, N. & Glue, P. 2020. Ketamine and neuroticism: a double-hit hypothesis of internalizing disorders. *Personality Neuroscience*, 3, e2. https://doi.org/10.1017/pen.2020.2

McNaughton, N., James, D. T. D., Stewart, J., Gray, J. A., Valero, I. & Drewnowski, A. 1977. Septal driving of hippocampal theta rhythm as a function of frequency in the male rat: effects of drugs. *Neuroscience*, 2, 1019–1027.

McNaughton, N., Kocsis, B. & Hajós, M. 2007. Elicited hippocampal theta rhythm: a screen for anxiolytic and procognitive drugs through changes in hippocampal function? *Behavioural Pharmacology*, 18, 329–346. https://doi.org/10.1097/FBP.0b013e3282ee82e3

McNaughton, N., Logan, B., Panickar, K. S., Kirk, I. J., Pan, W., Brown, N. T. & Heenan, A. 1995a. Contribution of synapses in the medial supramammillary nucleus to the frequency of hippocampal theta rhythm in freely moving rats. *Hippocampus*, 5, 534–545.

McNaughton, N., Logan, B., Panickar, K. S., Kirk, I. J., Pan, W. X., Brown, N. T. & Heenan, A. 1995b. Contribution of synapses in the medial supramammillary nucleus to the frequency of hippocampal theta rhythm in freely moving rats. *Hippocampus*, 5, 534–45.

McNaughton, N. & Mason, S. T. 1980. The neuropsychology and neuropharmacology of the dorsal ascending noradrenergic bundle - a review. *Progress in Neurobiology*, 14, 157–219. https://doi.org/10.1016/0301-0082(80)90021-0

McNaughton, N. & Morris, R. G. M. 1987. Chlordiazepoxide, an anxiolytic benzodiazepine, impairs place navigation in rats. *Behavioural Brain Research*, 24, 39–46.

McNaughton, N. & Morris, R. G. M. 1992. Buspirone produces a dose-related impairment in spatial navigation. *Pharmacology, Biochemistry and Behavior*, 43, 167–171.

McNaughton, N., Owen, S., Boarder, M. R., Gray, J. A. & Fillenz, M. 1984. Responses to novelty in rats with lesions of the dorsal noradrenergic bundle. *New Zealand Journal of Psychology*, 13, 16–24.

McNaughton, N., Panickar, K. S. & Logan, B. 1996b. The pituitary-adrenal axis and the different behavioral effects of buspirone and chlordiazepoxide. *Pharmacology, Biochemistry and Behavior*, 54, 51–56. https://doi.org/10.1016/0091–3057(95)02129–9

McNaughton, N., Richardson, J. & Gore, C. 1986. Reticular elicitation of hippocampal slow waves: common effects of some anxiolytic drugs. *Neuroscience*, 19, 899–903.

McNaughton, N., Ruan, M. & Woodnorth, M. A. 2006b. Restoring theta-like rhythmicity in rats restores initial learning in the Morris water maze. *Hippocampus*, 16, 1102–1110

McNaughton, N. & Sedgwick, E. M. 1978. Reticular stimulation and hippocampal theta rhythm in rats: effects of drugs. *Neuroscience*, 3, 629–632.

McNaughton, N., Swart, C., Neo, P. S., Bates, V. & Glue, P. wrong-b. Anti-anxiety drugs reduce conflict-specific "theta"—A possible human anxiety-specific biomarker. *Journal of Affective Disorders*, 148, 104–111. https://doi.org/10.1016/j.jad.2012.11.057i

McNaughton, N., Swart, C., Neo, P. S. H., Bates, V. & Glue, P. 2013. Anti-anxiety drugs reduce conflict-specific "theta" – a possible human anxiety-specific biomarker. *Journal of Affective Disorders*, 148, 104–111. https://doi.org/10.1016/j.jad.2012.11.0571

McNaughton, N. & Vann, S. D. 2022. Construction of complex memories via parallel distributed cortical-subcortical iterative integration *Trends in Neurosciences*, 45, 550–562. https://doi.org/10.1016/j.tins.2022.04.006

McNaughton, N. & Wickens, J. 2003. Hebb, pandemonium and catastrophic hypermnesia: the hippocampus as a suppressor of inappropriate associations. *Cortex*, 39, 1139–1163. https://doi.org/10.1016/S0010-9452(08)70882-7

McNaughton, N. & Zangrossi, H. 2008. Theoretical approaches to the modeling of anxiety in animals. *In:* Blanchard, R. J., Blanchard, D. C., Griebel, G. & Nutt, D. J. (eds.) *Handbook of anxiety and fear* (Vol. 17, Chapter 2.1, pp. 11–27). Oxford, UK: Elsevier B.V. https://ddoi.org/10.1016/S1569-7339(07)00002-1.

McNish, K. A., Gewirtz, J. C. & Davis, M. 1997. Evidence of contextual fear after lesions of the hippocampus: a disruption of freezing but not fear-potentiated startle. *The Journal of Neuroscience*, 17, 9353–9360.

Meck, W. H. 1988. Hippocampal function is required for feedback control of an internal clock's criterion. *Behavioral Neuroscience*, 102, 54–60.

Meck, W. H., Church, R. M., Wenk, G. L. & Olton, D. S. 1987. Nucleus basalis magnocellularis and medial septal area lesions differentially impair temporal memory. *The Journal of Neuroscience*, 7, 3505–3511.

Medford, N. & Critchley, H. D. 2010. Conjoint activity of anterior insular and anterior cingulate cortex: awareness and response. *Brain Structure and Function*, 214, 535–549. https://doi.org/10.1007/s00429-010-0265-x

Medina, J. H., Paladini, A. C. & Izquierdo, I. 1993. Naturally occurring benzodiazepines and benzodiazepine-like molecules in brain. *Behavioural Brain Research*, 58, 1–8.

Meibach, R. C. & Siegel, A. 1977. Subicular projections to the posterior cingulate cortex in rats. *Experimental Neurology*, 57, 264–274.

Meldrum, B. S. 1975. Epilepsy and gamma-aminobutyric acid-mediated inhibition. *International Review of Neurobiology*, 17, 1–36.

Menard, J. & Treit, D. 1998. The septum and the hippocampus differentially mediate anxiolytic effects of R(+)-8-OH-DPAT. *Behavioural Pharmacology*, 9, 93–101.

Menard, J. & Treit, D. 2001. The anxiolytic effects of intra-hippocampal midazolam are antagonized by intra-septal L-glutamate. *Brain Research*, 888, 163–166.

Mendez-Ruette, M., Linsambarth, S., Moraga-Amaro, R., Quintana-Donoso, D., Mendez, L., Tamburini, G., Cornejo, F., Torres, R. F. & Stehberg, J. 2019. The role of the rodent insula in anxiety. *Frontiers in Physiology*, 10, A330. https://doi.org/10.3389/fphys.2019.00330

Menon, V. & Uddin, L. Q. 2010. Saliency, switching, attention and control: a network model of insula function. *Brain Structure and Function*, 214, 655–667. https://doi.org/10.1007/s00429-010-0262-0

Meunier, M., Bachevalier, J., Mishkin, M. & Murray, E. A. 1993. Effects on visual recognition of combined and separate ablations of the entorhinal and perirhinal cortex in rhesus monkeys. *The Journal of Neuroscience*, 13, 5418–5432.

Meunier, M., Hadfield, W., Bachevalier, J. & Murray, E. A. 1996. Effects of rhinal cortex lesions combined with hippocampectomy on visual recognition memory in rhesus monkeys. *Journal of Neurophysiology*, 75, 1190–1205.

Meyer, A. 2017. A biomarker of anxiety in children and adolescents: a review focusing on the error-related negativity (ERN) and anxiety across development. *Developmental and Cognitive Neuroscience*, 27, 58–68. https://doi.org/10.1016/j.dcn.2017.08.001

Meyer, T. J., Miller, M. L., Metzger, R. L. & Borkovec, T. D. 1990. Development and validation of the Penn state worry questionnaire. *Behaviour Research and Therapy*, 28, 487–495.

Michelini, G., Palumbo, I. M., DeYoung, C. G., Latzman, R. D. & Kotov, R. 2021. Linking RDoC and HiTOP: a new interface for advancing psychiatric nosology and neuroscience. *Clinical Psychology Reviews*, 86, 102025. https://doi.org/10.1016/j.cpr.2021.102025

Miczek, K. A. 1973. Effects of scopolamine, amphetamine and benzodiazepines on conditioned suppression. *Pharmacology, Biochemistry and Behavior*, 1, 401–411.

Miczek, K. A., Weerts, E. M., Vivian, J. A. & Barros, H. M. 1995. Aggression, anxiety and vocalizations in animals: GABAA and 5 HT anxiolytics. *Psychopharmacology (Berl)*, 121, 38–56.

Middleton, H. C., Ashby, M. & Robbins, T. W. 1994. Reduced plasma noradrenaline and abnormal heart rate variability in resting panic disorder patients. *Biological Psychiatry*, 36, 847–849.

Middleton, S. J. & McHugh, T. J. 2020. CA2: a highly connected intrahippocampal relay. *Annual Review of Neuroscience*, 43, 55–72. https://doi.org/10.1146/annurev-neuro-080719–100343

Milak, M. S., Rashid, R., Dong, Z., Kegeles, L. S., Grunebaum, M. F., Ogden, R. T., Lin, X., Mulhern, S. T., Suckow, R. F., Cooper, T. B., Keilp, J. G., Mao, X., Shungu, D. C. & Mann, J. J. 2020. Assessment of relationship of ketamine dose with magnetic resonance spectroscopy of Glx and GABA responses in adults with major depression: a randomized clinical trial. *JAMA Network Open*, 3, e2013211. https://doi.org/10.1001/jamanetworkopen.2020.13211

Milani, H. & Graeff, F. G. 1987. GABA-Benzodiazepine modulation of aversion in the medial hypothalamus of the rat. *Pharmacology, Biochemistry and Behavior*, 28, 21–27.

Millan, M. J. 2003. The neurobiology and control of anxious states. *Progress in Neurobiology*, 70, 83–244.

Millenson, J. R. 1967. Principles of behavioral analysis. New York: Macmillan.

Miller, A. M. P., Jacob, A. D., Ramsaran, A. I., De Snoo, M. L., Josselyn, S. A. & Frankland, P. W. 2023. Emergence of a predictive model in the hippocampus. *Neuron*. https://doi.org/10.1016/j.neuron.2023.03.011

Miller, C. L., Bickford, P. C., Wiser, A. K. & Rose, G. M. 1995. Long-term potentiation disrupts auditory gating in the rat hippocampus. *The Journal of Neuroscience*, 15, 5820–5830.

Miller, G. A., Galanter, E. H. & Pribram, K. H. 1960. *Plans and the structure of behavior*. New York: Rinehart and Winston.

Miller, N. E. 1944. Experimental studies of conflict. *In:* Hunt, J. M. (ed.) *Personality and the behavioural disorders* (pp. 431–465 (cited by Kimble 1961)). New York: Ronald Press.

Miller, N. E. 1951. Learnable drives and rewards. *In:* Stevens, S. S. (ed.) *Handbook of experimental psychology* (pp. 435–472). New York: Wiley.

Miller, R. 1989. Cortico-hippocampal interplay: self-organizing phase-locked loops for indexing memory. *Psychobiology*, 17, 115–128.

Miller, R. 1991. *Cortico-hippocampal interplay and the representation of contexts in the brain*. Berlin: Springer-Verlag.

Miller, R. R. 2021. Failures of memory and the fate of forgotten memories. *Neurobiology of Learning and Memory*, 181, 107426. https://doi.org/https://doi.org/10.1016/j.nlm.2021.107426

Miller, V. M. & Best, P. J. 1980. Spatial correlates of hippocampal unit activity are altered by lesions of the fornix and entorhinal cortex. *Brain Research*, 194, 311–323.

Milner, B. 1963. Effects of different brian lesions on card sorting. *Archives of Neurology*, 9, 90–100.

Milner, B. 1964. Some effects of frontal lobectomy in man. *In:* Warren, J. M. & Akert, K. (eds.) *The frontal granular cortex and behavior* (pp. 313–331). New York: McGraw-Hill.

Milner, B. 1970. Memory and the medial temporal regions of the brain. *In:* Pribram, K. H. & Broadbent, D. E. (eds.) *Biology of memory* (pp. 29–50). New York: Academic Press.

Milner, B. 1971. Interhemispheric differences and psychological processes. *British Medical Bulletin*, 27, 272–277.

Milner, B. 1995. Aspects of human frontal lobe function. *Advances in Neurology*, 66, 67–84.

Milner, B., Corkin, S. & Teuber, H. L. 1968. Further analysis of the hippocampal amnesic syndrome: 14-year follow-up study of H.M. *Neuropsychologia*, 6, 215–234.

Mineka, S. 1992. Evolutionary memories, emotional processing, and the emotional disorders. *The Psychology of Learning and Motivation*, 28, 161–206.

Mineka, S. & Öhman, A. 2002. Phobias and preparedness: the selective, automatic and encapsulated nature of fear. *Biological Psychiatry*, 52, 927–937.

Mitchell, D. J., McNaughton, N., Flanagan, D. & Kirk, I. J. 2008. Frontal-midline theta from the perspective of hippocampal "theta". *Progress in Neurobiology*, 86, 156–185. https://doi.org/10.1016/j.pneurobio.2008.09.005

Mizumori, S. J. Y., Miya, D. Y. & Ward, K. E. 1994. Reversible inactivation of the lateral dorsal thalamus disrupts hippocampal place representation and impairs spatial learning. *Brain Research*, 644, 168–174.

Mizumori, S. J. Y. & Williams, J. D. 1993. Directionally-selective mnemonic properties of neurons in the lateral dorsal nucleus of the thalamus of rats. *The Journal of Neuroscience*, 13, 4015–4028.

Mobbs, D., Hagan, C. C., Dalgleish, T., Silston, B. & Prevost, C. 2015. The ecology of human fear: survival optimization and the nervous system. *Frontiers in Neuroscience*, 9, A055. https://doi.org/10.3389/fnins.2015.00055

Mobbs, D. & Kim, J. J. 2015. Neuroethological studies of fear, anxiety, and risky decision-making in rodents and humans. *Current Opinion in Behavioral Sciences*, 5, 8–15. https://doi.org/10.1016/j.cobeha.2015.06.005

Mobbs, D., Petrovic, P., Marchant, J. L., Hassabis, D., Weiskopf, N., Seymour, B., Dolan, R. J. & Frith, C. D. 2007. When fear is near: threat imminence elicits prefrontal-periaqueductal gray shifts in humans. *Science*, 317, 1079–1083.

Mobbs, D., Trimmer, P. C., Blumstein, D. T. & Dayan, P. 2018. Foraging for foundations in decision neuroscience: insights from ethology. *Nature Reviews Neuroscience*, 19, 419–427. https://doi.org/10.1038/s41583-018-0010-7

Modigh, K. 1990. The pharmacology of clomipramine in anxiety disorders. *In:* McNaughton, N. & Andrews, G. (eds.) *Anxiety* (pp. 93–100). Otago: Otago University Press.

Mohebi, A., Pettibone, J. R., Hamid, A. A., Wong, J.-M. T., Vinson, L. T., Patriarchi, T., Tian, L., Kennedy, R. T. & Berke, J. D. 2019. Dissociable dopamine dynamics for learning and motivation. *Nature*, 570, 65–70. https://doi.org/10.1038/s41586-019-1235-y

Möhler, H. & Okada, T. 1977. Benzodiazepine receptor: demonstration in the central nervous system. *Science (NY)*, 198, 849–851.

Molnar Szakacs, I. & Uddin, L. Q. 2022. Anterior insula as a gatekeeper of executive control. *Neuroscience & Biobehavioral Reviews*, 139, 104736. https://doi.org/https://doi.org/10.1016/j.neubiorev.2022.104736

Money, E. A., Kirk, R. C. & McNaughton, N. 1992. Alzheimer's dementia produces a loss of discrimination but no increase in rate of memory decay in delayed matching to sample. *Neuropsychologia*, 30, 133–145.

Moore, H., Sarter, M. & Bruno, J. P. 1995. Bidirectional modulation of cortical acetylcholine efflux by infusion of benzodiazepine receptor ligands into the basal forebrain. *Neuroscience Letters*, 189, 31–34.

Morecraft, R. J., Stilwell-Morecraft, K. S., Cipolloni, P. B., Ge, J., McNeal, D. W. & Pandya, D. N. 2012. Cytoarchitecture and cortical connections of the anterior cingulate and adjacent somatomotor fields in the rhesus monkey. *Brain Research Bulletin*, 87, 457–497. https://doi.org/10.1016/j.brainresbull.2011.12.005

Morecraft, R. J. & Van Hoesen, G. W. 1998. Convergence of limbic input to the cingulate motor cortex in the rhesus monkey. *Brain Research Bulletin*, 45, 209–232.

Morel, C., Fernandez, S. P., Pantouli, F., Meye, F. J., Marti, F., Tolu, S., Parnaudeau, S., Marie, H., Tronche, F., Maskos, U., Moretti, M., Gotti, C., Han, M. H., Bailey, A., Mameli, M., Barik, J. & Faure, P. 2018. Nicotinic receptors mediate stress-nicotine detrimental interplay via dopamine cells' activity. *Molecular Psychiatry*, 23, 1597–1605. https://doi.org/10.1038/mp.2017.145

Morris, J., Firth, C. D., Perrett, D. I., Rowland, D. I., Young, A. W., Calder, A. J. & Dolan, R. J. 1996a. A differential neural response in the human amygdala to fearful and happy facial expressions. *Nature*, 383, 812–815.

Morris, R. G., Miotto, E. C., Feigenbaum, J. D., Bullock, P. & Polkey, C. E. 1997. The effect of goal-subgoal conflict on planning ability after frontal- and temporal-lobe lesions in humans. *Neuropsychologia*, 35, 1147–1157.

Morris, R. G., Pickering, A., Abrahams, S. & Feigenbaum, J. D. 1996b. Space and the hippocampal formation in humans. *Brain Research Bulletin*, 40, 487–490.

Morris, R. G. M. 1981. Spatial localisation does not require the presence of local cues. *Learning and Motivation*, 12, 239–260.

Morris, R. G. M. 1984. Development of a water-maze procedure for the study of spatial learning in the rat. *Journal of Neuroscience Methods*, 11, 47–60.

Morris, R. G. M., Garrud, P., Rawlins, J. N. P. & O'Keefe, J. 1982. Place navigation impaired in rats with hippocampal lesions. *Nature*, 297, 681–683.

Morris, R. G. M., Schenk, F., Tweedie, F. & Jarrard, L. E. 1990. Ibotenate lesions of hippocampus and/or subiculum: dissociating components of allocentric spatial learning. *European Journal of Neuroscience*, 2, 1016–1028.

Moscovitch, M., Cabeza, R., Winocur, G. & Nadel, L. 2016. Episodic memory and beyond: the hippocampus and neocortex in transformation. *Annual Review of Psychology*, 67, 105–134. https://doi.org/10.1146/annurev-psych-113011-143733

Moscovitch, M. & Gilboa, A. 2021. Systems consolidation, transformation and reorganization: Multiple Trace Theory, Trace Transformation Theory and their competitors. *In:* Kahana, M. J. & Wagner, A. D. (eds.) *The Oxford Handbook of Human Memory*. Oxford: Oxford University Press, in press, https://osf.io/preprints/psyarxiv/yxbrs.

Moscovitch, M., Rosenbaum, R. S., Gilboa, A., Addis, D. R., Westmacott, R., Grady, C., McAndrews, M. P., Levine, B., Black, S., Winocur, G. & Nadel, L. 2005. Functional neuroanatomy of remote episodic, semantic and spatial memory: a unified account based on multiple trace theory. *Journal of Anatomy*, 207, 35–66.

Moser, M. B. & Moser, E. I. 1998. Functional differentiation in the hippocampus. *Hippocampus*, 8, 608–619.

Moser, P. C., Hitchcock, J. M., Lister, S. & Moran, P. M. 2000. The pharmacology of latent inhibition as an animal model of schizophrenia. *Brain Research Reviews*, 33, 275–307. https://doi.org/https://doi.org/10.1016/S0165-0173(00)00026-6

Moses, S. N., Winocur, G., Ryan, J. D. & Moscovitch, M. 2007. Environmental complexity affects contextual fear conditioning following hippocampal lesions in rats. *Hippocampus*, 17, 333–337. https://doi.org/https://doi.org/10.1002/hipo.20275

Motta, S. C., Carobrez, A. P. & Canteras, N. S. 2017. The periaqueductal gray and primal emotional processing critical to influence complex defensive responses, fear learning and reward seeking. *Neuroscience & Biobehavioral Reviews*, 76, 39–47. https://doi.org/10.1016/j.neubiorev.2016.10.012

Mowrer, O. H. 1960. *Learning theory and behavior*. New York, Wiley.

Muir, G. M., Brown, J. E., Carey, J. P., Hirvonen, T. P., Della Santina, C. C., Minor, L. B. & Taube, J. S. 2009. Disruption of the head direction cell signal after occlusion of the semicircular canals in the freely moving chinchilla. *Journal of Neuroscience*, 29, 14521–14533. https://doi.org/10.1523/jneurosci.3450-09.2009

Muller, J., Pentyala, S., Dilger, J. & Pentyala, S. 2016. Ketamine enantiomers in the rapid and sustained antidepressant effects. *Therapeutic Advances in Psychopharmacology*, 6, 185 –192. https://doi.org/10.1177/

Muller, R. U. & Kubie, J. L. 1987. The effects of changes in the environment on the spatial firing of hippocampal complex-spike cells. *The Journal of Neuroscience*, 7(7), 1951–1968.

Muller, R. U., Kubie, J. L. & Ranck, J. B., Jr. 1987. Spatial firing patterns of hippocampal complex-spike cells in a fixed environment. *The Journal of Neuroscience*, 7(7), 1935–1950.

Mumby, D. G. 1995. Assessing working memory for objects in rats: no one said it was easy. *Neuroreport*, 6, 1960–1962.

Mumby, D. G. & Pinel, J. P. J. 1994. Rhinal cortex lesions and object recognition in rats. *Behavioral Neuroscience*, 108 (1), 11–18.

Mumby, D. G., Wood, E. R. & Pinel, J. P. J. 1992. Object-recognition memory is only mildly impaired in rats with lesions of the hippocampus and amygdala. *Psychobiology*, 20, 18–27. https://doi.org/10.3758/BF03327156

Munn, R. G. K. & McNaughton, N. 2008. Effects of fluoxetine on hippocampal rhythmic slow activity and behavioural inhibition. *Behavioural Pharmacology*, 19, 257–64. https://doi.org/10.1097/FBP.0b013e3282ff130 00008877-200805000-00010 [pii]

Murkar, A., De Koninck, J. & Merali, Z. 2021. Cannabinoids: revealing their complexity and role in central networks of fear and anxiety. *Neuroscience & Biobehavioral Reviews*, 131, 30–46. https://doi.org/https://doi.org/10.1016/j.neubiorev.2021.09.002

Murray, E. A. 1996. What have ablation studies told us about the neural substrates of stimulus memory? *The Neurosciences*, 8, 13–22.

Murray, H., Grey, N., Warnock-Parkes, E., Kerr, A., Wild, J., Clark, D. M. & Ehlers, A. 2022. Ten misconceptions about trauma-focused CBT for PTSD. *Cognitive Behavior Therapy*, 15, e33. https://doi.org/10.1017/S1754470X22000307

Muttoni, S., Ardissino, M. & John, C. 2019. Classical psychedelics for the treatment of depression and anxiety: a systematic review. *Journal of Affective Disorders*, 258, 11–24. https://doi.org/10.1016/j.jad.2019.07.076

Myers, J. S. 1971. Some effects of noncontingent aversive stimulation. *In:* Brush, F. R. (ed.) *Aversive conditioning and learning*. New York: Academic Press.

Nachev, P., Kennard, C. & Husain, M. 2008. Functional role of the supplementary and pre-supplementary motor areas. *Nature Reviews Neuroscience*, 9, 856–869. https://doi.org/10.1038/nrn2478

Nachev, P., Rees, G., Parton, A., Kennard, C. & Husain, M. 2005. Volition and conflict in human medial frontal cortex. *Current Biology*, 15, 122–128. https://doi.org/10.1016/j.cub.2005.01.006

Nachev, P., Wydell, H., O'Neill, K., Husain, M. & Kennard, C. 2007. The role of the pre-supplementary motor area in the control of action. *NeuroImage*, 36, T155-T163. https://doi.org/10.1016/j.neuroimage.2007.03.034

Nadel, L. 1991. The hippocampus and space revisited. *Hippocampus*, 1, 221–229.

Nadel, L. 2008. The hippocampus and context revisited. *In:* Mizumori, S. J. (ed.) *Hippocampal place fields: relevance to learning and memory* (pp. 3–15). Oxford: Oxford University Press.

Nadel, L. & Jacobs, W. J. 1996. The role of the hippocampus in PTSD, panic and phobia. *In:* Kato, N. (ed.) *The hippocampus: functions and clinical relevance* (pp. 455–463). Elsevier Science B.V.

Nadel, L. & Maurer, A. P. 2020. Recalling Lashley and reconsolidating Hebb. *Hippocampus*, 30, 776–793. https://doi.org/https://doi.org/10.1002/hipo.23027

Nagelhus, A., Andersson, S. O., Cogno, S. G., Moser, E. I. & Moser, M. B. 2023. Object-centered population coding in CA1 of the hippocampus. *Neuron*, 111, 2091–2104. https://doi.org/10.1016/j.neuron.2023.04.008

Nagpal, J., Herget, U., Choi, M. K. & Ryu, S. 2019. Anatomy, development, and plasticity of the neurosecretory hypothalamus in zebrafish. *Cell and Tissue Research*, 375, 5–22. https://doi.org/10.1007/s00441-018-2900-4

Nambua, A., Tokunob, H. & Takada, M. 2002. Functional significance of the cortico-subthalamo-pallidal 'hyperdirect' pathway. *Neuroscience Research*, 43, 111–117.

Näring, G. W. B. & Van der Staak, C. P. F. 1995. Perception of heart rate and blood pressure: the role of alexithymia and anxiety. *Psychotherapy and Psychosomatics*, 63, 193–200.

Nauta, W. J. H. & Feirtag, M. 1986. *Fundamental Neuroanatomy*, New York, W.H. Freeman & Co.

Nelson, A. J. D., Kinnavane, L., Amin, E., O'Mara, S. M. & Aggleton, J. P. 2020. Deconstructing the direct reciprocal hippocampal-anterior thalamic pathways for spatial learning. *The Journal of Neuroscience*, 40, 6978–6990. https://doi.org/10.1523/jneurosci.0874-20.2020

Nemeroff, C. B. 2007. Prevalence and management of treatment-resistant depression. *Journal of Clinical Psychiatry*, 68, 17–25.

Neo, P. S. H. & McNaughton, N. 2011. Frontal theta power linked to neuroticism and avoidance. *Cognitive, Affective, & Behavioral Neuroscience*, 11, 396–403. https://doi.org/10.3758/s13415-011-0038-x

Neo, P. S. H., McNaughton, N. & Sellbom, M. 2021. Early and late signals of unexpected reward contribute to low extraversion and high disinhibition, respectively. *Personality Neuroscience*, 4, e5. https://doi.org/10.1017/pen.2021.4

Neo, P. S. H., Thurlow, J. & McNaughton, N. 2011. Stopping, goal-conflict, trait anxiety and frontal rhythmic power in the stop-signal task. *Cognitive Affective & Behavioral Neuroscience*, 11, 485–493. https://doi.org/10.3758/s13415-011-0046-x

Nerad, L. 1997. Lesions of the posterior insular cortex impair water maze performance in the rat. *International Journal of Neuroscience*, 90, 1–7.

Nerad, L. & McNaughton, N. 2006. The septal EEG suggests a distributed organization of the pacemaker of hippocampal theta in the rat. *European Journal of Neuroscience*, 24, 155–66.

Nerad, L., Ramirez-Amaya, V., Ormsby, C. E. & Bermudez-Rattoni, F. 1996. Differential effects of anterior and posterior insular cortex lesions on the acquisition of conditioned taste aversion and spatial learning. *Neurobiology of Learning and Memory*, 66, 44–50.

Nesse, R. M. & Klaas, R. 1994. Risk perception by patients with anxiety disorders. *Journal of Nervous and Mental Diseases*, 182, 465–470.

Newman, J. P. 1987. Reaction to punishment in extraverts and psychopaths: implications for the impulsive behaviour of disinhibited individuals. *Journal of Research in Personality*, 21, 464–480.

Nguyen, L., Thomas, K. L., Lucke-Wold, B. P., Cavendish, J. Z., Crowe, M. S. & Matsumoto, R. R. 2016. Dextromethorphan: an update on its utility for neurological and neuropsychiatric disorders. *Pharmacology & Therapeutics*, 159, 1–22. https://doi.org/https://doi.org/10.1016/j.pharmthera.2016.01.016

Nielsen, M., Braestrup, C. & Squires, R. F. 1978. Evidence for a late evolutionary appearance of brain-specific benzodiazepine receptors: an investigation of 18 vertebrate and 5 invertebrate species. *Brain Research*, 141, 342–346.

Nieuwenhuis, S. n., Slagter, H. A. e. A., von Geusau, N. J. A. J. A., Heslenfeld, D. J. J. & Holroyd, C. B. B. 2005. Knowing good from bad: differential activation of human cortical areas by positive and negative outcomes. *European Journal of Neuroscience*, 21, 3161–3168.

Nieuwenhuys, R. 2012. The insular cortex: a review. *Progress in Brain Research*, 195, 123–63. https://doi.org/10.1016/B978-0-444-53860-4.00007-6

Nilssen, E. S., Doan, T. P., Nigro, M. J., Ohara, S. & Witter, M. P. 2019. Neurons and networks in the entorhinal cortex: a reappraisal of the lateral and medial entorhinal subdivisions mediating parallel cortical pathways. *Hippocampus*, 29, 1238–1254. https://doi.org/https://doi.org/10.1002/hipo.23145

Nishikawa, H., Inoue, T., Izumi, T. & Koyama, T. 2007. Synergistic effects of tandospirone and selective serotonin reuptake inhibitors on the contextual conditioned fear stress response in rats. *European Neuropsychopharmacology*, 17, 643–650. https://doi.org/https://doi.org/10.1016/j.euroneuro.2007.02.010

Nolen-Hoeksema, S. 2001. Gender differences in depression. *Current Directions in Psychological Science*, 10, 173–176.

Nolen-Hoeksema, S., Wisco, B. E. & Lyubomirsky, S. 2008. Rethinking rumination. *Perspectives on Psychological Science*, 3, 400–424.

Noritake, A., Ninomiya, T. & Isoda, M. 2021. Subcortical encoding of agent-relevant associative signals for adaptive social behavior in the macaque. *Neuroscience & Biobehavioral Reviews*, 125, 78–87. https://doi.org/https://doi.org/10.1016/j.neubiorev.2021.02.018

Norman, Y., Raccah, O., Liu, S., Parvizi, J. & Malach, R. 2021. Hippocampal ripples and their coordinated dialogue with the default mode network during recent and remote recollection. *Neuron*, 109, 2767–2780. https://doi.org/https://doi.org/10.1016/j.neuron.2021.06.020

Novemsky, N. & Kahneman, D. 2005. The boundaries of loss aversion. *Journal of Marketing Research*, 42, 119–128.

Noyes, R., Jr., Burrows, G. D., Reich, J. H., Judd, F. K., Garvey, M. J., Norman, T. R., Cook, B. L. & Marriott, P. 1996. Diazepam versus alprazolam for the treatment of panic disorder. *Journal of Clinical Psychiatry*, 57, 349–355.

Noyes, R., Jr., Kathol, R., Clancy, J. & Crowe, R. R. 1981. Antianxiety Effects of Propranolol:A Review of Clinical Studies. *In:* Klein, D. F. & Rabkin, J. (eds.) *Anxiety: new research and changing concepts* (pp. 81–93). New York: Raven Press.

Nuno-Perez, A. & Mameli, M. 2020. In DA club of reinforcement: glutamate, it's your birthday. *Neuron*, 107, 765–767. https://doi.org/https://doi.org/10.1016/j.neuron.2020.07.036

Nutt, D., Erritzoe, D. & Carhart-Harris, R. 2020. Psychedelic psychiatry's brave new world. *Cell*, 181, 24–28. https://doi.org/10.1016/j.cell.2020.03.020

Nutt, D. J. 1996. The pharmacology of human anxiety. *Pharmacology and Therapeutics*, 47, 233–266.

Nutt, D. J. 2005. Overview of diagnosis and drug treatments of anxiety disorders. *CNS Spectrums*, 10, 49–56. https://doi.org/10.1017/S1092852900009901

Nutt, D. J. & Lister, R. G. 1987. The effect of the imidazodiazepine Ro 15-4513 on the anticonvulsant effects of diazepam, sodium pentobarbital and ethanol. *Brain Research*, 413, 193–196.

Nutt, D. J. & Malizia, A. L. 2001. New insights into the role of the GABAA-benzodiazepine receptor in psychiatric disorder. *British Journal of Psychiatry*, 179, 390–396.

O'Keefe, J. 1976. Place units in the hippocampus of the freely moving rat. *Experimental Neurology*, 51, 78–109.

O'Keefe, J. & Black, A. H. 1978. Single unit and lesion experiments on the sensory inputs to the hippocampal map. *In:* Elliott, K. & Whelan, J. (eds.) *Functions of the septo-hippocampal system. Ciba Foundation Symposium 50 (New Series)* (pp. 179–192). Amsterdam: Elsevier.

O'Keefe, J. & Burgess, N. 1996. Geometric determinants of the place fields of hippocampal neurons. *Nature*, 381, 425–428.

O'Keefe, J. & Conway, D. H. 1978. Hippocampal place units in the freely moving rat: why they fire where they fire. *Experimental Brain Research*, 31, 573–590. https://doi.org/10.1007/BF00239813

O'Keefe, J. & Dostrovsky, J. 1971. The hippocampus as a spatial map. Preliminary evidence from unit activity in the freely-moving rat. *Brain Research*, 34, 171–175.

O'Keefe, J. & Nadel, L. 1978. *The hippocampus as a cognitive map*, Oxford, Clarendon Press.

O'Keefe, J. & Speakman, A. 1987. Single unit activity in the rat hippocampus during a spatial memory task. *Experimental Brain Research*, 68, 1–27.

O'Mara, S. M. 1995. Spatially selective firing properties of hippocampal formation neurons in rodents and primates. *Progress in Neurobiology*, 45, 253–274.

O'Mara, S. M., Rolls, E. T., Berthoz, A. & Kesner, R. P. 1994. Neurons responding to whole-body motion in the primate hippocampus. *The Journal of Neuroscience*, 14, 6511–6523.

Ogden, J. & Corkin, S. 1991. Memories of H.M. *In:* Abraham, W. C., Corballis, M. & White, K. G. (eds.) *Memory mechanisms: a tribute to G.V. Goddard* (Chapter 10, pp. 195–215). New Jersey: Lawrence Erlbaum.

Ogle, C. M., Rubin, D. C. & Siegler, I. C. 2016. Accounting for posttraumatic stress disorder symptom severity with pre- and posttrauma measures: a longitudinal study of older adults. *Clinical and Psychological Science*, 4, 272–286. https://doi.org/10.1177/2167702615583227

Ogle, C. M., Siegler, I. C., Beckham, J. C. & Rubin, D. C. 2017. Neuroticism increases PTSD symptom severity by amplifying the emotionality, rehearsal, and centrality of trauma memories. *Journal of Personality*, 85, 702–715. https://doi.org/10.1111/jopy.12278

Öhman, A. 1979. Fear relevance, autonomic conditioning, and phobias: a laboratory model. *In:* Sjoden, P. O., Bates, S. & Dockens, W. W. (eds.) *Trends in behavior therapy* (pp. 107–133). New York: Academic Press.

Öhman, A. 2005. The role of the amygdala in human fear: automatic detection of threat. *Psychoneuroendocrinology*, 30, 953–8. https://doi.org/10.1016/j.psyneuen.2005.03.019

Öhman, A. 2009. Of snakes and faces: an evolutionary perspective on the psychology of fear. *Scandinavian Journal of Psychology*, 50, 543–52. https://doi.org/10.1111/j.1467-9450.2009.00784.x

Öhman, A. & Mineka, S. 2001. Fears, phobias, and preparedness: toward an evolved module of fear and fear learning. *Psychological Review*, 108, 483–522.

Öhman, A. & Mineka, S. 2003. The malicious serpent: snakes as a prototypical stimulus for an evolved module of fear. *Current Directions in Psychological Science*, 12, 5–9.

Ojala, K. E. & Bach, D. R. 2020. Measuring learning in human classical threat conditioning: translational, cognitive and methodological considerations. *Neuroscience & Biobehavioral Reviews*, 114, 96–112. https://doi.org/https://doi.org/10.1016/j.neubiorev.2020.04.019

Okaichi, Y. & Okaichi, H. 1994. Effects of fimbria-fornix lesions on avoidance tasks with temporal elements in rats. *Physiology and Behavior*, 56, 759–765.

Okasha, A., Bishry, Z., Khalil, A. H., Darwish, T. A., Seif El Dawla, A. & Shohdy, A. 1994. Panic disorder. An overlapping or independent entity. *British Journal of Psychiatry*, 164, 818–825.

Olaman, S. J. & McNaughton, N. 2001. Chlordiazepoxide specifically impairs nonspatial reference memory in the cued radial arm maze in rats. *Pharmacology, Biochemistry and Behavior*, 70, 133–139.

Oleksiak, C. R., Ramanathan, K. R., Miles, O. W., Perry, S. J., Maren, S. & Moscarello, J. M. 2021. Ventral hippocampus mediates the context-dependence of two-way signaled avoidance in male rats. *Neurobiology of Learning and Memory*, 183, 107458. https://doi.org/https://doi.org/10.1016/j.nlm.2021.107458

Olsen, R. W. 2018. GABAA receptor: positive and negative allosteric modulators. *Neuropharmacology*, 136, 10–22. https://doi.org/https://doi.org/10.1016/j.neuropharm.2018.01.036

Olsen, R. W., Greenlee, D., Van Ness, P. & Ticku, M. K. 1978a. Studies on the gamma-aminobutyric acid receptor/ionophore proteins in mammalian brain. *In:* Fonnum, F. (ed.) *Amino acids as chemical transmitters* (pp. 467–486). New York: Plenum Press.

Olsen, R. W., Ticku, M. K., Greenlee, D. & Van Ness, P. 1978b. GABA receptor and ionophore binding sites: interaction with various drugs. *In:* Krogsgaard-Larsen, P., Scheel Kruger, J. & Kofod, H. (eds.) *GABA-neurotransmitters* (pp. 165–178). New York: Academic Press.

Olton, D. S. 1978a. Characteristics of spatial memory. *In:* Hulse, S. H., Fowler, H. & Honig, W. K. (eds.) *Cognitive processes in animal behavior* (pp. 341–373). Hillsdale, N.J.: Erlbaum.

Olton, D. S. 1978b. The function of septo-hippocampal connections in spatially organized behaviour. *In:* Elliott, K. & Whelan, J. (eds.) *Functions of the septo-hippocampal system. Ciba Foundation Symposium 58 (New Series)* (pp. 327–342). Amsterdam: Elsevier.

Olton, D. S., Becker, J. T. & Handelmann, G. E. 1979a. Hippocampus, space and memory. *Behavioral and Brain Sciences*, 2, 313–322.

Olton, D. S., Becker, J. T. & Handelmann, G. E. 1979b. Hippocampus, space, and memory: authors' responses. *Behavioral and Brain Sciences*, 2, 352–359.

Olton, D. S., Branch, M. & Best, P. J. 1978a. Spatial correlates of hippocampal unit activity. *Experimental Neurology*, 58, 387–409.

Olton, D. S. & Isaacson, R. L. 1968. Hippocampal lesions and active avoidance. *Physiology and Behavior*, 3, 719–724.

Olton, D. S. & Papas, B. C. 1979. Spatial memory and hippocampal function. *Neuropsychologia*, 17, 669–682.

Olton, D. S., Walker, J. A. & Gage, F. H. 1978b. Hippocampal connections and spatial discrimination. *Brain Research*, 139, 295–308.

Olton, D. S. & Werz, M. A. 1978. Hippocampal function and behaviour: spatial discrimination and response inhibition. *Physiology and Behavior*, 20, 597–606.

Orenius, T. I., Raij, T. T., Nuortimo, A., Näätänen, P., Lipsanen, J. & Karlsson, H. 2017. The interaction of emotion and pain in the insula and secondary somatosensory cortex. *Neuroscience*, 349, 185–194. https://doi.org/10.1016/j.neuroscience.2017.02.047

Oscar-Berman, M. O. & Samuels, I. 1973. Stimulus-preference and memory factors in Korsakoff's syndrome. (A paper presented at the American Psychological Association meeting, Montreal.).

Oscar-Berman, M. O. & Samuels, I. 1977. Stimulus preference and memory factors in Korsakoff's syndrome. *Neuropsychologia*, 15, 99–106.

Ostlund, S. B. & Balleine, B. W. 2007. Orbitofrontal cortex mediates outcome encoding in Pavlovian but not instrumental conditioning. *The Journal of Neuroscience*, 27, 4819–4825. https://doi.org/10.1523/jneurosci.5443-06.2007

Ottaviani, C., Shapiro, D. & Fitzgerald, L. 2011. Rumination in the laboratory: what happens when you go back to everyday life? *Psychophysiology*, 48, 453–461.

Page, A. C. 1994. Distinguishing panic disorder and agoraphobia from social phobia. *Journal of Nervous and Mental Diseases*, 182, 611–617.

Page, H. J. I. & Jeffery, K. J. 2018. Landmark-based updating of the head direction system by retrosplenial cortex: a computational model. *Frontiers in Cellular Neuroscience*, 12, A191. https://doi.org/10.3389/fncel.2018.00191

Pan, W.-X. & McNaughton, N. 2004. The supramammillary area: its organization, functions and relationship to the hippocampus. *Progress in Neurobiology*, 74, 127–166. https://doi.org/10.1016/j.pneurobio.2004.09.003

Pan, W. & McNaughton, N. 1997. The medial supramammillary nucleus, spatial learning and the frequency of hippocampal theta activity. *Brain Research*, 764, 101–108.

Pan, W. & McNaughton, N. 2002. The role of the medial supramammillary nucleus in the control of hippocampal theta activity and behaviour in rats. *European Journal of Neuroscience*, 16, 1797–1809.

Pande, A. C., Feltner, D. E., Jefferson, J. W., Davidson, J. R. T., Pollack, M., Stein, M. B., Lydiard, R. B., Futterer, R. s., Robinson, P., Slomkowski, M., DuBoff, E., Phelps, M., Janney, C. A. & Werth, J. L. 2004. Efficacy of the novel anxiolytic pregabalin in social anxiety disorder. *Journal of Clinical Psychopharmacology*, 24, 141–149. https://doi.org/10.1097/01.jcp.0000117423.05703.e7

Pandya, D., Dye, P. & Butters, N. 1971. Efferent cortico-cortical projections of the prefrontal cortex in the Rhesus monkey. *Brain Research*, 31, 35–46.

Pandya, D. N. & Barnes, C. L. 1987. Architecture and connections of the frontal lobe. *In:* Perceman, E. (ed.) *The frontal lobe revisited* (pp. 41–72). New York: IRBN Press.

Panksepp, J. 1982. Towards a general psychobiological theory of emotions. *Behavioral and Brain Sciences*, 5, 407–468. https://doi.org/10.1017/S0140525X00012759

Papakostas, G. I., Trivedi, M. H., Alpert, J. E., Seifert, C. A., Krishen, A., Goodale, E. P. & Tucker, V. L. 2008. Efficacy of bupropion and the selective serotonin reuptake inhibitors in the treatment of anxiety symptoms in major depressive disorder: a meta-analysis of individual patient data from 10 double-blind, randomized clinical trials. *Journal of Psychiatric Research*, 42, 134–40. https://doi.org/10.1016/j.jpsychires.2007.05.012

Papez, J. W. 1937. A proposed mechanism of emotion. *Archives of Neurological Psychiatry*, 38, 725–743.

Papp, L. A., Klein, D. F. & Gorman, J. M. 1993. Carbon dioxide hypersensitivity, hyperventilation, and panic disorder. *American Journal of Psychiatry*, 150, 1149–1157.

Park, A. J., Harris, A. Z., Martyniuk, K. M., Chang, C.-Y., Abbas, A. I., Lowes, D. C., Kellendonk, C., Gogos, J. A. & Gordon, J. A. 2021. Reset of hippocampal–prefrontal circuitry facilitates learning. *Nature*, online. https://doi.org/10.1038/s41586-021-03272-1

Parkes, S. L., Ravassard, P. M., Cerpa, J. C., Wolff, M., Ferreira, G. & Coutureau, E. 2018. Insular and ventrolateral orbitofrontal cortices differentially contribute to goal-directed behavior in rodents. *Cerebral Cortex*, 28, 2313–2325. https://doi.org/10.1093/cercor/bhx132

Parkin, A. J., Rees, J. E., Hunkin, N. M. & Rose, P. E. 1994. Impairment of memory following discrete thalamic infarction. *Neuropsychologia*, 32, 39–51.

Parmeggiani, P. L., Azzaroni, A. & Lenzi, P. 1971. On the functional significance of the circuit of Papez. *Brain Research*, 30, 357–374.

Parmeggiani, P. L., Lenzi, P. L. & Azzaroni, A. 1974. Transfer of the hippocampal output by the anterior thalamic nuclei. *Brain Research*, 67, 269–278.

Passani, M. B., Lin, J. S., Hancock, A., Crochet, S. & Blandina, P. 2004. The histamine H3 receptor as a novel therapeutic target for cognitive and sleep disorders. *Trends in Pharmacological Sciences*, 25, 618–625.

Passingham, R. E. 1993. *The frontal lobes and voluntary action*, Oxford, Oxford University Press.

Paulus, M. P., Feinstein, J. S., Castillo, G., Simmons, A. N. & Stein, M. B. 2005. Dose-dependent decrease of activation in bilateral amygdala and insula by lorazepam during emotion processing. *Archives of General Psychiatry*, 62, 282–288. https://doi.org/10.1001/archpsyc.62.3.282

Paulus, M. P. & Stein, M. B. 2006. An insular view of anxiety. *Biological Psychiatry*, 60, 383–387. https://doi.org/10.1016/j.biopsych.2006.03.042

Pavlides, C., Donishi, T., Ribeiro, S., Mello, C. V., Blanco, W. & Ogawa, S. 2019. Hippocampal functional organization: a microstructure of the place cell network encoding space. *Neurobiology of Learning and Memory*, 161, 122–134. https://doi.org/https://doi.org/10.1016/j.nlm.2019.03.010

Pavlov, I. P. 1927. *Conditioned reflexes (trans. G. V. Anrep)*, London, Constable & Co. Ltd, Dover edition, by special arrangement with Oxford University Press.

Payne, J. D., Nadel, L., Britton, W. B. & Jacobs, J. 2004. The biopsychology of trauma and memory. *In:* Reisberg, D. & Hertel, P. (eds.) *Memory and emotion* (pp. 76–128). online: Oxford University Press.

Pelosi, G. G., Resstel, L. L., Soares, V. P., Zangrossi, H., Guimaraes, F. S. & Correa, F. M. 2009. Anxiolytic-like effect of noradrenaline microinjection into the dorsal periaqueductal gray of rats. *Behavioural Pharmacology*, 20, 252–9. https://doi.org/10.1097/FBP.0b013e32832c7098

Peng, K., Steele, S. C., Becerra, L. & Borsook, D. 2018. Brodmann area 10: collating, integrating and high level processing of nociception and pain. *Progress in Neurobiology*, 161, 1–22. https://doi.org/10.1016/j.pneurobio.2017.11.004

Penke, L., Denissen, J. J. A. & Miller, G. F. 2007. The evolutionary genetics of personality. *European Journal of Personality*, 21, 549–587. https://doi.org/10.1002/per.629

Perkins, A. & Corr, P. J. 2014. Anxiety as an adaptive emotion. *In:* Parrott, W. G. (ed.) *The positive side of negative emotions* (Chapter 2, pp. 37–54). New York: Guilford Press.

Perkins, A., Patrick, F., Wise, T., Meyer, N., Mazibuko, N., Oates, A., Bijl, A., Danjou, P., O'Connor, S., Doolin, E., Wooldridge, C., Rathjen, D., Macare, C., Williams, S. & Young, A. 2021. Cholinergic modulation of disorder-relevant human defensive behaviour in generalised anxiety disorder. *Translational Psychiatry*, 11, e13. https://doi.org/10.1038/s41398-020-01141-5

Perkins, A. M., Ettinger, U., Davis, R., Foster, R., Williams, S. C. R. & Corr, P. J. 2009. Effects of lorazepam and citalopram on human defensive reactions: ethopharmacological differentiation of fear and anxiety. *The Journal of Neuroscience*, 29, 12617–12624. https://doi.org/10.1523/jneurosci.2696-09.2009

Perkins, A. M., Ettinger, U., Weaver, K., Schmechtig, A., Schrantee, A., Morrison, P. D., Sapara, A., Kumari, V., Williams, S. C. & Corr, P. J. 2013. Advancing the defensive explanation for anxiety disorders: lorazepam effects on human defense are systematically modulated by personality and threat-type. *Translational Psychiatry*, 3, e246. https://doi.org/10.1038/tp.2013.20

Perkins, A. M. J., Cooper, A. B., Abdelall, M., Smillie, L. D. & Corr, P. J. 2010. Personality and defensive reactions: fear, trait anxiety, and threat magnification. *Journal of Personality*, 78, 1071–1090.

Pesold, C. & Treit, D. 1994. The septum and amygdala differentially mediate the anxiolytic effects of benzodiazepines. *Brain Research*, 638, 295–301.

Pesold, C. & Treit, D. 1995. The central and basolateral amygdala differentially mediate the anxiolytic effects of benzodiazepines. *Brain Research*, 671, 213–221.

Petersen, P. C. & Buzsáki, G. 2020. Cooling of medial septum reveals theta phase lag coordination of hippocampal cell assemblies. *Neuron*, 107, 731–744.e3. https://doi.org/https://doi.org/10.1016/j.neuron.2020.05.023

Petrides, M. 1994. Frontal lobes and working memory: evidence from investigations of the effects of cortical excisions in nonhuman primates. *In:* Boller, F. & Grafman, J. (eds.) *Handbook of neuropsychology* (Vol. 9, pp. 59–82). Montreal: Elsevier Science Publishers.

Petrides, M. & Pandya, D. N. 1994. Comparative architectonic analysis of the human and the macaque frontal cortex. *In:* Boller, F. & Grafman, J. (eds.) *Handbook of neurpsychology* (Vol. 9, pp. 17–58). Montreal: Elsevier Science Publishers.

Petrides, M. & Pandya, D. N. 2007. Efferent association pathways from the rostral prefrontal cortex in the macaque monkey. *Journal of Neuroscience*, 27, 11573–11586. https://doi.org/10.1523/jneurosci.2419-07.2007

Pettit, N. L., Yuan, X. C. & Harvey, C. D. 2022. Hippocampal place codes are gated by behavioral engagement. *Nature Neuroscience.* https://doi.org/10.1038/s41593-022-01050-4

Phillips, M. L., Young, A. W., Scott, S. K., Calder, A. J., Andrew, C., Giampietro, V., Williams, S. C. R., Bullmore, E. T., Brammer, M. & Gray, J. A. 1998. Neural responses to facial and vocal expressions of fear and disgust. *Proceedings of the Royal Society of London. B:Biological Sciences*, 265, 1809–1817.

Phillips, M. L., Young, A. W., Senior, C., Brammer, M., Andrew, C., Calder, A. J., Bullmore, E. T., Perrett, D. I., Rowland, D., Williams, S. C. R., Gray, J. A. & David, A. S. A. 1997. A specific neural substrate for perceiving facial expressions of disgust. *Nature*, 389, 495–498.

Phillips, R. G. & LeDoux, J. E. 1994. Lesions of the dorsal hippocampal formation interfere with background but not foreground contextual fear conditioning. *Learning and Memory*, 1, 34–44.

Pickering, A. 1997. The conceptual nervous system and personality: from Pavlov to neural networks. *European Psychologist*, 2, 139–163.

Pickering, A. D., Corr, P. J. & Gray, J. A. 1999. Interactions and reinforcement sensitivity theory: a theoretical analysis of Rusting & Larsen (1997). *Personality and Individual Differences*, 26, 357–365.

Pickering, A. D., Corr, P. J., Powell, J. H., Kumari, V., Thornton, J. C. & Gray, J. A. 1997. Individual differences in reactions to reinforcing stimuli are neither black nor white: to what extent are they gray? *In:* Nyborg, H. (ed.) *The scientific study of human nature: tribute to Hans J. Eysenck at eighty* (pp. 36–67). London: Elsevier.

Pickering, A. D. & Pesola, F. 2014. Modeling dopaminergic and other processes involved in learning from reward prediction error: contributions from an individual differences perspective. *Frontiers in Human Neuroscience*, 8. A740 https://doi.org/10.3389/fnhum.2014.00740

Pigott, S. & Milner, B. 1994. Capacity of visual short-term memory after unilateral frontal or anterior temporal-lobe resection. *Neuropsychologia*, 32, 969–981.

Pinel, J. P. J. 1997. *Biopsychology*, Boston, Allyn and Bacon.

Pinel, J. P. J. 2011. *Biopsychology (8th ed.*), Boston, Allyn and Bacon (Pearson).

Pinheiro, S. N., Del-Ben, C. M., Zangrossi Jr, H. & Graeff, F. G. 2008. Anxiolytic and panicolytic effects of escitalopram in the elevated T-maze. *Journal of Psychopharmacology*, 22, 132–137.

Pitman, R. K. 1989. Posttraumatic stress disorder hormones, and memory [editorial]. *Biological Psychiatry*, 26, 221–223.

Pitman, R. K., Orr, S. P. & Shalev, A. Y. 1993. Once bitten, twice shy: beyond the conditioning model of PTSD. *Biological Psychiatry*, 33, 145–146.

Pittendrigh, C. S. 1958. Adaptation, natural selection and behaviour. *In:* Roes, A. & Simpson, G. G. (eds.) *Behaviour and evolution* (Volume 1, Chapter 8, pp. 390–416). New Haven: Yale University Press.

Plutchik, R. 1962. *The emotions: facts, theories and a new model*, New York, Random House.

Pobbe, R. L. H., Zangrossi, H., Blanchard, D. C. & Blanchard, R. J. 2011. Involvement of dorsal raphe nucleus and dorsal periaqueductal gray 5-HT receptors in the modulation of mouse defensive behaviors. *European Neuropsychopharmacology*, 21, 306–315. https://doi.org/https://doi.org/10.1016/j.euroneuro.2010.05.004

Poltronieri, S. C., Zangrossi, H. & de Barros Viana, M. 2003. Antipanic-like effect of serotonin reuptake inhibitors in the elevated T-maze. *Behavioural Brain Research*, 147, 185–192. https://doi.org/https://doi.org/10.1016/S0166-4328(03)00151-7

Ponnusamy, R., Poulos, A. M. & Fanselow, M. S. 2007. Amygdala-dependent and amygdala-independent pathways for contextual fear conditioning. *Neuroscience*, 147, 919–927.

Ponserre, M., Peters, C., Fermani, F., Conzelmann, K.-K. & Klein, R. 2020. The insula cortex contacts distinct output streams of the central amygdala. *The Journal of Neuroscience*, 40, 8870–8882. https://doi.org/10.1523/jneurosci.0567-20.2020

Poucet, B., Thinus-Blanc, C. & Muller, R. U. 1994. Place cells in the ventral hippocampus of rats. *Neuroreport*, 5, 2045–2048.

Poulos, A. M., Ponnusamy, R., Dong, H. W. & Fanselow, M. S. 2010. Compensation in the neural circuitry of fear conditioning awakens learning circuits in the bed nuclei of the stria terminalis. *Proceedings of the National Academy of Sciences of the United States of America*, 107, 14881–6. https://doi.org/1005754107 [pii] 10.1073/pnas.1005754107

Poulton, R., Caspi, A. & Moffitt, T. E. 2023. Fear and anxiety: lessons learned from the Dunedin longitudinal study. *Neuroscience and Biobehavioral Reviews*, 148, 105118. https://doi.org/10.1016/j.neubiorev.2023.105118

Poulton, R. & Menzies, R. G. 2002a. Fears born *and* bred: toward a more inclusive theory of fear acquisition. *Behaviour Research and Therapy*, 40, 197–208.

Poulton, R. & Menzies, R. G. 2002b. Non-associative fear acquisition: a review of the evidence from retrospective and longitudinal research. *Behaviour Research and Therapy*, 40, 127–149.

Powell, G. E. 1979. *Brain and personality*, London, Saxon House.

Poythress, N. G., Skeem, J. L., Weir, J., Lilienfeld, S. O., Douglas, K. S., Edens, J. F. & Kennealy, P. J. 2008. Psychometric properties of Carver and White's (1994) BIS/BAS scales in a large sample of offenders. *Personality and Individual Differences*, 45, 732–737.

Preter, M. & Klein, D. F. 2008. Panic, suffocation false alarms, separation anxiety and endogenous opioids. *Progress in Neuro-Psychopharmacology and Biological Psychiatry*, 32, 603–612. https://doi.org/https://doi.org/10.1016/j.pnpbp.2007.07.029

Price, J. L. 2006. Connections of the orbital cortex. *In:* Zald, D. H. & Rauch, S. L. (eds.) *The orbital frontal cortex* (Chapter 3). Oxford: Oxford University Press.

Priestley, J. B., Bowler, J. C., Rolotti, S. V., Fusi, S. & Losonczy, A. 2022. Signatures of rapid plasticity in hippocampal CA1 representations during novel experiences. *Neuron*, 110, 1978–1992.e6. https://doi.org/https://doi.org/10.1016/j.neuron.2022.03.026

Prodan, A., Davies, H., Eneqvist, H., Mastroberardino, G., Wijayathunga, H., Wardlaw, K. & Morris, R. G. M. 2022. Memory recall: new behavioral protocols for examining distinct forms of context specific recall in animals. *Neurobiology of Learning and Memory*, 195, 107685. https://doi.org/https://doi.org/10.1016/j.nlm.2022.107685

Qi, S., Hassabis, D., Sun, J., Guo, F., Daw, N. & Mobbs, D. 2018. How cognitive and reactive fear circuits optimize escape decisions in humans. *Proceedings of the National Academy of Sciences*, 115, 3186–3191. https://doi.org/10.1073/pnas.1712314115

Quesseveur, G., Nguyen, H. T., Gardier, A. M. & Guiard, B. P. 2012. 5-HT2 ligands in the treatment of anxiety and depression. *Expert Opinion on Investigational Drugs*, 21, 1701–1725. https://doi.org/10.1517/13543784.2012.719872

Quilty, L. C., DeYoung, C. G., Oakman, J. M. & Bagby, R. M. 2014. Extraversion and behavioural activation: integrating the components of approach. *Journal of Personality Assessment*, 96, 87–94.

Quirk, G. J., Muller, R. U. & Kubie, J. L. 1990. The firing of hippocampal place cells in the dark depends on the rat's recent experience. *The Journal of Neuroscience*, 10, 2008–2017.

Quirk, G. J., Muller, R. U., Kubie, J. L. & Ranck, J. B., Jr. 1992. The positional firing properties of medial entorhinal neurons: description and comparison with hippocampal place cells. *The Journal of Neuroscience*, 12, 1945–1963.

Rachman, S. 1977. The conditioning theory of fear- acquisition: a critical examination. *Behaviour Research and Therapy*, 15, 375–387.

Rachman, S. 1978. An anatomy of obsessions. *Behaviour Analysis and Modification*, 2, 253–278.

Rachman, S. & Seligman, M. E. P. 1976. Unprepared phobias: be prepared. *Behaviour Research and Therapy*, 14, 333–338.

Rae, C. L., Hughes, L. E., Anderson, M. C. & Rowe, J. B. 2015. The prefrontal cortex achieves inhibitory control by facilitating subcortical motor pathway connectivity. *Journal of Neuroscience*, 35, 786–94. https://doi.org/10.1523/JNEUROSCI.3093-13.2015

Ragozzino, M. E. & Kesner, R. P. 1999. The role of the agranular insular cortex in working memory for food reward value and allocentric space in rats. *Behavioural Brain Research*, 98, 103–112.

Rahman, F., Nanu, R., Schneider, N. A., Katz, D., Lisman, J. & Pi, H.-J. 2021. Optogenetic perturbation of projections from thalamic nucleus reuniens to hippocampus disrupts spatial working memory retrieval more than encoding. *Neurobiology of Learning and Memory*, 179, 107396. https://doi.org/https://doi.org/10.1016/j.nlm.2021.107396

Rajbhandari, A. K., Octeau, C. J., Gonzalez, S., Pennington, Z. T., Mohamed, F., Trott, J., Chavez, J., Ngyuen, E., Keces, N., Hong, W. Z., Neve, R. L., Waschek, J., Khakh, B. S. & Fanselow, M. S. 2021. A basomedial amygdala to intercalated cells microcircuit expressing PACAP and its receptor PAC1 regulates contextual fear. *The Journal of Neuroscience*, 41, 3446–3461. https://doi.org/10.1523/jneurosci.2564-20.2021

Rajkowska, G. & Goldman-Rakic, P. S. 1995a. Cytoarchitectonic definition of prefrontal areas in the normal human cortex: I. Remapping of areas 9 and 46 using quantitative criteria. *Cerebral Cortex*, 5, 307–322.

Rajkowska, G. & Goldman-Rakic, P. S. 1995b. Cytoarchitectonic definition of prefrontal areas in the normal human cortex: II. Variability in locations of areas 9 and 46 and relationship to the Talairach coordinate system. *Cerebral Cortex*, 5, 323–337.

Rammsayer, T. H. 1998. Extraversion and dopamine: individual differences in response to changes in dopaminergic activity as a possible biological basis of extraversion. *European Psychologist*, 3, 37–50. https://doi.org/10.1027/1016-9040.3.1.37

Rampino, A., Torretta, S., Rizzo, G., Viscanti, G., Quarto, T., Gelao, B., Fazio, L., Attrotto, M. T., Masellis, R., Pergola, G., Bertolino, A. & Blasi, G. 2019. Emotional stability interacts with cortisol levels before fMRI on brain processing of fearful faces. *Neuroscience*, 416, 190–197. https://doi.org/https://doi.org/10.1016/j.neuroscience.2019.08.002

Ranck, J. B., Jr. 1973. Studies on single neurons in dorsal hippocampal formation and septum in unrestrained rats. *Experimental Neurology*, 41, 461–555.

Randall, L. O. & Kappell, B. 1973. Pharmacological activity of some benzodiazepines and their metabolites. *In:* Garattini, S., Mussini, E. & Randall, L. O. (eds.) *The benzodiazepines* (pp. 27–51). New York: Raven Press.

Randall, P. K., Bremner, J. D., Krystal, J. H., Nagy, L. M., Heninger, G. R., Nicolaou, A. L. & Charney, D. S. 1995. Effects of the benzodiazepine antagonist flumazenil in PTSD. *Biological Psychiatry*, 38, 319–324.

Rapoport, J. L. 1989. The biology of obsessions and compulsions. *Scientific American*, 260, 63–69.

Rassovsky, Y. & Kushner, M. G. 2003. Carbon dioxide in the study of panic disorder: issues of definition, methodology, and outcome. *Journal of Anxiety Disorders*, 17, 1–32. https://doi.org/https://doi.org/10.1016/S0887-6185(02)00181-0

Ravindran, L. N., Kim, D. S., Letamendi, A. M. & Stein, M. B. 2009. A randomized controlled trial of atomoxetine in generalized social anxiety disorder. *Journal of Clinical Psychopharmacology*, 29, 561–564. https://doi.org/10.1097/JCP.0b013e3181bf6303

Ravindran, L. N. & Stein, M. B. 2010. The pharmacologic treatment of anxiety disorders: a review of progress. *Journal of Clinical Psychiatry*, 71, 839–854. https://doi.org/10.4088/JCP.10r06218blu

Rawlins, J. N. P. 1977. *Behavioural and physiological correlates of limbic system activity*, Unpublished D.Phil. Thesis, University of Oxford.

Rawlins, J. N. P. 1985. Association across time: the hippocampus as a temporary memory store. *Behavioral and Brain Sciences*, 8, 479–496.

Rawlins, J. N. P., Lyford, G. L., Seferiades, A., Deacon, R. M. J. & Cassaday, H. J. 1993. Critical determinants of nonspatial working memory deficits in rats with conventional lesions of the hippocampus or fornix. *Behavioral Neuroscience*, 107, 420–433.

Rawlins, J. N. P. & Tsaltas, E. 1983. The hippocampus, time and working memory. *Behavioural Brain Research*, 10, 233–262.

Raymond, C. R. 2007. LTP forms 1, 2 and 3: different mechanisms for the 'long' in long term potentiation. *Trends in Neurosciences*, 30, 167–175.

Razran, G. 1971. *Mind in evolution*, Boston, Houghton Mifflin.

Reddy, L., Zoefel, B., Possel, J. K., Peters, J., Dijksterhuis, D. E., Poncet, M., van Straaten, E. C. W., Baayen, J. C., Idema, S. & Self, M. W. 2021. Human hippocampal neurons track moments in a sequence of events. *The Journal of Neuroscience*, 41, 6714–6725. https://doi.org/10.1523/jneurosci.3157-20.2021

Redgrave, P. & Dean, P. 1997. Does the PAG learn about emergencies from the superior colliculus? *In:* Depaulis, A. & Bandler, R. (eds.) *The midbrain periaqueductal gray matter* (pp. 199–209). New York: Plenum Press.

Redgrave, P. & Gurney, K. 2006. The short-latency dopamine signal: a role in discovering novel actions? *Nature Reviews Neuroscience*, 7, 967–975.

Redgrave, P., Vautrelle, N. & Reynolds, J. N. J. 2011. Functional properties of the basal ganglia's re-entrant loop architecture: selection and reinforcement. *Neuroscience*, 198, 138–151. https://doi.org/10.1016/j.neuroscience.2011.07.060

Reis, F. M. C. V., Lee, J. Y., Maesta-Pereira, S., Schuette, P. J., Chakerian, M., Liu, J., La-Vu, M. Q., Tobias, B. C., Ikebara, J. M., Kihara, A. H., Canteras, N. S., Kao, J. C. & Adhikari, A. 2021a. Dorsal periaqueductal gray ensembles represent approach and avoidance states. *eLife*, 10, e64934. https://doi.org/10.7554/eLife.64934

Reis, F. M. C. V., Liu, J., Schuette, P. J., Lee, J. Y., Maesta-Pereira, S., Chakerian, M., Wang, W., Canteras, N. S., Kao, J. C. & Adhikari, A. 2021b. Shared dorsal periaqueductal gray activation patterns during exposure to innate and conditioned threats. *The Journal of Neuroscience*, 41, 5399–5420. https://doi.org/10.1523/jneurosci.2450-20.2021

Reis, F. M. C. V., Mobbs, D., Canteras, N. S. & Adhikari, A. 2023. Orchestration of innate and conditioned defensive actions by the periaqueductal gray. *Neuropharmacology*, 109458. https://doi.org/https://doi.org/10.1016/j.neuropharm.2023.109458

Rempel-Clower, N. L., Zola, S. M., Squire, L. R. & Amaral, D. G. 1996. Three cases of enduring memory impairment after bilateral damage limited to the hippocampal formation. *The Journal of Neuroscience*, 16, 5233–5255.

Rendell, L. & Whitehead, H. 2001. Culture in whales and dolphins. *Behavioral and Brain Sciences*, 24, 309–324.

Ressler, R. L., Goode, T. D., Kim, S., Ramanathan, K. R. & Maren, S. 2021. Covert capture and attenuation of a hippocampus-dependent fear memory. *Nature Neuroscience*, 24, 677–684. https://doi.org/10.1038/s41593-021-00825-5

Reuter, M., Cooper, A. J., Smillie, L. D., Markett, S. & Montag, C. 2015. A new measure for the revised reinforcement sensitivity theory: psychometric criteria and genetic validation. *Frontiers for System Neuroscience*, 9, 38. https://doi.org/10.3389/fnsys.2015.00038

Reuter, M., Schmitz, A., Corr, P. J. & Hennig, J. 2006. Molecular genetics support Gray's personality theory: the interaction of COMT and DRD2 polymorphisms predicts the behavioral approach system. *International Journal of Neuropsychopharmacology*, 9, 155–166. https://doi.org/10.1017/S146114570500541

Revelle, W. 2007. Experimental approaches to the study of personality. *In:* Robins, B., Fraley, R. C. & Krueger, R. F. (eds.) *Handbook of research methods in personality psychology* (pp. 37–61). New York: Guilford Press.

Revusky, S. 1971. The role of interference in association over a delay. *In:* Honig, W. K. & James, P. H. R. (eds.) *Animal memory* (pp. 155–213). New York: Academic Press.

Reynolds, J. N. & Wickens, J. R. 2002. Dopamine-dependent plasticity of corticostriatal synapses. *Neural Networks*, 15, 507–521.

Reynolds, J. N. J., Hyland, B. I. & Wickens, J. R. 2001. A cellular mechanism of reward-related learning. *Nature*, 413, 67–70.

Reynolds, S. M. & Zahm, D. S. 2005. Specificity in the projections of prefrontal and insular cortex to ventral striatopallidum and the extended amygdala. *Journal of Neuroscience*, 25, 11757–11767.

Rhoads, D. E., Grimes, N., Kaushal, S., Mallari, J. & Orlando, K. 2012. Decision time and perseveration of adolescent rats in the T-maze are affected differentially by buspirone and independent of 5-HT-1A expression. *Pharmacology Biochemistry and Behavior*, 102, 58–63. https://doi.org/https://doi.org/10.1016/j.pbb.2012.03.024

Richards, G., Schoch, P. & Haefely, W. 1991. Benzodiazepine receptors: new vistas. *The Neurosciences*, 3, 191–203.

Rickels, K. & Rynn, M. 2002. Pharmacotherapy of generalized anxiety disorder. *Journal of Clinical Psychiatry*, 63, 9–16.

Rickert, E. J., Bennett, T. L., Lane, P. & French, J. 1978. Hippocampectomy and the attenuation of blocking. *Behavioural Biology*, 22, 147–160.

Ridley, R. M., Timothy, C. J., MacLean, C. J. & Baker, H. F. 1995. Conditional learning and memory impairments following neurotoxic lesion of the CA1 field of the hippocampus. *Neuroscience*, 67, 263–275.

Rigoli, F., Ewbank, M., Dalgleish, T. & Calder, A. 2016. Threat visibility modulates the defensive brain circuit underlying fear and anxiety. *Neuroscience Letters*, 612, 7–13. https://doi.org/10.1016/j.neulet.2015.11.026

Risold, P. Y. & Swanson, L. W. 1996. Structural evidence for functional domains in the rat hippocampus. *Science*, 272, 1484–1486.

Rivas, J., Gaztelu, J. M. & García-Austt, E. 1996. Changes in hippocampal cell discharge patterns and theta rhythm spectral properties as a function of walking velocity in the guinea pig. *Experimental Brain Research*, 108, 113–118.

Rizzi-Wise, C. A. & Wang, D. V. 2021. Putting together pieces of the lateral septum: multifaceted functions and its neural pathways. *eNeuro*, 8, ENEURO.0315-21.2021. https://doi.org/10.1523/eneuro.0315-21.2021

Robert, V., Therreau, L., Chevaleyre, V., Lepicard, E., Viollet, C., Cognet, J., Huang, A., Boehringer, R., Polygalov, D., McHugh, T. & Piskorowski, R. 2021. Local circuit allowing hypothalamic control of hippocampal area CA2 activity and consequences for CA1. *eLife*, 10, e63352. https://doi.org/10.7554/eLife.63352

Roberts, A. C. 1996. Comparison of cognitive function in human and non-human primates. *Cognitive Brain Research*, 3, 319–327.

Roberts, A. C., Robbins, T. W. & Everitt, B. J. 1988. The effects of intradimensional and extradimensional shifts on visual discrimination learning in humans and non-human primates. *Quarterly Journal of Experimental Psychology*, 40B, 321–341.

Roberts, C., Sahakian, B. J. & Robbins, T. W. 2020. Psychological mechanisms and functions of 5-HT and SSRIs in potential therapeutic change: lessons from the serotonergic modulation of action selection, learning, affect, and social cognition. *Neuroscience & Biobehavioral Reviews*, 119, 138–167. https://doi.org/https://doi.org/10.1016/j.neubiorev.2020.09.001

Robertson, H. A., Martin, I. L. & Candy, J. M. 1978. Differences in benzodiazepine receptor binding in Maudsley reactive and Maudsley nonreactive rats. *European Journal of Pharmacology*, 50, 455–457.

Robillard, G., Bouchard, S., Fournier, T. & Renaud, P. 2003. Anxiety and presence during VR immersion: a comparative study of the reactions of phobic and non-phobic participants in therapeutic virtual environments derived from computer games. *CyberPsychology & Behavior*, 6, 467–476. https://doi.org/10.1089/109493103769710497

Robinson, D. S. 1993. Serotonin receptor subtypes and affective disorders. *Clinical Neuropharmacology*, 16 Suppl. 3, S1–S5.

Robinson, J. & Brandon, M. 2021. Skipping ahead: a circuit for representing the past, present, and future. *eLife*, 10, e68795. https://doi.org/10.7554/eLife.68795

Robinson, J., Manseau, F., Ducharme, G., Amilhon, B., Vigneault, E., El Mestikawy, S. & Williams, S. 2016. Optogenetic activation of septal glutamatergic neurons drive hippocampal theta rhythms. *The Journal of Neuroscience*, 36, 3016–3023. https://doi.org/10.1523/jneurosci.2141-15.2016

Robinson, R. B. & Siegelbaum, S. A. 2003. Hyperpolarization-activated cation currents: from molecules to physiological function. *Annual Review of Physiology*, 65, 453–480. https://doi.org/10.1146/annurev.physiol.65.092101.142734

Rocchi, F., Oya, H., Balezeau, F., Billig, A. J., Kocsis, Z., Jenison, R. L., Nourski, K. V., Kovach, C. K., Steinschneider, M., Kikuchi, Y., Rhone, A. E., Dlouhy, B. J., Kawasaki, H., Adolphs, R., Greenlee, J. D. W., Griffiths, T. D., Howard, M. A. & Petkov, C. I. 2021. Common fronto-temporal effective connectivity in humans and monkeys. *Neuron*, 109, 852–868.e8. https://doi.org/https://doi.org/10.1016/j.neuron.2020.12.026

Rodgers, R. J. & Cole, J. C. 1993. Influence of social isolation, gender, strain, and prior novelty on plus-maze behaviour in mice. *Physiology and Behavior*, 54, 729–736.

Rodgers, R. J. & Cole, J. C. 1994. The elevated plus-maze: pharmacology, methodology and ethology. *In:* Cooper, S. J. & Hendrie, C. A. (eds.) *Ethology and psychopharmacology*. John Wiley and Sons Ltd.

Rodgers, R. J., Cole, J. C., Aboualfa, K. & Stephenson, L. H. 1995. Ethopharmacological analysis of the effects of putative 'Anxiogenic' agents in the mouse elevated plus-maze. *Pharmacology, Biochemistry and Behavior*, 52, 805–813.

Rodriguez, C. I., Kegeles, L. S., Levinson, A., Feng, T., Marcus, S. M., Vermes, D., Flood, P. & Simpson, H. B. 2013. Randomized controlled crossover trial of ketamine in obsessive-compulsive disorder: proof-of-concept. *Neuropsychopharmacology*, 38, 2475–2483. https://doi.org/10.1038/npp.2013.150

Roesler, R. & McGaugh, J. L. 2022. The entorhinal cortex as a gateway for amygdala influences on memory consolidation. *Neuroscience*, 497, 86–96. https://doi.org/https://doi.org/10.1016/j.neuroscience.2022.01.023

Rogers-Carter, M. M. & Christianson, J. P. 2019. An insular view of the social decision-making network. *Neuroscience & Biobehavioral Reviews*, 103, 119–132. https://doi.org/https://doi.org/10.1016/j.neubiorev.2019.06.005

Rogers-Carter, M. M., Varela, J. A., Gribbons, K. B., Pierce, A. F., McGoey, M. T., Ritchey, M. & Christianson, J. P. 2018. Insular cortex mediates approach and avoidance responses to social affective stimuli. *Nature Neuroscience*, 21, 404–414. https://doi.org/10.1038/s41593-018-0071-y

Rolle, C. E., Pedersen, M. L., Johnson, N., Amemori, K.-i., Ironside, M., Graybiel, A. M., Pizzagalli, D. A. & Etkin, A. 2021. The role of the dorsal–lateral prefrontal cortex in reward sensitivity during approach–avoidance conflict. *Cerebral Cortex*. https://doi.org/10.1093/cercor/bhab292

Rolls, E. T. 2023. Emotion, motivation, decision-making, the orbitofrontal cortex, anterior cingulate cortex, and the amygdala. *Brain Structure and Function*, 228, 1201–1257. https://doi.org/10.1007/s00429-023-02644-9

Rolls, E. T. & O'Mara, S. M. 1995. View-responsive neurons in the primate hippocampal complex. *Hippocampus*, 5, 409–424.

Roncon, C. M., Biesdorf, C., Santana, R. G., Zangrossi, H., Graeff, F. G. & Audi, E. A. 2012. The panicolytic-like effect of fluoxetine in the elevated T-maze is mediated by serotonin-induced activation of endogenous opioids in the dorsal periaqueductal gray. *Journal of Psychopharmacology*, 26, 525–531.

Ronel, Z. 2018. The lateral prefrontal cortex and selection/inhibition in ADHD. *Frontiers in Human Neuroscience*, 12, A65. https://doi.org/10.3389/fnhum.2018.00065

Röper, G. & Rachman, S. 1976. Obsessional-compulsive checking: experimental replication and development. *Behaviour Research and Therapy*, 14, 25–32.

Rose, J. D. 2002. The neurobehavioral nature of fishes and the question of awareness and pain. *Reviews in Fisheries Science*, 10, 1–38.

Rosenberg, R. & Jensen, P. N. 1994. Treatment of panic disorder with alprazolam and imipramine: clinical relevance of DSM III dysthymia. *European Journal of Psychiatry*, 9, 27–32.

Rosenfeld, D. S. & Furman, Y. 1994. Pure sleep panic: two case reports and a review of the literature. *Sleep*, 17, 462–465.

Rosenkilde, C. E. 1979. Functional heterogeneity of the prefrontal cortex in the monkey: a review. *Behavioral and Neural Biology*, 25, 301–345.

Rosenzweig, M. R., Bennett, E. L., Colombo, P. J., Lee, D. W. & Serrano, P. A. 1993. Short-term, intermediate-term, and long-term memories. *Behavioural Brain Research*, 57, 193–198.

Ross, R. T., Orr, W. B., Holland, P. C. & Berger, T. W. 1984. Hippocampectomy disrupts acquisition and retention of learned conditional responding. *Behavioral Neuroscience*, 98, 211–225.

Ross, T. W. & Easton, A. 2022. The hippocampal horizon: constructing and segmenting experience for episodic memory. *Neuroscience & Biobehavioral Reviews*, 132, 181–196. https://doi.org/https://doi.org/10.1016/j.neubiorev.2021.11.038

Rosso, M., Wirz, R., Loretan, A. V., Sutter, N. A., Pereira da Cunha, C. T., Jaric, I., Würbel, H. & Voelkl, B. 2022. Reliability of common mouse behavioural tests of anxiety: a systematic review and meta-analysis on the effects of anxiolytics. *Neuroscience & Biobehavioral Reviews*, 143, 104928. https://doi.org/https://doi.org/10.1016/j.neubiorev.2022.104928

Rowan, M. J., Cullen, W. K. & Moulton, B. 1990. Buspirone impairment of performance of passive avoidance and spatial learning tasks in the rat. *Psychopharmacology (Berl)*, 100, 393–398.

Roy-Byrne, P. 2015. Treatment-refractory anxiety; definition, risk factors, and treatment challenges. *Dialogues Clinical Neuroscience*, 17, 191–206.

Ruan, M., Young, C. K. & McNaughton, N. 2017. Bi-directional theta modulation between the septo-hippocampal system and the mammillary area in free-moving rats. *Frontiers in Neural Circuits*, 11, Article 62. https://doi.org/10.3389/fncir.2017.00062

Rubia, K., Smith, A. B., Brammer, M. J. & Taylor, E. 2003. Right inferior prefrontal cortex mediates response inhibition while mesial prefrontal cortex is responsible for error detection. *NeuroImage*, 20, 351–358.

Rucker, J. J. H., Iliff, J. & Nutt, D. J. 2018. Psychiatry & the psychedelic drugs. Past, present & future. *Neuropharmacology*, 142, 200–218. https://doi.org/https://doi.org/10.1016/j.neuropharm.2017.12.040

Rudolph, U. & Mohler, H. 2004. Analysis of GABAA receptor function and dissection of the pharmacology of benzodiazepines and general anesthetics through mouse genetics. *Annual Review of Pharmacology and Toxicology*, 44, 475–98.

Rudy, J. W. & Sutherland, R. J. 1989. The hippocampal formation is necessary for rats to learn and remember configural discriminations. *Behavioural Brain Research*, 34, 97–109.

Rudy, J. W. & Sutherland, R. J. 1992. Wait a minute, Jarrard and Davidson's data support configural association theory. *Hippocampus*, 2, 89–89.

Rushe, T. M., Morris, R. G., Miotto, E. C., Feigenbaum, J. D., Woodruff, P. W. R. & Murray, R. M. 1999. Problem-solving and spatial working memory in patients with schizophrenia and with focal frontal and temporal lobe lesions. *Schizophrenia Research*, 37, 21–33.

Russell, N. A., Horii, A., Smith, P., Darlington, C. L. & Bilkey, D. 2006. Lesions of the vestibular system disrupt hippocampal theta rhythm in the rat. *Journal of Neurophysiology*, 96, 4–14.

Ryan, P. J., Ma, S., Olucha-Bordonau, F. E. & Gundlach, A. L. 2011. Nucleus incertus--An emerging modulatory role in arousal, stress and memory. *Neuroscience & Biobehavioral Reviews*, 35, 1326–1341. https://doi.org/10.1016/j.neubiorev.2011.02.004

Sachdev, P. & Hay, P. 1996. Site and size of lesion and psychosurgical outcome in obsessive- compulsive disorder: a magnetic resonance imaging study. *Biological Psychiatry*, 39, 739–742.

Sachschal, J., Woodward, E., Wichelmann, J. M., Haag, K. & Ehlers, A. 2019. Differential effects of poor recall and memory disjointedness on trauma symptoms. *Clinical and Psychological Science*, 7, 1032–1041. https://doi.org/10.1177/2167702619847195

Sacks, O. 1985. *The man who mistook his wife for a hat, and other clinical tales.* London: Picador.

Sadeghi, S., McIntosh, J., Shadli, S. M., Healey, D., Rostami, R., Trani, P. & McNaughton, N. 2018. Does behavioural inhibition system dysfunction contribute to Attention Deficit Hyperactivity Disorder? *Personality Neuroscience*, 2, e5. https://doi.org/10.1017/pen.2019.5

Sadeh, T., Ozubko, J. D., Winocur, G. & Moscovitch, M. 2016. Forgetting patterns differentiate between two forms of memory representation. *Psychological Science*, 27, 810–820. https://doi.org/10.1177/0956797616638307

Sadeh, T. & Pertzov, Y. 2020. Scale-invariant characteristics of forgetting: toward a unifying account of hippocampal forgetting across short and long timescales. *Journal of Cognitive Neuroscience*, 32, 386–402. https://doi.org/10.1162/jocn_a_01491

Sah, P. 2017. Fear, anxiety, and the amygdala. *Neuron*, 96, 1–2. https://doi.org/10.1016/j.neuron.2017.09.013

Sah, P., Faber, E. S. L., Lopez De Armentia, M. & Power, J. 2003. The amygdaloid complex: anatomy and physiology. *Physiological Reviews*, 83, 803–834.

Sainsbury, R. S. & Montoya, C. P. 1984. The relationship between type 2 theta and behavior. *Physiology and Behavior*, 33, 621–626.

Saito, M., Toyoda, H., Kawakami, S., Sato, H., Bae, Y. C. & Kang, Y. 2012. Capsaicin induces theta-band synchronization between gustatory and autonomic insular cortices. *Journal of Neuroscience*, 32, 13470–87. https://doi.org/10.1523/JNEUROSCI.5906-11.2012

Sakimoto, Y. & Sakata, S. 2020. The role of the hippocampal theta rhythm in non-spatial discrimination and associative learning task. *Neuroscience & Biobehavioral Reviews*, 110, 92–99. https://doi.org/https://doi.org/10.1016/j.neubiorev.2018.09.016

Samson, R. D. e. D. & Pare, D. n. 2005. Activity-dependent synaptic plasticity in the central nucleus of the amygdala. *Journal of Neuroscience*, 25, 1847–1855.

Samuels, I. & Valian, V. 1968. Hippocampal lesions and redundant visual cues: effects on spatial reversal learning and subsequent visual discriminations. *Proceedings of the 76th Annual Convention of the American Psychological Association*, 3, 321–322.

Sanacora, G., Treccani, G. & Popoli, M. 2012. Towards a glutamate hypothesis of depression: an emerging frontier of neuropsychopharmacology for mood disorders. *Neuropharmacology*, 62, 63–77. https://doi.org/10.1016/j.neuropharm.2011.07.036

Sanders, H., Wilson, M. A. & Gershman, S. J. 2020. Hippocampal remapping as hidden state inference. *eLife*, 9, e51140. https://doi.org/10.7554/eLife.51140

Sanderson, W. C. & Wetzler, S. 1993. Observations on the cognitive behavioral treatment of panic disorder: impact of benzodiazepines. *Psychotherapy*, 30, 125–132.

Sandford, J. J., Argyropoulos, S. V. & Nutt, D. J. 2000. The psychobiology of anxiolytic drugs: part 1: basic neurobiology. *Pharmacology & Therapeutics*, 88, 197–212.

Sanfey, A. G., Loewenstein, G., McClure, S. M. & Cohen, J. D. 2006. Neuroeconomics: cross-currents in research on decision-making. *Trends in Cognitive Sciences*, 10, 108–116. https://doi.org/10.1016/j.tics.2006.01.009

Sanger, D. J. 1985. GABA and the behavioral effects of anxiolytic drugs. *Life Sciences*, 36, 1503–1513.

Sanger, D. J., Benavides, J., Perrault, G., Morel, E., Cohen, C., Joly, D. & Zivkovic, B. 1994. Recent developments in the behavioral pharmacology of benzodiazepine (omega) receptors: evidence for the functional significance of receptor subtypes. *Neuroscience & Biobehavioral Reviews*, 18, 355–372.

Sapolsky, R. M. 2001. Atrophy of the hippocampus in posttraumatic stress disorder: how and when? *Hippocampus*, 11, 90–91.

Sapolsky, R. M. 2004. *Why zebras don't get ulcers*, New York, Henry Holt and Company.

Sapolsky, R. M., Uno, H., Rebert, C. S. & Finch, C. E. 1990. Hippocampal damage associated with prolonged glucocorticoid exposure in primates. *The Journal of Neuroscience*, 10, 2897–2092.

Sara, S. J., Devauges, V. & Biegon, A. 1993. Maudsley rat strains, selected for differences in emotional responses, differ in behavioral response to clonidine and in [125I]clonidine binding in the locus coeruleus. *Behavioural Brain Research*, 57, 101–104.

Sartori, S. B. & Singewald, N. 2019. Novel pharmacological targets in drug development for the treatment of anxiety and anxiety-related disorders. *Pharmacology & Therapeutics*, 204, e107402. https://www.ncbi.nlm.nih.gov/pubmed/31470029

Sartory, G., MacDonald, R. & Gray, J. A. 1990. Effects of diazepam on approach, self-reported fear and psychophysiological responses in snake phobics. *Behaviour Research and Therapy*, 28, 273–282.s

Sassenberg, T. A., Burton, P. C., Mwilambwe-Tshilobo, L., Jung, R. E., Rustichini, A., Spreng, R. N. & DeYoung, C. G. 2023. Conscientiousness associated with efficiency of the salience/ventral attention network: replication in three samples using individualized parcellation. *Neuroimage*, 272, 120081.

Saucier, G. 2018. Culture, morality and individual differences: comparability and incomparability across species. *Philosohical Transactions of the Royal Society of London - B Biological Sciences*, 373. https://doi.org/10.1098/rstb.2017.0170

Sauer-Zavala, S., Southward, M. W. & Semcho, S. A. 2020. Integrating and differentiating personality and psychopathology in cognitive behavioral therapy. *Journal of Personality*, 90, 89-102. https://doi.org/https://doi.org/10.1111/jopy.12602

Schafe, G. E., Doyere, V. & LeDoux, J. 2005. Tracking the fear engram: the lateral amygdala is an essential locus of fear memory storage. *Journal of Neuroscience*, 25, 10010–10014.

Schallek, W., Schlosser, W. & Randall, L. O. 1972. Recent developments in the pharmacology of the benzodiazepines. *Advances in Pharmaceuticals for Chemotherapy*, 10, 119–181.

Scherrer, J. F., True, W. R., Xian, H., Lyons, M. J., Eisen, S. A., Goldberg, J., Lin, N. & Tsuang, M. T. 2000. Evidence for genetic influences common and specific to symptoms of generalized anxiety and panic. *Journal of Affective Disorders*, 57, 25–35.

Schmidt, M. V., Abraham, W. C., Maroun, M., Stork, O. & Richter-Levin, G. 2013. Stress-induced metaplasticity: from synapses to behavior. *Neuroscience*, 250, 112–120. https://doi.org/10.1016/j.neuroscience.2013.06.059

Schmitz, T. W., Correia, M. M., Ferreira, C. S., Prescot, A. P. & Anderson, M. C. 2017. Hippocampal GABA enables inhibitory control over unwanted thoughts. *Nature Communications*, 8, A01311. https://doi.org/10.1038/s41467-017-00956-z

Schneider, M., Broggini, A. C., Dann, B., Tzanou, A., Uran, C., Sheshadri, S., Scherberger, H. & Vinck, M. 2021. A mechanism for inter-areal coherence through communication based on connectivity and oscillatory power. *Neuron*, 109, 4050–4067.e12. https://doi.org/https://doi.org/10.1016/j.neuron.2021.09.037

Schoenbaum, G., Setlow, B., Saddoris, M. P. & Gallagher, M. 2003. Encoding predicted outcome and acquired value in orbitofrontal cortex during cue sampling depends upon input from basolateral amygdala. *Neuron*, 39, 855–867.

Schönbrodt, F. D. & Perugini, M. 2013. At what sample size do correlations stabilize? *Journal of Research in Personality*, 47, 609–612. https://doi.org/10.1016/j.jrp.2013.05.009

Schuckit, M. A. 1984. Clinical studies of buspirone. *Psychopathology*, 17, 61–68.

Schuette, P. J., Reis, F. M. C. V., Maesta-Pereira, S., Chakerian, M., Torossian, A., Blair, G. J., Wang, W., Blair, H. T., Fanselow, M. S., Kao, J. C. & Adhikari, A. 2020. Long-term characterization of hippocampal remapping during contextual fear acquisition and extinction. *The Journal of Neuroscience*, 40, 8329–8342. https://doi.org/10.1523/jneurosci.1022-20.2020

Schulkin, J. 1994. Melancholic depression and the hormones of adversity: a role for the amygdala. *Current Directions in Psychological Science*, 3, 41–44.

Schulkin, J., McEwen, B. S. & Gold, P. W. 1994. Allostasis, amygdala, and anticipatory angst. *Neuroscience & Biobehavioral Reviews*, 18, 385–396.

Schultz, W. 1998. Predictive reward signal of dopamine neurons. *Journal of Neurophysiology*, 80, 1–27. https://doi.org/10.1152/jn.1998.80.1.1

Schultz, W. 2002. Getting formal with dopamine and reward. *Neuron*, 36, 241–263.

Schultz, W. 2016. Dopamine reward prediction-error signalling: a two-component response. *Nature Reviews Neuroscience*, 17, 183–95. https://doi.org/10.1038/nrn.2015.26

Schultz, W., Dayan, P. & Montague, P. R. 1997. A neural substrate of prediction and reward. *Science*, 275, 1593–1599.

Schultz, W., Stauffer, W. R. & Lak, A. 2017. The phasic dopamine signal maturing: from reward via behavioural activation to formal economic utility. *Current Opinion in Neurobiology*, 43, 139–148. https://doi.org/10.1016/j.conb.2017.03.013

Schwartzkroin, P. A. 1994. Cellular electrophysiology of human epilepsy. *Epilepsy Research*, 17, 185–192. https://doi.org/https://doi.org/10.1016/0920-1211(94)90049-3

Schwob, M., Daniels, M., Robinson, D. & Berman, E. 1989. Adverse experiences reported following marketing of buspirone; period of report October 1984 February 1989. unpublished ms kindly supplied by Bristol-Myers.

Scottish Office 1996. *Neurosurgery for mental disorders*, Edinburgh, Her Majesty's Stationery Office.

Segal, M. 1977a. The effects of brainstem priming stimulation on interhemispheric hippocampal responses in the awake rat. *Experimental Brain Research*, 28, 529–541.

Segal, M. 1977b. Excitability changes in rat hippocampus during conditioning. *Experimental Neurology*, 55, 67–73.

Segal, M. & Bloom, F. E. 1974. The action of norepinephrine in the rat hippocampus. II. Activation of the input pathway. *Brain Research*, 72, 99–111.

Segal, M. & Bloom, F. E. 1976. The action of norepinephrine in the rat hippocampus. IV. The effects of locus coeruleus stimulation on evoked hippocampal unit activity. *Brain Research*, 107, 513–525.

Sekeres, M. J., Winocur, G., Moscovitch, M., Anderson, J. A. E., Pishdadian, S., Martin Wojtowicz, J., St-Laurent, M., McAndrews, M. P. & Grady, C. L. 2018. Changes in patterns of neural activity underlie a time-dependent transformation of memory in rats and humans. *Hippocampus*, 28, 745–764. https://doi.org/https://doi.org/10.1002/hipo.23009

Selden, N. R. W., Everitt, B. J., Jarrard, L. E. & Robbins, T. W. 1991. Complementary roles for the amygdala and hippocampus in aversive conditioning to explicit and contextual cues. *Neuroscience*, 42, 335–350.

Selemon, L. D., Goldman-Rakic, P. S. & Tamminga, C. A. 1995. Prefrontal cortex. *American Journal of Psychiatry*, 152, 5–5.

Seligman, M. E. P. 1971. Phobias and preparedness. *The Behaviour Therapist*, 2, 307–320.

Seligman, M. E. P. 1975. *Helplessness*, San Francisco, Freeman.

Sellbom, M. 2019. The MMPI-2-Restructured Form (MMPI-2-RF): assessment of personality and psychopathology in the twenty-first century. *Annual Review of Clinical Psychology*, 15, 149–177. https://doi.org/10.1146/annurev-clinpsy-050718-095701

Sellbom, M., Kremyar, A. J. & Wygant, D. B. 2021. Mapping MMPI-3 scales onto the hierarchical taxonomy of psychopathology. *Psychological Assessment*, in press. https://doi.org/10.1037/pas0001049

Senoussi, M., Verbeke, P., Desender, K., De Loof, E., Talsma, D. & Verguts, T. 2022. Theta oscillations shift towards optimal frequency for cognitive control. *Nature Human Behaviour*. https://doi.org/10.1038/s41562-022-01335-5

Seo, D.-o., Zhang, E. T., Piantadosi, S. C., Marcus, D. J., Motard, L. E., Kan, B. K., Gomez, A. M., Nguyen, T. K., Xia, L. & Bruchas, M. R. 2021. A locus coeruleus to dentate gyrus noradrenergic circuit modulates aversive contextual processing. *Neuron*, 109, 2116–2130.e6. https://doi.org/https://doi.org/10.1016/j.neuron.2021.05.006

Setem, J., Pinheiro, A. P., Motta, V. A., Morato, S. & Cruz, A. P. M. 1999. Ethopharmacological analysis of 5-HT ligands on the rat elevated plus maze. *Pharmacology, Biochemistry and Behavior*, 62, 515–521.

Shadli, S. M., Ando, L. C., McIntosh, J., Lodhia, V., Russell, B. R., Kirk, I. J., Glue, P. & McNaughton, N. 2021a. Right frontal anxiolytic-sensitive EEG 'theta' rhythm in the stop-signal task is a theory-based anxiety disorder biomarker. *Scientific Reports*, 11, 19746. https://doi.org/10.1038/s41598-021-99374-x

Shadli, S. M., Glue, P., McIntosh, J. & McNaughton, N. 2015. An improved human anxiety process biomarker: characterization of frequency band, personality and pharmacology. *Translational Psychiatry*, 5, e699. https://doi.org/10.1038/tp.2015.188

Shadli, S. M., Harrison, O. K., Russell, B. R., Lodhia, V., Kirk, I. J., Glue, P. & McNaughton, N. submitted. Source localisation of a theory-based anxiety disorder biomarker *Currently under revision*.

Shadli, S. M., High, O., Byers, B., Gibbs, P., Steller, R., Glue, P. & McNaughton, N. 2020a. Human anxiety-specific "theta" occurs with selective stopping and localizes to right inferior frontal gyrus. *Behavioral Neuroscience*, 134, 547–555. https://doi.org/10.1037/bne0000316

Shadli, S. M., Kawe, T., Martin, D., McNaughton, N., Neehoff, S. & Glue, P. 2018a. Ketamine effects on EEG during therapy of treatment-resistant generalized anxiety and social anxiety. *International Journal of Neuropsychopharmacology*, pyy032–pyy032. https://doi.org/10.1093/ijnp/pyy032

Shadli, S. M., Kawe, T., Martin, D., McNaughton, N., Neehoff, S. & Glue, P. 2018b. Ketamine effects on EEG during therapy of treatment-resistant generalized anxiety and social anxiety. *International Journal of Neuropsychopharmacology*, 21, 717–724. https://doi.org/10.1093/ijnp/pyy032

Shadli, S. M., McIntosh, J. & McNaughton, N. 2020b. Anxiety process "theta" biomarker in the stop signal task eliminated by a preceding relaxation test. *Behavioral Neuroscience*, 134, 556–561 https://doi.org/10.1037/bne0000328

Shadli, S. M., Smith, M. J., Glue, P. & McNaughton, N. 2016. Testing an anxiety process biomarker: generalisation from an auditory to a visual stimulus. *Biological Psychology*, 117, 50–55. https://doi.org/10.1016/j.biopsycho.2016.02.011

Shadli, S. M., Tewari, V., Holden, J. & McNaughton, N. 2021b. Laterality of an EEG anxiety disorder biomarker largely follows handedness. *Cortex*, 140, 210–221. https://doi.org/10.1016/j.cortex.2021.03.025

Shan, X., Contreras, M. P., Sawangjit, A., Dimitrov, S., Born, J. & Inostroza, M. 2023. Rearing is critical for forming spatial representations in pre-weanling rats. *Behavioural Brain Research*, 452, 114545. https://doi.org/10.1016/j.bbr.2023.114545

Sharp, P. E., Blair, H. T., Etkin, D. & Tzanetos, D. B. 1995. Influences of vestibular and visual motion information on the spatial firing patterns of hippocampal place cells. *The Journal of Neuroscience*, 15, 173–189.

Sharp, P. E. & Green, C. 1994. Spatial correlates of firing patterns of single cells in the subiculum of the freely moving rat. *The Journal of Neuroscience*, 14, 2339–2356.

Shear, M. K. & Maser, J. D. 1994. Standardized assessment for panic disorder research: a conference report. *Archives of General Psychiatry*, 51, 346–354.

Sheehan, D. V., Ballenger, J. & Jacobson, G. 1981. Relative efficacy of monoamine oxidase inhibitors and tricyclic antidepressants in the treatment of endogenous anxiety. *In:* Klein, D. F. & Rabkin, J. (eds.) *Anxiety new research and changing concepts* (pp. 47–67). New York: Raven Press.

Sheehan, D. V., Raj, A. B., Sheehan, K. H. & Soto, S. 1990. Is buspirone effective for panic disorders? *Journal of Clinical Psychopharmacology*, 10, 3–11.

Shekhar, A. 1993. GABA receptors in the region of the dorsomedial hypothalamus of rats regulate anxiety in the elevated plus-maze test. I. Behavioral measures. *Brain Research*, 627, 9–16.

Shekhar, A. 1994. Effects of treatment with imipramine and clonazepam on an animal model of panic disorder. *Biological Psychiatry*, 36, 748–758.

Shekhar, A., Sims, L. S. & Bowsher, R. R. 1993. GABA receptors in the region of the dorsomedial hypothalamus of rats regulate anxiety in the elevated plus-maze test. II. Physiological measures. *Brain Research*, 627, 17–24.

Shephard, E., Stern, E. R., van den Heuvel, O. A., Costa, D. L. C., Batistuzzo, M. C., Godoy, P. B. G., Lopes, A. C., Brunoni, A. R., Hoexter, M. Q., Shavitt, R. G., Reddy, Y. C. J., Lochner, C., Stein, D. J., Simpson, H. B. & Miguel, E. C. 2021. Toward a neurocircuit-based taxonomy to guide treatment of obsessive-compulsive disorder. *Molecular Psychiatry*, 26, 4583–4604. https://doi.org/10.1038/s41380-020-01007-8

Shepherd, E. H., Fournier, N. M., Sutherland, R. J. & Lehmann, H. 2021. Distributed learning episodes create a context fear memory outside the hippocampus that depends on perirhinal and anterior cingulate cortices. *Learning & Memory*, 28, 405–413. https://doi.org/10.1101/lm.053396.121

Shi, C. J. & Cassell, M. D. 1998. Cortical, thalamic, and amygdaloid connections of the anterior and posterior insular cortices. *Journal of Comparative Neurology*, 399, 440–468.

Shi, T. Y., Feng, S. F., Wei, M. X., Huang, Y., Liu, G., Wu, H. T., Zhang, Y. X. & Zhou, W. X. 2018. Kainate receptor mediated presynaptic LTP in agranular insular cortex contributes to fear and anxiety in mice. *Neuropharmacology*, 128, 388–400. https://doi.org/10.1016/j.neuropharm.2017.10.037

Shibata, S., Yamashita, K., Yamamoto, E., Ozaki, T. & Ueki, S. 1989. Effects of benzodiazepine and GABA antagonists on anticonflict effects of antianxiety drugs injected into the rat amygdala in a water-lick suppression test. *Psychopharmacology*, 98, 38–44.

Shinder, M. E. & Taube, J. S. 2014. Resolving the active versus passive conundrum for head direction cells. *Neuroscience*, 270, 123–138. https://doi.org/10.1016/j.neuroscience.2014.03.053

Sidman, M., Stoddard, L. & Mohr, J. 1968. Some additional quantitative observations of immediate memory in a patient with bilateral hippocampal lesions. *Neuropsychologia*, 6, 245–254.

Silva, C. & McNaughton, N. 2019. Are periaqueductal gray and dorsal raphe the foundation of appetitive and aversive control? A comprehensive review. *Progress in Neurobiology*, 177, 33–72. https://doi.org/https://doi.org/10.1016/j.pneurobio.2019.02.001

Silva, C., Young, C. K. & McNaughton, N. 2022. Prefrontal and hippocampal theta rhythm show anxiolytic-like changes during periaqueductal-elicited "panic" in rats. *Hippocampus*, 32, 679-694. https://doi.org/https://doi.org/10.1002/hipo.23459

Silveira, M. C. L. & Graeff, F. G. 1992. Defense reaction elicited by microinjection of kainic acid into the medial hypothalamus of the rat: antagonism by a GABA A receptor agonist. *Behavioral and Neural Biology*, 57, 226–232.

Simon, P. & Soubrié, P. 1979. Behavior studies to differentiate anxiolytic and sedative activity of the tranquilizing drugs. In: Boissier, J. R. (ed.) *Differential psychopharmacology of anxiolytics and sedatives. Modern problems of pharmacopsychiatry, Vol. 14* (pp. 99–142). Basel: Karger.

Simonov, P. V. 1974. On the role of the hippocampus in the integrative activity of the brain. *Acta Neurobiologica Experimentalis*, 34, 33–41.

Simonov, P. V. 1997. Brain mechanisms of emotions. *Neuroscience and Behavioral Physiology*, 27, 405–413.

Sinclair, L. & Nutt, D. 2007. Anxiolytics. *Psychiatry*, 6, 284–288. https://doi.org/https://doi.org/10.1016/j.mppsy.2007.04.007

Sinden, J. D., Rashid-Doubell, F., Kershaw, T. R., Nelson, A., Chadwick, A., Jat, P. S., Noble, M. D., Hodges, H. & Gray, J. A. 1997. Recovery of spatial learning by grafts of a conditionally immortalized hippocampal neuroepithelial cell line into the ischaemia-lesioned hippocampus. *Neuroscience*, 81, 599–608.

Sinha, M. & Narayanan, R. 2015. HCN channels enhance spike phase coherence and regulate the phase of spikes and LFPs in the theta-frequency range. *Proceedings of the National Academy of Sciences*, 112, E2207–E2216. https://doi.org/10.1073/pnas.1419017112

Sinha, S. S., Coplan, J. D., Pine, D. S., Martinez, J. A., Klein, D. F. & Gorman, J. M. 1999. Panic induced by carbon dioxide inhalation and lack of hypothalamic-pituitary-adrenal axis activation. *Psychiatry Research*, 86, 93–98.

Siok, C. J., Taylor, C. P. & Hajós, M. 2009. Anxiolytic profile of pregabalin on elicited hippocampal theta oscillation. *Neuropharmacology*, 56, 379–385. https://doi.org/10.1016/j.neuropharm.2008.09.013

Sirigu, A., Zalla, T., Pillon, B., Grafman, J., Agid, Y. & Dubois, B. 1995. Selective impairments in managerial knowledge following pre-frontal cortex damage. *Cortex*, 31, 301–316.

Skaggs, W. E. & McNaughton, B. L. 1996. Replay of neuronal firing sequences in rat hippocampus during sleep following spatial experience. *Science*, 271, 1870–1873.

Skaggs, W. E., McNaughton, B. L., Wilson, M. A. & Barnes, C. A. 1996. Theta phase precession in hippocampal neuronal populations and the compression of temporal sequences. *Hippocampus*, 6, 149–172.

Skinner, B. F. 1938. *The behavior of organisms.* New York: Appleton-Century.

Slade, T. I. M. & Watson, D. 2006. The structure of common DSM-IV and ICD-10 mental disorders in the Australian general population. *Psychological Medicine*, 36, 1593–1600. https://doi.org/10.1017/S0033291706008452

Slee, A., Nazareth, I., Bondaronek, P., Liu, Y., Cheng, Z. & Freemantle, N. 2019. Pharmacological treatments for generalised anxiety disorder: a systematic review and network meta-analysis. *The Lancet*, 393, 768–777. https://doi.org/10.1016/s0140-6736(18)31793-8

Smederevac, S., Mitrović, D., Čolović, P. & Nikolašević, Z. 2014. Validation of the measure of revised reinforcement sensitivity theory constructs. *Journal of Individual Differences*, 35, 12–21. https://doi.org/10.1027/1614-0001/a000121

Smederevac, S., Sadiković, S., Čolović, P., Vučinić, N., Milutinović, A., Riemann, R., Corr, P., Prinz, M. & Budimlija, Z. 2022. Quantitative behavioral genetic and molecular genetic foundations of the approach and avoidance strategies. *Current Psychology*. https://doi.org/10.1007/s12144-022-02724-9

Smillie, L. D., Cooper, A. J. & Pickering, A. D. 2011. Individual differences in reward-prediction-error: extraversion and feedback-related negativity. *Social Cognitive and Affective Neuroscience*, 6, 646–52. https://doi.org/10.1093/scan/nsq078

Smillie, L. D., Jach, H. K., Hughes, D. M., Wacker, J., Cooper, A. J. & Pickering, A. D. 2019. Extraversion and reward-processing: consolidating evidence from an electroencephalographic index of reward-prediction-error. *Biological Psychology*, 146, 107735. https://doi.org/10.1016/j.biopsycho.2019.107735

Smillie, L. D., Jackson, C. J. & Dalgleish, L. I. 2006. Conceptual distinctions between Carver and White's (1994) BAS scales: a reward-reactivity versus trait impulsivity perspective. *Personality and Individual Differences*, 40, 1039–1050.

Smith, D. M., Yang, Y. Y., Subramanian, D. L., Miller, A. M. P., Bulkin, D. A. & Law, L. M. 2022. The limbic memory circuit and the neural basis of contextual memory. *Neurobiology of Learning and Memory*, 187, 107557. https://doi.org/https://doi.org/10.1016/j.nlm.2021.107557

Smith, M. L. & Milner, B. 1984. Differential effects of frontal-lobe lesions on cognitive estimation and spatial memory. *Neuropsychologia*, 22, 697–705.

Smith, P. F. 2017. The vestibular system and cognition. *Current Opinion in Neurology*, 30, 84–89.

Smith, R. & Lane, R. D. 2015. The neural basis of one's own conscious and unconscious emotional states. *Neuroscience & Biobehavioral Reviews*, 57, 1–29. https://doi.org/https://doi.org/10.1016/j.neubiorev.2015.08.003

Smythe, J. W., Murphy, D., Bhatnagar, S., Timothy, C. & Costall, B. 1996. Muscarinic antagonists are anxiogenic in rats tested in the black-white box. *Pharmacology, Biochemistry and Behavior*, 54, 57–63.

Soares, M. C., Gerlai, R. & Maximino, C. 2018. The integration of sociality, monoamines and stress neuroendocrinology in fish models: applications in the neurosciences. *Journal of Fish Biology*, 93, 170–191. https://doi.org/doi:10.1111/jfb.13757

Sobanski, T. & Wagner, G. 2017. Functional neuroanatomy in panic disorder: status quo of the research. *World Journal of Psychiatry*, 7, 12–33. https://doi.org/10.5498/wjp.v7.i1.12

Sokolov, E. N. 1960. Neuronal models and the orienting reflex. *In:* Brazier, M. A. B. (ed.) *The central nervous system and behaviour, 3rd Conference* (pp. 187–276). New York: Josiah Macy Jr Foundation.

Sokolov, E. N. 1963. *Perception and the conditioned reflex*, Oxford, Pergamon Press.

Solomon, P. R. 1977. Role of the hippocampus in blocking and conditioned inhibition of the rabbit's nictating membrane response. *Journal of Comparative and Physiological Psychology*, 91, 407–417.

Solomon, P. R. & Moore, J. W. 1975. Latent inhibition and stimulus generalization of the classically conditioned nictating membrane response in rabbits following dorsal hippocampal ablation. *Journal of Comparative and Physiological Psychology*, 89, 1192–1203.

Solomon, P. R., Nichols, G. L., Kiernan Iii, J. M., Kamer, R. S. & Kaplan, L. J. 1980. Differential effects of lesions in medial and dorsal raphe of the rat: latent inhibition and septohippocampal serotonin levels. *Journal of Comparative and Physiological Psychology*, 94, 145–154. https://doi.org/10.1037/h0077655

Soma, S., Suematsu, N., Sato, A. Y., Tsunoda, K., Bramian, A., Reddy, A., Takabatake, K., Karube, F., Fujiyama, F. & Shimegi, S. 2021. Acetylcholine from the nucleus basalis magnocellularis facilitates the retrieval of well-established memory. *Neurobiology of Learning and Memory*, 183, 107484. https://doi.org/https://doi.org/10.1016/j.nlm.2021.107484

Somogyi, P., Katona, L., Klausberger, T., Lasztóczi, B. & Viney, T. J. 2014. Temporal redistribution of inhibition over neuronal subcellular domains underlies state-dependent rhythmic change of excitability in the hippocampus. *Philosophical Transactions of the Royal Society B: Biological Sciences*, 369, 20120518. https://doi.org/10.1098/rstb.2012.0518

Sosa, R., Mata-Luévanos, J. & Buenrostro-Jáuregui, M. 2021. The role of the lateral habenula in inhibitory learning from reward omission experiences. *eNeuro*, ENEURO.0016-21.2021. https://doi.org/10.1523/eneuro.0016-21.2021

Soubrié, P. 1986. Reconciling the role of central serotonin neurons in human and clinical behavior. *Behavioral and Brain Sciences*, 9, 319–319.

Southwick, S. M., Bremner, D., Krystal, J. H. & Charney, D. S. 1994. Psychobiologic research in post-traumatic stress disorder. *Psychiatric Clinics of North America*, 17, 251–264.

Souza, T. M. E., Rodrigues, C., Souza, M. M., Vinadé, E., Coitinho, A., Choi, H. & Izquierdo, I. 2001. Involvement of the serotonergic type 1A (5-HT1A) receptor in the agranular insular cortex in the consolidation of memory for inhibitory avoidance in rats. *Behavioural Pharmacology*, 12, 349–353.

Spielberger, C. D., Gorusch, R. L., Lushene, R., Vagg, P. R. & Jacobs, G. A. 1983. *Manual for the STATE-TRAIT ANXIETY INVENTORY (Form Y)*, Palo Alto, CA94306, Consulting Psychologists Press.

Spivak, B., Strous, R. D., Shaked, G., Shabash, E., Kotler, M. & Weizman, A. 2006. Reboxetine versus fluvoxamine in the treatment of motor vehicle accident-related posttraumatic stress disorder: a double-blind, fixed-dosage, controlled trial. *Journal of Clinical Psychopharmacology*, 26, 152–6. https://doi.org/10.1097/01.jcp.0000203195.65710.f0

Squire, L. R., Amaral, D. G. & Press, G. A. 1990. Magnetic resonance imaging of the hippocampal formation and mammillary nuclei distinguish medial temporal lobe and diencephalic amnesia. *The Journal of Neuroscience*, 10, 3106–3117.

Squire, L. R. & Cave, C. B. 1991. The hippocampus, memory and space. *Hippocampus*, 1, 269–271.

Squire, L. R. & Zola-Morgan, S. 1984. The neuropsychology of memory: new links between humans and experimental animals. *Annals of the New York Academy of Sciences*, 444, 137–149.

Squire, L. R. & Zola-Morgan, S. 1991. The medial temporal lobe memory system. *Science*, 253, 1380–1386.

Stachenfeld, K. L., Botvinick, M. M. & Gershman, S. J. 2017. The hippocampus as a predictive map. *Nature Neuroscience*, 20, 1643–1653. https://doi.org/10.1038/nn.4650 https://www.nature.com/articles/nn.4650#supplementary-information

Stackman, R. W., Golob, E. J., Bassett, J. P. & Taube, J. S. 2003. Passive transport disrupts directional path integration by rat head direction cells. *Journal of Neurophysiology*, 90, 2862–2874. https://doi.org/10.1152/jn.00346.2003

Stanton, M. E. 2000. Multiple memory systems, development and conditioning. *Behavioural Brain Research*, 110, 25–37.

Steckler, T. & Muir, J. L. 1996. Measurement of cognitive function: relating rodent performance with human minds. *Cognitive Brain Research*, 3, 299–308.

Stein, D. J., Hollander, E., Mullen, L. S., DeCaria, C. M. & Liebowitz, M. R. 1992. Comparison of clomipramine, alprazolam and placebo in the treatment of obsessive-compulsive disorder. *Human Psychopharmacology*, 7, 389–395. https://doi.org/10.1002/hup.470070604

Stein, D. J., Vythilingum, B. & Seedat, S. 2004. Pharmacotherapy of phobias. *In:* Maj, M. (ed.) *Evidence & experience in psychiatry. Vol. 7* (Chapter 3). *Phobias*. John Wiley & Sons, Ltd.

Stein, M. B. 1998. Neurobiological perspectives on social phobia: from affiliation to zoology. *Biological Psychiatry*, 44, 1277–1285.

Stein, M. B., Asmundson, G. J. G. & Chartier, M. 1994a. Autonomic responsivity in generalized social phobia. *Journal of Affective Disorders*, 31, 211–221.

Stein, M. B., Koverola, C., Hanna, C., Torchia, M. G. & McClarty, B. 1997. Hippocampal volume in women victimized by childhood sexual abuse. *Psychological Medicine*, 27, 951–959.

Stein, M. B., Walker, J. R. & Forde, D. R. 1994b. Setting diagnostic thresholds for social phobia: considerations from a community survey of social anxiety. *American Journal of Psychiatry*, 151, 408–412.

Steinberg, E. E., Gore, F., Heifets, B. D., Taylor, M. D., Norville, Z. C., Beier, K. T., Földy, C., Lerner, T. N., Luo, L., Deisseroth, K. & Malenka, R. C. 2020. Amygdala-midbrain connections modulate appetitive and aversive learning. *Neuron*, 106, 1026–1043.e9. https://doi.org/https://doi.org/10.1016/j.neuron.2020.03.016

Steinmetz, J. E. 2000. Brain substrates of classical eyeblink conditioning: a highly localized but also distributed system. *Behavioural Brain Research*, 110, 13–24.

Stephan, H. & Andy, O. J. 1969. Quantitative comparative neuroanatomy of primates: an attempt at a phylogenetic interpretation. *Annals of the New York Academy of Sciences*, 167, 370–387. https://doi.org/10.1111/j.1749-6632.1969.tb20457.x

Sternson, S. M. 2013. Hypothalamic survival circuits: blueprints for purposive behaviors. *Neuron*, 77, 810–824. https://doi.org/10.1016/j.neuron.2013.02.018

Stevens, J. C. & Pollack, M. H. 2005. Benzodiazepines in clinical practice: consideration of their long-term use and alternative agents. *Journal of Clinical Psychiatry*, 66, 21–27.

Stevenson, M. & McNaughton, N. 2013. A comparison of phenylketonuria with attention deficit hyperactivity disorder: do markedly different aetiologies deliver common phenotypes? *Brain Research Bulletin*, 99, 63–83. https://doi.org/10.1016/j.brainresbull.2013.10.003

Stewardson, H. & Sambrook, T. D. 2023. Valence precedes value in neural encoding of prediction error. *Psychophysiology*, e14266. https://doi.org/10.1111/psyp.14266

Stewart, S. H. & Conrod, P. J. (eds.) 2008. *Anxiety and substance use disorders: the vicious cycle of comorbidity*. New York: Springer Science+Business Media, Inc.

Stouffer, S. A., Lumsdaine, A. A., Lumsdaine, M. H., Williams, R. M., Smith, M. B., Janis, I. L., Star, S. A. & Cottrell, L. S. 1949. *Studies in social psychology in world war II: Vol 2. The American soldier: combat and its aftermath*, Princeton, Princeton University Press, cited by Broadhurst, P. L. (1960) page 37.

Strange, B. A., Witter, M. P., Lein, E. S. & Moser, E. I. 2014. Functional organization of the hippocampal longitudinal axis. *Nature Reviews Neuroscience*, 15, 655–669. https://doi.org/10.1038/nrn3785

Strauss, C. V. A., Maisonnette, S. S., Coimbra, N. C. & Zangrossi, H. 2003. Effects of N-methyl-d-aspartate-induced amygdala lesion in rats submitted to the elevated T-maze test of anxiety. *Physiology & Behavior*, 78, 157–163. https://doi.org/https://doi.org/10.1016/S0031-9384(02)00960-5

Strawn, J. R. & Geracioti, T. D., Jr. 2007. The treatment of generalized anxiety disorder with pregabalin, an atypical anxiolytic. *Neuropsychiatric Disease and Treatment*, 3, 237–243.

Ström-Olsen, R. & Carlisle, R. 1971. Bi-frontal stereotactic tractotomy: a follow-up study of its effects on 210 patients. *British Journal of Psychiatry*, 118, 141–154.

Sugar, J., Witter, M., van Strien, N. & Cappaert, N. 2011. The retrosplenial cortex: intrinsic connectivity and connections with the (para)hippocampal region in the rat. An interactive connectome. *Frontiers in Neuroinformatics*, 5, A7. https://doi.org/10.3389/fninf.2011.00007

Sumner, R. L., Spriggs, M. J., Muthukumaraswamy, S. D. & Kirk, I. J. 2020. The role of Hebbian learning in human perception: a methodological and theoretical review of the human Visual Long-Term Potentiation paradigm. *Neuroscience & Biobehavioral Reviews*, 115, 220–237. https://doi.org/https://doi.org/10.1016/j.neubiorev.2020.03.013

Suryanarayana, S. M., Pérez-Fernández, J., Robertson, B. & Grillner, S. 2020. The evolutionary origin of visual and somatosensory representation in the vertebrate pallium. *Nature Ecology & Evolution,* 4, 639-651. https://doi.org/10.1038/s41559-020-1137-2

Sutherland, N. S. & Mackintosh, N. J. 1971. *Mechanisms of animal discrimination learning.* London: Academic Press.

Sutherland, R. J., Lee, J. Q., McDonald, R. J. & Lehmann, H. 2020. Has multiple trace theory been refuted? *Hippocampus*, 30, 842–850. https://doi.org/10.1002/hipo.23162

Sutherland, R. J. & Rudy, J. W. 1989. Configural association theory: the role of the hippocampal formation in learning, memory and amnesia. *Psychobiology*, 17, 129–144.

Suzdak, P., Glowa, J. R., Crawley, J. N., Schwartz, R. D., Skolnick, P. & Paul, S. M. 1986. A selective imidabenzodiazepine antagonist of ethanol in the rat. *Science*, 234, 1243–1247.

Suzuki, W. A. & Amaral, D. G. 1994. Topographic organization of the reciprocal connections between the monkey entorhinal cortex and the perirhinal and parahippocampal cortices. *The Journal of Neuroscience*, 14, 1856–1877.

Suzuki, W. A., Zola-Morgan, S., Squire, L. R. & Amaral, D. G. 1993. Lesions of the perirhinal and parahippocampal cortices in the monkey produce long-lasting memory impairment in the visual and tactual modalities. *The Journal of Neuroscience*, 13, 2430–2451.

Swanson, L. W. 1995. Mapping the human brain: past, present, and future. *Trends in Neuroscience*, 18, 471–474.

Swanson, L. W. 2018. Brain maps 4.0—Structure of the rat brain: an open access atlas with global nervous system nomenclature ontology and flatmaps. *Journal of Comparative Neurology*, 526, 935–943. https://doi.org/10.1002/cne.24381

Swayze, V. W., II 1995. Frontal leukotomy and related psychosurgical procedures in the era before antipsychotics (1935-1954): a historical overview. *American Journal of Psychiatry*, 152, 505–515.

Szadzinska, W., Danielewski, K., Kondrakiewicz, K., Andraka, K., Nikolaev, E., Mikosz, M. & Knapska, E. 2021. Hippocampal inputs in the prelimbic cortex curb fear after extinction. *The Journal of Neuroscience*, 41, 9129–9140. https://doi.org/10.1523/jneurosci.0764-20.2021

Takahashi, K., Lin, J. S. & Sakai, K. 2006. Neuronal activity of histaminergic tuberomammillary neurons during wake-sleep states in the mouse. *Journal of Neuroscience*, 26, 10292–10298.

Takamiya, S., Shiotani, K., Ohnuki, T., Osako, Y., Tanisumi, Y., Yuki, S., Manabe, H., Hirokawa, J. & Sakurai, Y. 2021. Hippocampal CA1 neurons represent positive feedback during the learning process of an associative memory task. *Frontiers in Systems Neuroscience*, 15, A718619. https://doi.org/10.3389/fnsys.2021.718619

Takeuchi, T., Duszkiewicz, A. J., Sonneborn, A., Spooner, P. A., Yamasaki, M., Watanabe, M., Smith, C. C., Fernandez, G., Deisseroth, K., Greene, R. W. & Morris, R. G. 2016. Locus coeruleus and dopaminergic consolidation of everyday memory. *Nature*, 537, 357–362. https://doi.org/10.1038/nature19325

Talalaenko, A. N., Pankrat'ev, D. V. & Goncharenko, N. V. 2003. Neurochemical characteristics of the ventromedial hypothalamus in mediating the antiaversive effects of anxiolytics in different models of anxiety. *Neuroscience and Behavioral Physiology*, 33, 255–261.

Tallman, J. F., Paul, S. M., Skolnick, P. & Gallager, D. W. 1980. Receptors for the age of anxiety: pharmacology of the benzodiazepines. *Science*, 267, 274–281.

Tan, E., Marks, I. M. & Marset, P. 1971. Bimedial leucotomy in obsessive compulsive neurosis: a controlled serial enquiry. *British Journal of Psychiatry*, 118, 155–164.

Tan, S., Kirk, R. C., Abraham, W. C. & McNaughton, N. 1990. Chlordiazepoxide reduces discriminability but not rate of forgetting in delayed conditional discrimination. *Psychopharmacology (Berl)*, 101, 550–554.

Tanaka, D. & Goldman, P. S. 1976. Silver degeneration and autoradiographic evidence for a projection from the principal sulcus to the septum in the Rhesus monkey. *Brain Research*, 103, 535–540.

Tanila, H., Shapiro, M. L. & Eichenbaum, H. 1997. Discordance of spatial representation in ensembles of hippocampal place cells. *Hippocampus*, 7, 613–623.

Tapper, A. R. & Molas, S. 2020. Midbrain circuits of novelty processing. *Neurobiology of Learning and Memory*, 176, 107323. https://doi.org/https://doi.org/10.1016/j.nlm.2020.107323

Taquet, M., Geddes, J. R., Husain, M., Luciano, S. & Harrison, P. J. 2021. 6-month neurological and psychiatric outcomes in 236 379 survivors of COVID-19: a retrospective cohort study using electronic health records. *The Lancet Psychiatry*, 8, P416-427. https://doi.org/10.1016/s2215-0366(21)00084-5

Taube, J. S. 2007. The head direction signal: origins and sensory-motor integration. *Annual Review of Neuroscience*, 30, 181–207. https://doi.org/10.1146/annurev.neuro.29.051605.112854

Taube, J. S., Goodridge, J. P., Golob, E. J., Dudchenko, P. A. & Stackman, R. W. 1996. Processing the head direction cell signal: a review and commentary. *Brain Research Bulletin*, 40, 477–486.

Taube, J. S., Muller, R. U. & Ranck, J. B., Jr. 1990a. Head-direction cells recorded from the postsubiculum in freely moving rats. I. Description and quantitative analysis. *The Journal of Neuroscience*, 10, 420–435.

Taube, J. S., Muller, R. U. & Ranck, J. B., Jr. 1990b. Head-direction cells recorded from the postsubiculum in freely moving rats. II. Effects of environmental manipulations. *The Journal of Neuroscience*, 10, 436–447.

Taxidis, J., Pnevmatikakis, E. A., Dorian, C. C., Mylavarapu, A. L., Arora, J. S., Samadian, K. D., Hoffberg, E. A. & Golshani, P. 2020. Differential emergence and stability of sensory and temporal representations in context-specific hippocampal sequences. *Neuron*, 108, 984–998.e9. https://doi.org/https://doi.org/10.1016/j.neuron.2020.08.028

Taylor, J. 1953. A personality scale of manifest anxiety. *Journal of Abnormal Social Psychology*, 48, 285–290. https://doi.org/10.1037/h0056264

Teaford, M., Keller, K. & Merfeld, D. M. 2022. The contribution of interoceptive signals to spatial orientation: a mini-review. *Neuroscience & Biobehavioral Reviews*, 143, 104943. https://doi.org/https://doi.org/10.1016/j.neubiorev.2022.104943

Teasdale, J. D. 1977. Psychological treatment of phobias. *In:* Sutherland, N. S. (ed.) *Tutorial essays in psychology, Vol. 2* (pp. 137–163). Hillsdale, N.J.: Erlbaum.

Teicher, M. H. 1988. Biology of anxiety. *Medical Clinics of North America*, 72, 791–814.

Teixeira, R. C., Zangrossi, H., Jr. & Graeff, F. G. 2000. Behavioral effects of acute and chronic imipramine in the elevated T-maze model of anxiety. *Pharmacology, Biochemistry and Behavior*, 65, 571–576.

Tervo, D. G. R., Kuleshova, E., Manakov, M., Proskurin, M., Karlsson, M., Lustig, A., Behnam, R. & Karpova, A. Y. 2021. The anterior cingulate cortex directs exploration of alternative strategies. *Neuron*, 109, 1876–1887.e6. https://doi.org/https://doi.org/10.1016/j.neuron.2021.03.028

Teyler, T. & Discenna, P. 1986. The hippocampal memory indexing theory. *Behavioral Neuroscience*, 100, 147–154.

Teyler, T. J. & Rudy, J. W. 2007. The hippocampal indexing theory and episodic memory: updating the index. *Hippocampus*, 17, 1158–1169. https://doi.org/https://doi.org/10.1002/hipo.20350

Thaler, D., Chen, Y. C., Nixon, P. D., Stern, C. E. & Passingham, R. E. 1995. The functions of the medial premotor cortex. I. Simple learned movements. *Experimental Brain Research*, 102, 445–460.

Theves, S., Fernández, G. & Doeller, C. F. 2020. The hippocampus maps concept space, not feature space. *The Journal of Neuroscience*, 40, 7318–7325. https://doi.org/10.1523/jneurosci.0494-20.2020

Theves, S., Neville, D. A., Fernández, G. & Doeller, C. F. 2021. Learning and representation of hierarchical concepts in hippocampus and prefrontal cortex. *The Journal of Neuroscience*, 41, 7675–7686. https://doi.org/10.1523/jneurosci.0657-21.2021

Thew, G. R., Wild, J. & Ehlers, A. 2023. Early intervention in post-traumatic stress disorder without exposure to trauma memories using internet-delivered cognitive therapy: a pilot case series. *British Journal of Clinical Psychology*. https://doi.org/10.1111/bjc.12419

Thomas, R. K. 1996. Investigating cognitive abilities in animals: unrealized potential. *Cognitive Brain Research*, 3, 157–166.

Thompson, B., Santopetro, N. J., Brush, C. J., Foti, D. & Hajcak, G. 2023. Neural deficits in anticipatory and consummatory reward processing are uniquely associated with current depressive symptoms during adolescence. *Psychophysiology*, n/a, e14257. https://doi.org/https://doi.org/10.1111/psyp.14257

Thompson, R. F. 1986. The neurobiology of learning and memory. *Science*, 233, 941–947.

Thompson, S. A., Duncan, J. S. & Smith, S. J. M. 2000. Partial seizures presenting as panic attacks. *British Medical Journal*, 321, 1002–1003.

Ticku, M. K. & Olsen, R. W. 1978. Interaction of barbiturates with dihydropicrotoxinin binding sites related to the GABA receptor-ionophore system. *Life Sciences*, 22, 1643–1652.

Tiedemann, L. J., Alink, A., Beck, J., Büchel, C. & Brassen, S. 2020. Valence encoding signals in the human amygdala and the willingness to eat. *The Journal of Neuroscience*, 40, 5264–5272. https://doi.org/10.1523/jneurosci.2382-19.2020

Timmermann, C., Roseman, L., Schartner, M., Milliere, R., Williams, L. T. J., Erritzoe, D., Muthukumaraswamy, S., Ashton, M., Bendrioua, A., Kaur, O., Turton, S., Nour, M. M., Day, C. M.,

Leech, R., Nutt, D. J. & Carhart-Harris, R. L. 2019. Neural correlates of the DMT experience assessed with multivariate EEG. *Scientific Reports*, 9, 16324. https://doi.org/10.1038/s41598-019-51974-4

Toczek, S. 1960. Disturbances of inhibitory processes due to lesions in the frontal area of the brain in man. *Acta Biologica Experimentalis*, 20, 103–119.

Tom, S. M., Fox, C. R., Trepel, C. & Poldrack, R. A. 2007. The neural basis of loss aversion in decision-making under risk. *Science*, 315, 515–517.

Tomaz, C., Dickinson-Anson, H., McGaugh, J. L., Souza-Silva, M. A., Viana, M. B. & Graeff, F. G. 1993. Localization in the amygdala of the amnestic action of diazepam on emotional memory. *Behavioural Brain Research*, 58, 99–105.

Torgersen, S. 1979. The nature and origin of common phobic fears. *British Journal of Psychiatry*, 134, 343–351.

Torrubia, R., Ávila, C., Moltó, J. & Caseras, X. 2001. The sensitivity to punishment and sensitivity reward questionnaire (SPSRQ) as a measure of Gray's anxiety and impulsivity dimensions. *Personality and Individual Differences*, 31, 837–862.

Torrubia, R. & Tobena, A. 1984. A scale for the assessment of "susceptibility to punishment" as a measure of anxiety: preliminary results. *Personality and Individual Differences*, 5, 371–375.

Towe, A. L. & Luschei, E. S. 1981. Preface. *In:* Towe, A. L. & Luschei, E. S. (eds.) *Motor coordination* (pp. vii–viii). New York: Plenum Press.

Trask, S., Shipman, M. L., Green, J. T. & Bouton, M. E. 2020. Some factors that restore goal-direction to a habitual behavior. *Neurobiology of Learning and Memory*, 169, 107161. https://doi.org/https://doi.org/10.1016/j.nlm.2020.107161

Treit, D., Pesold, C. & Rotzinger, S. 1993a. Noninteractive effects of diazepam and amygdaloid lesions in two animal models of anxiety. *Behavioral Neuroscience*, 107, 1099–1105.

Treit, D., Robinson, A., Rotzinger, S. & Pesold, C. 1993b. Anxiolytic effects of serotonergic interventions in the shock-probe burying test and the elevated plus mase. *Behavioural Brain Research*, 54, 23–34.

Treynor, W., Gonzalez, R. & Nolen-Hoeksema, S. 2003. Rumination reconsidered: a psychometric analysis. *Cognitive Therapy and Research*, 27, 247–259.

Trimble, M. R. 1990. Benzodiazepines in clinical practice. *In:* Wheatley, D. (ed.) *The anxiolytic jungle: where next* (pp. 9–21). Chichester: John Wiley & Sons.

Trivedi, M. A. & Coover, G. D. 2004. Lesions of the ventral hippocampus, but not the dorsal hippocampus, impair conditioned fear expression and inhibitory avoidance on the elevated T-maze. *Neurobiology of Learning and Memory*, 81, 172–184.

Trut, L. 1999. Early canid domestication: the farm-fox experiment. *American Scientist*, 87, retrieved from https://web.archive.org/web/20110623153014/http://www.americanscientist.org:80/issues/id.813,y.1999,no.2,content.true,page.2,css.print/issue.aspx.

Tsang, E., Orlandini, C., Sureka, R., Crevenna, A. H., Perlas, E., Prankerd, I., Masferrer, M. E. & Gross, C. T. 2023. Induction of flight via midbrain projections to the cuneiform nucleus. *PLoS One*, 18, e0281464. https://doi.org/10.1371/journal.pone.0281464

Tsanov, M., Chah, E., Vann, S. D., Reilly, R. B., Erichsen, J. T., Aggleton, J. P. & O'Mara, S. M. 2011. Theta-modulated head direction cells in the rat anterior thalamus. *Journal of Neuroscience*, 31, 9489–9502. https://doi.org/10.1523/JNEUROSCI.0353-11.2011

Tsujimoto, T., Ogawa, M., Tsukada, H., Kakiuchi, T. & Sasaki, K. 1999. Activation of the insular and opercular regions of the monkey by drinking are revealed by positron emission tomography. *Neuroscience Letters*, 261, 135–138.

Tucker, P. M. & Czapla, C. S. 2020. Post-COVID stress disorder: another emerging consequence of the global pandemic. *Psychiatric Times*, October 6, online.

Tully, J. L., Dahlen, A. D., Haggarty, C. J., Schioth, H. B. & Brooks, S. 2022. Ketamine treatment for refractory anxiety: a systematic review. *British Journal of Clinical Pharmacology*, 8, 4412–4426. https://doi.org/10.1111/bcp.15374

Tulving, E. 1985. On the classification problem in learning and memory. *In:* Nilsson, L. G. & Archer, T. (eds.) *Perspectives on learning and memory* (pp. 67–94). New Jersey: Lawrence Erlbaum Associates, Publishers.

Tversky, A. & Kahneman, D. 1991. Loss aversion in riskless choice: a reference dependent model. *The Quarterly Journal of Economics*, 106, 1039–1061.

Uddin, L. Q. 2015. Salience processing and insular cortical function and dysfunction. *Nature Reviews Neuroscience*, 16, 55–61. https://doi.org/10.1038/nrn3857

Umbach, G., Kantak, P., Jacobs, J., Kahana, M., Pfeiffer, B. E., Sperling, M. & Lega, B. 2020. Time cells in the human hippocampus and entorhinal cortex support episodic memory. *Proceedings of the National Academy of Sciences*, 117, 28463–28474. https://doi.org/10.1073/pnas.2013250117

Urban, D. J., Zhu, H., Marcinkiewcz, C. A., Michaelides, M., Oshibuchi, H., Rhea, D., Aryal, D. K., Farrell, M. S., Lowery-Gionta, E., Olsen, R. H. J., Wetsel, W. C., Kash, T. L., Hurd, Y. L., Tecott, L. H. & Roth, B. L. 2015. Elucidation of the behavioral program and neuronal network encoded by dorsal raphe serotonergic neurons. *Neuropsychopharmacology*, 41, 1404–1415. https://doi.org/10.1038/npp.2015.293

Urban, J. H., Van de Kar, L. D., Lorens, S. A. & Bethea, C. L. 1986. Effect of the anxiolytic drug buspirone on prolactin and corticosterone secretion in stressed and unstressed rat. *Pharmacology, Biochemistry and Behavior*, 25, 457–462.

Urban, M. M., Stingl, M. R. & Meinhardt, M. W. 2023. Mini-review: the neurobiology of treating substance use disorders with classical psychedelics. *Frontiers in Neuroscience*, 17, A1156319. https://doi.org/10.3389/fnins.2023.1156319

Urrutia Desmaison, J. D., Sala, R. W., Ayyaz, A., Nondhalee, P., Popa, D. & Lena, C. 2023. Cerebellar control of fear learning via the cerebellar nuclei-Multiple pathways, multiple mechanisms? *Frontiers in System Neuroscience*, 17, 1176668. https://doi.org/10.3389/fnsys.2023.1176668

Ursin, H. 1980. Affective and instrumental aspects of fear and aggression. *In:* Koukkou, M., Lehmann, D. & Agnst, J. (eds.) *Functional states of the brain: their determinants* (pp. 119–130). Elsevier/North-Holland Biomedical Press.

Ursin, H. 1985. The instrumental effects of emotional behavior. *In:* Bateson, P. P. G. & Klopfer, P. H. (eds.) *Perspectives in ethology* (pp. 45–62). Plenum Publishing Corporation.

Vahid-Ansari, F., Daigle, M., Manzini, M. C., Tanaka, K. F., Hen, R., Geddes, S. D., Béïque, J.-C., James, J., Merali, Z. & Albert, P. R. 2017. Abrogated Freud-1/Cc2d1a repression of 5-HT1A autoreceptors induces fluoxetine-resistant anxiety/depression-like behavior. *The Journal of Neuroscience*, 37, 11967–11978. https://doi.org/10.1523/jneurosci.1668-17.2017

Vaidya, S. P. & Johnston, D. 2013. Temporal synchrony and gamma-to-theta power conversion in the dendrites of CA1 pyramidal neurons. *Nature Neuroscience*, 16, 1812–1820. https://doi.org/10.1038/nn.3562

Valero, I., Stewart, J., McNaughton, N. & Gray, J. A. 1977. Septal driving of the hippocampal theta rhythm as a function of frequency in the male rat: effects of adreno-pituitary hormones. *Neuroscience*, 2, 1029–1032.

Vamvakopoulou, I. A., Narine, K. A. D., Campbell, I., Dyck, J. R. B. & Nutt, D. J. 2022. Mescaline: the forgotten psychedelic. *Neuropharmacology*, 109294. https://doi.org/https://doi.org/10.1016/j.neuropharm.2022.109294

Van Ameringen, M., Mancini, C. & Streiner, D. 1994. Sertraline in social phobia. *Journal of Affective Disorders*, 31, 141–145.

van Groen, T., Kadish, I. & Wyss, J. M. 2002. The role of the laterodorsal nucleus of the thalamus in spatial learning and memory in the rat. *Behavioural Brain Research*, 136, 329–337. https://doi.org/https://doi.org/10.1016/S0166-4328(02)00199-7

Van Hoesen, G. W. & Pandya, D. N. 1975. Some connections of the entorhinal (area 28) and perirhinal (area 35) cortices of the Rhesus monkey. I. Temporal lobe afferents. *Brain Research*, 95, 1–24.

Van Hoesen, G. W., Pandya, D. N. & Butters, N. 1972. Cortical afferents to the entorhinal cortex of the Rhesus monkey. *Science (NY)*, 175, 1471–1473.

Van Hoesen, G. W., Pandya, D. N. & Butters, N. 1975. Some connections of the entorhinal (area 28) and perirhinal (area 35) cortices of the Rhesus monkey. II. Frontal lobe afferents. *Brain Research*, 95, 25–38.

Van Hoesen, G. W., Rosene, D. L. & Mesulam, M. M. 1979. Subicular input from temporal cortex in the Rhesus monkey. *Science (NY)*, 205, 608–610.

Van Houtem, C. M., Laine, M. L., Boomsma, D. I., Ligthart, L., van Wijk, A. J. & De Jongh, A. 2013. A review and meta-analysis of the heritability of specific phobia subtypes and corresponding fears. *Journal of Anxiety Disorders*, 27, 379–388. https://doi.org/10.1016/j.janxdis.2013.04.007

van Loenen, I., Scholten, W., Muntingh, A., Smit, J. & Batelaan, N. 2022. The effectiveness of virtual reality exposure-based cognitive behavioral therapy for severe anxiety disorders, obsessive-compulsive disorder, and posttraumatic stress disorder: meta-analysis. *Journal of Medical Internet Research*, 24, e26736. https://doi.org/10.2196/26736

van Marwijk, H., Allick, G., Wegman, F., Bax, A. & Riphagen, II 2012. Alprazolam for depression. *Cochrane Database of Systematic Reviews*, Art. No.: CD007139. https://doi.org/10.1002/14651858.CD007139.pub2

van Oers, K., van den Heuvel, K. & Sepers, B. 2023. The epigenetics of animal personality. *Neuroscience & Biobehavioral Reviews*, 150, 105194. https://doi.org/10.1016/j.neubiorev.2023.105194

Vanderwolf, C. H. 1969. Hippocampal electrical activity and voluntary movement in the rat. *Electroencephalography and Clinical Neurophysiology*, 26, 407–418.

Vanderwolf, C. H. 1995. Does a history of convulsions increase the amnestic effect of temporal region brain lesions? *Physiology and Behavior*, 57, 193–197.

Vanderwolf, C. H. 2003. *An odyssey through the brain, behavior and the mind.* Boston, MA: Springer US.

Vann, S. D. 2013. Dismantling the Papez circuit for memory in rats. *eLife*, 2, e00736. https://doi.org/10.7554/eLife.00736

Varga, V., Hangya, B., Kránitz, K., Ludányi, A., Zemankovics, R., Katona, I., Shigemoto, R., Freund, T. F. & Borhegyi, Z. 2008. The presence of pacemaker HCN channels identifies theta rhythmic GABAergic neurons in the medial septum. *Journal of Physiology*, 586, 3893–3915.

Varley, T., Carhart-Harris, R., Roseman, L., Menon, D. & Stamatakis, E. 2019. Serotonergic psychedelics LSD & psilocybin increase the fractal dimension of cortical brain activity in spatial and temporal domains. *Preprint.* https://doi.org/10.1101/517847

Velazquez-Hernandez, G. & Sotres-Bayon, F. 2021. Lateral habenula mediates defensive responses only when threat and safety memories are in conflict. *eneuro*, in press, ENEURO.0482-20.2021. https://doi.org/10.1523/eneuro.0482-20.2021

Veltman, D. J., Van Zijderveld, G. A. & Van Dyck, R. 1996. Epinephrine infusions in panic disorder: a double-blind placebo-controlled study. *Journal of Affective Disorders*, 39, 133–140.

Venner, A., Mochizuki, T., De Luca, R., Anaclet, C., Scammell, T. E., Saper, C. B., Arrigoni, E. & Fuller, P. M. 2019. Reassessing the role of histaminergic tuberomammillary neurons in arousal control. *The Journal of Neuroscience*, 39, 8929–8939. https://doi.org/10.1523/jneurosci.1032-19.2019

Veraart, J. K. E., van Westenbrugge, M., van Wulfften Palthe, J. E., van der Meij, A., Schoevers, R. A. & de Jong, J. 2023. Repeated oral esketamine in patients with treatment resistant depression and comorbid posttraumatic stress disorder. *Heliyon*, 9, e15883. https://doi.org/10.1016/j.heliyon.2023.e15883

Verbanac, J. S., Commissaris, R. L., Altman, H. J. & Pitts, D. K. 1994. Electrophysiological characteristics of locus coeruleus neurons in the Maudsley reactive (MR) and non-reactive (MNRA) rat strains. *Neuroscience Letters*, 179, 137–140.

Verbanac, J. S., Commissaris, R. L. & Pitts, D. K. 1995. An electrophysiological evaluation of serotonergic dorsal raphe neurons in Maudsley rats. *Life Sciences*, 56, 245–250.

Verbruggen, F. & Logan, G. D. 2008. Response inhibition in the stop-signal paradigm. *Trends in Cognitive Science*, 12, 418–424. https://doi.org/10.1016/j.tics.2008.07.005

Vertes, R. P., Colom, L. V., Fortin, W. J. & Bland, B. H. 1993. Brainstem sites for the carbachol elicitation of the hippocampal theta rhythm in the rat. *Experimental Brain Research*, 96, 419–429.

Vertes, R. P. & Kocsis, B. 1997. Brainstem-diencephalo-septohippocampal systems controlling the theta rhythm of the hippocampus. *Neuroscience*, 81, 893–926.

Vesuna, S., Kauvar, I. V., Richman, E., Gore, F., Oskotsky, T., Sava-Segal, C., Luo, L., Malenka, R. C., Henderson, J. M., Nuyujukian, P., Parvizi, J. & Deisseroth, K. 2020. Deep posteromedial cortical rhythm in dissociation. *Nature*, 96, 87–94. https://doi.org/10.1038/s41586-020-2731-9

Viallet, F., Vuillon-Cacciuttolo, G., Legallet, E., Bonnefoi-Kyriacou, B. & Trouche, E. 1995. Bilateral and side-related reaction time impairments in patients with unilateral cerebral lesions of a medial frontal region involving the supplementary motor area. *Neuropsychologia*, 33, 215–223.

Viana, M. B., Tomaz, C. & Graeff, F. G. 1994. The elevated T-maze: a new animal model of anxiety and memory. *Pharmacology, Biochemistry and Behavior*, 49, 549–554.

Vicario, C. M., Salehinejad, M. A., Felmingham, K., Martino, G. & Nitsche, M. A. 2019. A systematic review on the therapeutic effectiveness of non-invasive brain stimulation for the treatment of anxiety disorders. *Neuroscience & Biobehavioral Reviews*, 96, 219–231. https://doi.org/https://doi.org/10.1016/j.neubiorev.2018.12.012

Victor, M., Adams, R. D. & Collins, G. H. 1971. *The Wernicke-Korsakoff syndrome*. Oxford: Blackwell.

Vidailhet, P., Danion, J. M., Kauffmann-Muller, F., Grangé, D., Giersch, A., Van Der Linden, M. & Imbs, J. L. 1994. Lorazepam and diazepam effects on memory acquisition in priming tasks. *Psychopharmacology (Berl)*, 115, 397–406.

Vieira, J. B., Schellhaas, S., Enström, E. & Olsson, A. 2020. Help or flight? Increased threat imminence promotes defensive helping in humans. *Proceedings of the Royal Society B: Biological Sciences*, 287, 20201473. https://doi.org/doi:10.1098/rspb.2020.1473

Vinogradova, O. S. 1975. Functional organization of the limbic system in the process of registration of information: facts and hypotheses. *In:* Isaacson, R. I. & Pribram, K. H. (eds.) *The hippocampus (volume 2)* (pp. 3–69). New York: Plenum Press.

Vinogradova, O. S., Brazhnik, E. S., Karanov, A. M. & Zhadina, D. 1980. Neuronal activity of the septum following various types of deafferentation. *Brain Research*, 187, 353–368.

Vinogradova, O. S. & Brazhnik, P. S. 1978. Neuronal aspects of septo-hippocampal relations. *In:* Elliott, K. & Whelan, J. (eds.) *Functions of the septo-hippocampal system. Ciba Foundation Symposium 58 (New Series)* (pp. 145–171). Amsterdam: Elsevier.

Virley, D., Ridley, R. M., Sinden, J. D., Kershaw, T. R., Harland, S., Rashid, T., French, S., Sowinski, P., Gray, J. A., Lantos, P. L. & Hodges, H. 1999. Primary CA1 and conditionally immortal MHP36 cell grafts restore conditional discrimination learning and recall in marmosets after excitotoxic lesions of the hippocampal CA1 field. *Brain*, 122, 2321–2335.

Vnek, N. & Rothblat, L. A. 1996. The hippocampus and long-term object memory in the rat. *The Journal of Neuroscience*, 16, 2780–2787.

Vo, B. N., Marron Fernandez de Velasco, E., Rose, T. R., Oberle, H., Luo, H., Hopkins, C. R. & Wickman, K. 2021. Bidirectional influence of limbic GIRK channel activation on innate avoidance behavior. *The Journal of Neuroscience*, 41, 5809–5821. https://doi.org/10.1523/jneurosci.2787-20.2021

Vogel, S. & Schwabe, L. 2019. Stress, aggression, and the balance of approach and avoidance. *Psychoneuroendocrinology*, 103, 137–146. https://doi.org/https://doi.org/10.1016/j.psyneuen.2019.01.020

Vogt, B. 2009. *Cingulate neurobiology and disease*. Oxford: Oxford University Press.

Vogt, B. A. 1985. Cingulate cortex. *In:* Peters, A. & Jones, E. G. (eds.) *Cerebral cortex: association and auditory cortices* (pp. 89–149). New York: Plenum Press.

Vollenweider, F. X. & Preller, K. H. 2020. Psychedelic drugs: neurobiology and potential for treatment of psychiatric disorders. *Nature Reviews Neuroscience*, 611–624. https://doi.org/10.1038/s41583-020-0367-2

Wacker, J. & Smillie, L. D. 2015. Trait extraversion and dopamine function. *Social and Personality Psychology Compass*, 9, 225–238. https://doi.org/10.1111/spc3.12175

Wagner, A. R. 1963. Conditioned frustration as a learned drive. *Journal of Experimental Child Psychology*, 66, 142–148.

Wagner, A. R. 1966. Frustration and punishment. *In:* Haber, R. M. (ed.) *Current research on motivation* (pp. 229–239). New York: Holt, Rinehart, Winston.

Wagner, A. R. 1969. Frustrative nonreward: a variety of punishment? *In:* Campbell, B. A. & Church, R. M. (eds.) *Punishment and aversive behavior* (pp. 157–181). New York: Appleton-Century-Crofts.

Wagner, A. R. 1978. Experiences and the priming of STM. *In:* Hulse, S. H., Fowler, H. & Honig, W. K. (eds.) *Cognitive processes in animal behaviour* (pp. 177–209). Hillsdale, NJ.: Lawrence Erlbaum.

Walker, J. A. & Olton, D. S. 1979. Spatial memory deficit following fimbria-fornix lesions: independent of time for stimulus processing. *Physiology and Behavior*, 23, 11–15.

Walsh, Z., Mollaahmetoglu, M., Rootman, J., Golsof, S., Keeler, J., Marsh, B., Nutt, D. & Morgan, C. 2022. Ketamine for the treatment of mental health and substance use disorders: comprehensive systematic review. *BJPsych Open*, 8, e19. https://doi.org/10.1192/bjo.2021.1061

Wan, R. Q., Pang, K. & Olton, D. S. 1994. Hippocampal and amygdaloid involvement in nonspatial and spatial working memory in rats: effects of delay and interference. *Behavioral Neuroscience*, 108, 866–882.

Wang, L., Chen, Irene Z. & Lin, D. 2015. Collateral pathways from the ventromedial hypothalamus mediate defensive behaviors. *Neuron*, 85, 1344–1358. https://doi.org/10.1016/j.neuron.2014.12.025

Wang, M., Foster, D. J. & Pfeiffer, B. E. 2020. Alternating sequences of future and past behavior encoded within hippocampal theta oscillations. *Science*, 370, 247–250. https://doi.org/10.1126/science.abb4151

Wang, W., Schuette, P. J., Nagai, J., Tobias, B. C., Cuccovia V. Reis, F. M., Ji, S., de Lima, M. A. X., LaVu, M. Q., Maesta-Pereira, S., Chakerian, M., Leonard, S. J., Lin, L., Severino, A. L., Cahill, C. M., Canteras, N. S., Khakh, B. S., Kao, J. C. & Adhikari, A. 2021. Coordination of escape and spatial navigation circuits orchestrates versatile flight from threats. *Neuron*, 109, 1848–1860.e8. https://doi.org/https://doi.org/10.1016/j.neuron.2021.03.033

Wang, Y., McCane, B., McNaughton, N., Huang, Z., Shadli, S. M. & Neo, P. 2019. AnxietyDecoder: an EEG-based anxiety predictor using a 3-D convolutional neural network. *2019 International Joint Conference on Neural Networks (IJCNN)* (pp. 1–8). Budapest, Hungary: IEEE.

Wang, Y. M., Xia, C. Y., Jia, H. M., He, J., Lian, W. W., Yan, Y., Wang, W. P., Zhang, W. K. & Xu, J. K. 2022. Sigma-1 receptor: a potential target for the development of antidepressants. *Neurochemistry International*, 159, 105390. https://doi.org/10.1016/j.neuint.2022.105390

Wang, Z. W., Valdes, J., Noyes, R., Zoega, T. & Crowe, R. R. 1998. Possible association of a cholecystokinin promotor polymorphism (CCK-36CT) with panic disorder. *American Journal of Medical Genetics*, 81, 228–234. https://doi.org/10.1002/(SICI)1096-8628(19980508)81:3<228::AID-AJMG5>3.0.CO;2-S

Ward, A., Lyubomirsky, S., Sousa, L. & Nolen-Hoeksema, S. 2003. Can't quite commit: rumination and uncertainty. *Personality and Social Psychology Bulletin*, 29, 96–107.

Wardle, J., Hayward, P., Higgit, A., Stabl, M., Blizard, R. & Gray, J. A. 1994. Effects of concurrent diazepam treatment on the outcome of exposure therapy on agoraphobia. *Behaviour Research and Therapy*, 32, 203–215.

Warrington, E. K. & Weiskrantz, L. 1968. A study of learning and retention in amnesic patients. *Neuropsychologia*, 6, 283–291.

Warrington, E. K. & Weiskrantz, L. 1970. Amnesic syndrome: consolidation or retrieval? *Nature*, 228, 628–630.

Warrington, E. K. & Weiskrantz, L. 1974. The effect of prior learning on subsequent retention in amnesic patients. *Neuropsychologia*, 12, 419–428.

Warrington, E. K. & Weiskrantz, L. 1978. Further analysis of the prior learning effect in amnesic patients. *Neuropsychologia*, 16, 169–177.

Watabe-Uchida, M., Eshel, N. & Uchida, N. 2017. Neural circuitry of reward prediction error. *Annual Review of Neuroscience*, 40, 373–394. https://doi.org/10.1146/annurev-neuro-072116-031109

Watanabe, M. 1996. Reward expectancy in primate prefrontal neurons. *Nature*, 382, 629–632.

Watrous, A. J., Fried, I. & Ekstrom, A. D. 2011. Behavioral correlates of human hippocampal delta and theta oscillations during navigation. *Journal of Neurophysiology*, 105, 1747–1755.

Watson, D., Clark, L. A. & Harkness, A. R. 1994. Structures of personality and their relevance to psychopathology. *Journal of Abnormal Psychology*, 103, 18–31.

Watson, D., Levin-Aspenson, H. F., Waszczuk, M. A., Conway, C. C., Dalgleish, T., Dretsch, M. N., Eaton, N. R., Forbes, M. K., Forbush, K. T., Hobbs, K. A., Michelini, G., Nelson, B. D., Sellbom, M., Slade, T., South, S. C., Sunderland, M., Waldman, I., Witthöft, M., Wright, A. G. C., Kotov, R., Krueger, R. F. & Workgroup, H. U. 2022. Validity and utility of Hierarchical Taxonomy of Psychopathology (HiTOP): III. Emotional dysfunction superspectrum. *World Psychiatry*, 21, 26–54. https://doi.org/https://doi.org/10.1002/wps.20943

Watson, J. B. & Rayner, B. 1920. Conditioned emotional reactions. *Journal of Experimental Child Psychology*, 3, 1–14.

Waziri, R. 1990. Psychosurgery for anxiety and obsessive-compulsive disorders. *In:* Noyes, R., Roth, M. & Burrows, G. D. (eds.) *Handbook of anxiety, Vol 4* (pp. 519–535). Amsterdam: Elsevier.

Webster, D. B. & Voneida, T. J. 1964. Learning deficits following hippocampal lesions in split-brain cats. *Experimental Neurology*, 10, 170–182.

Wechsler, T. F., Kumpers, F. & Muhlberger, A. 2019. Inferiority or even superiority of virtual reality exposure therapy in phobias? A systematic review and quantitative meta-analysis on randomized controlled trials specifically comparing the efficacy of virtual reality exposure to gold standard in vivo exposure in agoraphobia, specific phobia, and social phobia. *Frontiers in Psychology*, 10, A1758. https://doi.org/10.3389/fpsyg.2019.01758

Weera, M. M., Shackett, R. S., Kramer, H. M., Middleton, J. W. & Gilpin, N. W. 2021. Central amygdala projections to lateral hypothalamus mediate avoidance behavior in rats. *The Journal of Neuroscience*, 41, 61–72. https://doi.org/10.1523/jneurosci.0236-20.2020

Weess, H. G., Steinberg, R. & Pritzel, M. 1994. Mnestic disorders in long-term high-dose diazepam abuse: a pilot study. *European Journal of Psychiatry*, 9, 254–259.

Wehrli, J. M., Xia, Y., Gerster, S. & Bach, D. R. 2022. Measuring human trace fear conditioning. *Psychophysiology*, 59, e14119. https://doi.org/https://doi.org/10.1111/psyp.14119

Weinstock, L. M. & Whisman, M. A. 2006. Neuroticism as a common feature of the depressive and anxiety disorders: a test of the revised integrative hierarchical model in a national sample. *Journal of Abnormal Psychology*, 115, 68–74. https://doi.org/10.1037/0021-843X.115.1.68

Weisberg, S. M. & Ekstrom, A. D. 2021. Hippocampal volume and navigational ability: the map(ping) is not to scale. *Neuroscience & Biobehavioral Reviews*, 126, 102–112. https://doi.org/https://doi.org/10.1016/j.neubiorev.2021.03.012

Weiskrantz, L. 1978. A comparison of hippocampal pathology in man and other animals. *In:* Elliott, K. & Whelan, J. (eds.) *Functions of the septo-hippocampal system. Ciba Foundation Symposium 58 (New Series)* (pp. 373–387). Amsterdam: Elsevier.

Weiskrantz, L. & Warrington, E. K. 1975. The problem of the amnesic syndrome in man and animals. *In:* Isaacson, R. L. & Pribram, K. H. (eds.) *The hippocampus, Vol. 2. Neurophysiology and behaviour* (pp. 411–428). New York: Plenum Press.

Weiskrantz, L. & Warrington, E. K. 1979. Conditioning in amnesic patients. *Neuropsychologia*, 17, 187–194.

Weiss, C., Kronforst-Collins, M. A. & Disterhoft, J. F. 1996. Activity of hippocampal pyramidal neurons during trace eyeblink conditioning. *Hippocampus*, 6, 192–209.

Weiss, K. R., Friedman, R. & McGregor, S. 1974. Effects of septal lesions of latent inhibition and habituation of the orienting response in rats. *Acta Neurobiologica Experimentalis*, 34, 491–504.

Wells, C. E., Amos, D. P., Jeewajee, A., Douchamps, V., Rodgers, J., O'Keefe, J., Burgess, N. & Lever, C. 2013. Novelty and anxiolytic drugs dissociate two components of hippocampal theta in behaving rats. *The Journal of Neuroscience*, 33, 8650–8667. https://doi.org/10.1523/jneurosci.5040-12.2013

Welter, M. L., Burbaud, P., Fernandez-Vidal, S., Bardinet, E., Coste, J., Piallat, B., Borg, M., Besnard, S., Sauleau, P., Devaux, B., Pidoux, B., Chaynes, P., Tezenas du Montcel, S., Bastian, A., Langbour, N., Teillant, A., Haynes, W., Yelnik, J., Karachi, C. & Mallet, L. 2011. Basal ganglia dysfunction in OCD: subthalamic neuronal activity correlates with symptoms severity and predicts high-frequency stimulation efficacy. *Translational Psychiatry*, 1, e5. https://doi.org/10.1038/tp.2011.5

Westenberg, H. G. M. 1999. Facing the challenge of social anxiety disorder. *European Neuropsychopharmacology*, 9, S93–S99. https://doi.org/10.1016/S0924-977X(99)00029-2

Westra, H. A., Stewart, S. H. & Conrad, B. E. 2002. Naturalistic manner of benzodiazepine use and cognitive behavioral therapy outcome in panic disorder with agoraphobia. *Anxiety Disorders*, 16, 233–246.

Wheatley, D. 1990. The new alternatives. *In:* Wheatley, D. (ed.) *In the anxiolytic jungle: where next?* (pp. 163–184). Chichester: John Wiley.

Whelan, M. 2020. *Embodying a computational model of hippocampal replay for robotic reinforcement learning.* M Phil, The University of Sheffield.

Whishaw, I. Q. 1998. Place learning in hippocampal rats and the path integration hypothesis. *Neuroscience & Biobehavioral Reviews*, 22, 209–220.

Whishaw, I. Q. 1999. The hippocampus and path integration. *Behavioral and Brain Sciences*, 22, 467–479.

Whishaw, I. Q., Cassel, J. C. & Jarrard, L. E. 1995. Rats with fimbria-fornix lesions display a place response in a swimming pool: a dissociation between getting there and knowing where. *The Journal of Neuroscience*, 15, 5779–5788.

Whishaw, I. Q. & Tomie, J. A. 1991. Acquisition and retention by hippocampal rats of simple, conditional, and configual tasks using tactile and olfactory cues: implications for hippocampal function. *Behavioral Neuroscience*, 105(6), 787–797.

Whishaw, I. Q. & Tomie, J. A. 1995. Rats with fimbria-fornix lesions can acquire and retain a visual-tactile transwitching (configural) task. *Behavioral Neuroscience*, 109, 607–612.

Whishaw, I. Q. & Tomie, J. A. 1997. Perseveration on place reversals in spatial swimming pool tasks: further evidence for place learning in hippocampal rats. *Hippocampus*, 7, 361–370.

Whishaw, I. Q. & Vanderwolf, C. H. 1973. Hippocampal EEG and behavior: changes in amplitude and frequency of RSA (theta rhythm) associated with spontaneous and learned movement patterns in rats and cats. *Behavioral Biology*, 8, 461–484.

White, J. 2000. Bites and stings from venomous animals: a global overview. *Therapeutic Drug Monitoring*, 22, 65–68.

White, K. G. 1985. Characteristics of forgetting functions in delayed matching to sample. *Journal of the Experimental Analysis of Behaviour*, 44, 15–34.

Wickens, D. D. 1970. Encoding categories of words: an empirical approach to meaning. *Psychological Review*, 77, 1–15.

Wickens, J. R., Reynolds, J. N. J. & Hyland, B. I. 2003. Neural mechanisms of reward-related motor learning. *Current Opinion in Neurobiology*, 13, 685–690.

Widiger, T. A. & Oltmanns, J. R. 2017. Neuroticism is a fundamental domain of personality with enormous public health implications. *World Psychiatry*, 16, 144–145. https://doi.org/10.1002/wps.20411

Wiecki, T. V. & Frank, M. J. 2013. A computational model of inhibitory control in frontal cortex and basal ganglia. *Psychological Review*, 120, 329–355. https://doi.org/10.1037/a0031542.supp

Wiener, S. I. 1996. Spatial, behavioral and sensory correlates of hippocampal CA1 complex spike cell activity: implications for information processing functions. *Progress in Neurobiology*, 49, 335–361.

Wiener, S. I. & Korshunov, V. A. 1996. Place-independent behavioural correlates of hippocampal neurones in rats. *Neuroreport*, 7, 183–188.

Wikenheiser, A. M., Gardner, M. P. H., Mueller, L. E. & Schoenbaum, G. 2021. Spatial representations in rat orbitofrontal cortex. *The Journal of Neuroscience*, 41, 6933–6945. https://doi.org/10.1523/jneurosci.0830-21.2021

Wikenheiser, A. M. & Schoenbaum, G. 2016. Over the river, through the woods: cognitive maps in the hippocampus and orbitofrontal cortex. *Nature Reviews Neuroscience*, 17, 513–523. https://doi.org/10.1038/nrn.2016.56

Wikinski, S., Lombardo, M., Medina, J. H. & Rubio, M. C. 1994. Lack of anxiolytic effect of diazepam in pre-anaesthetic medication. *British Journal of Anaesthesiology*, 72, 694–696.

Willett, R. 1960. The effects of psychosurgical procedures on behaviour. *In:* Eysenck, H. J. (ed.) *Handbook of abnormal psychology* (pp. 566–610). London: Pitman.

Williams, J., Gray, J. A., Snape, M. & Holt, L. 1989. Long-term effects of septohippocampal stimulation on behavioural responses to anxiogenic stimuli. *In:* Tyrer, P. (ed.) *Psychopharmacology of anxiety* (pp. 80–108). Oxford: Oxford University Press.

Williams, T., McCaul, M., Schwarzer, G., Cipriani, A., Stein, D. J. & Ipser, J. 2020. Pharmacological treatments for social anxiety disorder in adults: a systematic review and network meta-analysis. *Acta Neuropsychiatrica*, 32, 169–176. https://doi.org/10.1017/neu.2020.6

Williamson, M. J., Paul, S. M. & Skolnick, P. 1978. Labelling of benzodiazepine receptors in vivo. *Nature*, 275, 551–553.

Willner, P. J. & Crowe, R. 1977. Effect of chlordiazepoxide on the partial reinforcement extinction effect. *Pharmacology, Biochemistry and Behavior*, 7, 4779–4782.

Wilmerding, L. K., Kondratyev, I., Ramirez, S. & Hasselmo, M. E. 2023. Route-dependent spatial engram tagging in mouse dentate gyrus. *Neurobiology of Learning and Memory*, 200, 107738. https://doi.org/10.1016/j.nlm.2023.107738

Wilson, G. D., Barrett, P. T. & Gray, J. A. 1989. Human reactions to reward and punishment: a questionnaire examination of Gray's personality theory. *British Journal of Psychology*, 80, 509–515. https://doi.org/10.1111/j.2044-8295.1989.tb02339.x

Wilson, G. D., Gray, J. A. & Barrett, P. T. 1990. A factor analysis of the Gray-Wilson personality questionnaire. *Personality and Individual Differences*, 11(10), 1037–1045. https://doi.org/10.1016/0191-8869(90)90131-A

Wilson, M. A. & McNaughton, B. L. 1993. Dynamics of the hippocampal ensemble code for space. *Science*, 261, 1055–1058.

Wilson, M. A. & McNaughton, B. L. 1994. Reactivation of hippocampal ensemble memories during sleep. *Science*, 265, 676–679.

Winocur, G. 1979. Effects of interference on discrimination learning and recall by rats with hippocampal lesions. *Physiology and Behavior*, 22, 339–345.

Winocur, G. 1981. The amnesic syndrome: a deficit in cue utilization. *In:* Cermak, L. (ed.) *Human memory and amnesia* (pp. 139–169). Hillsdale, N.J.: Erbaum.

Winocur, G. 1985. The hippocampus and thalamus: their roles in short- and long-term memory and the effects of interference. *Behavioural Brain Research*, 16, 135–152.

Winocur, G. 1992. A comparison of normal old rats and young adult rats with lesions to the hippocampus or prefrontal cortex on a test of matching-to-sample. *Neuropsychologia*, 30, 769–781.

Winocur, G. & Kinsbourne, M. 1978. Contextual cueing as an aid to Korsakoff amnesics. *Neuropsychologia*, 16, 671–682.

Winocur, G. & Mills, J. A. 1970. Transfer between related and unrelated problems following hippocampal lesions in rats. *Journal of Comparative and Physiological Psychology*, 73, 162–169.

Winocur, G. & Moscovitch, M. 2011. Memory transformation and systems consolidation. *Journal of the International Neuropsychological Society*, 17, 766–780. https://doi.org/10.1017/S1355617711000683

Winocur, G., Moscovitch, M. & Bontempi, B. 2010. Memory formation and long-term retention in humans and animals: convergence towards a transformation account of hippocampal–neocortical interactions. *Neuropsychologia*, 48, 2339–2356. https://doi.org/https://doi.org/10.1016/j.neuropsychologia.2010.04.016

Winocur, G., Moscovitch, M., Fogel, S., Rosenbaum, R. S. & Sekeres, M. 2005. Preserved spatial memory after hippocampal lesions: effects of extensive experience in a complex environment. *Nature Neuroscience*, 8, 273–275. https://doi.org/10.1038/nn1401

Winocur, G., Moscovitch, M. & Sekeres, M. 2007. Memory consolidation or transformation: context manipulation and hippocampal representations of memory. *Nature Neuroscience*, 10, 555–557. https://doi.org/10.1038/nn1880

Winocur, G. & Olds, J. 1978. Effects of context manipulation on memory and reversal learning in rats with hippocampal lesions. *Journal of Comparative and Physiological Psychology*, 92, 312–321.

Winocur, G. & Weiskrantz, L. 1976. An investigation of paired-associate learning in amnesic patients. *Neuropsychologia*, 14, 97–110.

Winter, J. C. & Petti, D. T. 1987. The effects of 8-Hydroxy-2-(di-n-propylamino)tetralin and other serotonergic agonists on performance in a radial maze: a possible role for 5-HT1A receptors in memory. *Pharmacology, Biochemistry and Behavior*, 27, 625–628.

Wise, S. P. 2008. Forward frontal fields: phylogeny and fundamental function. *Trends in Neurosciences*, 31, 599–608. https://doi.org/https://doi.org/10.1016/j.tins.2008.08.008

Wittchen, H. U., Zhao, S., Kessler, R. C. & Eaton, W. W. 1994. DSM-III-R generalized anxiety disorder in the National Comorbidity Survey. *Archives of General Psychiatry*, 51, 355–364.

Wixted, J. T. 2004. The psychology and neuroscience of forgetting. *Annual Review of Psychology*, 55, 235–269. https://doi.org/10.1146/annurev.psych.55.090902.141555

Wohlgemuth, M. J., Yu, C. & Moss, C. F. 2018. 3D hippocampal place field dynamics in free-flying echolocating bats. *Frontiers in Cellular Neuroscience*, 12, A270. https://doi.org/10.3389/fncel.2018.00270

Wolfson, P. E., Andries, J., Feduccia, A. A., Jerome, L., Wang, J. B., Williams, E., Carlin, S. C., Sola, E., Hamilton, S., Yazar-Klosinski, B., Emerson, A., Mithoefer, M. C. & Doblin, R. 2020. MDMA-assisted psychotherapy for treatment of anxiety and other psychological distress related to life-threatening illnesses: a randomized pilot study. *Scientific Reports*, 10, 20442. https://doi.org/10.1038/s41598-020-75706-1

Woodnorth, M.-A. & McNaughton, N. 2005. Different systems in the posterior hypothalamic nucleus of rats control theta frequency and trigger movement. *Behavioural Brain Research*, 163, 107–114.

Woodnorth, M. A., Kyd, R. J., Logan, B. J., Long, M. A. & McNaughton, N. 2003. Multiple hypothalamic sites control the frequency of hippocampal theta rhythm. *Hippocampus*, 13, 361–374.

Woodnorth, M. A. & McNaughton, N. 2002a. Benzodiazepine receptors in the medial-posterior hypothalamus mediate the reduction of hippocampal theta frequency by chlordiazepoxide. *Brain Research*, 954, 194–201.

Woodnorth, M. A. & McNaughton, N. 2002b. Similar effects of medial supramammillary or systemic injection of chlordiazepoxide on both theta frequency and fixed-interval responding. *Cognitive, Affective, & Behavioural Neuroscience*, 2, 76–83.

World Health Organisation. 2010. *International Statistical Classification of Diseases and Related Health Problems 10th revision.* [Online]. http://apps.who.int/classifications/icd10/browse/2010/en [Accessed 20 July 2021].

World Health Organization 1992. *The ICD-10 classification of mental and behavioural disorders.* Geneva: World Health Organization.

World Health Organization. 2021. *International Statistical Classification of Diseases and Related Health Problems 11th Revision* [Online]. https://icd.who.int/browse11/l-m/en [Accessed 20 July 2021].

World Health Organization. 2023. *International Statistical Classification of Diseases and Related Health Problems 11th Revision* [Online]. https://icd.who.int/browse11/l-m/en [Accessed 14 April 2023].

Wright, A. A. 1994. Primacy effects in animal memory and human nonverbal memory. *Animal Learning and Behaviour*, 22, 219–223.

Wright, A. G. C., Creswell, K. G., Flory, J. D., Muldoon, M. F. & Manuck, S. B. 2019. Neurobiological functioning and the personality-trait hierarchy: central serotonergic responsivity and the stability metatrait. *Psychological Science*, 30, 1413–1423. https://doi.org/10.1177/0956797619864530

Wu, C., Wang, Y., He, Y., Wu, S., Xie, Z., Zhang, J., Shen, J., Wang, Z. & He, L. 2020. Sub-anesthetic and anesthetic ketamine produce different long-lasting behavioral phenotypes (24 h post-treatment) via inducing different brain-derived neurotrophic factor (BDNF) expression level in the hippocampus. *Neurobiology of Learning and Memory*, 167, e107136. https://doi.org/https://doi.org/10.1016/j.nlm.2019.107136

Xiao, C., Wei, J., Zhang, G. W., Tao, C., Huang, J. J., Shen, L., Wickersham, I. R., Tao, H. W. & Zhang, L. I. 2023. Glutamatergic and GABAergic neurons in pontine central gray mediate opposing valence-specific behaviors through a global network. *Neuron*, 111, 1496–1503. https://doi.org/10.1016/j.neuron.2023.02.012

Yadin, E., Thomas, E., Strickland, C. E. & Grishkat, H. L. 1991. Anxiolytic effects of benzodiazepines in amygdala-lesioned rats. *Psychopharmacology*, 103, 473–479.

Yamaguchi, T. & Lin, D. 2018. Functions of medial hypothalamic and mesolimbic dopamine circuitries in aggression. *Current Opinion in Behavioral Sciences*, 24, 104–112. https://doi.org/10.1016/j.cobeha.2018.06.011

Yee, B. K. & Rawlins, J. N. P. 1994. The effects of hippocampal formation ablation or fimbria- fornix section on performance of a nonspatial radial arm maze task by rats. *The Journal of Neuroscience*, 14, 3766–3774.

Yee, D. M., Crawford, J. L., Lamichhane, B. & Braver, T. S. 2021. Dorsal anterior cingulate cortex encodes the integrated incentive motivational value of cognitive task performance. *The Journal of Neuroscience*, 41, 3707–3720. https://doi.org/10.1523/jneurosci.2550-20.2021

Yeragani, V. K., Srinivasan, K., Balon, R., Ramesh, C. & Berchou, R. 1994. Lactate sensitivity and cardiac cholinergic function in panic disorder. *American Journal of Psychiatry*, 151, 1226–1228.

Yeterian, E. H., Pandya, D. N., Tomaiuolo, F. & Petrides, M. 2012. The cortical connectivity of the prefrontal cortex in the monkey brain. *Cortex*, 48, 58–81. https://doi.org/https://doi.org/10.1016/j.cortex.2011.03.004

Yeung, M., Treit, D. & Dickson, C. T. 2012. A critical test of the hippocampal theta model of anxiolytic drug action. *Neuropharmacology*, 62, 155–160.

Yeung, N., Botvinick, M. M. & Cohen, J. D. 2004. The neural basis of error detection: conflict monitoring and the error-related negativity. *Psychological Review*, 111, 931–959

Yoder, R. M., Clark, B. J., Brown, J. E., Lamia, M. V., Valerio, S., Shinder, M. E. & Taube, J. S. 2011. Both visual and idiothetic cues contribute to head direction cell stability during navigation along complex routes. *Journal of Neurophysiology*, 105, 2989–3001. https://doi.org/10.1152/jn.01041.2010

Yonelinas, A. P., Ranganath, C., Ekstrom, A. D. & Wiltgen, B. J. 2019. A contextual binding theory of episodic memory: systems consolidation reconsidered. *Nature Reviews Neuroscience*, 20, 364–375. https://doi.org/10.1038/s41583-019-0150-4

Young, B. & McNaughton, N. 2000. Common firing patterns of hippocampal cells in a differential reinforcement of low rates of response schedule. *Journal of Neuroscience*, 20, 7043–7051.

Young, B. J. & McNaughton, N. 1997. Activity of hippocampal neurons in rats during DRL performance. *Society for Neuroscience Abstracts*, 23, 503–503.

Young, C. K. & McNaughton, N. 2009. Coupling of theta oscillations between anterior and posterior midline cortex and with the hippocampus in freely behaving rats. *Cerebral Cortex*, 19, 24–40. https://doi.org/10.1093/cercor/bhn055

Young, G. 2022. Broadening defense mechanisms: literature review and discussion. *In:* Young, G. (ed.) *Causality and neo-stages in development: toward unifying psychology* (Chapter 11, pp. 309–351). Cham: Springer International Publishing.

Young, W. S. & Kuhar, M. J. 1980. Radiohistochemical localization of benzodiazepine receptors in rat brain. *Journal of Pharmacology and Experimental Therapeutics*, 212, 337–346.

Zak, P. J. 2004. Neuroeconomics. *Philosophical Transactions of the Royal Society of London: B*, 359, 1737–1748.

Zangrossi, H., Jr. & Graeff, F. G. 1997. Behavioral validation of the elevated T-maze, a new animal model of anxiety. *Brain Research Bulletin*, 44, 1–5.

Zanos, P. & Gould, T. D. 2018. Mechanisms of ketamine action as an antidepressant. *Molecular Psychiatry*, 23, 801–811. https://doi.org/10.1038/mp.2017.255

Zanotti, A., Arban, R., Perazzolo, M. & Giusti, P. 1994. Diazepam impairs place learning in naive but not in maze- experienced rats in the Morris water maze. *Psychopharmacology (Berl)*, 115, 73–78.

Zarate, C. A., Jr., Mathews, D., Ibrahim, L., Chaves, J. F., Marquardt, C., Ukoh, I., Jolkovsky, L., Brutsche, N. E., Smith, M. A. & Luckenbaugh, D. A. 2013. A randomized trial of a low-trapping nonselective N-methyl-D-aspartate channel blocker in major depression. *Biological Psychiatry*, 74, 257–264. https://doi.org/10.1016/j.biopsych.2012.10.019

Zarate Jr, C. A., Singh, J. B., Carlson, P. J., Brutsche, N. E., Ameli, R., Luckenbaugh, D. A., Charney, D. S. & Manji, H. K. 2006. A randomized trial of an N-methyl-D-aspartate antagonist in treatment-resistant major depression. *Archives of General Psychiatry*, 63, 856–864. https://doi.org/10.1001/archpsyc.63.8.856

Zeidler, Z., Hoffmann, K. & Krook-Magnuson, E. 2020. HippoBellum: acute cerebellar modulation alters hippocampal dynamics and function. *The Journal of Neuroscience*, 40, 6910–6926. https://doi.org/10.1523/jneurosci.0763–20.2020

Zeithamova, D. & Bowman, C. R. 2020. Generalization and the hippocampus: more than one story? *Neurobiology of Learning and Memory*, 175, 107317. https://doi.org/https://doi.org/10.1016/j.nlm.2020.107317

Zhang, J., Whitehurst, L. N. & Mednick, S. C. 2022. The role of sleep for episodic memory consolidation: stabilizing or rescuing? *Neurobiology of Learning and Memory*, 191, 107621. https://doi.org/https://doi.org/10.1016/j.nlm.2022.107621

Zhang, K. & Hashimoto, K. 2018. An update on ketamine and its two enantiomers as rapid-acting antidepressants. *Expert Review of Neurotherapeutics*, 19, 83–92. https://doi.org/10.1080/14737175.2019.1554434

Zhang, X.-Y., Peng, S.-Y., Shen, L.-P., Zhuang, Q.-X., Li, B., Xie, S.-T., Li, Q.-X., Shi, M.-R., Ma, T.-Y., Zhang, Q., Wang, J.-J. & Zhu, J.-N. 2020a. Targeting presynaptic H3 heteroreceptor in nucleus accumbens to improve anxiety and obsessive-compulsive-like behaviors. *Proceedings of the National Academy of Sciences*, 117, 32155–32164. https://doi.org/10.1073/pnas.2008456117

Zhang, X., Kim, J. & Tonegawa, S. 2020b. Amygdala reward neurons form and store fear extinction memory. *Neuron*, 105, 1077–1093.e7. https://doi.org/https://doi.org/10.1016/j.neuron.2019.12.025

Zhao, H., Zhang, B.-L., Yang, S.-J. & Rusak, B. 2015. The role of lateral habenula–dorsal raphe nucleus circuits in higher brain functions and psychiatric illness. *Behavioural Brain Research*, 277, 89–98. https://doi.org/https://doi.org/10.1016/j.bbr.2014.09.016

Zhao, X., Hsu, C.-L. & Spruston, N. 2022. Rapid synaptic plasticity contributes to a learned conjunctive code of position and choice-related information in the hippocampus. *Neuron*, 110, 96–108.e4. https://doi.org/https://doi.org/10.1016/j.neuron.2021.10.003

Zhu, X. O. & McNaughton, N. 1994a. A comparison of the acute effects of a tricyclic and a MAOI antidepressant on septal driving of hippocampal rhythmical slow activity. *Psychopharmacology (Berl)*, 114, 337–344.

Zhu, X. O. & McNaughton, N. 1994b. The interaction of serotonin depletion with anxiolytics and antidepressants on reticular-elicited hippocampal RSA. *Neuropharmacology*, 33, 1597–1605.

Zhu, X. O. & McNaughton, N. 1995a. Effects of long-term administration of phenelzine on reticular-elicited hippocampal rhythmical slow activity. *Neuroscience Research*, 21, 311–316.

Zhu, X. O. & McNaughton, N. 1995b. Similar effects of buspirone and chlordiazepoxide on a fixed interval schedule with long-term, low-dose administration. *Journal of Psychopharmacology*, 9, 326–330.

Zinbarg, R. E. 1990. Animal research and behaviour therapy part I: behaviour therapy is not what you think it is. *The Behaviour Therapist*, 13, 171–175.

Zinbarg, R. E. & Mineka, S. 1991. Animal models of psychopathology: II. simple phobia. *The Behaviour Therapist*, 14, 61–65.

Zola-Morgan, S., Squire, L. R. & Amaral, D. G. 1986. Human amnesia and the medial temporal region: enduring memory impairment following a bilateral lesion limited to field CA1 of the hippocampus. *The Journal of Neuroscience*, 6, 2950–2967.

Zola-Morgan, S., Squire, L. R., Amaral, D. G. & Suzuki, W. A. 1989. Lesions of perirhinal and parahippocampal cortex that spare the amygdala and hippocampal formation produce severe memory impairment. *The Journal of Neuroscience*, 9, 4355–4370.

Zola-Morgan, S., Squire, L. R. & Ramus, S. J. 1994. Severity of memory impairment in monkeys as a function of locus and extent of damage within the medial temporal lobe memory system. *Hippocampus*, 4, 483–495.

Zorowitz, S., Rockhill, A. P., Ellard, K. K., Link, K. E., Herrington, T., Pizzagalli, D. A., Widge, A. S., Deckersbach, T. & Dougherty, D. D. 2019. The neural basis of approach-avoidance conflict: a model based analysis. *eNeuro*, 6, ENEURO.0115-19.2019. https://doi.org/10.1523/eneuro.0115-19.2019

Zutshi, I., Brandon, M. P., Fu, M. L., Donegan, M. L., Leutgeb, J. K. & Leutgeb, S. 2018. Hippocampal neural circuits respond to optogenetic pacing of theta frequencies by generating accelerated oscillation frequencies. *Current Biology*, 28, P1179–1188.e3. https://doi.org/10.1016/j.cub.2018.02.061

Index

For the benefit of digital users, indexed terms that span two pages (e.g., 52–53) may, on occasion, appear on only one of those pages.

Tables and figures are indicated by *t* and *f* following the page number